Clinician's Handbook of Child Behavioral Assessment

Clinician's Handbook of Child Behavioral Assessment

EDITED BY

MICHEL HERSEN
Pacific University
Forest Grove, Oregon

ELSEVIER

AMSTERDAM • BOSTON • HEIDELBERG • LONDON
NEW YORK • OXFORD • PARIS • SAN DIEGO
SAN FRANCISCO • SINGAPORE • SYDNEY • TOKYO

Academic Press is an imprint of Elsevier

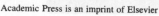

AP

Elsevier Academic Press
30 Corporate Drive, Suite 400, Burlington, MA 01803, USA
525 B Street, Suite 1900, San Diego, California 92101-4495, USA
84 Theobald's Road, London WC1X 8RR, UK

This book is printed on acid-free paper. ♾

Library of Congress Cataloging-in-Publication Data
Clinician's handbook of child behavioral assessment / edited by Michel Hersen.
p. cm.
Includes bibliographical references and index.
ISBN 0-12-343014-3 (pbk. : alk. paper) 1. Behavioral assessment of children—Handbooks, manuals, etc. 2. Psychological tests for children—Handbooks, manuals, etc. I. Hersen, Michel. II. Title.
RJ503.7.B42C55 2006
618.92'89075—dc22 2005014580

British Library Cataloguing in Publication Data
A catalogue record for this book is available from the British Library

ISBN13: 978-0-12-343014-4
ISBN10: 0-12-343014-3

For all information on all Elsevier Academic Press publications
visit our Web site at www.books.elsevier.com

Printed and bound by CPI Group (UK) Ltd, Croydon, CR0 4YY

Transferred to Digital Print 2011

CONTENTS

PART I

GENERAL ISSUES

1

OVERVIEW OF BEHAVIORAL ASSESSMENT WITH CHILDREN

DAVID REITMAN

2

DEVELOPMENTAL CONSIDERATIONS

SUSAN TINSLEY LI AND SANDRA ROGERS

3

PSYCHOMETRIC CONSIDERATIONS

DANIEL M. BAGNER, MICHELLE D. HARWOOD, AND SHEILA M. EYBERG

4

ANALOGUE AND VIRTUAL REALITY ASSESSMENT

SARI D. GOLD AND BRIAN P. MARX

5

BEHAVIORAL INTERVIEWING OF PARENTS

WILLIAM G. SHARP, CARA B. REEVES, AND ALAN M. GROSS

6

ACTIVITY MEASUREMENT

MARK D. RAPPORT, MICHAEL J. KOFLER, AND CARMEN HIMMERICH

7

STRUCTURED AND SEMISTRUCTURED INTERVIEWS

HELEN ORVASCHEL

8

CHILD SELF-REGULATION

MARTIN AGRAN AND MICHAEL L. WEHMEYER

9

PSYCHOPHYSIOLOGICAL ASSESSMENT

FRANK H. WILHELM, SILVIA SCHNEIDER, AND BRUCE H. FRIEDMAN

10

PEER SOCIOMETRIC ASSESSMENT

ELIAS MPOFU, JOLYNN CARNEY, AND MICHAEL C. LAMBERT

PART II

EVALUATION OF SPECIFIC DISORDERS AND PROBLEMS

11

ANXIETY AND FEAR

JANET WOODRUFF-BORDEN AND OVSANNA T. LEYFER

12

DEPRESSION

WILLIAM M. REYNOLDS

13

SOCIAL SKILLS DEFICITS

MEGAN M. MCCLELLAND AND CORI SCALZO

14

ALCOHOL AND DRUG ABUSE

BRAD C. DONOHUE, JENNIFER KARMELY, AND MARILYN J. STRADA

15

PEER RELATIONSHIP PROBLEMS

LINDA A. LEBLANC, RACHAEL A. SAUTTER, AND DAWN J. DORE

16

ATTENTION-DEFICIT/HYPERACTIVITY DISORDER

MARK D. RAPPORT, THOMAS M. TIMKO, JR., AND RACHEL WOLFE

17

EATING DISORDERS

MICHELLE HEFFNER MACERA AND J. SCOTT MIZES

18

MENTAL RETARDATION

V. MARK DURAND AND KRISTIN V. CHRISTODULU

19

CONDUCT DISORDERS

KURT A. FREEMAN AND JENNIFER M. HOGANSEN

20

PERVASIVE DEVELOPMENT DISORDERS

LAURA SCHREIBMAN, AUBYN C. STAHMER, AND NATACHA AKSHOOMOFF

21

HABIT DISORDERS

MICHAEL B. HIMLE, CHRISTOPHER A. FLESSNER, JORDAN T. BONOW, AND DOUGLAS W. WOODS

PART III

SPECIAL ISSUES

22

CHILD ABUSE ASSESSMENT

DEBORAH WISE

23

CLASSROOM ASSESSMENT

JANINE P. STICHTER AND TIMOTHY J. LEWIS

24

PEDIATRIC BEHAVIORAL NEUROPSYCHOLOGY

EILEEN B. FENNELL

25

ACADEMIC SKILLS PROBLEMS

EDWARD S. SHAPIRO AND MILENA A. KELLER

26

ETHICAL AND LEGAL ISSUES

CATHERINE MILLER

CONTRIBUTORS

Numbers in parentheses indicate the pages on which the authors' contributions begin.

Martin Agran (181), Department of Special Education, University of Wyoming, Laramie, Wyoming 82071

Natacha Akshoomoff (503), Child and Adolescent Services Research Center, Department of Psychiatry, School of Medicine, University of California, San Diego, California 92123-4282

Daniel M. Bagner (63), Department of Clinical and Health Psychology, University of Florida, Gainesville, Florida 32610-0165

Jordan T. Bonow (527), Department of Psychology, University of Wisconsin, Milwaukee, Wisconsin 53211

JoLynn Carney (233), Department of Counselor Education, Counseling Psychology and Rehabilitation Services, The Pennsylvania State University, University Park, Pennsylvania 16802-3110

Kristin V. Christodulu (459), Department of Psychology, State University of New York, Albany, New York 12222

Brad C. Donohue (337), Department of Psychology, University of Nevada, Las Vegas, Las Vegas, Nevada 89154-5030

Dawn J. Dore (377), Department of Psychology, Western Michigan University, Kalamazoo, Michigan 49008

V. Mark Durand (459), University of South Florida, St. Petersburg, Florida 33701-5016

Sheila M. Eyberg (63), Department of Clinical and Health Psychology, University of Florida, Gainesville, Florida 32610-0165

Eileen B. Fennell (587), Department of Clinical and Health Psychology, University of Florida, Gainesville, Florida 32610-1065

Christopher A. Flessner (527), Department of Psychology, University of Wisconsin, Milwaukee, Wisconsin 53211

Kurt A. Freeman (477), Child Development and Rehabilitation Center, Oregon Health and Science University, Portland, Oregon 97239

Bruce H. Friedman (201), Department of Psychology, Virginia Polytechnic Institute and State University, Blacksburg, Virginia 24061-0436

Sari D. Gold (81), Department of Psychology, Temple University, Philadelphia, Pennsylvania 19122

Alan M. Gross (103), Department of Psychology, The University of Mississippi, University, Mississippi 38677

Michelle D. Harwood (63), Department of Clinical and Health Psychology, University of Florida, Gainesville, Florida 32610-1065

Michael B. Himle (527), Department of Psychology, University of Wisconsin, Milwaukee, Wisconsin 53211

Carmen Himmerich (125), Department of Psychology, University of Central Florida, Orlando, Florida 32816-1390

Jennifer M. Hogansen (477), Child Development and Rehabilitation Center, Oregon Health and Science University, Eugene, Oregon 97403

Jennifer Karmely (337), Department of Psychology, University of Nevada, Las Vegas, Las Vegas, Nevada 89154-5030

Milena A. Keller (605), School Psychology Program, Lehigh University, Bethlehem, Pennsylvania 18015

Michael J. Kofler (125), Department of Psychology, University of Central Florida, Orlando, Florida 32816-1390

Michael C. Lambert (233), Department of Human Development and Family Services, University of Missouri, Columbia, Missouri 65203

Linda A. LeBlanc (377), Department of Psychology, Western Michigan University, Kalamazoo, Michigan 49008

Timothy J. Lewis (569), Special Education, University of Missouri, Columbia, Missouri 65211

Ovsanna T. Leyfer (267), Department of Psychological and Brain Sciences, University of Louisville, Louisville, Kentucky 40292

Michelle Heffner Macera (437), Center for Hope of the Sierras, Reno, Nevada 89509

Brian P. Marx (81), Department of Psychology, Temple University, Philadelphia, Pennsylvania 19122

Megan M. McClelland (313), Department of Human Development and Family Sciences, Oregon State University, Corvallis, Oregon 97331

Catherine Miller (631), School of Professional Psychology, Pacific University, Forest Grove, Oregon 97116-2328

J. Scott Mizes (437), Department of Behavioral Medicine and Psychiatry, School of Medicine, West Virginia University, Morgantown, West Virginia 26505-2854

Elias Mpofu (233), Department of Counselor Education, Counseling Psychology and Rehabilitation Services, The Pennsylvania State University, University Park, Pennsylvania 16802-3110

Helen Orvaschel (159), Center for Psychological Studies, Nova Southeastern University, Fort Lauderdale, Florida 33314-7721

Mark D. Rapport (125, 401), Department of Psychology, University of Central Florida, Orlando, Florida 32816-1390

Cara B. Reeves (103), Department of Psychology, The University of Mississippi, University, Mississippi 38677

David Reitman (3), Center for Psychological Studies, Nova Southeastern University, Fort Lauderdale, Florida 33314

William M. Reynolds (291), Department of Psychology, Humboldt State University, Arcata, California 95521-8299

Sandra Rogers (25), School of Occupational Therapy, Pacific University, Forest Grove, Oregon 97116

Rachael A. Sautter (377), Department of Psychology, Western Michigan University, Kalamazoo, Michigan 49008

Cori Scalzo (313), Cognitive Assessment Services, Inc., Bronxville, New York 10708

Silvia Schneider (201), Department of Clinical Child and Adolescent Psychology, Institute for Psychology, University of Basel, CH-4055 Basel, Switzerland

Laura Schreibman (503), Psychology Department, University of California, San Diego, La Jolla, California 92093-0109

Edward S. Shapiro (605), Department of Education and Human Services, Center for Promoting Research to Practice, Lehigh University, Bethlehem, Pennsylvania 18015

William G. Sharp (103), Department of Psychology, The University of Mississippi, University, Mississippi 38677

Aubyn C. Stahmer (503), Child and Adolescent Services Research Center, Children's Hospital and Health Center of San Diego, San Diego, California 92123-4282

Janine P. Stichter (569), Special Education, University of Missouri, Columbia, Missouri 65211

Marilyn J. Strada (337), Department of Psychology, University of Nevada, Las Vegas, Las Vegas, Nevada 89154-5030

Thomas M. Timko, Jr. (401), Department of Psychology, University of Central Florida, Orlando, Florida 32816-1390

Susan Tinsley Li (25), School of Professional Psychology, Pacific University, Portland, Oregon 97205

Michael L. Wehmeyer (181), Beach Center, University of Kansas, Lawrence, Kansas 66045-7534

Frank H. Wilhelm (201), Health Psychophysiology Laboratory, Institute for Psychology, University of Basel, CH-4055 Basel, Switzerland

Deborah Wise (549), School of Professional Psychology, Pacific University, Portland, Oregon 97205-2732

Rachel Wolfe (401), Department of Psychology, University of Central Florida, Orlando, Florida 32816-1390

Janet Woodruff-Borden (267), Department of Psychological and Brain Sciences, University of Louisville, Louisville, Kentucky 40292

Douglas W. Woods (527), Department of Psychology, University of Wisconsin, Milwaukee, Wisconsin 53211

PREFACE

Several texts and handbooks on behavioral assessment have been published, most of them now outdated. Many new developments in this field cut across strategies, computerization, virtual reality techniques, and ethical and legal issues. Over the years many new assessment strategies have either been developed, and existing ones have been refined. In addition, it is now important to include a functional assessment and to document case conceptualization and its relation to assessment and treatment planning. In general, texts and tomes on behavioral assessment tend to give short shrift to child assessment, with proportionately fewer chapters allotted to this issue. Moreover, developmental considerations tend to be overlooked in many instances. Such omissions represent a gap in the literature, making for an unbalanced view of this lively assessment field. Many of the existing texts are either theoretical/research in focus or clinical in nature. Nowhere are the various aspects of behavioral assessment placed in a comprehensive research/clinical context, nor is there much integration as to conceptualization and treatment planning. This *Clinician's Handbook of Child Behavioral Assessment* was undertaken to correct these deficiencies of coverage in a single reference work.

This volume on child behavioral assessment contains 26 chapters, beginning with general issues, followed by evaluation of specific disorders and problems, and closing with special issues. To ensure cross-chapter consistency in the coverage of disorders, these chapters follow a similar format, including an introduction, assessment strategies, research basis, clinical utility, conceptualization and treatment planning, a case study, and summary. Special issue coverage includes child abuse assessment, classroom assessment, behavioral neuropsychology, academic skills problems, and ethical-legal issues.

Many individuals have contributed to the development of this work. First, I thank the contributors for sharing their expertise with us. Second, I thank Carole Londeree, my excellent editorial assistant, and Cynthia Polance and Gregory May, my graduate student assistants, for their technical expertise. And finally, but hardly least of all, I thank Nikki Levy, my editor at Elsevier, for understanding the value and timeliness of this project.

Michel Hersen
Forest Grove, Oregon

PART I

General Issues

1

Overview of Behavioral Assessment with Children

DAVID REITMAN

Center for Psychological Studies
Nova Southeastern University
Fort Lauderdale, Florida

INTRODUCTION

Publication of the *Clinician's Handbook of Child Behavioral Assessment* follows some 30 years after the appearance of the first text devoted entirely to behavioral assessment (Hersen & Bellack, 1976). Since that time, knowledge about child behavioral assessment (CBA) has increased greatly. Growth in CBA can be traced through texts devoted to the subject. In 1976, only 2 of 18 assessment chapters were dedicated to children, one on "behavioral excesses" and another on "behavioral deficits." In 1984, *Child Behavioral Assessment* (Ollendick & Hersen, 1984) featured three chapters on general assessment issues, seven chapters on behavioral assessment methodology, and chapters on integrating assessment and treatment and ethics. Of the general assessment chapters, one examined developmental concerns and, amazingly, only a single chapter focused on "diagnostic issues" (Ollendick & Hersen, 1984). In 1993, the *Handbook of Child and Adolescent Assessment* provided a comprehensive view of child assessment that spoke to a broader audience, with nine chapters devoted to diagnostic issues (Ollendick & Hersen, 1993). The present 26-chapter book suggests a field that is becoming more inclusive and at the same time more highly specialized. This book contains 10 chapters on general child assessment (e.g., methods, models), 11 chapters largely devoted to child and adolescent problems featured in the *Diagnostic and Statistical Manual of Mental Disorders* (DSM), and five chapters concerned with special topics, such as assessment in legal and educational settings.

This overview of CBA offers a refined definition of behavioral assessment that incorporates recent conceptual advances and examines trends in behavioral assessment from that perspective. The recent history of CBA is then reviewed and current trends are highlighted. The overview closes with a discussion of the current challenges that face contemporary child behavioral assessors and their implications for the future of the field.

CHILD BEHAVIORAL ASSESSMENT DEFINED

Ollendick and Hersen (1984, 1993) defined child behavioral assessment as "an exploratory hypothesis-testing process in which a range of specific procedures is used in order to understand a given child, group, or social ecology and to formulate and evaluate specific intervention strategies" (p. 6). This definition continues to be widely endorsed by leaders in the field (Johnston & Murray, 2003), yet given the diverse actions that occur under the umbrella of behavioral assessment today, some refinement of this definition may be needed. Notably, while most contemporary approaches to behavioral assessment can be described as data based or empirical, the nature of "hypothesis testing" and the types of "understanding" that arise in the context of present-day CBA appear conceptually distinct.

Conceptual advances in behavioral theory may have implications for defining behavioral assessment. One such conceptual advance may be Hayes, Follette, and Follette's (1995) distillation of the methodological and contextual behavioral traditions within contemporary behavioral theory. The methodological tradition consists of a mechanistic/structural or "neobehavioral" view pioneered by Watson, Wolpe, and Beck. This tradition matured in the context of adult outpatient practice and is today most readily identified with cognitive and cognitive behavioral therapies. By contrast, the contextualist or radical behavioral view was elaborated by Skinner, Baer, and Risley. This tradition evolved in child populations and adult (institutional) settings and is identified as applied behavior analysis. Both behavioral traditions regard individualized assessment and cross-situational variability as important theoretical assumptions (Mash & Terdal, 1988). On the other hand, based on experiences derived from the operant laboratory, radical behaviorists also value data derived from repeated observations and direct manipulation of consequences (contingencies). Not surprisingly, given the demands of working with adults with internalizing problems, such as anxiety and depression, methodological behaviorists are less inclined to insist on direct observation and more inclined to rely on self-reports. Because contingency control and access to clients are limited, methodological behaviorists are also more tolerant of inference and, perhaps, more sensitive to the challenges associated with gathering data in outpatient settings.

Following from the foregoing discussion, it is suggested that the term *diagnostic assessment* be applied when behavioral assessors seek information intended to inform diagnosis. Further, when the nature of the hypothesis testing

TABLE 1.1 Varieties of Behavioral Assessment: Diagnostic and Functional

	Type of Behavioral Assessment	
	Diagnostic	Functional
Purpose	Identify categorical taxonomy(s) that best fit symptom presentation	Identify environmental influences (broadly construed) on behavior, in context
Commonly used methods	Utilize diagnostic interview, rating scales (frequency/intensity—compared to appropriate norm group), observations/self-monitoring (with emphasis on presence or absence of symptoms)	Utilize diagnostic interview (to identify setting events, antecedents, behavior, and consequences; ABCs), rating scales (less common), observations/self-monitoring (with emphasis on identifying manipulatable ABCs and setting events)
Outcomes	Outcomes utilized at post-treatment to evaluate success (pre–post)	Outcomes obtained (more frequently) to evaluate effectiveness and to guide clinical decision making (at each session)
Treatment logic	Diagnosis dictates treatment. Manualized therapies based on diagnosis. Some treatments are quite flexible and more "modular." Opportunities exist to subdivide some diagnostic categories in terms of function (e.g., school refusal).	Interventions designed to meet functional needs, teach or shape skills that permit acquisition of reinforcement in socially acceptable manner (balance of needs of person with needs of others). Rather than manualized treatment (tx), tx selection tends to be based on techniques that influence setting events, discriminative stimuli, or motivational operations

concerns not which diagnosis is most appropriate but, rather, the purpose, cause, or function of behavior, this activity may be called *functional assessment*. Functional assessment is distinguished from *functional analysis* (Table 1.1) because no attempt is made to manipulate sources of control in the former case (Alberto & Troutman, 2003). The aforementioned assessment endeavors can thus be included under the larger domain of "behavioral assessment." A third dimension of CBA, outcome evaluation, is discussed at the conclusion of the chapter.

FOUNDATIONS OF BEHAVIORAL ASSESSMENT

Although a recent study of assessment practices (Cashel, 2002) among APA-member clinicians found that almost 60% of child and adolescent clinicians described themselves as cognitive behavioral (51.9%) or behavioral (7.4%), behavioral assessment has not always enjoyed wide acceptance. Indeed, behavioral assessment arose out of, and in opposition to, a more established tradition within psychological assessment that concerned itself primarily with the evaluation of traits such as intelligence and personality (Ollendick & Hersen, 1984). Assessment efforts within that tradition sought to identify latent traits that explained or caused current functioning (e.g., poor academic performance was viewed as caused by low intelligence). By contrast, behavioral assessment has historically "been directed toward a description of current behavior and a specification of organismic and environmental conditions that occasion and maintain it" (Ollendick & Hersen, 1984, p. 4). An important question addressed in this overview concerns how well that description applies to CBA as it is practiced today.

Since the mid-1980s debates about how to define behavioral assessment and evaluate its adequacy have been numerous (Haynes, 1998; R. O. Nelson, 1983). For example, drawing on publication trends in assessment methods and research designs over an 18-year period in *Behavior Therapy*, Gross (1990) noted substantial drift from earlier definitions of behavioral research and practice. For Gross (1990), behavioral assessment implied individualized, direct assessment of behavior that made few assumptions about cross-situational behavioral consistency and minimized inference. Behavioral assessment was also characterized by the development of hypotheses about the function of behavior, with repeated, ongoing assessment to ensure that incorrect analyses would be modified to achieve treatment goals (for details see Table 1.2; Mash & Terdal, 1988; Silva, 1993).

TABLE 1.2 Distinguishing Between Traditional and Behavioral Assessment

	Traditional Assessment	Behavioral Assessment
Purpose/use of data	Identify underlying personality traits; to describe personality, diagnose/classify or predict (prognosis)	Identify antecedent and consequent events; to describe target behavior; to select, evaluate, and revise treatments
View of personality/ behavior	Stable across situations	Temporal and cross-situational consistency not expected
Test items	Selection based on how well items reflect a priori theory about underlying personality factors	Test items are instances of the behavior itself across multiple situations
Level of inference	Response is a "sign" of latent personality trait	Low level of inference; behavior is "sampled"
Methods/timing of assessment	Use of indirect methods; emphasis on pre- or post-treatment	Use of direct methods (e.g., direct observations, behavioral tests), ongoing assessment

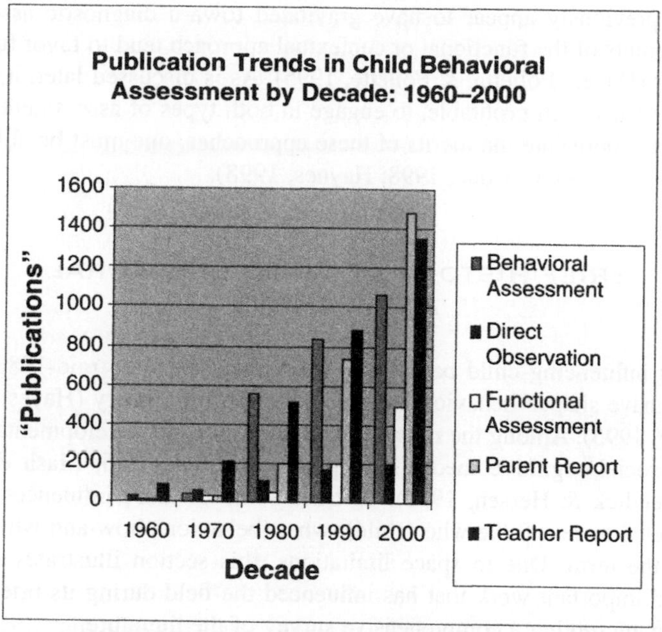

FIGURE 1.1 Publication trends in behavioral assessment, by decade. (*Note*: 2000–2004 publication data were doubled to estimate most recent decade.)

Trends in behavioral assessment and CBA are also reflected in the last half-century of published research (here defined to include dissertations, books and book chapters, and journals). Specifically, an electronic database (PsycInfo) search of the terms *behavioral assessment, direct observation, functional assessment or functional analysis, parent report or parent rating, teacher report or teacher rating*, and *child-related synonyms* (e.g., child, children, adolescent) revealed remarkable growth in CBA research overall and some interesting relative trends (see Figure 1.1). For example, while growth in entries including the term *direct observation* (a frequently identified core element of behavioral assessment) have not kept pace with *behavioral assessment*, there has been substantial growth in publications involving parent and teacher report and functional approaches to assessment. Overall, while essentially invisible prior to 1960, growth in publications in child behavioral assessment appear to have outpaced growth in general child assessment by roughly 5 to 1. By way of comparison, during that same period, publication growth in projective assessment was flat.

Recent years have seen a significant increase in diagnostically focused assessment, which tends toward a more topographical description of child behavior problems and places relatively less emphasis on contingency analysis and context than was characteristic of earlier approaches to behavioral assessment (see Mash & Terdal, 1988). Practitioners and scientists holding the methodological view described previously appear to have gravitated toward diagnostic assessment, while adherents of the functional or contextual approach tend to favor functional assessment (Hayes, Follette, & Follette, 1995). As is discussed later, it is possible, and perhaps even profitable, to engage in both types of assessment activity. However, to appreciate the merits of these approaches, one must be able to distinguish between them (Cone, 1998; Haynes, 1998).

BRIEF HISTORY OF CHILD BEHAVIORAL ASSESSMENT

Factors influencing child behavioral assessment since the mid-1980s mirror those that have shaped behavior therapy and behavioral theory (Hayes, Follette, & Follette, 1995). Among the most influential factors are developmental, cognitive, and social-cognitive theory (Kamphaus & Frick, 1996; Mash & Terdal, 1988; Ollendick & Hersen, 1993). To trace some of these influences, CBA is deconstructed to reveal the who (child), what (behavior), how and why (assessment) of the term. Due to space limitations, this section illustrates landmark events and important work that has influenced the field during its brief history, rather than attempting a comprehensive survey of the literature.

WHOSE BEHAVIOR IS BEING ASSESSED?

Early CBA efforts began with careful specification of target behaviors, setting events, antecedents, and consequent conditions (see Hawkins, 1986). However, despite some portrayals of CBA as narrow and simplistic, the assessment of context can be shown to have been an important facet of much of the earliest behavioral work with children. Indeed, although formal assessment of family factors was not common, the development of parent-directed interventions (Patterson, 1965) and clinical work with children in institutions, such as schools and hospitals, has long demanded a high level of concern about the environment (e.g., Van Houten et al., 1988). For example, in a case study of a highly noncompliant and antisocial boy, Patterson and Reid (1970) hypothesized about numerous contextual factors (e.g., family stress, poverty) that might contribute to maintenance and generalization failures. And by the 1980s, Forehand and colleagues (e.g., Forehand & McCombs, 1988) were conducting pioneering research on the impact of maternal depression and marital relations on treatment outcome, thus setting the stage for assessment of a much broader range of child-, parent-, and family-level variables (Chronis et al., 2004).

An important facet of contemporary CBA is to ensure that developmentally sensitive normative comparisons serve as the foundation for assigning a diagnosis (APA, 1994; Kamphaus & Frick, 1996). Today, there is wide agreement that assessment practices must be sensitive to the developmental level of the child, but early CBA did not typically employ nomothetic comparisons, leaving clinicians and researchers to determine for themselves the appropriateness of various social and behavioral acts (Kazdin, 1983). As noted by Hawkins (1986), "during this phase of our field's development, we often moved rather quickly from vague complaints of clients (or other referring agents) to a listing of behaviors to be changed, operating in an intuitive manner and with little conception of the process we used or its assumptions" (p. 333). Fortunately, for most externalizing and internalizing problems, it is now possible for child clinicians and researchers to utilize measures with relatively well-developed, representative norms that permit the acquisition of data from parents, teachers, and children. Often, these ratings can be compared to a cross section of similar children with respect to developmental status, gender, and, to a lesser degree, ethnicity and socioeconomic status [e.g., Achenbach & Rescorla, 2001, Child Behavior Checklist (CBCL); Conners, 1997, Conners' Rating Scales—Revised (CRS-R); C. R. Reynolds & Kamphaus, 1992, Behavior Assessment System for Children (BASC)].

Methodologically speaking, parent and teacher ratings tend to dominate contemporary child assessment (see Figure 1.1; Cashel, 2002), thus one might argue that focus of behavioral assessment remains on the child. However, there now appears to be greater awareness of the reciprocal relations between child behavior and the behavior of parents, teachers, peers, and siblings. One impact of this perspective has been that assessment is increasingly more likely to involve gathering information about raters themselves. That is, because parental psychopathology, substance abuse, and marital problems all appear to influence parent ratings of child behavior (see Patterson, Reid, & Dishion, 1992; Chronis et al., 2004), the possibility that ratings reflect variation in these factors rather than changes in the child's behavior have become more prominent in clinical decision making. Thus CBAs have become more sensitive to sources of bias in the system and more aware of how child behavior may serve as an antecedent for specific parenting practices (e.g., reprimands), rather than being viewed exclusively as a function of them. One prominent example of this phenomenon was a study demonstrating that changes in medication status (and, presumably, child behavior) produced changes in parenting practices (Barkley, 1989).

WHAT "BEHAVIOR" IS BEING ASSESSED?

Since the late 1960s, behavioral assessment has expanded in focus to include elements of the triple response system (i.e., motor, cognitive, and physiological responses; Nay, 1979). Consequently, the range of assessment targets has increased from those that are observable or potentially observable (e.g., heart rate, galvanic skin response) to include measures of beliefs, attitudes, and emotional states that require significantly greater inference (Cone, 1998; Hayes, Follette, & Follette, 1995). However, as long as measures of constructs and behavior are evaluated relative to appropriate standards (Barrios & Hartmann, 1986; Cone, 1998), most any measure of motor, cognitive, or physiological activity could serve as an appropriate target for behavioral assessment. Over time, interest in the triple response system has blended with psychometric considerations, resulting in widespread acceptance of multimodal assessment strategies for conducting psychological assessments with children (Reitman et al., 1998).

Despite the broad appeal of multimodal assessment models, few authors recommend attempting to assess all response systems in all clinical cases. Thus, guidance as to what behaviors and response systems to assess continues to present a challenge to CBAs (Fonseca & Perrin, 2001). Though not writing about child or family assessment per se, Bornstein, Bornstein, and Dawson (1984) offer pertinent criticisms about some well-known systems of combining assessment information. For example, they noted that the S-O-R-K-C (stimulus, organism, response, contingency, consequence) model (Kanfer & Saslow, 1969) "may be so thorough that it becomes impractical. . . . [T]he information obtained is still interpreted in a subjective manner" and most importantly, the "model does not really aid in the selection of a treatment strategy" (p. 230). Although decisions about what behaviors and response systems to assess and what to do with such information will remain complex, the implications of multimodal assessment for diagnosis have been more apparent.

In contrast to early conceptualizations, which tended to be based on more focal presenting problems, multimodal, comprehensive CBAs have revealed that children rarely experience a single problem and that, in fact, multiple diagnoses (i.e., comorbidity) are the rule rather than the exception. For example, children diagnosed with ADHD—Combined subtype, have a high likelihood of being diagnosed with Conduct Disorder or Oppositional Defiant Disorder (Plitszka, 2000). With respect to ADHD and aggressive behavior, screening for "comorbidity" may be of more than just diagnostic interest, because comorbid aggression appears to predict poorer treatment outcome for children with ADHD (Kuhne, Schachar, & Tannock, 1997). It has also become clear that for conduct disorder, age of onset appears to predict risk of sustained negative long-term outcomes (e.g., dropping out of school, incarceration) (Moffit & Caspi, 2001). In contrast to diagnostic assessment, multimodal assessment issues in functional assessment have just begun to receive attention (Sasso et al., 2001; Miltenberger, 2000).

HOW IS BEHAVIOR ASSESSED?

As the range of behavioral "systems" has expanded, the number of methods used to assess them has also increased. As noted previously, interviews and rating scales have become staples of the behavioral assessment process. However, the modality most commonly associated with behavioral assessment, direct observation, has been among the most controversial (Mash & Terdal, 1988; R. O. Nelson, 1983). Direct observation may occur in the natural environment or be obtained via clinical analogues. Direct observation is valued because the clinician has a greater likelihood of observing antecedents and consequences that may play a role in the evoking and maintaining of the problem behavior. However, many authors advise that the benefits of direct observation are offset by the cost of training raters, transportation, time required to conduct extended observations in the school or home, and time required to record and code data (see Haynes, 1998). Nevertheless, others argue that in vivo assessments are less costly than suggested (Reid et al., 1987), and Reitman et al. (1998) noted that the costs of misdiagnosis and/or misguided treatment selection must also be factored into any cost–benefit analysis involving direct observation.

Like direct observation, analogue assessment (an assessment technique created to simulate important aspects of the natural environment) has been controversial. Clinic-based analogues of child behavior in the classroom, such as the Restricted Academic Situation, may conserve time and resources compared with school-based observations (see Barkley, 1990), but it is unclear how widespread adoption has been outside of academic research centers. Finally, the generalizability of data obtained from clinic analogues has also been questioned (Danforth, Barkley, & Stokes, 1991).

An interesting review by Haynes (1998) has outlined the many ways in which technology can reduce barriers to conducting clinical behavioral assessments. For example, interviewing can be made more efficient by allowing clients to enter their own data, and computerized branching technology can significantly reduce the time and effort required to administer structured interviews. Computer technology can also facilitate the acquisition of observational data by trained raters, and handheld devices, such as cell phones, PDAs, and hybrids, will significantly expand the range of options available to behavioral assessors interested in real-time data collection. In summary, opportunities to collect data relevant to behavioral assessment will be greatly expanded in the years to come (Sturges, 1998).

A possible drawback associated with the introduction of new technologies is the likelihood that psychometric studies will be unable to keep pace with innovation. However, in as much as "accuracy" (see Cone, 1998) appears to be one of the most, if the not the most important dimensions of a valid behavioral assessment measure, data gathered via new technologies may quickly come to be viewed as the gold standard (incontrovertible index) applied to other methods. As computer processing speeds increase, software innovations continue, and costs decrease further, even the electronic transfer of video may become routine. Haynes (1998) summarized the many possible benefits of new technology for behavioral assessment by noting: "Technological advances in assessment (1) increase the standardization of assessment instruments, (2) increase the efficiency of assessment, (3) reduce many sources of measurement error, (4) facilitate the acquisition of data in the natural environment, (5) facilitate the multimodal and multimethod assessment strategies, and (6) facilitate clinical judgments" (p. 10).

WHY IS THE BEHAVIOR BEING ASSESSED?

Assessment can be described as having one of three general purposes: diagnosis, treatment selection, or treatment evaluation (Johnston & Murray, 2003). Functional assessment and treatment are frequently presented as closely linked within the functional assessment paradigm (see R. O. Nelson & Hayes, 1986), but the relationship between diagnosis and treatment is sometimes misrepresented. For example, Schulte (1996) notes: "One major goal of medical research has been to find and develop treatments for different diseases, and in medical practice a specific treatment is, in principle, indicated and determined once this disease has been diagnosed (indicatio morbis)" (p. 119). Although the extent to which a psychiatric diagnosis permits determination of treatment has been challenged (see Eifert, 1996), the development of manualized treatments that prescribe treatment on the basis of diagnostic status contrasts with the view that diagnostic assessment *can not* lead to effective intervention. In summary, whether assessment is geared toward improving diagnostic accuracy or to producing a more refined functional assessment, *both* efforts are directed at improving treatment selection and are therefore concerned with treatment outcomes. Because of the importance of this issue, the chapter closes with more detailed consideration of incremental validity (Johnston & Murray, 2003; Nelson-Gray, 2003) and the cost-benefits of various approaches to assessment (Yates & Taub, 2003).

CONTEMPORARY CHILD BEHAVIORAL ASSESSMENT

Although Mash and Terdal (1988) identify a multitude of characteristics of behavioral assessment, contemporary CBA appears to be distinguished by a diagnostic-empirical focus and increasing specialization. Recently, greater attention has been paid to contextual factors, but it remains to be seen how well functional assessments can be integrated into child behavioral assessment practices outside of research settings (Sasso et al., 2001).

Since the introduction of DSM-III (APA, 1980), the DSM has enjoyed greater acceptance with each revision. A landmark in this evolution concerns the addition of a separate section in the DSM-III focusing on "disorders usually first diagnosed in infancy, childhood, or adolescence" and acknowledgment in DSM-III and the research literature that "adult" forms of psychopathology, such as depression and anxiety, might also be observed in children. Concern about the implications of widespread acceptance of DSM and the medical model among behavioral practitioners has certainly waned since the inception of behavior therapy (Follette & Hayes, 1992). Indeed, one consequence of the increased acceptance of the DSM nosology has been to blur the distinction between traditional assessment and behavioral assessment (see Table 1.2). In addition to economic pressures to adopt the system, several factors have contributed to DSM's greater acceptance among CBAs, including DSM's "atheoretical approach" (but see Krasner, 1992, for another view), improvements in interrater reliability, greater attention to developmental factors, and reductions in the level of inference required to identify symptoms (Mash & Wolfe, 2005).

Another trend in contemporary CBA is greater specialization. For example, child practitioners recognize a distinction between internalizing and externalizing problems, and many describe their expertise in such terms (e.g., child-externalizing). Yet subspecialization is also apparent, and distinct assessment practices are beginning to develop within these ever-narrower categories. In the externalizing domain, interviews and rating scales tend to dominate lists of assessment practices for the disruptive behavior disorders (e.g., Attention-Deficit Hyperactivity Disorder, Oppositional Defiant Disorder, and Conduct Disorder), but state-of-the-art ADHD assessment is likely also to include direct observation (either analogue or naturalistic), supplemented by laboratory tests and self-report data (Gordon, 1997; Reitman & Hupp, 2003). By contrast, because of concerns about parents' ability to provide useful information and adolescents' willingness to supply it, file reviews and permanent product records (e.g., disciplinary records, classroom attendance logs) (Patterson, Reid, & Dishion, 1992) have become more important in the diagnostic assessment of Conduct Disorder. Choice of assessment targets and measurement strategies may also be influenced by research. For example, developmental psychopathologists have found that aggressive behavior may be expressed differently among boys and girls and that outcomes associated with conduct problems may be related to time of onset (Robins & Rutter, 1990). Many of the changes in the forthcoming DSM-V will attempt to redress shortcomings in the DSM's treatment of developmental issues (Pine et al., 2002).

In the internalizing domain, specifically with anxiety disorders, parents may be limited in their ability to provide diagnostic information, and children may be reluctant or unable to talk about their fears. As a result, behavioral avoidance tests (BATs) have been utilized to provide clearer evidence of impaired functioning than can typically be acquired via pencil-and-paper assessments. In some cases, BATs go beyond diagnostic considerations and are used to obtain functional assessment data (Silverman & Kurtines, 1996). Since mood and anxiety disorders among adults have been largely diagnosed on the basis of self-reports (e.g., Beck Depression Inventory, State-Trait Anxiety Inventory), measures of cognition and affect have been readily assimilated into assessment practices with children and adolescents (see W. M. Reynolds, 1994; Velting, Setzer, & Albano, 2004). In contrast to research and clinical work in the internalizing area, consideration of cognitive and affective variables has been less common with externalizing children (see Pelham, Wheeler, & Chronis, 1998).

Communication problems prevalent among children with developmental disabilities have helped functional behavioral analyses to become a staple of assessment practices in this population. Since the mid-1990s, functional analyses have been used almost to the exclusion of other methods, although rating scales and interviews are sometimes utilized (see O'Neill et al., 1997). Functional analyses involve direct manipulation of setting events, antecedents, or consequences (in analogue or in vivo situations) to test hypothesized relations between these manipulations and behavior change. Importantly, brief, modified versions of functional analysis are now being adapted to suit the demands of children with typically developing functional capacity and wider range of behavioral challenges (e.g., Northup & Gulley, 2001). Functional assessments that do not involve direct manipulation of the child's environment are increasingly utilized for higher functioning children, particularly as part of functional behavioral assessments mandated under IDEA-97 (Individuals with Disabilities Education Act, 1997) (Alberto & Troutman, 2003; Noell, 2003). Finally, increasing attention has been given to functional assessment in the area of school refusal behavior, and one study demonstrated that prescriptive treatments based on the function of school refusal appeared more effective than nonprescriptive treatments in which a standard treatment was applied without matching treatment to function (Kearney & Silverman, 1999).

TRAINING AND PRACTICE IN CHILD BEHAVIORAL ASSESSMENT

A complete analysis of contemporary CBA requires consideration of training programs and clinical practice. With respect to internship training, Elbert and Holden (1987) reported that child clinical interns were far more likely to utilize projective tests (75–88%) than either behavioral interviews (44–58%) or behavioral checklists (11–33%). A more recent survey of training directors indicated that they perceived training in cognitive-behavioral therapy as valuable. But, strangely, the authors did not assess the extent to which training in behavioral assessment methods was beneficial (Stedman, Hatch, & Shoenfeld, 2001). In contrast, a study of practicing behavior therapists (Elliot et al., 1996) revealed that the top five assessment practices (defined as the percentage of clients that received it) were interviews (94%), direct observation (52%), rating scales (49%), self-monitoring (44%), and interview with significant others (42%). Although results were not broken out by population treated (i.e., child vs. adult), it is notable that academics were more likely than practitioners to report that clients completed standardized rating scales (67% versus 48%). Also, both practitioners and academics reported use of "direct observation" with over 50% of their clients, but the details about the nature of the observations were not provided.

In the school system, interest in functional assessment has been boosted by legislation that requires it to meet due process requirements associated with changes in a child's educational placement (Noell, 2003). Nevertheless, while an increasingly strong database supports the efficacy of functional assessment when used with persons with developmental disabilities, limited data support the clinical utility of functional assessment with higher-functioning children in school settings (Gresham, 2004; Nelson-Gray, 2003; Noell, 2003). Leaders in school-based assessment have voiced concern about widespread dissemination of functional assessment practices in advance of solid empirical data and have called for more research (see Gresham, 2004; Sasso et al., 2001). Toward that end, a recently published study attempted to adapt functional assessment procedures to the school setting by developing function-based interviews and rating scales for teachers. Data from this preliminary study revealed that interrater agreement on a rank order of behavioral function was low (Kwak et al., 2004). By contrast, another study suggested that agreement across measurement methods (e.g., interview and ratings) was acceptable and that treatment response was enhanced when informed by functional assessment (Newcomer & Lewis, 2004).

It is difficult to imagine a future for CBA without economic support for practice. Yet anecdotal reports from CBAs suggest that reimbursement for traditional clinic-based testing has been limited in recent years (Kelley, 2003). McGlough and Clarkin (2004) note that many third-party payers distinguish between *evaluation* or *assessment* (defined in terms of a biopsychosocial interview) and *testing* (defined as norm-based, standardized evaluation intended to inform treatment planning or clarify complex diagnostic questions), with significant limitations being placed on the latter, more time- and resource-intensive efforts. So far, at least two studies suggest that practitioners working with children and adolescents feel that their ability to practice has been seriously constrained by managed care (Cashel, 2002; Piotrowski, Belter, & Keller, 1998).

Although not specific to CBA, one implication of testing limitations imposed by managed care is a reduction in the utilization of tests with limited or suspect psychometric qualities. Thus, while still popular, the use of projective tests, especially the Rorschach, appears to be declining. Notably, sharp reductions in the utilization of IQ and achievement tests are also evident (Cashel, 2002). While this may reflect reductions in unnecessary or superfluous psychoeducational testing (e.g., as part of a battery of tests given without regard to presenting problems), it also seems possible that some necessary testing is now foregone. Given that well over half the children diagnosed with common externalizing problems such as ADHD may have academic problems or learning disabilities (Lyon, Fletcher, & Barnes, 2003), reductions in psychoeducational assessment may reflect a real threat to the hypothesis-testing approach endorsed by Ollendick and Hersen (1993). Without some form of psychoeducational assessment, the ability of the clinician to rule out the contribution of academic difficulties (e.g., poor tool skills) to behavioral problems may be hampered significantly (see Witt & Beck, 1999).

In contrast to restrictions on traditional testing, use of behavioral rating scales (e.g., the CPRS/CTRS and CBCL/TRF) by a theoretically diverse group of APA-member clinicians working with children and adolescents appears to be on the rise (Cashel, 2002). When asked about HMO-related changes and the likely impact on their assessment practices, only rating scales (e.g., BASC, CBCL, CPRS, and TRF) were expected to be utilized more frequently in future assessments. Cashel (2002) points out that ease of use and interpretation may explain *both* the rising interest in behavioral rating scales and continuing popularity of some forms of projective testing (e.g., Draw-A-Person, Sentence Completion, Bender-Gestalt). Users of behavioral assessment methods such as rating scales noted benefits in tracking client progress, modifying treatment focus, and a desire to be in compliance with ethical guidelines concerning assessment and treatment (see Hatfield & Ogles, 2004; Lambert & Hawkins, 2004). Widely available, well-normed, easily administered, and resource-efficient measurement tools appear to have value for both third-party payers and clinicians.

Overall, the net impact of managed care on CBA seems mixed. Diagnostic assessments utilizing readily available, efficient measures stand to gain, while traditional testing and more labor- and cost-intensive approaches, including functional assessment, may be in jeopardy. In school settings, the use of functional assessment is likely to continue, as dictated by federal law and local implementation policy. However, preliminary data suggest that implementation and assessment integrity are problematic (Sasso et al., 2001). Interestingly, restrictions or limitations placed on psychoeducational testing by HMOs could represent an opportunity for curriculum-based instruction, a system of assessment and intervention that is solidly based on a behavioral approach to instruction (see Shinn, 1989). Some curriculum-based techniques are similar to procedures employed in functional analysis, in that they manipulate academic performance parameters (e.g., task difficulty) to clarify the function of behavioral problems in the classroom (O'Neill et al., 1997). Many curriculum-based approaches also offer significant time savings relative to traditional psychoeducational testing (Witt & Beck, 1999). However, unless the utility of these procedures can be clearly established, it seems improbable that third-party payers will authorize payment for these services. For CBAs to take advantage of new technologies, efforts must be directed to educating both consumers and third-party payers about the empirically supported benefits of diagnostic *and* functional assessment.

CHALLENGES AHEAD

Whether diagnostic or functional, it seems inevitable that greater empirical scrutiny will be brought to bear on assessment in clinical practice. There appears to be a strong synergy between interest in outcome assessment, the evidence-based treatment movement, demands for accountability outside of and within the mental health system, and efforts to establish the validity of behavioral assessment (Lambert & Hawkins, 2004). Interest in outcome assessment among behavioral and cognitive-behavior therapists working with children may be higher than among other clinicians. Hatfield and Ogles (2004) reported that among a heterogeneous sample of 874 APA-member child clinicians, only 37% reported routinely utilizing some form of measurement to track outcomes. However, that number rose to 50% among cognitive-behavioral therapists and to 54% among child clinicians in general (it was likely even higher among child clinicians with a cognitive-behavioral orientation, but these data were not reported). One important use of outcome evaluation data concerns the validation of assessment itself. Efforts to accomplish this formidable task are described next.

As noted previously, diagnostically focused assessment has become the dominant assessment model employed by contemporary CBAs. However, little work has been done to establish what Nelson-Gray (2003) calls "the treatment utility of assessment" for diagnostic assessment. Defined as "the degree to which assessment is shown to contribute to beneficial treatment outcome," the treatment utility of assessment derives from the concept of *incremental validity* (see Hayes, Nelson, & Jarrett, 1987). To justify any evaluation practice, assessment methods and procedures must result in greater or more rapid treatment success than either no assessment or an established assessment practice. Alternatively, an assessment approach might attain results similar to an established procedure, but do so using fewer resources. A key feature of determining the treatment utility of assessment concerns the need to *experimentally manipulate* (see Nelson-Gray, 2003, for details) some aspect of the assessment process (e.g., who has access to functional assessment data). Only then can the incremental validity of a given behavioral assessment practice be established.

With respect to diagnostic assessment in CBA, some hold that refinements in DSM taxonomies might produce more homogeneous groupings that could improve outcomes for structured, manualized, diagnosis-driven treatment approaches (Acierno, Hersen, & Van Hasselt, 1998). If outcomes did improve, this would provide indirect evidence of treatment utility. On that point, Cone (1998) suggests that topographical behavioral assessments (what is here called diagnostic assessment) "could be subjected to functional evaluation. If assessment produced data describing topography that was then used successfully for some purpose, the assessment would be seen as functionally useful" (p. 41), even if it was not derived from a functional assessment. Similarly, Nelson-Gray (2003) notes that even personality assessment (e.g., conscientiousness) could be shown to have treatment utility. For example, a parent's "low conscientiousness" score might predict dropout or poor compliance with homework assignments associated with participation in a manualized treatment. If a group of "low scorers" was so distinguished, received a modified form of treatment based on their conscientiousness score, and demonstrated improved treatment outcome, the addition of that assessment data could be said to have treatment utility (Nelson-Gray, 2003, terms this "the methodology of obtained differences," p. 522). Nelson-Gray (2003) has also suggested that when diagnostic groupings do not achieve homogeneity, there may be a greater need for functional assessment methodologies.

Because many manualized treatments are based on a diagnosis-to-treatment model, the treatment utility of diagnostic assessment should be evaluated in that context (Acierno, Hersen, & Van Hasselt, 1998). For example, major empirically supported parent-training models are relatively silent on the topic of functional behavioral assessment and appear to take a "structural" approach to treating externalizing problems (e.g., Hembree-Kigin & McNeil, 1995). Put another way, many manualized empirically supported parent-training programs neither teach functional assessment principles nor advise altering one's treatment approach based on the function of the behavioral problems displayed by the child. This is not an indictment of parent-training approaches, but it raises questions about the merits of diagnostic and functional assessment in contemporary behavioral practice with families. Mischel (1979) (as cited in Ollendick & Hersen, 1984, p. 740) once raised concerns about personality assessment that seem relevant in the present context:

> My intentions . . . were not to undo personality but to defend individuality and the uniqueness of each person against what I saw as the then prevalent form of clinical hostility: the tendency to use a few behavioral signs to categorize people enduringly into fixed slots on the assessor's favorite nomothetic trait dimensions and to assume that these slot positions were sufficiently informative to predict specific behavior and to make extensive decisions about a person's whole life.

With diagnostic assessment substituted for personality, is it unreasonable to ask whether the same state of affairs does not exist today? Specifically, does diagnostic assessment produce data sufficient to "make extensive decisions" such as developing treatment plans and making placement recommendations that may strongly affect a young person and their family? If diagnostic assessment and the treatment-from-diagnosis logic underlying many manualized treatments are not sufficient to produce positive outcomes, can functional assessment be presented as an alternative or supplemental approach? If so, it must be acknowledged that the treatment utility of functional assessment for persons not diagnosed with developmental disabilities has yet to be established.

Questions about incremental validity can also be extended to multimodal assessment. Consensus regarding the need for multimodal assessments have become so uniform that the relative lack of attention given to the utilization or efforts to combine information is striking, particularly for information that is inconsistent across raters (e.g., parents, teachers, and self-report). Notably, concerns about combining information exist in both functional and diagnostic assessment traditions (Miltenberger, 2000; Youngstrom, Loeber, & Stouthamer-Loeber, 2000). Beyond questions of "disagreement," critical questions also remain about the incremental validity of specific behavioral assessment practices utilized with children, including the computerized assessment of attention (Reitman et al., 1998), direct observation (Tyron, 1998), and teacher ratings (Handwerk et al., 1999; J. R. Nelson et al., 2002). Validity concerns also pertain to other assessment domains reviewed in this volume, including neuropsychological variables, psychophysiological measures (e.g., biofeedback), sociometric ratings (e.g., peer nomination), activity measurement, and responses obtained through virtual-reality assessment. As with assessment practices in general, the case for expanding the range of behavioral assessment methods with children will need to be made in terms of incremental validation. Finally, anecdotally, it appears that almost all studies evaluating combinations of information from multimodal assessments are concerned with the incremental value of the information for establishing diagnosis, rather than informing incremental validity as described here.

Although functional and diagnostic approaches can be distinguished, efforts have been made to combine them. One approach to blending diagnostic and functional approaches was introduced by Hawkins (1979), who argued that child assessment be conceptualized as a funnel. At the wide end of the funnel, child functioning is evaluated broadly, followed by a progressively more focused behavioral assessment. Scotti et al. (1996) later elaborated on this approach in light of the growing acceptance of the DSM model. Scotti et al. (1996) argued that Axes I and II were nicely suited to diagnostic assessment but that functional assessment was not served well by the existing axial format. Instead, they argued that Axes III and IV should be reformulated to allow for refinement of problem targets (i.e., symptoms) and to facilitate a more detailed account of setting events, antecedents, and consequences. Finally, Axis V would make better use of empirically supported measures to track outcomes. While it is presently unclear whether this blend of traditional (diagnostic) and behavioral assessment (functional, in present terms) is common practice among CBAs, it behooves proponents of any assessment model to establish incremental validity. In the absence of clear empirical data to guide clinical decision making, the consensus approach among CBAs seems to begin with treatment based on a largely diagnostic approach (e.g., treatment from diagnosis). If treatment results are unsatisfactory, functional assessment may then be utilized to "enhance" standard care (see Reitman & Hupp, 2003).

SUMMARY

Contemporary CBA can be thought of as involving two distinct, but potentially complementary approaches to hypothesis testing. One approach involves assigning individuals to categories (i.e., establishing differential diagnosis and/or comorbidity). Some authors have identified this approach as "taxonomic diagnosis" (Mash & Wolfe, 2005). The other approach, here described as functional assessment, involves identifying environmental influences on behavior (broadly construed, for many, as including organismic variables). This sense of the term *diagnosis* can also be understood as a "problem-solving analysis." In this overview, it has been argued that CBA is a multidimensional approach to data collection and analysis in which a range of procedures is used to facilitate clinical decision making for children or groups of children. It has been suggested that diagnostic and functional assessment constitute two different but potentially complementary approaches to clinical decision making. The increasingly important third variety of behavioral assessment concerns outcomes. Outcome evaluation can be used to measure the clinical utility of diagnostic or functional assessment or, more generally, to assess behavioral interventions or systems of care designed for children. Current trends in public policy and health care suggest that outcome evaluation will become an increasingly important subtype of behavioral assessment in the years ahead.

REFERENCES AND RESOURCES

Achenbach, T. M., & Rescorla, L. A. (2001). *Manual for ASEBA school-age forms and profiles.* Burlington, VT: University of Vermont, Research Center for Children, Youth, and Families.

Acierno, R., Hersen, M., & Van Hasselt, V. B. (1998). Prescriptive assessment and treatment. In A. S. Bellack & M. Hersen (Eds.), *Behavioral assessment: A practical handbook* (4th ed.). Boston: Allyn & Bacon.

Alberto, P., & Troutman, A. (2003). *Applied behavior analysis for teachers* (6th ed.). New York: Prentice Hall.

American Psychiatric Association. (1980). *Diagnostic and statistical manual of mental disorders* (3rd ed.). Washington, DC: Author.

American Psychiatric Association. (1994). *Diagnostic and statistical manual of mental disorders* (4th ed.). Washington, DC: Author.

Barkely, R. A. (1989). Hyperactive girls and boys: Stimulant drug effects on mother–child observations. *Journal of Child Psychology and Psychiatry, 30,* 379–390.

Barkley, R. A. (1990). *Attention deficit hyperactivity disorder: A handbook for diagnosis and treatment.* New York: Guilford Press.

Barrios, B. A., & Hartmann, D. P. (1986). The contributions of traditional assessment: Concepts, issues, and methodologies. In R. O. Nelson & S. C. Hayes (Eds.), *Conceptual foundations of behavioral assessment.* New York: Guilford Press.

Bornstein, P. H., Bornstein, M. T., & Dawson, B. (1984). Integrated assessment and treatment. In T. H. Ollendick & M. Hersen (Eds.), *Child behavioral assessment: Principles and procedures.* New York: Pergamon Press.

Cashel, M. L. (2002). Child and adolescent psychological assessment: Current clinical practices and the impact of managed care. *Professional Psychology: Research and Practice, 33,* 446–453.

Chronis, A. M., Chako, A., Fabiano, G. A., Wymbs, B. T., & Pelham, W. E. (2004). Enhancements to the behavioral parent training paradigm for families of children with ADHD: Review and future directions. *Journal of Child and Family Psychology Review, 7,* 1–27.

Cone, J. D. (1998). Psychometric considerations: Concepts, contents, and methods. In A. S. Bellack & M. Hersen (Eds.), *Behavioral assessment: A practical handbook* (4th ed.). Boston: Allyn & Bacon.

Conners, C. K. (1997). *Conners' Rating Scales—Revised Technical Manual.* North Tonawanda, NY: Multi-health Systems.

Danforth, J. S., Barkley, R. A., & Stokes, T. F. (1991). Observations of parent–child interactions with hyperactive children: Research and clinical implications. *Clinical Psychology Review, 11,* 703–727.

Dumas, J. E. (1989). Let's not forget the context in behavioral assessment. *Behavioral Assessment, 11,* 231–247.

Eifert, G. H. (1996). More theory-driven and less diagnosis-based behavior therapy. *Journal of Behavior Therapy and Experimental Psychiatry, 27,* 75–86.

Elbert, J. C., & Holden, E. W. (1987). Child diagnostic assessment: Current training practices in clinical psychology internships. *Professional Psychology: Research and Practice, 18,* 587–596.

Elliot, A. J., Miltenberger, R. G., Kaster-Bundgaard, J., & Lumley, V. (1996). A national survey of assessment and therapy techniques used by behavior therapists. *Cognitive and Behavioral Practice, 3,* 107–125.

Follette, W. C., & Hayes, S. C. (1992). Behavioral assessment in the DSM era. *Behavioral Assessment, 14,* 293–295.

Fonseca, A. C., & Perrin, S. (2001). Clinical phenomenology, classification and assessment of anxiety disorders in children and adolescents. In W. K. Silverman & P. D. A. Treffers (Eds.), *Anxiety disorders in children and adolescents: Research, assessment, and intervention.* New York: Cambridge University Press.

Forehand, R., & McCombs, A. (1988). Unraveling antecedent–consequence conditions in maternal depression and adolescent functioning. *Behavioral Research and Therapy, 26,* 399–405.

Gordon, M. (1997). *How to operate an ADHD clinic or subspecialty practice* (Rev. 1st ed.). DeWitt, NY: GSI Publications.

Gresham, F. M. (2004). Current status and future directions of school-based behavioral interventions. *School Psychology Review, 33,* 326–343.

Gross, A. M. (1990). An analysis of measures and design strategies in research in behavior therapy: Is it still behavioral? *The Behavior Therapist, 13,* 203–209.

Handwerk, M. J., Larzerlere, R. E., Soper, S. H., & Friman, P. C. (1999). Parent and child discrepancies in reporting severity of problem behaviors in three out-of-home settings. *Psychological Assessment, 11,* 14–23.

Hatfield, D. R., & Ogles, B. M. (2004). The use of outcome measures by psychologists in clinical practice. *Professional Psychology: Research and Practice, 35,* 485–491.

Hawkins, R. P. (1979). The functions of assessment: Implications for selection and development of devices for assessing repertoires in clinical, educational, and other settings. *Journal of Applied Behavior Analysis, 12,* 501–516.

Hawkins, R. P. (1986). Selection of target behaviors. In R. O. Nelson & S. C. Hayes (Eds.), *Conceptual foundations of behavioral assessment.* New York: Guilford Press.

Hayes, S. C., Follette, W. C., & Follette, V. M. (1995). Behavior therapy: A contextual approach. In A. S. Gurman & S. B. Messer (Eds.), *Essential psychotherapies: Theory and practice.* New York: Guilford Press.

Hayes, S. C., Nelson, R. O., & Jarrett, R. B. (1987). The treatment utility of assessment: A functional approach to evaluating assessment quality. *American Psychologist, 42,* 963–974.

Haynes, S. N. (1998). The changing nature of behavioral assessment. In A. S. Bellack & M. Hersen (Eds.), *Behavioral assessment: A practical handbook* (4th ed.). Boston: Allyn & Bacon.

Hembree-Kigin, T. L., & McNeil, C. B. (1995). *Parent–child interaction therapy.* New York: Plenum Press.

Hersen, M., & Bellack, A. S. (1976). Preface. In M. Hersen & A. S. Bellack (Eds.), *Behavioral assessment: A practical handbook.* New York: Pergamon Press.

Individuals with Disabilities Education Act Amendments of 1997 (Pub. L. No. 105-17). 20 U.S.C. 1400 *et seq.*

Johnston, C., & Murray, C. (2003). Incremental validity in the psychological assessment of children and adolescents. *Psychological Assessment, 15,* 496–507.

Kamphaus, R. W., & Frick, P. (1996). *Clinical assessment of child and adolescent personality and behavior.* Needham Heights, MA: Allyn & Bacon.

Kanfer, F. H. (1979). A few comments on the current status of behavioral assessment. *Behavioral Assessment, 1,* 37–40.

Kanfer, F. H., & Saslow, G. (1969). Behavioral diagnosis. In C. M. Franks (Ed.), *Behavior therapy: Appraisal and status.* New York: McGraw-Hill.

Kazdin, A. E. (1983). Psychiatric diagnosis, dimensions of dysfunction, and child behavior therapy. *Behavior Therapy, 14,* 73–99.

Kearney, C. A., & Silverman, W. K. (1999). Functionally based prescriptive and nonprescriptive treatment for children and adolescents with school refusal behavior. *Behavior Therapy, 30,* 673–695.

Kelley, M. L. (2003). Assessment of children's behavior in the school setting: An overview. In M. L. Kelley, D. Reitman, & G. H. Noell (Eds.), *Practitioner's guide to empirically based measures of school behavior.* AABT Clinical Assessment Series. New York: Kluwer Academic/Plenum.

Krasner, L. (1992). The concepts of syndrome and functional analysis: Compatible or incompatible? *Behavioral Assessment, 14,* 307–321.

Kuhne, M., Schachar, R., & Tannock, R. (1997). Impact of comorbid oppositional or conduct problems on attention-deficit hyperactivity disorder. *Journal of the American Academy of Child and Adolescent Psychiatry, 36,* 1715–1725.

Kwak, M. M., Ervin, R. A., Anderson, M. Z., & Austin, J. (2004). Agreement of function across methods used in school-based functional assessment with preadolescent and adolescent students. *Behavior Modification, 28,* 375–401.

Lambert, M. J., & Hawkins, E. J. (2004). Measuring outcome in professional practice: Considerations in selecting and using brief outcome instruments. *Professional Psychology: Research and Practice, 35,* 492–499.

Lyon, G. R., Fletcher, J. M., & Barnes, M. C. (2003). Learning disabilities. In E. J. Mash & R. A. Barkley (Eds.), *Child psychopathology* (2nd ed., pp. 520–586). New York: Guilford Press.

Mash, E. J., & Terdal, L. G. (1988). Behavioral assessment of child and family disturbance. In E. J. Mash & L. G. Terdal (Eds.), *Behavioral assessment of childhood disorders: Selected core problems* (2nd ed.). New York: Guilford Press.

Mash, E. J., & Wolfe, D. A. (2005). *Abnormal child psychology* (3rd ed.). Belmont, CA: Thompson Wadsworth.

McGlough, J. F., & Clarkin, J. F. (2004). Personality disorders. In M. Hersen (Ed.), *Psychological assessment in clinical practice: A pragmatic guide.* New York: Brunner-Routledge.

Miltenberger, R. G. (2000). Strategies for clarifying ambiguous functional analysis outcomes: Comments on Kennedy. *Journal of Positive Behavioral Interventions, 2,* 202–204.

Mischel, W. (1979). On the interface of cognition and personality: Beyond the person situation debate. *American Psychologist, 34,* 740–754.

Moffit, T. E., & Caspi, A. (2001). Childhood predictors differentiate life-course persistent and adolescent-limited antisocial pathways among males and females. *Development and Psychopathology, 13,* 355–375.

Nay, W. R. (1979). *Multimethod clinical assessment.* New York: Gardner Press.

Nelson, J. R., Benner, G. J., Reid, R. C., Epstein, M. H., & Currin, D. (2002). The convergent validity of office discipline referrals with the CBCL-TRF. *Journal of Emotional and Behavioral Disorders, 10,* 181–188.

Nelson, R. O. (1983). Behavioral assessment: Past, present, and future. *Behavioral Assessment, 5,* 195–206.

Nelson, R. O., & Hayes, S. C. (1986). The nature of behavioral assessment. In R. O. Nelson & S. C. Hayes (Eds.), *Conceptual foundations of behavioral assessment.* New York: Guilford Press.

Nelson-Gray, R. O. (2003). Treatment utility of psychological assessment. *Psychological Assessment, 15,* 521–531.

Newcomer, L. L., & Lewis, T. J. (2004). Functional behavioral assessment: An investigation of reliability and effectiveness of function-based interventions. *Journal of Emotional and Behavioral Disorders, 12,* 168–181.

Noell, G. H. (2003). Functional assessment of school-based concerns. In M. L. Kelley, D. Reitman, & G. H. Noell (Eds.), *Practitioner's guide to empirically based measures of school behavior.* AABT Clinical Assessment Series. New York: Kluwer Academic/Plenum.

Northup, J., & Gulley, V. (2001). Some contributions of functional analysis to the assessment of behaviors associated with attention deficit hyperactivity disorder and the effects of stimulant medication. *School Psychology Review, 30,* 227–238.

Ollendick, T. H., & Hersen, M. (1984). An overview of child behavioral assessment. In T. H. Ollendick & M. Hersen (Eds.), *Child behavioral assessment: Principles and procedures.* New York: Pergamon Press.

Ollendick, T. H., & Hersen, M. (1993). Child and adolescent behavioral assessment. In T. H. Ollendick & M. Hersen (Eds.), *Handbook of child and adolescent assessment.* Needham Heights, MA: Allyn & Bacon.

O'Neil, R. E., Horner, R. H., Albin, R.W., Sprague, J. R., Storey, K., & Newton, J. S. (1997). *Functional assessment and program development for problem behavior: A practical handbook* (2nd ed.). Pacific Grove, CA: Brooks/Cole.

Patterson, G. R. (1965). Responsiveness to social stimuli. In L. Krasner & L. Ullman (Eds.), *Research in behavior modification.* New York: Holt, Rinehart, & Winston.

Patterson, G. R. (1993). Orderly change in a stable world: The antisocial trait as a chimera. *Journal of Consulting and Clinical Psychology, 61,* 911–919.

Patterson, G. R., & Reid, J. B. Reciprocity and coercion: Two facets of social systems. In C. Neuringer & J. L. Michael (1970). *Behavior modification in clinical psychology.* New York: Appleton-Century-Crofts.

Patterson, G. R., Reid, J. B., & Dishion, T. R. (1992). Antisocial boys. Eugene, OR: Castalia.

Pelham, W. E., Wheeler, T., & Chronis, A. (1998). Empirically supported psychosocial treatments for attention deficit hyperactivity disorder. *Journal of Clinical Child Psychology, 27,* 190–205.

Pine, D. S., Alegria, M., Cook, E. H., Costello, E. J., Dahl, R. E., Koretz, D., Merikangas, K. R., Reiss, A. L., & Vitiello, B. (2002). Advances in developmental sciences and DSM-V (pp. 85–122). In D. J. Kupfer (Ed.), *A research agenda for DSM-IV.* Washington, DC: American Psychiatric Association.

Piotrowski, C., Belter, R. W., & Keller, J. W. (1998). The impact of managed care on the practice of psychological testing: Preliminary findings. *Journal of Personality Assessment, 70,* 441–447.

Plitszka, S. R. (2000). Patterns of psychiatric comorbidity with attention-deficit/hyperactivity disorder. *Child and Adolescent Psychiatric Clinics of North America, 9,* 525–540.

Reid, J. B., Baldwin, D. V., Patterson, G. R., & Dishion, T. J. (1987). Some problems relating to assessment of childhood disorders: A role for observational data. In M. Rutter, A. H. Tuma, & I. Lann (Eds.), *Assessment and diagnosis in child psychology.* New York: Guilford Press.

Reitman, D., & Hupp, S. D. A. (2003). Behavior problems in the school setting: Synthesizing structural and functional assessment. In M. L. Kelley, D. Reitman, & G. H. Noell (Eds.), *Practitioner's guide to empirically based measures of school behavior.* AABT Clinical Assessment Series. New York: Kluwer Academic/Plenum.

Reitman, D., Hummel, R., Franz, D. Z., & Gross, A. M. (1998). A review of methods and instruments for assessing externalizing disorders: Theoretical and practical considerations in rendering a diagnosis. *Clinical Psychology Review, 18,* 555–584.

Reynolds, C. R., & Kamphaus, R. W. (1992). *Manual: Behavior assessment system for children.* Circle Pines, MN: American Guidance Service.

Reynolds, W. M. (1994). Assessment of depression in children and adolescents by self-report. In W. M. & H. F. Johnston (Eds.), *Handbook of depression in children and adolescents* (pp. 209–234). New York: Plenum Press.

Robbins, L. N., & Rutter, M. (1990). *Straight and devious pathways from childhood to adulthood.* New York: Cambridge University Press.

Sasso, G. M., Conroy, M. A., Peck-Stichter, J., & Fox, J. J. (2001). Slowing down the bandwagon: The misapplication of functional assessment for students with emotional or behavioral disorders. *Behavioral Disorders, 26,* 282–296.

Scotti, J. R., Morris, T. L., McNeil, C. B., & Hawkins, R. P. (1996). DSM-IV and disorders of childhood and adolescence: Can structural criteria be functional? *Journal of Consulting and Clinical Psychology, 64,* 1177–1191.

Schulte, D. (1996). Tailor-made and standardized therapy: Complementary tasks in behavior therapy: A contrarian view. *Journal of Behavior Therapy and Experimental Psychiatry, 27,* 119–126.

Shinn, M. (1989). *Curriculum-based measurement: Assessing special children.* New York: Guilford Press.

Silva, F. (1993). *Foundations of behavioral assessment.* New York: Sage.

Silverman, W. K., & Kurtines, W. M. (1996). *Anxiety and phobic disorders: A pragmatic approach.* New York: Plenum Press.

Stedman, J. M., Hatch, J. P., & Shoenfeld, L. S. (2001). Internship directors' valuation of preinternship preparation in test-based assessment and psychotherapy. *Professional Psychology: Research & Practice, 32,* 421–424.

Sturges, J. W. (1998). Practical use of technology in professional practice. *Professional Psychology: Research & Practice, 29,* 183–188.

Tryon, W. W. (1998). Behavioral observation. In A. S. Bellack & M. Hersen (Eds.), *Behavioral assessment: A practical handbook* (4th ed.). Boston: Allyn & Bacon.

Van Houten, R., Axelrod, S., Bailey, J. S., Favell, J. E., Foxx, R. M., Iwata, B. A., & Lovaas, O. I. (1988). The right to effective behavioral treatment. *The Behavior Analyst, 11,* 111–114.

Velting, O. N., Setzer, N. J., & Albano, A. M. (2004). Update on advances in assessment and cognitive-behavioral treatment of anxiety disorders in children and adolescents. *Professional Psychology: Research and Practice, 35,* 42–54.

Witt, J. C., & Beck, R. (2000). *One-minute academic functional assessment and interventions: "Can't" do it . . . or "won't" do it?* Longmont, CO: Sopris West.

Yates, B. T., & Taub, J. (2003). Assessing the costs, benefits, cost-effectiveness, and cost-benefit of psychological assessment: We should, we can, and here's how. *Psychological Assessment, 15,* 478–495.

Youngstrom, E., Loeber, R., & Stouthamer-Loeber, M. (2000). *Journal of Consulting and Clinical Psychology, 68,* 1038–1050.

2

Developmental Considerations

Susan Tinsley Li
School of Professional Psychology
Pacific University
Portland, Oregon

Sandra Rogers

School of Occupational Therapy
Pacific University, Forest Grove, Oregon

INTRODUCTION

The ecology of the child includes complex nested systems of influence (Bronfenbrenner & Morris, 1998). One of the most important of these influences is the developmental context. Developmental considerations affect the assessment process with children and adolescents in multiple ways; thus, effective child assessment is based on a foundation and understanding of basic child developmental theories and processes. Core knowledge should include an understanding of why the developmental context matters and how development proceeds across basic dimensions.

THE IMPORTANCE OF THE DEVELOPMENTAL CONTEXT FOR ASSESSING CHILDREN

Why is knowledge of child development essential for assessment? The reasons for including development as a primary consideration span issues such as competent practice, establishment of a normative baseline, and measurement. Several of these arguments are articulated in the following discussion.

1) *An understanding of child development provides a context from which to determine whether a child's current behaviors are developmentally typical or atypical.* The fact that a child has started using two-word utterances has a dis-

tinctly different meaning in a 1-year-old, a 2-year-old, and a 3-year-old child. In the 1-year-old, this behavior may suggest advanced skills, in the 2-year-old, age appropriate behaviors, and in the 3-year-old, a possible language delay. Thus, the same behavior implies a different level of language acquisition when one considers what the typical level of language development should be for a given child's developmental age.

2) *Child development makes the comparison of scores to the normative group theoretically meaningful.* Related to the first point is the effective interpretation and comparison of a child's scores to the norm group of a particular test. Is it really conceptually meaningful that a child scored in the average range when compared to other 12-year-olds? Or is there an underlying assumption that 12-year-olds in general possess certain cognitive abilities and that the particular child being evaluated has visual spatial constructive abilities that are consistent with that developmental level? This assertion is basically the between-group, or *norm-referenced comparison*. When one compares a given child's performance to the normative group, the assumption is that one is comparing the individual child's score to the scores of children who theoretically have attained a similar level of development and, in this case, visual spatial constructive development.

3) *Information on basic developmental milestones is one aspect of a complete evaluation that improves the ability to make hypotheses about current problems.* No assessment is complete without a full multi-informant interview (i.e., child, primary caregiver, school personnel, etc.). A significant portion of that interview should be developmentally based. There are numerous examples of the best way to ask questions regarding a child's early development. However, the underlying issue that is often being addressed is whether the child reached his or her developmental milestones within normative limits or whether there is a pattern of delay. A complete developmental history places the child's current performance in context. For the child who displayed typical development, a present pattern of delay represents a departure. Similarly, an early delayed pattern provides confirmation of a different, yet stable and consistent, pattern of current and historical atypical development.

4) *Child development provides a within subject point of reference.* There is an inherent assumption that development proceeds in a linear fashion and that the developmental trajectory for most children increases over time. Although the life span perspective suggests that development is both multidirectional and multidimensional (Berk, 2004; Feldman, 2005), most professionals expect children to progress developmentally toward increased skills, with some minor periods of discontinuity. Thus, if a significant and persistent regression occurs within a child's scores, it becomes a marker or indicator of possible abnormality. This type of comparison, also called *time-referenced comparison* (Gilliam, 1999), answers the question of what the child's trajectory of functioning is with age, time, and maturation. There are some disorders of childhood and infancy that have regressions in development as one of the diagnostic criteria. For example, Rett's disorder is characterized by a prolonged developmental regression that is preceded by a period of normal development (APA, 2000).

5) *Theories of development can affect the interpretation of test results and the examiner's approach to test administration.* Stage theories of development assume that cognitive skills are discontinuous and that changes are qualitative in nature. There are implications of adherence to a continuous or discontinuous model of development for interpreting change in children's test scores. For example, one implication of a stage model of development is that retesting a child in six months could lead to vastly different scores or constant scores, depending on whether the child's "stage" of development has changed. Thus, the stability of test scores (i.e., what we typically consider test–retest reliability) may no longer be considered an important psychometric indicator. Similarly, an examiner who is a proponent of Lev Vygotsky's theory and his concept of the zone of proximal development (Vygotsky, 1978) may view "testing the limits" very differently following a standardized administration. Testing the limits and adding teaching tasks before administering cognitive measures may create a zone in which the child is able to demonstrate the skill.

In summary, taking developmental considerations into account is essential for competent evaluation and assessment of children and adolescents. This is not a new argument, for other authors have asserted the necessity of a developmental framework when interviewing (Greenspan & Greenspan, 2003) and designing treatment interventions for child and adolescent populations (Eyberg, Schuhmann, & Rey, 1998; Holmbeck, Greenley, & Franks, 2003; Weisz & Hawley, 2002).

Frequently, authors employ a developmental psychopathology framework as a way of conceptualizing the interplay of developmental factors with mental health issues from a theoretical perspective. The developmental psychopathology literature is founded on the concept that the expression of symptomatology and psychopathology in children and adolescents cannot be separated from their developmental level (Cicchetti & Rogosch, 2002). How an individual child responds adaptively or maladaptively to particular stressors at a given life stage determines the development of problematic or normative behavior (Forehand & Wierson, 1993). Such understanding of the interplay of physical, cognitive, and emotional development can easily be applied to the assessment and evaluation literature. Developmental assessment, like developmental psychopathology, takes developmental knowledge and research into account in a substantial way and does not assume that, because a particular measure has been normed with a given age group, it captures developmental processes and changes.

DIMENSIONS OF DEVELOPMENT

So what level of developmental expertise is required to be effective and competent in child assessment? At a minimum, knowledge of basic developmental theories is essential, in addition to familiarity with general terms frequently used in the developmental literature. Typically, at a gross level, the life span is broken into roughly seven periods of development: infancy, early childhood, middle childhood, adolescence, young adulthood, middle adulthood, and late adulthood. In this chapter we are concerned with the first part of the life span, or infancy, childhood, and adolescence. The qualifiers "early" and "late" are often added in the literature for overlap (e.g., early and late adolescence) but really do not provide much more than rudimentary categories. Short of picking up a developmental textbook (e.g., Feldman, 2005) and reading it in its entirety, the following sections provide an overview of some of the basic dimensions of children's development, including development of motor control, cognitive development, and emotional development.

This is not a comprehensive review but, rather, a brief synopsis to enable the reader to have a resource of general guidelines regarding changes in development across domains. Similar sources of this type of information have been provided by Holmbeck et al. (2003) and Forehand and Wierson (1993). Greenspan and Greenspan (2003) also provide a unique review of developmental changes that is dynamically oriented and clinically focused. It includes both age- and phase-appropriate categories for patterns of relationships, overall mood or emotional tone, affects, anxieties and fears, and thematic expression (Greenspan & Greenspan, 2003, Table 3.1). Within the realm of child psychology and psychiatry, occupational and physical therapists contribute to a comprehensive assessment by providing in-depth information about neuro-motor, sensory processing, and functional or adaptive skill analysis. Therapists will often use neuro-motor, developmental assessments and, increasingly, qualitative assessments based on dynamic systems theory to enable them to quantify abilities, document subtle changes over time, and provide information on the qualitative aspects of movement as well as to evaluate these developing motor skills.

DEVELOPMENT OF MOTOR CONTROL

MOTOR SKILLS

Motor development involves a child's ability to perform in object play and manipulation, self-care, mobility, and social functions.

General developmental considerations are based on either a neuro-maturation theory or a dynamic systems theory. If using a neuro-maturation theory, the following are assumed. (1) Movement progresses from primitive reflex patterns to voluntary controlled movement (i.e., involuntary grasp when an object is placed in the hand to purposefully reaching and grasping for an object. (2) The sequence and rate of development are consistent between children, and thus a normative developmental sequence can be employed. (3) Low-level skills are acquired before more complex skills, or, rather, skills are acquired from the mass to specific and from a proximal to distal sequence (i.e., gross palmar grasp precedes a pincer grasp, and head control occurs before reaching). Assuming a strict hierarchical approach is no longer acceptable in light of motor development research, however, neuro-maturation processes are helpful as general guidelines for the identification of specific areas of delay and in anticipation of their development. The use of the neuro-maturation theories is still evident in many motor evaluations.

The dynamical systems approach acknowledges that while most healthy 5-month-old children are able to reach toward an object purposefully, the patterns each child uses is quite unique. Some infants will make a slow, cautious approach, whereas others make a ballistic arm movement to reach and obtain the object. Although all first attempts are circuitous, the amount of corrections made to obtain the object, the speed at which the attempts are made, and the angle of arm movements are significantly different. Given the highly variable nature of viewing children through this lens, in dynamical systems motor behavior is not prescribed, but emerges through external and internal variables or constraints. These variables provide information or, rather, limit the boundaries for a child's behaviors across time. These variables come from within the child, the environment, and the task at hand. This theory emphasizes three stages of developing new skills and occupations. The first stage is exploratory activity. In this stage a child learns about self and the environment; the child would experiment with objects and tasks using different systems, new combinations, and new sequences of action. In the second stage or phase of learning the child uses feedback, and behavior is reinforced through exploration. Movement patterns vary less during this stage, but variation occurs in less dramatic ways. The final stage features the child who selects the most effective pattern to achieve a goal. Selection of a single pattern is self-organizing, but this pattern remains adaptable. High adaptability is always characteristic of a well-learned task. Action patterns are economical and will lead to new opportunities to explore the environment.

POSTURAL CONTROL

Postural control requires development of antigravity movements and proximal muscle control. Such control leads to an interaction between patterns of cocontraction and mature equilibrium responses, which in turn leads to dynamic control over both trunk and extremity movement. Current systems theories seem to explain motor development most accurately. Systems theories acknowledge that muscle strength, body size, sensory system functioning, cognitive skills, and environmental context will all contribute to motor and postural development. This section describes development of the motor milestones as antigravity movement, postural reactions, sensory processing, and anticipatory postural control develop.

Typical first-year-of-life development unfolds in a hierarchical scheme, moving from supine to prone to sitting, crawling, creeping, cruising, and finally

TABLE 2.1 Age of Postural Reaction Acquisition

Balance Reactions	Age, in Months
Righting reactions	
Neck on body	
Immature	Birth
Mature	4–5
Body on body	
Immature	Birth
Mature	4–5
Body on head	
Prone	1–2
Mature	4–5
Supine	5–6
Landau	
Immature	3
Mature	6–10
Flexion	
Partial (head in line)	3–4
Mature (head forward)	6–7
Vertical	
Partial (head in line)	2
Mature (head forward)	6
Protective reactions	
Forward	6–7
Lateral	6–11
Backward	9–12
Equilibrium reactions	
Prone	5–6
Supine	7–8
Sitting	7–10
Quadruped	9–12
Standing	12–21

walking. While this hierarchical model often describes development, it ignores the fact that there is a wide range of ages when these skills develop for many children. These models also do not account for those typically developing children who miss one or two of the milestones. In any case this scheme is useful for generating an overall view of a child's development. Postural control milestones are listed in Tables 2.1 and 2.2. The influences over postural control include the specific range of joint motion, strength, and muscle tone specific to each child. It is the integration of these factors with vision, cognition, and the desire to move that influences postural development and ultimately gross motor skills.

TABLE 2.2 Acquisition Ages of Early Motor Milestones

Motor Milestones	Age, in months
Head control	
Prone	
Lifts head to 45°	2
Lifts head to 90°	4
Supine	
Maintains head in midline	2
Lifts head in midline	6
Rolling	
Prone to supine	
Without rotation	4–6
With rotation	6–9
Supine to prone	
Without rotation	5–7
With rotation	6–9
Sitting	
Upright briefly with arm support	4–5
Sustained with arm support	5–6
Upright briefly without arm support	6–7
Sustained without arm support	7–9
Mobility	
Crawls	7–9
Creeps	9–11
Cruises	9–13
Walks	12–14
Walks backward	15–21
Stands briefly on one leg	18–24
Walks up steps without support	19–24
Walks down steps without support	25–30
Stands from supine using a sit-up	30–33
Stands on one foot for 5 seconds	30–36
Hops, changes feet, hops on alternate foot	49–54
Skips	55–60
Running	
Walks hurriedly	14–18
Runs well	18–24
Runs and avoids obstacles	24–30
Runs 15 yards in 6 seconds	37–42
Runs and stops without falling	43–48
Gallops	49–54
Jumping	
Jumps forward without falling	19–24
Jumps up	25–30
Jumps over string	31–36
Jumps with both feet, forward 2 feet	37–42
Jumps and turns body	49–54
Jumps back and forth over a line	55–60

(*continues*)

TABLE 2.2 *(continued)*

Fine-Motor Milestones	Age, in months
Reach/approach	
Reaches both arms in full range of motion	6–12
Reaches to midline, extended elbow	6–12
Reaches across midline	12–24
Grasp and prehension	
Closes fingers in tight grasp	0–2
Grasps rattle	0–2
Grasps and picks up rattle	3–5
Grasps toy string and pulls to obtain toy	3–5
Ulnar palmar grasp	3–5
Full palmar grasp	4–6
Picks up two cubes	6–8
Rakes tiny object	6–8
Radial digital grasp	7–9
Standard pincer grasp	9–11
Spherical grasp	12–24
Intrinsic plus grasp	12–24
Places tiny objects in bottle	15–23
Power grasp	36+
Voluntary release	
Releases objects freely	6–12
Releases 1-inch cube into container	12–24
Releases tiny object into small hole	12–24
Bilateral and midline skills	
Clasps hands while looking at objects	3–5
Places both hands on bottle	3–5
Retains objects in each hand	5–6
Holds or carries large ball	6–12
Unwraps toys	10–12
Places objects into a container	12–14
Stirs with spoon in cup	12–14
Places large shapes into holes	15–18
Uses both hands in midline; one holds and one manipulates objects	15–18
Demonstrates occasional hand preference	19–24
Demonstrates consistent hand preference	37–42
Prewriting and writing	
Grasps crayon with whole fist	11–12
Holds crayon with thumb and finger	23–25
Holds pencil with thumb and finger	36–48
Handwriting appropriate for grade	60+
Block construction	
Stacks cubes (2–4)	15–18
Stacks 8–10 cubes	25–30
Builds with 3 blocks	31–36

TABLE 2.2 (*continued*)

Fine-Motor Milestones	Age, in months
Paper activities	
Crumbles paper	6–8
Imitates scribble	10–12
Marks with crayon	12–14
Scribbles spontaneously	14–18
Paints within paper borders	19–24
Draws vertical line	19–24
Folds paper	19–24
Draws horizontal line	25–30
Snips with scissors	25–30
Draws a circle	31–36
Snips on line with scissors	28–35
Cuts paper in two with scissors	37–42
Draws a cross	37–42
Cuts out simple shapes with scissors	48–60
Cuts out complex shapes	60+
Rotates pencil to use eraser and rotates it back	60+
Manipulative prehension	
Finger-to-palm translation, small object	12–24
Points with index finger	12–16
Turns book pages one at a time	19–24
Removes screw cap lid from bottle	25–30
Strings 1-inch beads	25–30
Rolls clay into ball	36–42
Laces 3 holes with shoelace	37–42
Touches fingers to thumb	49–54
Uses a variety of in-hand manipulation skills	55+
Visual-motor	
Tracks objects, midline, to 90° side to side	0–2
Extends arms to toy	3–5
Touches fingers	3–5
Looks at distant objects	5–6
Bangs cup on table	6–8
Bangs two cubes	9–11
Removes pegs from pegboard	9–11
Opens book	12–14
Places peg in pegboard	12–14
Places multiple pegs in pegboard	16–19

FINE MOTOR MOVEMENT

Effective use of hands and arms to engage in a wide variety of manipulative activities in daily occupation is essential to development and depends on the coordination of foundational motor skills, cognition, and visual perception. Fine motor control relies on the foundational development and integration of postural-control, cognitive, and visual skills and includes reach, grasp, carry, release, and more complex skills, such as in-hand manipulation and bilateral hand use. As children develop, they coordinate and combine hand skills with visual skills. These skills allow children to engage in increasingly complex activities. Many dimensions of development, aside from motor skills, influence effective hand use; these include vision, visual-perceptual development, social and cultural influences, and somatosensory (tactile) functions.

Two developmental principles apply to hand skills development that are especially important to consider: mass-to-specific and proximal and distal. The mass-to-specific principle indicates that a less differentiated movement pattern will precede discrete, highly specialized skills. An infant will learn to use the whole hand to rake or bat at objects prior to using a pincer grasp to pick up a small pellet. The second principle of proximal and distal development implies that development will occur proximally (toward the trunk and head) and then gradually progress to the extremities and hand. It is important to note here that while this principle does document the overall progression of hand skills in development, it is not useful in guiding treatment. It is common to interpret this relationship to mean that hand skills can only develop after proximal control is gained. However, children can develop hand skills despite a lack of proximal control; this is achieved from the motor system pattern of innervation. One motor system is responsible for postural control and originates from the brainstem; in contrast, the second motor pathway originates from the corticospinal tract and is responsible for coordinated fine motor movement. Development of proximal and distal mechanisms is critical to achieving good fine motor skills. Refined movement of the hand also relies on the ability to effectively combine both stability and mobility. The child must develop the ability to stabilize the trunk and maintain an upright posture while manipulating objects. For the most optimal functioning, joints must be able to stabilize at any point within the normal range of movement and to move within small or large segments of the range. During some arm–hand activities, the hand (distal portion) is more active and the proximal limb is stable; an example of this is the grasping of objects. However, during carrying of objects, the hand is stable and the more proximal portion of the arm is moving. Another principle is that of straight movement patterns that develop prior to the emergence of controlled rotational movement patterns. At the shoulder, the ability to move in flexion and extension precedes the ability to control internal and external rotation. Asymmetrical movements are typically developed prior to symmetric movements, and reflexive patterns often precede coordination. A child will often use both sides asymmetrically and gradually develop coordination of both arms and then the skilled use of symmetric and asymmetric movements (for handwriting, as an example).

Table 2.3 shows the relationship between hand skill development and approximate chronological age.

TABLE 2.3 Developmental Sequence of Sample Self-Care Skills

Skill	Types of Tasks Within Skill	Approximate Age
Feeding	• Nursing or bottle-feeding of formula	0–6 months
	• Continues to nurse or bottle-feed • Takes cereal or pureed food from a spoon	5–7 months
	• Attempts to hold bottle, but may not retrieve it if it falls • Needs to be monitored for safety	6–8 months
	• Holds and tries to eat cracker, but sucks on it more than bites • Consumes soft foods that dissolve in the mouth • Grabs at spoon, but bangs it or sucks on either end of it	6–9 months
	• Finger-feeds self a portion of each meal • Meals consist of soft table foods (macaroni, peas, dry cereal) • Eats cooperatively, with adult feeding	9–13 months
	• Dips spoon in food • Brings spoon to mouth, but spills food by inverting spoon before it goes into mouth	12–14 months
	• Scoops food with spoon, and brings it to mouth	15–18 months
	• Demonstrates interest in using fork • May stab at food pieces • Proficient at spoon use, and eats cereal with milk or rice with gravy	2–3 years
	• Manages a greater variety of foods with appropriate utensil • Sips soups • Eats a variety of foods • Cuts with side of fork	3–5 years
	• Cuts with knife • Opens food packages • Follows table manners	6–9 years
Toileting	• Indicates discomfort when wet or soiled • Has regular bowel movements	1 year
	• Sits on the toilet when placed for short periods and supervised	1½ years
	• Urinates regularly in toilet	2 years
	• Achieves regulated toileting with occasional accidents • Bowel trained • Tells someone he/she needs to use the bathroom • May need reminders to go to the bathroom	2½ years
	• Goes to the bathroom independently • Seats self on toilet • Needs help wiping • Needs assistance with fasteners or difficult clothing	3 years
	• Independent in toileting, including tearing toilet paper, flushing, washing hands, managing clothing	4–5 years
Dressing	• Cooperates with dressing by holding out arms and legs • Pulls off clothing • Pulls off socks and shoes • Pushes arms through sleeves and legs through pants	1 year
	• Removes unfastened coat • Removes shoes if laces are untied	2 years

(continues)

TABLE 2.3 (*continued*)

Skill	Types of Tasks Within Skill	Approximate Age
Dressing (*cont.*)	• Helps pull down pants	
	• Finds arm holes in over-the-head shirts	
	• Pulls down elastic-waist pants	$2\frac{1}{2}$ years
	• Assists in pulling on socks	
	• Puts on front-buttoning coat or shirt	
	• Unbuttons large buttons	
	• Puts on over-the-head shirt with minimal assistance	3 years
	• Puts on shoes without fasteners (may be wrong foot)	
	• Puts on socks (may have heel on top)	
	• Independently pulls down pants	
	• Zips and unzips jacket once on track	
	• Needs assistance to remove over-the-head shirt	
	• Buttons large front buttons	
	• Finds front of clothing	$3\frac{1}{2}$ years
	• Snaps or hooks front fastener	
	• Unzips zipper on jacket	
	• Puts on mittens	
	• Buttons series of 3 or 4 large buttons	
	• Unbuckles shoes or belt	
	• Dresses with supervision	
	• Removes pullover garment independently	4 years
	• Buckles shoes or belt	
	• Zips jacket zipper	
	• Puts on socks correctly	
	• Puts on shoe, with assistance in lace tying	
	• Laces shoes	
	• Consistently identifies the front and back of garment	
	• Puts belt in belt loops	
	• Ties and unties knots	5 years
	• Dresses unsupervised	
	• Closes back zipper	6 years
	• Ties bow	
	• Buttons back buttons	
	• Snaps back snaps	
Home management	• Imitates housework	13 months
	• Picks up and puts toys away with parental reminders	2 years
	• Copies parents' domestic activities	
	• Carries things without dropping them	3 years
	• Dusts with help	
	• Gardens with help	
	• Puts toys away, with reminders	
	• Wipes spills	
	• Fixes dry cereal and snacks	4 years
	• Helps with sorting laundry	
	• Puts toys away neatly	5 years
	• Makes a sandwich	
	• Takes out trash	

TABLE 2.3 (*continued*)

Skill	Types of Tasks Within Skill	Approximate Age
Home management (*cont.*)	• Makes bed • Puts dirty clothes away • Answers telephone directly • Does simple errands	6 years
	• Does household chores without redoing • Cleans sink • Crosses street safely • Begins to cook simple meal • Puts clean clothes away • Hangs up clothes • Manages small amounts of money • Uses telephone correctly	7–9 years
	• Cooks simple meal with supervision • Does simple repairs with appropriate tools • Begins doing laundry • Sets table • Cares for pet with reminders	10–12 years
	• Cooks meals • Does laundry	13–14 years

ADAPTIVE SKILLS FOR SELF-CARE

Adaptive skills for self-care tasks include basic tasks like grooming, bathing, toileting, dressing, feeding, and functional mobility in the home and community. These tasks are really the expression of the child's underlying cognitive, motor, and communication skills. As a child develops, performance of these tasks are expected to be socially appropriate for the child's chronological age. These tasks are often richly embedded in cultural, social, and family routines as well as in the physical or contextual environment. In general, development of these skills will occur at more widely variable rates than either cognitive or motor skills and have cycles of expected regression and unpredictable behavior. For example, a child previously consistent in using the toilet will suddenly regress and begin to have repeated accidents, for no apparent medical or emotional reason. Active participation in a child's self-care routine has several benefits, including improving motor skills, processing skills, or cognitive skills, and will promote mastery of tasks that are both meaningful and important socially. Children typically develop self-care and adaptive skills in a sequence, as they do with both motor and cognitive skills, as overall competency increases. Understanding the sequence of self-care development helps therapists and families form realistic expectations for children and helps to determine the appropriate time to introduce new tasks or challenges.

Some tasks take on greater importance during a family's life cycle. In early childhood, feeding is usually of utmost importance because infants depend completely on parents or caregivers for nutrition. By 3 years of age, a child's ability to self-feed, dress, and toilet are usually the most important issues. As a child enters school, at the age of 5 or 6, the abilities to navigate in a school, dress him/herself (including fasteners and outerwear), toilet independently, socialize with peers, and groom become increasingly important. At this time, simple household tasks may be appropriate; for example, setting and clearing the table, making a sandwich, washing the table, making a bed, and feeding a pet may all be expected. During adolescence, independence with self-care, social skills, participation in chores and family events, sexuality, safety, caring for clothing, shopping, and managing money may all be critical to development. Table 2.3 highlights some of the most critical adaptive skills and provides a range of ages for expected success at these tasks.

COGNITIVE DEVELOPMENT

Cognitive development covers a wide range of functions and is intricately tied to the amazing changes in brain development that occur during childhood and adolescence. The frontal lobe is the area of the brain most critically involved in cognitive and intellectual changes in development, and it is the last brain structure to mature. Major periods of growth occur in the frontal cortex from birth to the second year of life and from 4 to 7 years of age; however, maturation is not complete until young adulthood. Part of the significant change in brain weight that occurs from birth onward is accounted for by glial cells and myelination. Myelination of important synaptic pathways continues into adolescence, while at the same time synaptic pruning occurs to make cognitive processing more efficient. These critical changes in brain development are necessary precursors to the complex cognitive skills that emerge in middle childhood and early adolescence and continue into adulthood.

But when and how do children acquire these cognitive skills? This question is the greatest source of fascination for developmental psychologists. Modern researchers are concerned with topics such as children's theory of mind, speed of processing, the ability to resist interference and cognitive inhibition, metacognition, and metastrategic knowing. This specificity of interest is in contrast to classical theories that have often attempted to address broad changes in children's thinking by creating stages to describe a progression of skills. Two of these classic theories, Piaget's stages of cognitive development and Selman's stages of perspective taking, provide an early look at conceptual models of children's cognitions.

Classical theories of cognitive development include Piaget's cognitive-developmental theory (Piaget, 1952, 1967; Piaget & Inhelder, 1969). Piaget postulated four stages, including the sensorimotor stage, which covers the period from birth to age 2, the preoperational stage (ages 2–6), concrete operations (ages 7–11), and formal operations (12–adult). Within Piaget's model, children begin to form mental representations based on repetitive actions that are initially reflexes. These mental representations allow children to hold objects in memory; thus, object permanence emerges in the middle of the first year. In the preoperational stage, children's cognitions are characterized by magical thinking and imaginary play. Logical thought is limited, and children in this stage exhibit difficulty reversing mental operations and focusing on multiple aspects of a problem. By the concrete operational stage, children are assumed to have mastered the essential skills of conservation, seriation, and classification. They exhibit better spatial reasoning than at younger ages. Finally, children are considered to enter formal operations, where they are able to engage in hypothetico-deductive reasoning. As has been widely noted, Piaget's theory has a number of limitations; however, it still remains prominent in the developmental psychology literature (Moshman, 1998; Keating, 1990). Table 2.4 provides a review of Piaget's stages and compares them with Selman's stages of perspective-taking (Selman, 1980). In Selman's (1980) model, a child's ability to take the perspective of peers or adult figures is hypothesized to increase from a level at which the child is unable to separate the thoughts and feelings of the self from those and others, to being able to imagine the perspective that a third person might have about a situation that the child had just encountered. Both Piaget's and Selman's theories are appealing in the way that they capture qualitative aspects of children's thinking about the world. But neither theory is amenable to reduction, in terms of identifying brain changes that accompany the proposed stages of development.

In contrast to the qualitative and discontinuous nature of Piaget's and Selman's theories, the information-processing model assumes gradual, quantitative increases in children's attention, memory, and mental operations. Beginning in infancy, children must learn both to inhibit reactions and to resist the interference of nonessential stimuli. Anyone who has observed a 6-month-old or a 6-year-old knows that these aspects of cognitive regulation are poorly developed in children, relative to adults. And yet, the abilities of the 6-year-old are phenomenal when compared to those of the 6-month-old. The processes of cognitive development continue such that by middle childhood, there is a significant increase in information-processing capacity, cognitive inhibition, and attention/planning (Dempster & Corkill, 1999; Kail, 2000; Lin, Hsiao, & Chen, 1999; Smith et al., 1998).

Three important concepts in the cognitive developmental literature that have particular relevance for assessment are speed of processing, metacognition, and cognitive inhibition. Speed of processing is a component in the current version of the Wechsler Intelligence Scale for Children (WISC-IV; Wechsler, 2004) and was present in the previous version (WISC-III; Wechsler, 1991). Conceptualized in the WISC-IV as one of the four broad factors underlying the global IQ score,

TABLE 2.4 Comparison of Classical Theories of Cognitive Development, Perspective-Taking, and Moral Reasoning

Piaget	Selman	Kohlberg
Piaget's stages of cognitive development • Stage 1: sensorimotor (birth–2 years) • Stage 2: preoperations (2–6 years) • Stage 3: concrete operations (7–11 years) • Stage 4: formal operations (12 years to adulthood) • Stage 5: postformal thought	Selman's theory of perspective-taking • Level 0 (3–6 years): undifferentiated ◦ Confuse feelings of self and other • Level 1 (4–9 years): social-informational ◦ People have access to different information, thus different perspectives • Level 2 (7–12 years): self-reflective ◦ Can "walk in another's shoes" • Level 3 (10–15 years): third-party or person ◦ Can imagine view of third person • Level 4 (14–adult): societal ◦ Third-party perspective influenced by society	Kohlberg's stages of moral development • Preconventional (morality externally controlled) ◦ Stage 1: punishment and obedience orientation ◦ Stage 2: instrumental purpose orientation • Conventional ◦ Stage 3: "good boy–good girl" orientation ◦ Stage 4: social-order-maintaining orientation • Postconventional/principled ◦ Stage 5: social contract orientation ◦ Stage 6: universal ethical principle orientation
Preoperational	Social-informational	Preconventional stage 1
Concrete operational	Self-reflective	Preconventional stage 2
Early formal operational	Third-party	Conventional stage 3
Formal operational	Societal	Conventional stage 4

speed of processing is thought to underlie the abilities to think, reason, and remember. Speed of processing increases from infancy to adulthood, with young adults responding at a rate that is 5 to 6 standard deviations faster than 8- to 10-year-olds. Speed of processing can even be assessed in infants; in fact, infant processing speed, as measured by visual tracking and habituation, may be a better predictor of later IQ than global mental and motor scales such as the Bayley Scales of Infant Development (Bayley, 1993). Although the exact nature of what causes increases in processing speed is a subject of debate, at present it appears that a global mechanism such as increased neuronal communication may be responsible. As speed of processing improves, this creates a "developmental cascade" leading to improvements in working memory and other aspects of cognition, such as cognitive self-evaluation, the use of cognitive strategies, and metastrategic knowing (Fry & Hale, 1996).

Metacognition and children's theory of mind are important contributors to developmental considerations in assessment. *Theory of mind* involves children's early understanding of the mind, metacognition, and ways of knowing (Flavell, 1979, 1981; Flavell, Miller, & Miller, 1993). *Metacognition* involves the ability to think about one's thinking and reflect on one's own knowledge (Kuhn, 2000). Metacognition develops throughout childhood but can be seen in its most basic forms in early childhood, when, even by age 3, children have some awareness that they and others "know" things. By age 4, they have an understanding of false beliefs or the idea that someone can come to an incorrect conclusion because they believe something that the child knows to be untrue, illustrating the beginning of metastrategic knowing.

The development of metamemory, or specifically knowledge about one's own memory, is an important marker because it enables children to think about how they remember information and what they might do to make their memory better (i.e., memory strategies) (Kuhn, 2000). Conceptually, remembering how to do something and remembering fact-based information is different; therefore, there is a distinction between memory strategies for procedural memory (i.e., metastrategic knowing for how to) and strategies for declarative memory (i.e., metacognitive knowing for facts) (Kuhn, 2000). As children mature, they are able to apply appropriate strategies with greater accuracy and inhibit ineffective strategies for remembering and retrieving information.

The development of strategies to improve performance and memory is most directly related to assessment in the area of test-taking strategies. Some children have a wide repertoire of skills in this area, and various assessment measures provide particular sections in which the examiner can record the child's spontaneous use of strategies (e.g., Wechsler Individual Achievement Test—Second Edition, WIAT-II, Wechsler, 1992). In order to be effective users or consumers of memory strategies, children must possess knowledge about their memory functions as well as be motivated to use effective strategies (Pierce & Lange, 2000).

Metastrategic knowing also has implications for parental coaching or teaching to the test, which can be a problem when achievement tests are used as the criteria for entry to desirable programs or services. Children who are taught compensatory and performance enhancement strategies may do better than non-coached peers. However, when the parental coaching is removed, the children may not be able to sustain the strategies if they have not changed their thinking about those strategies (Kuhn, 2000). Furthermore, the use of memory strategies may be culturally dependent (Pierce & Lange, 2000), in that some cultures emphasize the effort that children put into remembering, as compared to emphasizing or teaching the use of memory strategies.

A metamemory assessment may be a useful post-test that should correlate with children's executive functioning and predict improvements over time. In fact, children with strong metamemory skills and strategies may be the most likely to demonstrate practice effects, in that their ability to respond to the test items in more flexible ways may increase with exposure to the test, as compared to those whose metamemory skills are less advanced and who thus respond to the test in the same way each time it is given.

A third factor in cognitive development, *cognitive inhibition*, is related to attention and concentration, and it places a boundary on how effective particular strategies will be for the child. Inhibition, or the ability to resist interference, appears to be associated with frontal lobe development such that there is a general increase in the ability to inhibit reactions with maturation. The management of interference is important because it affects the use of stored information/knowledge, the availability of cognitive resources, and working memory capacity (Dempster & Corkill, 1999). Developmental trends in sustained and focused attention show marked changes in early childhood (Ruff & Lawson, 1990; Ruff & Rothbart, 1996). In general, it is expected that young children will to some degree exhibit inhibitory deficits, have less ability to resist interference, and be more likely to perseverate. However, when these problems are evidenced in an older child, it is often considered a cause for concern. Specific disorders such as Attention-Deficit/Hyperactivity Disorder have as a hallmark poor cognitive inhibition that is not consistent with the child's age or developmental level; the assessment of this disorder is the topic of a subsequent chapter. Thus, developmental differences in inhibition vary across individuals, and some children are at risk for greater difficulties in this area (Dempster & Corkill, 1999). The importance given to evaluating attention and concentration factors in child and adolescent assessments has increased substantially since the mid-1990s. This trend can be seen in the tendency to embed scales and subtests to evaluate attention and concentration factors as a separate domain in newer measures of memory, nonverbal intelligence, and executive functioning (e.g., Children's Memory Scale, Leiter International Performance Scale—Revised, and the NEPSY) (CMS: Cohen, 1997; NEPSY: Korkman, Kirk, & Kemp, 1998; Leiter-R: Roid & Miller, 1997).

EMOTIONAL DEVELOPMENT

Emotional development comprises another important domain of functioning, in addition to physical and cognitive advances. Accumulated research on aspects of emotional development is quite diverse. Notable changes are highlighted later in several key areas, including understanding of emotions, emotion knowledge and competence, and emotion regulation strategies.

The ability to interpret and predict one's own and another's emotional reactions is a foundational skill for interpersonal relationships. Early in development, children become aware of the six basic emotions: happy, angry, sad, scared, loving, and surprise (Shaver, Schwartz, Kirson, & O'Connor, 1987), and a developmental transition occurs in children's ability to identify and predict emotions in themselves and others. Early work on emotional development by Harter (1983) suggested a progression from the ability to predict single emotions to the ability to predict multiple simultaneous emotions that can be the same or different in valence. Wintre and Vallance (1994) found that even 4-year-olds can predict one emotion of varying intensity. By age 6, children comprehend that multiple emotions with variable intensity can occur together, but they assume that all of the feelings must be of the same valence. For example, children at that age understand that someone could feel very sad and a little angry at the same time, but they do not think the person could feel both happy *and* angry. An understanding of multiple emotions of variable intensity and of opposite valence does not occur until approximately 8 years of age (Wintre & Vallance, 1994), when children are able to comprehend that the same experience or target can elicit multiple feelings with opposite valence (i.e., both good and bad feelings). Thus, one might expect that a typical 9-year-old, in contrast to a 6-year-old, should be able to self-report his emotional state and capture some of the complexity of his emotional experience. The 9-year-old who is unable to conceive that he could feel both positively and negatively might be exhibiting a decreased level of emotional competence relative to his age level.

Emotional development can be separated into three basic phases: acquisition, refinement, and transformation (Haviland-Jones, Gebelt, & Stapley, 1997). All children are able to demonstrate emotional reactions; however, it is during the acquisition phase that children first begin to label these reactions. A "feeling vocabulary" begins early; by 2 years of age, most children are talking to their caregivers about feelings (Eisenberg, Fabes, & Losoya, 1997). In the refinement stage, children learn containment and enhancement strategies that shape and mold emotional expressions to be congruent with social expectations. Refinement in adolescence is particularly interesting, in that emotional signals may be awkward and exaggerated, with less of the subtlety found in adults. Unlike younger children, adolescents are able to plan for their emotional needs and to think about how to take care of themselves emotionally. Finally, in the transformation stage, children become aware of their emotions as a state or system. Although mood changes are common across childhood and are frequently associated with early adolescence and puberty, the awareness of mood changes is not developed until middle or late adolescence. Children are able to report changes (i.e., highs and lows) in positive emotions before negative ones and have trouble tracking variability in negative emotions.

Emotional competence is a complex construct that includes awareness of one's emotional state, the ability to discern others' emotions, using emotion vocabulary and terms, having a capacity for empathic and sympathetic emotional experiences, and understanding that one's inner emotions and outer expressions are not always congruent (Saarni, 1997). One aspect of emotional competence is emotional knowledge, or the child's fund of information about emotional experience in the self and others (Brenner & Salovey, 1997). Although children begin to scan others' facial expressions in infancy, it is not until about 7–8 years of age that children have basic competence in reading the emotions of others in familiar situations. It is about this time that children are able to use display rules common to their culture to guide their overt expression of emotion. Thus, by school age, children should have a complete range of emotional displays and labels as well as the ability to suppress undesirable displays of emotion (Haviland-Jones et al., 1997).

Saarni's (1997) skills of emotional competence also include the capacity for adaptive coping. Emotion regulation is one aspect of self-regulation and includes "the ability to manage one's actions, thoughts, and feelings in adaptive and flexible ways across a variety of contexts" (Saarni, 1997, p. 39). Studying children's coping is one way we learn about the development of emotion regulation. There are several general trends in children's coping that are not surprising, given the changes in cognitive development discussed earlier. As children mature, they are able to generate a greater number of coping alternatives (Brenner & Salovey, 1997; Saarni, 1997; Saarni, Mumme, & Campos, 1998). Use of cognitively oriented strategies and internal strategies increases with age, such that by age 10 most children have developed emotion-focused strategies and are improving in their problem-solving skills. In addition, solitary coping strategies increase, such that there is less of a reliance on caregivers to provide solace and social support and to cue the child to enact coping behaviors. Although younger children may have internal strategies available to them, they may not be able to access or utilize them without parental coaching. Indeed, parents are important in the development and modeling of coping strategies (Kliewer, Fearnow, & Miller, 1996).

There are individual differences in temperament and environmental factors that affect emotion regulation (Thompson, 1990). Individual differences, including high levels of negative emotionality and low regulation, tend to be fairly stable across childhood and are predictive of poorer outcomes and decreased social functioning at home and at school (Eisenberg et al., 1997).

What are the implications of emotional development for the assessment of children and adolescents? Milestones in this area have the most direct relevance for the assessment of emotional and behavioral functioning. Certainly, clinicians and researchers have identified that children with a range of disorders, such as ADHD, conduct disorder, nonverbal learning disorders, Autism/Asperger's, and depression have a decreased ability to identify their own and others' emotions when compared to same-age peers, misinterpret social cues, and have a decreased repertoire of adaptive self-regulation strategies. Evidence of deficiencies in these areas is indirectly provided by reviewing the content of child and adolescent treatment programs, such as Kendall's Coping Cat, Kazdin's problem solving, or Clarke and Lewinsohn's Coping with Depression course, which frequently target the skills noted earlier. (For further treatment description, see Clarke, Debar, & Lewinsohn, 2003; Kazdin, 2003; Kendall, Aschenbrand, & Hudson, 2003.)

Although broadband measures such as the Behavior Assessment System for Children (BASC; Reynolds & Kamphaus, 1992) and the Child Behavior Checklist (CBCL; Achenbach, 1991) are helpful and have clinical utility for the assessment of specific symptom clusters, they do little to provide a framework for evaluating a child's level of development or progression in specific areas of emotional functioning. In general, emotional development, as compared to cognitive development, is not readily considered a factor that affects performance on intelligence tests. However, when considering questions from the WISC-IV, such as "How are happy and sad alike?," emotional knowledge and emotional competence may be involved. Facial recognition and memory for faces such as those present on the Children's Memory Scale (CMS; Cohen, 1997) may be easier for children adept at interpreting facial cues.

ADDITIONAL CHANGES IN SOCIAL EMOTIONAL AND SOCIAL COGNITIVE DEVELOPMENT

Advancements in emotional and cognitive capacities interact with one another and are intricately tied to the development of interpersonal understanding and social relationships. The experience of emotions is integrated with an understanding of the self and others. This section addresses the relationship between the self and others, empathy, interpersonal relationships, moral reasoning, and extreme self-focus characteristic of early adolescent social cognition (e.g., adolescent egocentrism).

SELF AND OTHER

There are four basic stages in the development of an individual sense of self and separate other (Hoffman, 2000). In the first stage, the distinction between the self and other is unclear or confused. Later in infancy, there is an awareness of self and other as physically separate, but confusion about internal differences remains. As children mature, they become aware that they and others (i.e., caregivers and friends) not only are distinct physically but also experience separate and different internal states. Finally, adolescents are capable of understanding the uniqueness of each individual's history and how this affects internal experiences.

INTERPERSONAL RELATIONSHIPS: PEERS AND FRIENDS

In addition to family influences, peers and close friends are significant determinants of child and adolescent developmental outcomes. Peers and friendships affect school performance and engagement and may be a foundation for the formation of romantic relationships (Furman, 1999). Like emotional competence, peer competence is an important skill that predicts positive adjustment. Although the meaning of friendship is similar across the life span, including an emphasis on reciprocity (Vaughn, Colvin, Azria, Caya, & Krzysik, 2001), interpersonal interactions show a developmental progression (Hartup & Stevens, 1999). In preschool and early childhood, the goal is to engage with others and participate successfully in group activities (Sroufe, Egeland, & Carlson, 1999). Toddlers and young children define their relationships in terms of time spent together; and as early as ages 3–4, they have preferences for specific children, usually of the same gender (Hartup & Stevens, 1999; Vaughn et al., 2001). Beginning in middle childhood and continuing into adolescence, youngsters show an increased reliance for support on peers as well as primary caregivers (Hetherington, 1999). One of the tasks of middle childhood is the formation of specific friendships. Having friends and the quality of friendship are linked to adaptive outcomes (Hartup, 1996). On average, school-age children have between three and five close friends (Hartup & Stevens, 1999). Adolescent friendships are characterized by common activities and self-disclosure. Interpersonal relationships are an important developmental consideration, given that the time spent with peers and friends during middle childhood and adolescence is the greatest across the life span.

EMPATHY

Differences in the awareness of self and other affect the development of empathic behaviors. Infancy is characterized by egocentric empathic distress, in which the infant has difficulty distinguishing between her own and another's distress (i.e., you cry, I cry). This stage is followed by quasi-egocentric empathic distress, in which the young child thinks she and others feel the same (i.e., you cry, I help with what *I* would want for comfort). As the sense of an independent and unique self becomes solidified, empathy behaviors become more complex. When children are able to empathize accurately with another's feelings that differ from their own, they are able to engage in veridical empathic distress (feeling what is appropriate to the other's situation), which is usually present around age 6–7. Finally, metaempathic awareness, or a self-reflective metacognitive awareness of empathic distress, emerges that is characteristic of mature empathy (Hoffman, 2000).

MORAL REASONING

Cognitive changes such as perspective-taking and problem solving, combined with empathic behaviors and emotional knowledge, lead to changes in moral behavior. In Kohlberg's classic theory of moral reasoning, changes in children's moral development occur in stagelike fashion. Like Piaget, Kohlberg (Kohlberg, 1969; Kohlberg, Levine, & Hewer, 1983) described a theory of development in which qualitative differences characterized moral reasoning at three broad stages, the preconventional, conventional, and postconventional (see Table 2.4). Each major stage has two substages that reflect transitional developments in moral thinking. Recent research has confirmed a developmental progression in moral reasoning and supports some of Kohlberg's basic stages (Dawson, 2002; Gibbs, 2003).

Moral reasoning may be related to children's performance on the comprehension subtest of the WISC-IV. Responding in societally acceptable ways and using moral reasoning is likely to earn the child a higher score on this subtest. However, little research has investigated relations between moral development and intellectual performance.

SOCIAL COGNITION

Social-cognitive changes include perspective-taking and self-monitoring. An increased ability to self-monitor both thoughts and feelings may spark the change in self-focus or increased egocentrism associated with adolescence. The concepts of the imaginary audience and personal fable are associated with the work of Elkind (Elkind, 1967; Elkind & Bowen, 1979) and include an inability to differentiate one's own concerns from those of others (imaginary audience) and exaggerated feelings of personal uniqueness (personal fable). It is almost as if the adolescent has regressed in his understanding of self and other. However, the temporary increase in these cognitions seen in early adolescence appears to be related to changes in social perspective-taking (see Selman's theory, presented earlier) (Vartanian & Powlishta, 1996) and reflect social-cognitive development. Although in early adolescence there is a general increase of imaginary audience and personal fable beliefs, these beliefs decrease from early to late adolescence and co-occur with a corresponding decline in self-monitoring (Lapsley, Jackson, Rice, & Shadid, 1988).

DEVELOPMENTAL PROFILE

When a child is evaluated, aspects of psychopathology, symptoms, or atypical development become the focus of clinical attention. However, as has been articulated earlier, it is important to take developmental considerations into account. Thus, we advocate the creation of a developmental profile that aids the clinician in maintaining a focus on developmental factors. Imagine you are designing a computer program that provides an interpretive summary or developmental profile based on a client's age and gender. The goal of a developmental profile is to place the child in a normative developmental context. What types of normative developmental information would be helpful to receive on the profile? For example, according to major developmental theorists, what are the unique developmental issues associated with this period? This could include important stages or theories that explain developmental processes at this age. According to patterns of physical and motor development, what is this individual likely to be experiencing? What characterizes individuals of this age in terms of physical growth and postural and fine-motor control? Are specific aspects of cognitive development being highlighted in this period? Are specific skills being gained, lost, or maintained? What characterizes emotional development at this age?

The following developmental profile (Table 2.5) has been created for a 6-year-old female child to illustrate how a developmental profile might be constructed. Later in the chapter, we use this developmental profile as a context for a 6-year-old clinical case.

MULTIDISCIPLINARY MODELS AND TEAMING

This chapter was written conjointly by a child clinical psychologist and a pediatric occupational therapist, with the purpose of providing a developmental foundation for the assessment process with children. As this partnership illustrates, there is a fundamental need for multidisciplinary collaboration when evaluating children. As academicians, we recognize the importance of training students to think broadly about evaluations and to consult with colleagues within and outside of their discipline.

The who, what, where, and when of a multidisciplinary evaluation is determined by the context in which the evaluation occurs and the diagnostic complexity of the case. Shortly, we present a case example in which we articulate various procedures and measures that may be involved in the evaluation of a child with spina bifida (myelomeningocele or meningomyelocele). We hope by this illustration to provide students and practitioners with a picture of the various roles that different professionals might play with respect to a comprehensive developmental evaluation.

When combining expertise across disciplines, it is important to consider ways to communicate effectively and facilitate sharing of information across professions. Every profession has its own culture and vocabulary. Briggs (1999) provides some useful advice with regard to giving and receiving feedback in multidisciplinary teams. Given the importance of effective collaboration, Bagnato and Neisworth (1999) present a set of common standards for assessment evaluations that are more likely to lead to cooperation and teamwork among multiple professionals.

ILLUSTRATIVE CASE: "MARCIE," A CHILD WITH SPINA BIFIDA

Marcie is a 6-year-old child born at term to her 23-year-old mother, who did not receive consistent prenatal care. At the time of birth, a thoracic-level spina bifida with meningomyelocele was evident. It was surgically closed at 2 days of age, and a ventriculoperitoneal shunt was inserted at 8 days of age to correct the

TABLE 2.5 Developmental Profile

Name: Case 1
Age: 6 years
Gender: female
Developmental period: early childhood

- Classic theories or theorists
  - Erik Erikson's psychosocial stage = initiative versus guilt (3–6 years)
  - Sigmund Freud's psychosexual stage = phallic (3–6 years)
  - Jean Piaget's cognitive development stage = preoperational (2–7 years), which is characterized by magical thinking, animism, make-believe play, egocentrism, irreversibility, inability to conserve, and centration
  - Selman's perspective-taking stage = undifferentiated (3–6 years)
  - Kohlberg's moral reasoning stage = preconventional stage (punishment-and-obedience orientation)
- Physical and motor development
  - Decreased growth rate compared to infancy but still a period of rapid change
  - Continued myelination, leading to improved attention, memory, and motor control; corpus callosum grows rapidly (3–6 years), enhancing ability for complex processing; continued lateralization of right and left cerebral hemispheres
  - Frontal cortex undergoes significant growth (4–7 years)
  - Handwriting should be appropriate for grade; should have in-hand manipulation skills and the ability to cut complex shapes
  - Adaptive skills involve the ability to navigate in a school, dress and groom oneself (including fasteners and outerwear), and toilet independently; simple household tasks may be appropriate as chores
- Cognitive development
  - Information-processing theory states that cognitive abilities improve and change due to increases in attention, memory, and metacognition
- Refinements in attentional skills, increased capacity, and improved memory strategies (i.e., rehearsal) lead to "central conceptual structures"
  - According to Piaget, make-believe play also helps children to create mental representations
  - Speed of information processing increases steadily; however, it is far lower than at older ages
  - Relative to older children, children at this age lack sophisticated metacognitive skills, have poor cognitive self-regulation and cognitive inhibition
- Social/emotional development
  - Emotion knowledge includes recognition that more than one emotion can be experienced at the same time, but precludes these emotions being of opposite valence
  - Emotional refinement should include an emerging ability to inhibit undesirable and socially unacceptable emotional expressions
  - Basic coping strategies are developed, with a smaller repertoire than at older ages and more often external than internal in nature. Continues to rely on primary caregivers for social support as a coping strategy. More likely to use coping strategies when cued by adults
  - Understands that self and other are distinct, with different internal experiences; however, an individual's unique history is not taken into account
  - Both family processes and peer relationships are important and influential contexts for school-age children; should have approximately three to five close friends

hydrocephalus associated with her Chiari II malformation (common in children with meningomyelocele, the brainstem and cerebellum are displaced downward). At age 4, she needed to have her shunt surgically corrected for a blockage. She did require a vesicostomy to treat the recurrent urinary tract infection, allowing urine to drain into her diaper continuously at 1 year of age, and it is anticipated that she will continue to require use of a catheter. Scoliosis is common, and it is anticipated that Marcie will require orthotics and surgical intervention to prevent scoliosis and the development of further impairments.

During her first year, Marcie received early intervention services, including physical and occupational therapies, speech and language instruction, and an early childhood development program. She made good progress, and at 12 months she was speaking several single words, sitting independently, and crawling by propelling herself with her arms. She was able to stand using a parapodium (an external flexible skeleton). By 3 years of age, Marcie was independently using the parapodium for mobility; she is still using this for mobility, but it is anticipated that as she grows she will require a wheelchair.

Fine motor impairments include difficulty with handwriting and in-hand manipulation skills. She is able to use a tripod grasp but is unable to maintain her grasp and frequently drops her pencil and quickly moves to other tasks. She forms all of her letters, but her handwriting quickly becomes illegible. She is able to feed herself independently, with assistance for cutting foods. She is age appropriate and independent in dressing her upper body, brushing her teeth and hair, and bathing with adapative equipment. She requires maximum assistance with lower extremities and management of her bowel and bladder functions and for transfers. She enjoys watching sports with her father, watching movies, and making art projects. Her artwork adorns many rooms in the house.

EVALUATION OF MOTOR CONTROL

Occupational therapists are instrumental in helping parents and children learn how to modify tasks and routines so that children use self-care and other typical occupations on a daily basis. Physical therapists are instrumental in helping children achieve mobility. A typical occupational therapy evaluation and treatment strategy for Marcie would include the initial and then ongoing evaluation of her needed, wanted, and desired success in a balance of play, school, and self-care areas. This evaluation would include her family's priorities for achieving these occupations. A typical physical therapy assessment would include a detailed examination of Marcie's motor skills. Thus, an evaluation would include assessment of postural motor skills, fine motor skills, cognitive skills, and self-care skills (see Table 2.6). How Marcie masters and completes tasks would be the focus of the evaluation. Each portion of the evaluation would be interpreted to identify how independence is being either supported or hindered by the motor or cognitive skills. The motor portion of the evaluation might be conducted jointly by an occupational therapist and a physical therapist, since many of the

TABLE 2.6 Commonly Used Assessments for Motor, Sensory, and Functional Skills

Domain	Assessment	Age	Purpose/Description
Developmental motor	Alberta Infant Motor Scale (Piper & Darrah, 1994)	0–18 months	Norm-referenced test measuring gross motor movements and the quality of those movements. Consists of 58 items. Child is observed in several positions. Takes 30 min. to administer. Identifies motor delays.
	Toddler and Infant Motor Evaluation (Miller & Roid, 1994)	4 months to 3.5 years	Norm-referenced test. Eight subtests measure mobility, stability, motor organization, functional performance, social/emotional abilities, movement component analysis, movement quality, and atypical positions. Administered in 1 hour. Comprehensive assessment of motor abilities.
	Test of Infant Motor Performance (Campbell, Osten, Kolobe, & Fisher, 1993)	0–4 months	Criterion-referenced test consists of 28 observed items and 25 elicited items measuring postures and movements in preterm and full-term infants. Takes 30 min. to administer.
	Peabody Developmental Motor Scales-2 (Folio & Fewell, 2000)	1 month to 6 years	Norm-referenced test based on common developmental milestones measuring fine and gross motor skills. Consists of two motor scales. Takes 60 min. to administer.
	Bruininks–Oseretsky Test of Motor Proficiency (Bryden, Singh, Steenhuis, & Clarkson, 1994)	4.5–14.5 years	Norm-refenced test measuring fine and gross motor skills. Consists of nine subtests. Takes 45 min. to administer.
	Milani–Comparetti Motor Development Screening Test (Milani Comparetti & Gidoni, 1967)	1 month to 2 years	Norm-referenced test designed to diagnose developmental delays. Consists of 27 items measuring primitive reflexes, tilting, righting, and protective reactions, spontaneous posture, and movement. Takes 10–15 min. to administer.
	Posture and Fine Motor Assessment of Infants (Case-Smith & Bigsby, 2000)	2–12 months	Criterion-referenced test measuring whether motor skills are normal and appropriate for age. Two scales measure posture and fine motor skills. Requires 25–30 minutes to administer.
	Evaluation Tool of Children's Handwriting (Amundson, 1995)	6–11 years	Criterion-referenced evaluation is designed to measure the manuscript and cursive handwriting skills within a classroom context. Legibility components and hand skill with a pencil are included. Administration takes 15–25 min.

(*continues*)

TABLE 2.6 *(continued)*

Domain	Assessment	Age	Purpose/Description
Sensory	Sensory Integration and Praxis Tests (Ayres, 1989)	4 years to 8 years 11 months	Norm-referenced test consisting of 17 tests measuring visual perception, praxis, tactile processing, vestibular processing, and sensory motor skills. Computer scored. Requires 4 hours to administer.
	Sensory Profile, infant/toddler or adolescent (Brown & Dunn, 2002; Dunn, 1999)	3–18 years	Questionnaire requires caregivers or adolescents to rate behaviors that measure sensory processing. Requires 15–20 minutes to complete.
Functional	Hawaii Early Learning Profile (Fununo, O'Reilly, Hosaka, Zeisloft, & Allman, 1994)	Birth to 36 months	Criterion-referenced assessment tool on five domains of social, cognitive, communication, self-help, gross and fine motor, and visual motor skills. Takes 45 min. to administer.
	School Function Assessment (Coster, Deeney, Haltiwanger, & Haley, 1998)	5–11 years	Judgment-based questionnaire for measuring a child's performance, level of participation, and need for assistance in school activities. Consists of both physical and cognitive tasks on three scales.
Combined	Miller Assessment for Preschoolers (Miller, 1988)	2 years 9 months to 5 years 8 months	Norm-referenced test measuring sensory and motor abilities, balance, coordination, cognitive and language skills over 18 items. Requires 30–45 min. to administer.
	First STEP (Miller, 1993)	3–5 years	Norm-referenced screening tool used to identify children at risk for developmental problems. Consist of tasks that measure cognition, communication, motor, social-emotional, and adaptive behavior. Takes 15–25 min. to administer.
	Assessment of Motor and Process Skills School Version (Fisher, 1997, 1999)	8 years to adult and school version	Criterion-referenced test that consists of ADL performance on five to six tasks selected from a calibrated list of 56. Measures cognitive and motor skills within a context and is used to predict performance.

underlying motor skills would be of interest to both therapies. An occupational therapist might only be interested in how the motor function either inhibits or supports Marcie's ability to brush her hair and dress independently. In Marcie's case, the therapist would use both a remedial approach (i.e., focus on the development of more mature hand skills) and a modification approach (make adaptive clothing so that pants are easier to put on). The therapist would use observations of motor performance as well as standardized assessments. The standardized assessments for Marcie would likely include the Functional Independence Measure for Children (WeeFIM), which is a functional activity of daily living evaluation for children with disabilities. For a more formal evaluation of fine motor skills, the Erhardt Developmental Prehension Assessment (Revised) would be used to assess the relative contribution of prehension patterns to success in skills such as handwriting. Other assessments might include the School Function Assessment to determine the relative contribution of motor skills to achieving success in the classroom. In Marcie's case, treatment would focus on developing age-appropriate play, school, and self-care skills. For example, in self-care between 5 and 9 years of age, Marcie would be developing the ability to care for herself by doing pressure-relief pushups when she has been sitting for long periods and be able to perform skin checks for skin breakdown with verbal cues. She would care for her personal adaptive devices with reminders and would be able to catheterize herself at home or school. She might be working on using a keyboard with a laptop fitted with a specialized keyguard to allow greater accuracy and less continual gripping required for homework assignments. A therapist might help Marcie explore a greater range of social and leisure pursuits to foster a better balance of sedentary and more active play. Her school environment would be carefully examined to help improve attending in the classroom, for example, providing Marcie with a quiet location to complete assignments or finish her work without the typical classroom distractions. She may need to have a willing peer to give her cues; placement of objects may make attending easier for Marcie. She would likely benefit from a combined treatment approach, with many disciplines providing support within her regular classroom. Treatment might include both an individual and a consultative role by the therapist, giving opportunities to practice a greater range and variation of hand skills while providing information to the classroom teacher to adapt the environment to foster Marcie's participation.

EVALUATION OF COGNITIVE DOMAINS OF DEVELOPMENT

Given that Spina Bifida is often detected before birth, developmental evaluations would begin as early as is feasible, given Marcie's perinatal surgeries. Infant developmental evaluations often combine motor and cognitive domains within a single test, such as the Bayley Scales of Infant Development (BSID-II; Bayley, 1993). Another key transition time at which an evaluation is likely to occur is prior to school entry. In this particular case, Marcie had psychoeducational testing prior to school entry at 5 years of age, which indicated that she fell in the average range of intellectual functioning (an IQ score of 90). An average to low-average IQ score is not uncommon among children with Spina Bifida; however, more subtle neurocognitive and learning impairments are often present (Fletcher, Dennis, & Northrup, 2000).

By age 6 or 7, greater specificity in evaluating cognitive skills is often desired as academic problems become apparent. Fortunately, a larger range of evaluation measures are normed for children in this age group. A recommended battery of tests for Marcie might include the measures listed in Table 2.7. This would provide information about multiple domains of functioning, including intellectual abilities, academic achievement, memory, verbal, and spatial skills, and executive functions. Children with Spina Bifida exhibit an increased incidence of deficits in complex visual-spatial processing, language content, and rapid and accurate word finding. Thus, targeted testing in these areas would be warranted. Unfortunately, limited research has addressed memory and executive functioning

TABLE 2.7 Example Evaluation Measures[a] for Cognitive and Emotional Functioning of Marcie: A Child with Spina Bifida

Cognitive Domain	Evaluation Measure
General intellectual	• Wechsler Preschool and Primary Scales of Intelligence (WPPSI-III) • Wechsler Intelligence Scale for Children (WISC-IV)
Memory	• Wide Range Assessment of Memory and Learning (WRAML-II) • Children's Memory Scales (CMS)
Executive functioning	• NEPSY
Academic achievement	• Woodcock Johnson Tests of Achievement (WJR-III) • Wechsler Individual Achievement Test (WIAT-II)
Attention/concentration	• Subscales from the Leiter-R, CMS, NEPSY, WISC-IV, etc.
Visual-spatial skills	• Beery Test of Visual Motor Integration—5th edition • Leiter Test of Nonverbal Intelligence
Emotional Functioning	**Evaluation Measure**
Self-esteem	• Peirs–Harris • Harter Basic Concept Scale
Internalizing symptoms (child report)	• Children's Depression Inventory; Reynold's Anxiety Scale, Revised Manifest Anxiety Scale for Children; Fear Survey for Children
Internalizing and externalizing symptoms (multi-informant)	• Child Behavior Checklist (CBCL); Behavior Assessment Scale for Children (BASC); Connor's Rating Scales

[a]See Sattler (2001, 2002, 2004) for a review of each of the measures included in this table.

in this population in order to establish a common profile for children with spina bifida (Fletcher et al., 2000).

Based on a comprehensive evaluation, Marcie's learning impairments included a short attention span, lack of frustration tolerance, and difficulty with spatial relationships and organizational skills. Executive functions, including the abilities to plan, initiate, sequence, sustain and pace work, were impairing her school performance. Academic skills were below grade level in reading and arithmetic.

Integrating the developmental profile places the preceding evaluations in context. Although Marcie exhibits deficits in metacognitive skills, cognitive self-regulation, and attention relative to same-age peers, these skills are developing and are far from being mastered in this age group. Early intervention may have different benefits for skills that are progressing developmentally relative to skills that should have been acquired by this age. Interventions to improve these skills may be beneficial to all children in Marcie's class and may not need to be targeted solely to an individual child to be effective. As noted earlier, developmental changes in motor speed also influence the assessment of processing-speed rates (i.e., time it takes to push a button). The WISC-IV has fewer motor-dependent tasks, with fewer subtests in which bonus points can be received for quick performance and fewer subtests with timed tasks, as compared to the previous version. This should be particularly helpful to Marcie, given her fine motor impairments.

EVALUATION OF SOCIAL AND EMOTIONAL DOMAINS OF DEVELOPMENT

Marcie's emotional functioning should be evaluated, including internalizing and externalizing symptomatology, such as withdrawal/depression, anxiety, self-esteem, hyperactivity/inattention, and conduct problems. When evaluating children, it is particularly important to draw information from multiple sources. In Marcie's case, parents, teachers, peers, her therapists, and ongoing medical professionals would all be appropriate sources of information. It is recommended practice to include as many sources and methods as feasible, keeping in mind that low agreement among sources is a documented effect (Achenbach, McConaughy, & Howell, 1987).

In terms of her social and emotional development, Marcie's medical concerns and impairments have challenged her both emotionally and socially. While Marcie is outgoing and has a positive affect, she has few friends, and she interacts with peers as a younger child. Peer sociometric ratings are one of the most common assessment techniques used to measure peer acceptance, rejection, and likeability. Most children Marcie's age are just beginning the process of forming close, stable friendships. Marcie's level of emotional competence and her abilities to interpret and predict the emotions of others and to engage in veridical empathic distress may be below the level of same-age peers, making her seem like a younger child. Emotion-regulation strategies and her use of adaptive coping in the face of peer teasing may protect Marcie's self-esteem and reduce the risks associated with peer rejection.

SUMMARY

Developmental considerations are essential for competent and comprehensive child and adolescent evaluations. This chapter has attempted to provide an overview of the foundational developmental skills in a number of domains, including sensory/motor, cognitive, and social/emotional functioning, to provide the clinician, student, or academic with a quick reference to developmental ages within these domains. The interdisciplinary team of professionals who provide services to children needs to consider the functioning of the whole individual. An effective evaluation team might include psychologists, physical and occupational therapists, and other professionals who share some of the same concerns but who differ considerably in their approach to treatment and assessment. Understanding how foundational components, which include a comprehensive assessment of cognitive, social/emotional, sensory, and motor processing, can elucidate causative or concurrent factors in development is critical to conceptualizing appropriate treatment. A complete evaluation improves the ability to form hypotheses about current problems and affords the clinician with a mechanism to identify areas of normative performance as strengths and to indicate areas of developmental delay. A comprehensive evaluation also establishes a baseline of functioning from which a clinician can document progress. In subsequent chapters, a developmental approach is assumed to influence the specific assessment topics with children and adolescents, regardless of whether social skills deficits or child abuse is the particular area of evaluation under consideration.

REFERENCES AND RESOURCES

Achenbach, T. M. (1991). *Manual for the child behavior checklist and 1991 profile*. Burlington, VT: University Associates in Psychiatry.

Achenbach, T. M., McConaughy, S. H., & Howell, C. T. (1987). Child/adolescent behavioral and emotional problems: Implications of cross-informant correlations for situational specificity. *Psychological Bulletin, 101*, 213–232.

American Psychiatric Association. (2000). *Diagnostic and statistical manual of mental disorders* (4th ed. text revision). Washington, DC: Author.

Amundson, S. J. (1995). *Evaluation tool of children's handwriting*. Homer, AK: OT Kids.

Ayres, A. J. (1989). *Sensory Integration and Praxis Test*. Los Angeles: Western Psychological Services.

Bagnato, S. J., & Neisworth, J. T. (1999). Collaboration and teamwork in assessment for early intervention. In L. C. Mayes & W. S. Gilliam (Eds.), *Child and adolescent psychiatric clinics of North America: Comprehensive psychiatric assessment of young children*. Philadelphia: W. B. Saunders.

Bard, C., Fleury, M., & Hay, L. (Eds.). (1990). *Development of eye–hand coordination across the life span*. Columbia, SC: University of South Carolina Press.

Bartlett, D. (1997). Primitive reflexes and early motor development. *Developmental and Behavioral Pediatrics, 18*(1), 151–156.

Batshaw, M. L. (Ed.). (2002). *Children with disabilities* (5th ed.). Baltimore: Brooks.

Bayley, N. (1993). *Bayley Scales of Infant Development* (2nd ed.). San Antonio, TX: Psychological Corporation.

Berk, L. E. (2004). *Development through the life span* (3rd ed.). Boston: Allyn & Bacon.

Brenner, E. M., & Salovey, P. (1997). Emotion regulation during childhood: Developmental, interpersonal, and individual considerations. In P. Salovey & D. J. Sluyter (Eds.), *Emotional development and emotional intelligence: Educational implications*. New York: Basic Books.

Briggs, M. H. (1999). Systems for collaboration: Integrating multiple perspectives. In L. C. Mayes & W. S. Gilliam (Eds.), *Child and adolescent psychiatric clinics of North America: Comprehensive psychiatric assessment of young children*. Philadelphia: W. B. Saunders.

Bronfenbrenner, U., & Morris, P. A. (1998). The ecology of developmental processes. In W. Damon & R. M. Lerner (Eds.), *Handbook of child psychology: Vol. 1. Theoretical models of human development* (5th ed., pp. 993–1028). New York: Wiley.

Brown, C. J., & Dunn, W. (2002). *Sensory profile*. San Antonio, TX: Psychological Corporation.

Bryden, M. P., Singh, M., Steenhuis, R. E., & Clarkson, K. L. (1994). A behavioral measure of hand preference as opposed to hand skill. *Neuropsychologia, 32*(8), 991–999.

Campbell, S. K., Osten, E. T., Kolobe, T. H. A., & Fisher, A. G. (1993). Development of the Test of Infant Motor Performance. *Physical Medicine & Rehabilitation Clinics of North America, 4*(3), 541–550.

Case-Smith, J. (1995). The relationships among sensorimotor components, fine motor skill, and functional performace in preschool children. *American Journal of Occupational Therapy, 49*(7), 645–652.

Case-Smith, J. (1996). Analysis of current motor development theory and recently published infant motor assessments. *Infants & Young Children, 9*(1), 29–41.

Case-Smith, J. (2005). *Occupational Therapy for Children*. St. Louis, MO: Mosby.

Case-Smith, J., & Bigsby, R. (2000). *Posture and fine motor assessment of infants*. San Antonio, TX: Psychological Corporation.

Case-Smith, J., Bigsby, R., & Clutter, J. (1998). Perceptual–motor coupling in the development of grasp. *American Journal of Occupational Therapy, 52*(2), 102–110.

Case-Smith, J., & Rogers, S. (1999). Physical and occupational therapy. In L. C. Mayes & W. S. Gilliam (Eds.), *Child and adolescent psychiatric clinics of North America: Comprehensive psychiatric assessment of young children*. Philadelphia: W. B. Saunders.

Cech, D., & Martin, S. (Eds.). (2002). *Functional movement development across the life span*. Philadelphia: W. B. Saunders.

Christiansen, C. H., & Matuska, K. M. (2004). *Ways of living: Adaptive strategies for special needs* (3rd ed.). Bethesda, MD: AOTA Press.

Cicchetti, D., & Rogosch, F. A. (2002). A developmental psychopathology perspective on adolescence. *Journal of Consulting and Clinical Psychology, 70*, 6–20.

Clarke, G. N., DeBar, L. L., & Lewinsohn, P. M. (2003). Cognitive-behavioral group treatment for adolescent depression. In A. E. Kazdin & J. R. Weisz (Eds.), *Evidence-based psychotherapies for children and adolescents* (pp. 120–134). New York: Guilford Press.

Cohen, M. (1997). *Children's Memory Scale*. San Antonio, TX: Psychological Corporation.

Collins, W. A., & Laursen, B. (1999). *Relationships as developmental contexts: The Minnesota symposia on child psychology: Vol. 30*. Mahwah, NJ: Erlbaum.

Coster, W. J., Deeney, T., Haltiwanger, J., & Haley, S. (1998). *School Function Assessment*. San Antonio, TX: Psychological Corporation.

Dawson, T. L. (2002). New tools: new insights: Kohlberg's moral judgment stages revisited. *International Journal of Behavioral Development, 26*, 154–166.

Dempster, F. N., & Corkill, A. J. (1999). Interference and inhibition in cognition and behavior: Unifying themes for educational psychology. *Educational Psychology Review, 11,* 1–88.

Dunn, W. (1999). *Sensory Profile: Users manual.* San Antonio, TX: Psychological Corporation.

Eisenberg, N., Fabes, R. A., & Losoya, S. (1997). Emotional responding: Regulation, social correlates, and socialization. In P. Salovey & D. J. Sluyter (Eds.), *Emotional development and emotional intelligence: Educational implications.* New York: Basic Books.

Elkind, D. (1967). Egocentrism in adolescence. *Child Development, 38,* 1025–1034.

Elkind, D., & Bowen, R. (1979). Imaginary audience behavior in children and adolescents. *Developmental Psychology, 15,* 38–44.

Eyberg, S., Schuhmann, E., & Rey, J. (1998). Psychosocial treatment research with children and adolescents: Developmental issues. *Journal of Abnormal Child Psychology, 26,* 71–81.

Feldman, R. S. (2005). *Development across the life span* (3rd ed.). Upper Saddle River, NJ: Pearson Education.

Fisher, A. G. (1997). *School AMPS: School version of the assessment of motor and process skills.* Fort Collins, CO: Three Star Press.

Fisher, A. G. (1999). *Assessment of motor and process skills* (3rd ed.). Fort Collins, CO: Three Star Press.

Flavell, J. (1979). Metacognition and cognitive monitoring: A new area of cognitive-developmental inquiry. *American Psychologist, 34,* 906–911.

Flavell, J. H. (1981). Monitoring social cognitive enterprises: Something else that may develop in the area of social cognition. In J. H. Flavell & L. Ross (Eds.), *Social cognitive development: Frontiers and possible futures.* Cambridge, England: Cambridge University Press.

Flavell, J. H., Miller, P. M., & Miller, S. A. (1993). *Cognitive development* (3rd ed.). Englewood Cliffs, NJ: Prentice Hall.

Fletcher, J. M., Dennis, M., & Northrup, H. (2000). Hydrocephalus. In K. O. Yeates, M. D. Ris, & H. G. Taylor (Eds.), *Pediatric neuropsychology: Research, theory, and practice* (pp. 25–46). New York: Guilford Press.

Folio, R., & Fewell, R. (2000). *The Peabody Developmental Motor Scales (manual)* (2nd ed.). Austin, TX: Pro Ed.

Forehand, R., & Wierson, M. (1993). The role of developmental factors in planning behavioral interventions for children: Disruptive behavior as an example. *Behavior Therapy, 24,* 117–141.

Fry, A. F., & Hale, S. (1996). Processing speed, working memory, and fluid intelligence: Evidence for a developmental cascade. *Psychological Science, 7,* 237–241.

Fununo.S., O'Reilly, K., Hosaka, C. M., Zeisloft, B., & Allman, T. Q. (1994). *Hawaii Early Learning Profile.* Palo Alto, CA: Vort.

Furman, W. (1999). Friends and lovers: The role of peer relationships in adolescent romantic relationships. In W. A. Collins & B. Laursen (Eds.). *Relationships as developmental contexts: The Minnesota symposia on child psychology: Vol. 30.* Mahwah, NJ: Erlbaum.

Gibbs, J. C. (2003). *Moral development and reality: Beyond the theories of Kohlberg and Hoffman.* Thousand Oaks, CA: Sage.

Gilliam, W. S. (1999). Developmental assessment: Its role in comprehensive psychiatric assessment of young children. In L. C. Mayes & W. S. Gilliam (Eds.), *Child and adolescent psychiatric clinics of North America: Comprehensive psychiatric assessment of young children.* Philadelphia: W. B. Saunders.

Greenspan, S. I., & Greenspan, N. T. (2003). *The clinical interview of the child* (3rd ed.). Washington, DC: American Psychiatric Publishing.

Haley, S. M., Ludlow, L. H., & Coster, W. J. (1993). Pediatric Evaluation of Disability Inventory. *Physical Medicine and Rehabilitation Clinics of North America, 4*(3), 529–540.

Haley, S. M., Coster, W. J., Ludlow, L. H., Haltiwanger, J. T., & Andrellos, P. J. (1992). *Pediatric Evaluation of Disability Inventory.* Boston, MA: PEDI Research Group.

Harter, S. (1983). Children's understanding of multiple emotions: A cognitive-developmental approach. In W. F. Overton (Ed.), *The relationship between social and cognitive development* (pp. 147–194). Hillsdale, NJ: Erlbaum.

Harter, S. (1998). The development of self-representations. In N. Eisenberg (Ed.), *Handbook of child psychology: Vol. 3. Social, emotional, and personality development* (5th ed.). New York: Wiley.

Hartup, W. W. (1996). The company they keep: Friendships and their development significance. *Child Development, 67,* 1–13.

Hartup, W. W., & Stevens, N. (1999). Friendships and adaptation across the life span. *Current Directions in Psychological Science, 8,* 76–79.

Haviland-Jones, J., Gebelt, J. L., & Stapley, J. C. (1997). The questions of development in emotions. In P. Salovey & D. J. Sluyter (Eds.), *Emotional development and emotional intelligence: Educational implications.* New York: Basic Books.

Henderson, A., & Pehoski, C. (Eds.). (1994). *Hand function in the child.* St. Louis, MO: Mosby.

Hetherington, E. M. (1999). Social capital and the development of youth from nondivorced, divorced, and remarried families. In W. A. Collins & B. Laursen (Eds.). *Relationships as developmental contexts: The Minnesota symposia on child psychology: Vol. 30.* Mahwah, NJ: Erlbaum.

Hoffman, M. L. (2000). *Empathy and moral development: Implications for caring and justice.* Cambridge, England: Cambridge University Press.

Holmbeck, G. N., Greenley, R. N., & Franks, E. A. (2003). Developmental issues and considerations in research and practice. In A. E. Kazdin & J. R. Weisz (Eds.), *Evidence-based psychotherapies for children and adolescents* (pp. 120–134). New York: Guilford Press.

Kail, R. (2000). Speed of information processing: Developmental change and links to intelligence. *Journal of School Psychology, 38,* 51–61.

Kail, R., & Hall, L. K. (1994). Processing speed, naming speed, and reading. *Developmental Psychology, 30,* 949–954.

Kail, R., & Park, Y. (1994). Global developmental change in processing time. *Merrill-Palmer Quarterly, 38,* 525–541.

Kamm, K., Thelen, E., & Jensen, J. (1990). A dynamical systems approach to motor development. *Physical Therapy, 70*(12), 763–775.

Kazdin, A. E. (2003). Problem-solving skills training and parent management training for conduct disorder. In A. E. Kazdin & J. R. Weisz (Eds.), *Evidence-based psychotherapies for children and adolescents* (pp. 120–134). New York: Guilford Press.

Keating, D. P. (1990). Adolescent thinking. In S. S. Feldman & G. R. Elliott (Eds.), *At the threshold: The developing adolescent* (pp. 54–89). Cambridge, MA: Harvard University Press.

Kendall, P. C., Aschenbrand, S. G., & Hudson, J. L. (2003). Child-focused treatment of anxiety. In A. E. Kazdin & J. R. Weisz (Eds.), *Evidence-based psychotherapies for children and adolescents* (pp. 81–100). New York: Guilford Press.

Kliewer, W., Fearnow, M. D., & Miller, P. A. (1996). Coping socialization in middle childhood: Tests of maternal and paternal influences. *Child Development, 67,* 2339–2357.

Kohlberg, L. (1969). Stage and sequence: The cognitive-developmental approach to socialization. In D. A. Goslin (Ed.), *Handbook of socialization theory and research* (pp. 347–480). Chicago: Rand McNally.

Kohlberg, L., Levine, C., & Hewer, A. (1983). *Moral stages: A current formulation and a response to critics.* Basel, Switzerland: Karger.

Korkman, M., Kirk, U., & Kemp, S. (1998). *NEPSY: A developmental neuropsychological assessment.* San Antonio, TX: Psychological Corporation.

Kramer, P., & Hinjosa, J. (1999). *Frames of reference for pediatric occupational therapy.* Philadelphia: W. B. Saunders.

Kuhn, D. (2000a). Metacognitive development. *Current Directions in Psychological Science, 9,* 178–181.

Lapsley, D. K., Jackson, S., Rice, K., & Shadid, G. E. (1988). Self-monitoring and the "new look" at the imaginary audience and personal fable: An ego-developmental analysis. *Journal of Adolescent Research, 3,* 17–31.

Lin, C. C., Hsiao, C. K., & Chen, W. J. (1999). Development of sustained attention assessed using the continuous performance test among children 6–15 years. *Journal of Abnormal Child Psychology, 27,* 403–412.

Milani Comparetti, A., & Gidoni, E. A. (1967). Routine developmental examination in normal and retarded children. *Developmental Medicine and Child Neurology, 9,* 631–638.

Miller, L. J. (1988). *Miller Assessment for Preschoolers (MAP) manual.* San Antonio, TX: Psychological Corporation.

Miller, L. J. (1993). *The first step.* San Antonio, TX: Psychological Corporation.

Miller, L. J., & Roid, G. H. (1994). *The T.I.M.E. Toddler and Infant Motor Evaluation.* Tucson, AZ: Therapy Skill Builders.

Moshman, D. (1998). Cognitive development beyond childhood. In D. Kuhn & R. S. Siegler (Eds.), *Handbook of child psychology: Vol. 2. Cognition, perception and language* (pp. 957–978). New York: Wiley.

Piaget, J. (1952). *The origins of intelligence in children.* New York: W. W. Norton. (Original work published 1936).

Piaget, J. (1967). *Six psychological studies.* New York: Random House.

Piaget, J., & Inhelder, B. (1969). *The psychology of the child.* New York: Basic Books.

Pierce, S. H., & Lange, G. (2000). Relationships among metamemory, motivation, and memory performance in young school-age children. *British Journal of Developmental Psychology, 18,* 121–135.

Piper, M. C., & Darrah, J. (1994). *Motor assessment of the developing infant.* Philadelphia: W. B. Saunders.

Reynolds, C. R., & Kamphaus, R. W. (1992). *The Behavior Assessment System for Children.* Circle Pines, MN: American Guidance Service.

Roid, G. H., & Miller, L. J. (1997). *Leiter International Performance Scale—Revised.* Wood Dale, IL: Stoelting.

Ruff, H. A., & Lawson, K. R. (1990). Development of sustained, focused attention in young children during free play. *Developmental Psychology, 26,* 85–93.

Ruff, H. A., & Rothbart, M. K. (1996). *Attention in early development.* New York: Oxford University Press.

Saarni, C. (1997). Emotional competence and self-regulation in childhood. In P. Salovey & D. J. Sluyter (Eds.), *Emotional development and emotional intelligence: Educational implications.* New York: Basic Books.

Saarni, C. (1999). *The development of emotional competence.* New York: Guilford Press.

Saarni, C., Mumme, D. L., & Campos, J. J. (1998). Emotional development: Action, commonwealth, and understanding. In W. Damon & R. M. Lerner (Eds.), *Handbook of child psychology* (5th ed., pp. 237–309). New York: Wiley.

Sattler, J. M. (2001). *Assessment of children: Cognitive applications* (Vol. I, 4th ed.). San Diego, CA: Sattler.

Sattler, J. M. (2002). *Assessment of children: Behavioral and clinical applications* (Vol. II, 4th ed.). San Diego, CA: Sattler.

Sattler, J. M. (2004). *Assessment of children: WISC-IV and WPPSI-III supplement.* San Diego, CA: Sattler.

Schnieder, W., & Pressley, M. (1997). *Memory development between two and twenty* (2nd ed.). Mahwah, NJ: Erlbaum.

Selman, R. L. (1980). *The growth of interpersonal understanding.* New York: Academic Press.

Shaver, P., Schwartz, J., Kirson, D., & O'Connor, C. (1987). Emotion knowledge: Further explorations of a prototype approach. *Journal of Personality and Social Psychology, 52,* 1061–1086.

Sheslow, D., & Adams, W. (2004). *Wide Range Assessment of Memory and Learning* (2nd ed.). Wilmington, DE: Wide Range.

Smith, A. E., Jussim, L., Eccles, J., VanNoy, M., Madon, S., & Palumbo, P. (1998). Self-fulfilling prophecies, perceptual biases, and accuracy at the individual and group levels. *Journal of Experimental Social Psychology, 34,* 530–561.

Sparrow, S., Balla, D., & Cicchetti, D. (1984). *Vineland Adaptive Behavior Scales*. Circle Pines, MN: American Guidance Services.

Sroufe, L. A., Egeland, B., & Carlson, E. A. (1999). One social world: The integrated development of parent–child and peer relationships. In W. A. Collins & B. Laursen (Eds.), *Relationships as developmental contexts: The Minnesota symposia on child psychology: Vol. 30*. Mahwah, NJ: Erlbaum.

Thelen, E. (1995). Motor development. A new synthesis. *American Psychologist, 50*(2), 79–95.

Thelen, E., Corbetta, D., & Spencer, J. P. (1996). Development of reaching during the first year: Role of movement speed. *Journal of Experimental Psychology: Human Perception & Performance, 22*(5), 1059–1076.

Thompson, R. A. (1990). Emotion and self-regulation. In *Socioemotional development*, Nebraska Symposium on Motivation 1988 (pp. 367–467).

Vartanian, L. R., & Powlishta, K. K. (1996). A longitudinal examination of the social-cognitive foundations of adolescent egocentrism. *Journal of Early Adolescence, 16,* 157–158.

Vaughn, B. E., Colvin, T. N., Azria, M. R., Caya, L., & Krzysik, L. (2001). Dyadic analyses of friendship in a sample of preschool-age children attending Head Start: Correspondence between measures and implications for social competence. *Child Development, 72,* 862–878.

Vygotsky, L. (1978). *Mind in society: The development of higher mental processes*. Cambridge, MA: Harvard University Press.

Wechsler, D. (1991). *Wechsler Intelligence Scale for Children* (3rd ed.). San Antonio, TX: Psychological Corporation.

Wechsler, D. (2004). *Wechsler Intelligence Scale for Children* (4th ed.). San Antonio, TX: Psychological Corporation.

Weisz, J. R., & Hawley, K. M. (2002). Developmental factors in the treatment of adolescents. *Journal of Consulting and Clinical Psychology, 70,* 21–43.

Wintre, M. G., & Vallance, D. D. (1994). A developmental sequence in the comprehension of emotions: Intensity, multiple emotions, and valence. *Developmental Psychology, 30,* 509–514.

Woodcock, R. W., McGrew, K. S., & Mather, N. (2001). *The Woodcock–Johnson III*. Itasca, IL: Riverside.

Woollacott, M., & Shumway-Cook, A. (Eds.). (1989). *Development of posture and gait across the life span*. Columbia, SC: University of South Carolina Press.

3

PSYCHOMETRIC CONSIDERATIONS

DANIEL M. BAGNER
MICHELLE D. HARWOOD
SHEILA M. EYBERG

Department of Clinical and Health Psychology
University of Florida
Gainesville, Florida

INTRODUCTION

Child behavioral assessment has been defined as a procedure in which multiple empirically validated assessment tools are used to investigate hypotheses and draw conclusions about a child's functioning and subsequently to implement an appropriate treatment plan (Ollendick & Hersen, 1993). Behavioral observation is the hallmark of behavioral assessment, but comprehensive behavioral assessment also includes interviews, rating scales, and other standardized instruments (Eyberg, 1985). The primary advantage of behavioral observation is that it provides measurement that is not biased by the perceptions of individuals involved in the child's life (Hops, Davis, & Longoria, 1995). Behavioral assessment differs from more traditional psychological assessment, in that its goal is to describe and specify behaviors rather than personality and trait characteristics in conceptualizing dysfunction (Ollendick & Hersen).

In contrast to adult assessment, the child brings unique developmental concerns to behavioral assessment, including the rapidly changing developmental expectations for child behavior and the associated need to account for developmental changes during repeated measurement (Eyberg, Schuhmann, & Rey, 1998). The child's behavior is also highly situation-specific, requiring assessment information from multiple informants (e.g., mothers, fathers, teachers) and multiple settings to provide a comprehensive picture of child functioning.

Results from the child behavioral assessment have significant consequences not only for the child but also for the child's family (Haynes, Nelson, & Blaine, 1999). They may indicate the need for additional educational or mental health services for the child, change long-term expectations for the child's functioning, and lead to special planning for the child's future. The magnitude of these consequences points to the importance of reliable and valid measures that form the basis for these conclusions.

Psychometrics, or psychometry, is defined as the science of psychological assessment. It involves inspection of psychological instruments for their reliability and validity, the two core dimensions of psychometric evaluation (Haynes et al., 1999). These psychometric properties indicate the extent to which an instrument approximates true measurement of a construct of interest. *True measurement* refers to accurate and precise evaluation of objective information that occurs independent of the specific assessor or assessment instrument (Lachenmeyer, 1974). The term *construct* refers to the variable one intends to measure (Kazdin, 1998). Constructs frequently measured within child assessment include intellectual ability, developmental level, academic achievement, specific mental disorders (e.g., major depressive disorder), specific behavior problems (e.g., noncompliance), and parenting constructs such as discipline style and parenting stress.

In this chapter, we examine the core dimensions of psychometric evaluation, reliability and validity, as they relate to child behavioral assessment. Strategies used to evaluate these psychometric properties are discussed, with examples from common child behavioral assessment instruments. The section on reliability addresses research and clinical issues related to test–retest reliability, interrater reliability, alternate-form reliability, internal consistency, and internal structure. The section on validity addresses issues related to face validity, content validity, and criterion validity as well as the more specific types of validity within the general category of criterion validity (i.e., discriminative, concurrent, and predictive validity). We conclude with research and clinical implications for psychometric issues in child behavioral assessment.

RELIABILITY

Reliability refers to the consistency of an assessment measure across time, raters, settings, and items. Measurement reliability is particularly important in the assessment of child behavior because the rapid developmental changes that occur during childhood affect the consistency of child behavior itself (Yule, 1993). Measurements taken at different times and in different settings must take these changes into account. The importance of measurement reliability is also highlighted in child assessment because of the extensive reliance placed on secondary sources (e.g., parents and teachers). These sources provide information on child behavior that may vary greatly, in part because of different expectations for child behavior by different adults in the child's life.

TEST–RETEST RELIABILITY

Test–retest reliability, also known as *temporal stability*, refers to the consistency of a score on an instrument over time (Haynes et al., 1999). It is assessed by the correlation of scores obtained on a single measure administered to a sample at two points in time. The degree of consistency over time is affected both by the length of time between the two administrations and by the type of information measured. For example, characteristics assumed to be stable, such as IQ and temperament, would be expected to have high test–retest reliability over an extended interval of time. In contrast, characteristics that are more fluid in children, such as depressed mood, would be expected to have lower correlations, especially over long intervals of time.

In some instances, test–retest reliability over an extended interval of time is particularly important. For example, in randomized controlled trials of child behavior therapy, the outcome measures must be stable for the length of the treatment period to ensure that any differences between the treatment and the control groups at the second administration of the measure (post-treatment) is a result of the treatment itself and not of measurement error. In addition, scores for individual children in a no-treatment control group are expected to remain in the same rank order relative to one another between the two test administrations, because there has been no intervention that might differentially affect the control children. This correlation between the two test administrations for the control group represents the test–retest reliability, or the temporal stability, of the measure.

One instrument used to assess child disruptive behavior with high test–retest reliability is the Eyberg Child Behavior Inventory (ECBI; Eyberg & Pincus, 1999). The ECBI is a parent report instrument containing 36 behaviors that are rated on two scales: On the Intensity Scale, parents rate the frequency of the behaviors from *Never* (1) to *Always* (7), yielding a measure of severity of child disruptive behavior; on the *Yes-No* Problem Scale, parents indicate whether the behaviors are a problem for themselves, yielding a measure of parent tolerance for the child's behavior. This instrument has shown test–retest reliability coefficients of .80 and .85 across 12 weeks and .75 and .75 across 10 months on the Intensity and Problem Scales, respectively (Funderburk, Eyberg, Rich, & Behar, 2003). The high degree of stability over these extended time intervals suggests that changes observed in ECBI scores during treatment reflect actual changes in child behavior rather than measurement error. Thus, instruments with high test–retest reliability assessed over time intervals comparable to treatment length lend confidence to treatment-outcome data obtained using those instruments.

INTERRATER RELIABILITY

Interrater reliability refers to the degree to which an instrument provides consistent results when completed by multiple raters or observers (Eyberg & Pincus, 1999). Evaluating interrater reliability is important for determining the extent to which scores on an instrument reflect true variance in the intended construct (Haynes et al., 1999). That is, high interrater reliability suggests that the instrument can objectively measure the construct of interest and is not simply a reflection of rater subjectivity. For rating scale measures, interrater reliability indicates how much the ratings made by two or more informants about the same child agree. For observational measures, interrater reliability (often called interobserver reliability or intercoder reliability) indicates the extent of agreement between two or more observers independently recording (coding) the same behaviors during the same observation period.

In clinical assessment, behavioral observation often includes measurement of both the child's behaviors and the behaviors of others (e.g., parents, teachers, and peers) that maintain the child's behaviors. Observational measurement systems specify the situations and the interval of time in which relevant behaviors of the child and others are measured as well as the exact behaviors that define the constructs of interest. Interobserver reliability is calculated separately for each coded behavior to provide evidence of the consistency in coding each individual measure/behavior from which conclusions are drawn. It is assumed that other observers using the observational system, if trained in a similar way, can use the measurement system with similar consistency.

Interobserver reliability can be measured using percent agreement, kappa, bivariate correlations, or intraclass correlations (Kazdin, 1998). Percent agreement is typically used for categorical data (i.e., the behavior occurred or did not). It is estimated using a simple calculation of the number of agreements on the occurrence of the behavior at a specific time divided by the number of agreements plus disagreements between observers. A limitation of percent agreement is that it may overestimate interrater reliability, particularly when chance agreements are high (Molina, Pelham, Blumenthal, & Galiszewski, 1998). In contrast, kappa provides a more conservative estimate of interobserver reliability for categorical data by using a complex formula that accounts for chance agreement. For continuous variables, simple correlations between pairs of observers on the frequency of occurrence of a behavior across children provide an estimate of agreement. Because correlations do not account for disagreements on specific occurrences of a behavior between observers, intraclass correlations provide a more accurate estimate of interobserver reliability for continuous variables (Molina et al.). Similar to kappa, intraclass correlation coefficients account for random error variation.

The Dyadic Parent–Child Interaction Coding System (DPICS; Eyberg, McDiarmid, Duke, & Boggs, 2005) is a behavioral observation system developed for use in assessment of disruptive behavior disorders in young children. The DPICS includes 12 parent and 12 child behavior categories to measure the quality of parent–child interaction during three 5-minute standard situations that vary in the degree of parental control required. Kappa estimates of the DPICS categories ranged from .53 to .88 in a study of children with oppositional defiant disorder and their mothers (McDiarmid, Boggs, & Eyberg, 2004). The strength of interobserver agreement may be influenced by factors such as the number of observers, number of behavior categories in the system, frequency of occurrence and complexity of the observed behaviors, specificity of coding guidelines, and overlap among categories (Hops et al., 1995). Ongoing coder training is essential for maintaining reliability of complex coding systems.

The interrater reliability of child behavior rating scales (also called *interscorer reliability*) is calculated as the correlation between scores of different raters, such as mothers and fathers, rating the same child (Kazdin, 1998). Interscorer reliability provides information on the consistency of the obtained score when the scale is completed by different informants. For example, the Behavior Assessment System for Children (BASC; Reynolds & Kamphaus, 1992) consists of rating scales designed to assess emotional disorders, personality characteristics, and behavioral problems in children and adolescents. The system includes rating scales for teachers (Teacher Rating Scale [TRS]), parents (Parent Rating Scale [PRS]), and children (Self-Report of Personality [SRP]). Interscorer reliability for the PRS, calculated as the correlation between scores of mothers and of fathers, ranged from .46 to .71; for the TRS, interscorer reliability coefficients between different teachers rating the same child ranged from .42 to .93 (Reynolds & Kamphaus). Assessing agreement between raters on such scales provides evidence as to whether the scale items are explicit enough to be rated consistently by different informants of the same child (Kamphaus, 2003).

ALTERNATE-FORM RELIABILITY

Alternate-form reliability, also known as *equivalent-* or *parallel-form reliability*, refers to the correlation between two different versions (i.e., different items intended to measure the same construct) of the same testing instrument when administered to the same population (Kazdin, 1998). For alternate forms of an instrument to be considered reliable, their score means and variances should be approximately equal for the same population, and the correlation between the two forms given to the same population should be at least .80 (Sattler, 2001). Alternate forms for measures are used primarily to allow for testing the same person twice without repeating exact items from the previous administration. Alternate-form reliability is most useful for performance-based measures that will be administered twice in close succession. For example, to evaluate the outcome of a brief, intensive tutoring program for academic skills, the use of alternate forms of an achievement test would help prevent improved scores due to practice effects alone.

The Peabody Picture Vocabulary Test (PPVT-III; Dunn & Dunn, 1997) is a commonly used measure of receptive language requiring a child to point to one of four pictures that corresponds to a word orally presented by the examiner. There are two forms (A and B) of this measure, developed so that pictures from each form are matched by content categories (e.g., actions, foods, tools) and designed to provide item equivalency between forms. The two forms are highly correlated with each other at the various age groups (median $r = .94$; Dunn & Dunn, 1997), providing evidence of equivalence between forms A and B. Although alternate forms reduce practice effects, repeated testing of similar constructs may still lead to improved scores on performance-based psychological instruments (Uchiyama, D'Elia, Dellinger, & Becker, 1995).

INTERNAL CONSISTENCY

Internal consistency is defined as the magnitude of consistency or homogeneity among the individual items of a scale (Haynes et al., 1999; Kazdin, 1998) and is an important estimate of reliability on behavioral rating scale measures. Internal consistency coefficients indicate the extent to which the individual items in a scale are related to each other, or consistent with each other, in reflecting the construct that the scale is intended to measure (Haynes et al.). Internal consistency is a cost-effective method of establishing scale reliability because it requires only one test administration to a single population. Although not equivalent to test–retest reliability, internal consistency can often provide a good estimate of test–retest reliability (Kamphaus, Dowdy, & Kroncke, 2003).

Different formulas are used to measure the internal consistency of a rating scale, including Cronbach's alpha, split-half reliability, and Kuder–Richardson 20, depending on the characteristics of the items and on the response format. Cronbach's alpha, for example, is the mean correlation of all possible sets of half the items within a scale (Achenbach & Rescorla, 2001). Scales with more items allow for a more stable measurement of Cronbach's alpha due to the increased number of sets included within the overall correlation. For instance, a scale with 10 items would include 126 correlations, whereas a scale with 20 items would include 92,378 correlations contributing to Cronbach's alpha reliability.

Scales that measure a unitary, higher-order construct should have strong internal consistency across all items. A *higher-order construct* refers to a broad, inclusive category comprising multiple components that all contribute to, or define, the construct. For example, the Childhood Autism Rating Scale (CARS; Schopler, Reichler, & Renner, 1990) is a 15-item clinician rating scale developed to identify children with autism and to distinguish them from developmentally handicapped children without autism. It consists of one higher-order construct, autism, and each item is given equal weight in the total score (Saemundsen, Magnússon, Smári, & Sigurdardóttir, 2003). Internal consistency in the standardization sample was high ($\alpha = .94$; Schopler et al.), indicating strong homogeneity among the 15 items that represent the autism construct.

It is not always appropriate to examine internal consistency as an estimate of scale reliability. Internal consistency should not be examined when covariance among the elements of the scale is not assumed to exist (Haynes et al., 1999). For example, survey instruments are often used to assess the occurrence of a range of behaviors and experiences. The Life Events Checklist (LEC; Johnson & McCutcheon, 1980) is a self-report instrument for children and adolescents to identify the number and perception of stressful life events during the past year. In the LEC, there is no theoretical reason for different life stressors to be related to each other to form a higher-order construct. Thus, internal consistency is not a relevant psychometric property for the LEC. Instead, test–retest reliability is a more appropriate estimate of reliability for this type of scale and has been demonstrated adequately for the LEC (Brand & Johnson, 1982).

INTERNAL STRUCTURE

Internal structure, or *factor structure*, reflects the covariance among latent constructs within an assessment instrument (Haynes et al., 1999). For instruments assumed to have multiple constructs included within them, factor analyses are often used to divide a higher-order construct into smaller interrelated sets of constructs (Marcoulides & Hershberger, 1997). Ideally, theory drives development of an instrument containing multiple constructs, and the reliability of these constructs is assessed via factor analysis. An *exploratory factor analysis*, or *principal components analysis*, is initially used to investigate the factor structure of an assessment instrument, whereas *confirmatory factor analytic* strategies substantiate these identified factors in additional samples. Using these multiple statistical procedures makes it possible to identify the reliability of the factor structure across populations.

The Child Behavior Checklist (CBCL/1½–5) (Achenbach & Rescorla, 2001) is a parent-report instrument that contains multiple constructs, or factors, to assess various aspects of psychopathology in young children ages 1½ to 5 years. Achenbach and Rescorla conducted exploratory and confirmatory factor analyses to determine the seven factors ("syndromes") of the 99 items that constitute this version of the CBCL. The syndrome scales include: Emotionally Reactive, Somatic Complaints, Sleep Problems, Aggressive Behavior, Anxious/Depressed, Withdrawn, Attention Problems, and Aggressive Behavior. Patterns of association among the seven syndromes were also examined via factor analysis to determine "higher-order factors" within the domain of psychopathology. The Aggressive Behavior and Attention Problems syndromes were most highly correlated with each other and were combined into a higher-order factor labeled the Externalizing factor. The Emotionally Reactive, Anxious/Depressed, Somatic Complaints, and Withdrawn syndromes correlated most highly with each other and were labeled the Internalizing factor. The Sleep Problems syndrome did not correlate highly with either group of syndromes and was therefore not included in either the Internalizing or Externalizing factor, but all seven syndromes were included in the Total Problems scale of psychopathology.

An instrument's internal structure should be examined for all populations in which the instrument will be used. For example, to ensure appropriateness of the CBCL/1½–5 for both boys and girls, Achenbach and Rescorla (2001) conducted all factor analyses separately for each gender and for both genders combined. Additional factor analytic research has been conducted to determine the applicability of the CBCL for children with unique characteristics that might influence the factor structure. For example, in the assessment of disruptive behavior disorders in children with mental retardation (MR), it is important to ensure that the pattern of symptoms measured by the CBCL/4–18 (Achenbach, 1991) is consistent with that of normally developing children. Borthwick-Duffy, Lane, and Widaman (1997) subjected the CBCL/4–18 to confirmatory factor analysis in a sample of children and adolescents with MR. Although the five individual factors of the CBCL/4–18 were not confirmed in this sample, the higher-order factors (Internalizing and Externalizing) were similar to those in Achenbach's (1991) normative sample of children. These results support the use of the higher-order factors of the CBCL/4–18 with this population, but suggest that drawing conclusions from individual syndrome scores may be inappropriate for children with MR. Thus, studies examining the consistency of an instrument's internal structure provide information on the generalizability of the instrument to children from diverse populations.

VALIDITY

Validity refers to the accuracy with which an instrument measures the intended construct (Haynes et al., 1999). Examination of validity is important both in the development of child behavioral assessment instruments and in the selection of appropriate instruments for measuring child behavior. An important consideration in assessing validity is that an instrument must first demonstrate that it can be consistently measured (i.e., reliability) before it is possible to determine if the instrument accurately measures its intended construct (i.e., validity; Singleton & Straits, 2005). There are several types of validity. *Construct validity* refers to the broad category of validity that encompasses all other types of validity (Kazdin, 1998). It includes face validity, content validity, and criterion validity. Criterion validity includes discriminative validity, concurrent validity, and predictive validity (Kazdin, 1998), and concurrent validity encompasses convergent and discriminant validity (Butcher, 1999). In this chapter we describe the types of validity according to this hierarchical structure (see Figure 3.1).

FACE VALIDITY

Face validity is defined as the extent to which an assessment instrument appears to measure the intended construct (Kazdin, 1998). That is, when we look at the items in the instrument, they seem like items that would relate to the construct of interest. Although face validity can provide useful qualitative data (Popovic, Milne, & Barrett, 2003), it is based on individual interpretation and is not considered a formal psychometric property (Hausknecht, Day, & Thomas, 2004). Face validity may have utility in the early stages of instrument development for creating the item pool but has limited value in instrument evaluation. The Children's Depression Inventory (CDI) is a child self-report instrument

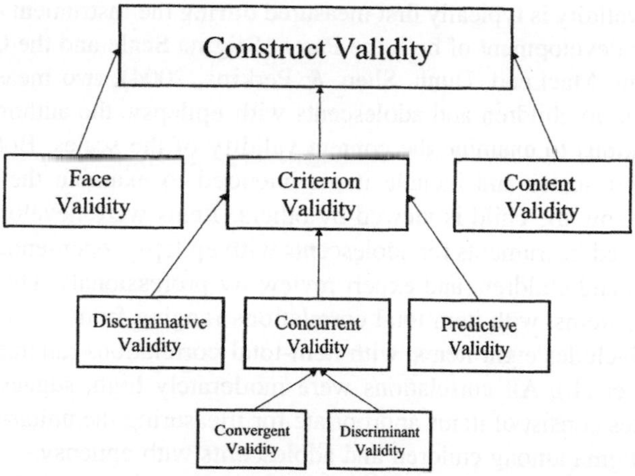

FIGURE 3.1 Hierarchical organization of validity indices.

designed to assess symptoms of depression in children and adolescents ages 7–17 (Kovacs, 1992). The brevity of the CDI provides an efficient assessment of depressive symptomatology, although the CDI may be insufficient to detect children with depression (Fristad, Emery, & Beck, 1997). The high face validity of the CDI seems to limit its effectiveness at identification due to the influence of social desirability. Research has shown a relation between low scores on the CDI (indicating fewer depressive symptoms) and high scores on a measure of defensiveness (Steele, Phipps, & Srivastava, 1999). Thus, evidence suggests that the CDI should not be used for screening or as a single diagnostic indicator of childhood depression. Instead, it should be used for its originally developed purpose (Kovacs, 1992), as an indicator of child distress and an important component of a comprehensive behavioral assessment (Jones-Hiscock, 2004). This issue highlights the importance of considering face validity in selecting instruments that address the intended construct while at the same time examining other indices of validity.

CONTENT VALIDITY

Like face validity, content validity refers to the extent to which the elements of an assessment instrument represent the intended construct (Haynes et al., 1999). However, content validity differs from face validity in that it involves a more comprehensive examination of those elements and uses quantitative data. Item-total scale correlations provide an estimate of content validity by accounting for each item's ability to represent the overall construct of the instrument. Establishing content validity requires both inclusion of items that address relevant aspects of the intended construct and exclusion of items that provide information extraneous to the core construct (Haynes & Lench, 2003).

Content validity is typically first measured during the instrument development stage. In the development of both the Parent Stigma Scale and the Child Stigma Scale (Austin, MacLeod, Dunn, Shen, & Perkins, 2004), two measures of perceived stigma in children and adolescents with epilepsy, the authors used item-total correlations to examine the content validity of the scales. Both scales use 5-point Likert scales and include items intended to examine the influence of epilepsy on how the child is viewed by others. Items were developed based on previously used instruments for adolescents with epilepsy, open-ended interviews with parents and children, and expert review by professionals. The parent scale includes five items, with item-total correlations ranging from .43 to .70, and the child scale includes eight items, with item-total correlations ranging from .44 to .65 (Austin et al.). All correlations were moderately high, suggesting that the Stigma Scales consist of items appropriate for measuring the unitary construct of perceived stigma among children and adolescents with epilepsy.

CRITERION VALIDITY

Criterion validity refers to the association between the instrument of interest and previously validated instruments or "gold standard" assessment strategies in evaluating the accuracy of that instrument (Haynes, 1999). *Gold standard assessment strategies* refer to either comprehensive behavioral assessment comprised of expert evaluation using interviews, observations, and psychometrically validated instruments (Zolotor & Mayer, 2004) or a separate criterion that is considered to be completely accurate (Rich & Eyberg, 2001), such as a child abuse report or being held back a grade in school. Criterion validity encompasses three types of validity: discriminative, concurrent, and predictive validity.

Discriminative Validity

Discriminative validity refers to the ability of an instrument to classify children into contrasting groups based on the behavior assessed by that instrument (Robins, Schoff, Glutting, & Abelkop, 2003). If an instrument will be used to make a categorical decision, such as whether or not a child has significant depression (the construct that is measured) and should be treated, the instrument's discriminative validity is highly important. However, if the instrument will be used as a continuous scale to determine, for example, how much change in depression (the construct that is measured) occurred during treatment, discriminative validity may be less relevant.

Evidence of high discriminative validity helps ensure the appropriateness of a measure for inclusion in child assessment involving clinical decision making. A brief screening instrument, the General Behavior Inventory (GBI; Depue, 1987), exemplifies a behavioral self-report instrument with strong discriminative validity for identifying unipolar and bipolar depressive disorders in children and adolescents. In a sample of 10- to 17-year-olds previously diagnosed according to a well-established diagnostic interview schedule, investigators found that the

GBI accurately distinguished between the youngsters with and without mood disorders, youngsters with mood disorders from those with disruptive behavior disorders, and youngsters with unipolar depression from those with bipolar depression (Danielson, Youngstrom, Findling, & Calabrese, 2003). Although no instrument should be used alone for making important diagnostic decisions, the brevity and discriminative validity of the GBI lend strong support for its utility in behavioral child assessment.

Concurrent Validity

Concurrent validity is defined as the correlation between two instruments, administered at the same point in time, that measure either similar or dissimilar constructs. Although sometimes used interchangeably with convergent validity, concurrent validity encompasses both convergent and divergent validity (Butcher, 1999). The purpose of concurrent validity is to determine how well an instrument measures the construct of interest in comparison to an established instrument that has been shown to measure the same construct (shown by a significant correlation between the two instruments) or to measure a different construct (shown by a nonsignificant or negligible correlation between the two instruments).

Convergent Validity

Convergent validity is used to examine the degree of overlap between two instruments intended to assess the same or similar constructs. The strength of the correlation between two instruments should be related to the extent of covariance between scores (Haynes et al., 1999). For example, convergent validity between two instruments designed to assess self-esteem is expected to be higher than convergent validity between an instrument designed to assess self-esteem and an instrument designed to assess popularity. More confidence can be placed in instruments that are significantly correlated with established instruments measuring the same construct.

There are a number of issues to consider in examining the comparison measure used to establish convergent validity. The Conners' Rating Scales—Revised (CRSR; Conners, 1997) include three instruments (a parent rating scale, teacher rating scale, and adolescent self-rating scale) that measure child and adolescent symptoms of ADHD and commonly associated problems. To permit brief screening, Conners created a short-form of each instrument that includes the three most clinically relevant subscales from the corresponding long form: the Oppositional, Cognitive Problems, and Hyperactivity subscales. From each instrument, items on the three subscales with the highest factor loadings were selected for inclusion on the short-form instrument. The convergent validity of each short form was investigated by examining the correlations between the short-form subscales and the corresponding long-form subscales. For example, the Oppositional subscale of the Conners' Parent Rating Scale—Revised: Short Form (CPRS-R: S) was compared with the Oppositional subscale of the Conners' Parent Rating Scales-Revised: Long Form (CPRS-R: L). The corresponding Oppositional subscale on the short and long forms of the CPRS are intended to measure identical constructs and, therefore, should be highly correlated with each other. The correlation was .98 for boys and .97 for girls, demonstrating excellent convergent validity for the short-form Oppositional subscale (Conners). These results suggest that the CPRS-R: S may be used as an efficient measure of oppositional behavior associated with ADHD.

For the CRSR, convergent validity was also examined by comparing related, but not identical, constructs. For example, the convergent validity of the CPRS-R: L was examined by comparing intercorrelations of all subscales of this parent-report measure and the Continuous Performance Test (CPT) Overall index, a computerized performance measure of inattention. Moderate correlations with the CPT were found for the Cognitive Problems subscale and DSM-IV Inattentive subscale of the CPRS-R: L (Conners, 1997). These findings suggest that the CPRS-R: L measures a similar construct as the CPT, providing evidence that scores on the CPRS-R: L are capturing the intended construct of inattention.

Discriminant Validity

Discriminant validity (also called *divergent validity*) is used to examine the relationship between the instrument of interest and an instrument measuring a different construct (Kazdin, 1998). Evidence of discriminant validity is shown by the absence of a significant correlation between two instruments (Kazdin). Measurement of discriminant validity is important because it ensures that an instrument uniquely measures a single construct without measuring aspects of another, unrelated, construct. Evidence of discriminant validity is particularly valuable when examining one instrument in comparison to another instrument that measures a construct that potentially could overlap but is intended to be different.

For example, anxiety and depression are two distinct disorders that commonly co-occur and have some related symptoms that may complicate diagnostic specificity (Endler & Macrodimitris, 2003). Thus, it is critical to have an instrument that can allow for distinct diagnosis of either condition. For instance, the Multidimensional Anxiety Scale for Children (MASC; March, Parker, Sullivan, Stallings, & Conners, 1997), a 39-item child and adolescent self-report rating scale, is intended to measure symptoms of general, social, and separation anxiety and not symptoms of depression. March et al. examined the correlations of the MASC subscales with the Revised Children's Manifest Anxiety Scale (RCMAS; Reynolds & Richmond, 1979) and the CDI (Kovacs, 1992). The MASC total score was significantly correlated with the RCMAS ($r = .63, p < .01$) but not with the CDI ($r = .19, p > .05$), suggesting that the MASC is able to measure the construct of anxiety accurately and to distinguish anxious from depressed children, despite frequently overlapping symptoms between these two disorders. The discriminant validity of the MASC increases confidence that this scale can be used to identify anxiety, even in children who may also be depressed.

Predictive Validity

Predictive validity refers to the relation between performance on the measure of interest at one point in time and performance on a criterion measure at a later point in time (Kazdin, 1998). Like concurrent validity, predictive validity is assessed by a correlation between scores on two separate measures, but predictive validity is distinguished from concurrent validity by the different administration times.

In child behavioral assessment, predictive validity is important for instruments used to identify children for preventive intervention programs. For example, if a measure of child disruptive behavior were found to predict later delinquency, that instrument would be useful (cost effective) in selecting children for a delinquency prevention program.

The importance of predictive validity can be illustrated with the Child Abuse Potential Inventory (CAPI; Milner, 1986). The CAPI is a 160-item parent self-report screening instrument of child physical abuse potential with good predictive validity. Its intent is to examine the risk of a future event of child maltreatment with items related to the primary risk factors: parental rigidity, family problems, and parent distress. For a construct of this kind, it is the predictive validity of the measure that is essential. Using future child protective services abuse reports as the criterion measure, Chaffin and Valle (2003) demonstrated that the CAPI Abuse Scale has stronger predictive validity than case demographic and historical data. Studies such as this highlight the value of establishing predictive validity to provide convincing evidence of the feasibility of cost-effective screening for identification of families in need of preventive services.

SUMMARY

This chapter has examined the core dimensions of psychometric analysis—reliability and validity—as they relate to behavioral assessment instruments used with children and adolescents. Demonstration that an instrument is reliable and valid for its intended purpose is essential to provide meaningful assessment results. However, not all types of reliability or all types of validity are relevant or necessary for a given instrument.

We examined several types of measurement reliability, including test–retest reliability, alternate-form reliability, interrater reliability, internal consistency, and internal structure. Test–retest reliability is particularly important for treatment-outcome instruments because they must demonstrate stability without intervention in order to provide meaningful evidence that change has occurred because of treatment. Interobserver reliability must be demonstrated for direct observation measures to ensure that the results do not reflect the idiosyncratic coding of a particular observer. Interrater reliability is important for rating scales in which similar scores would be expected across multiple informants. Alternate-form reliability should be examined for performance-based constructs in which two versions of the instrument are needed because multiple administrations of the instrument could lead to practice effects. Internal consistency is essential for rating scales intended to measure a single construct. For instruments containing multiple constructs, a demonstration of the instrument's internal structure is needed for all populations for which the instrument will be used.

In this chapter, we also examined several types of validity important to consider in child behavioral assessment instruments, including face validity, content validity, and criterion validity, which collectively may provide evidence of an instrument's construct validity. Face validity has some utility during the development of psychological instruments, but it is not a formal psychometric property and can detract from an instrument due to social desirability. Content validity provides a more in-depth examination of whether its elements comprehensively assess the intended construct while excluding items that are extraneous to the intended construct.

Criterion validity serves to identify the accuracy of an assessment instrument by comparing it to previously validated assessment strategies. It encompasses three subcomponents of validity: discriminative, concurrent, and predictive validity. Discriminative validity is particularly important for instruments used for diagnostic decision making. Concurrent validity may be most useful in the development of more cost-effective instruments for which an established method of assessing the construct exists. It subsumes both convergent and discriminant (divergent) validity. Convergent validity demonstrates that an instrument appropriately measures the intended construct by comparing it to another instrument measuring the same or a similar construct. Discriminant validity, on the other hand, demonstrates that an instrument can effectively differentiate between the intended construct and an unrelated construct. Predictive validity is particularly important for instruments used to predict future behavior, for which early detection would allow preventive interventions to alter the predicted course of events.

The core dimensions of psychometric analysis, reliability and validity, must be considered in the selection of appropriate measurement instruments for use in child behavioral assessment for research or clinical purposes. The critical psychometric properties to consider will depend on both the nature (e.g., rating scale, behavioral observation) and purpose of the assessment tool. Careful consideration of psychometric properties will help to ensure objective and comprehensive measurement within child behavioral assessment.

REFERENCES AND RESOURCES

Achenbach, T. M. (1991). *Manual for the Child Behavior Checklist/4-18 and 1991 profile*. Burlington, VT: University of Vermont Department of Psychiatry.

Achenbach, T. M., & Rescorla, L. A. (2001). *Manual of the ASEBA School-Age Forms & Profiles.* Burlington, VT: University of Vermont, Research Center for Children, Youth, & Families.

Austin, J. K., MacLeod, J., Dunn, D. W., Shen, J., & Perkins, S. M. (2004). Measuring stigma with children with epilepsy and their parents: Instrument development and testing. *Epilepsy and Behavior, 5,* 472–482.

Borthwick-Duffy, S. A., Lane, K. L., & Widaman, K. F. (1997). Measuring problem behaviors in children with mental retardation: Dimensions and predictors. *Research in Developmental Disabilities, 18,* 415–433.

Brand, A. H., & Johnson, J. H. (1982). Note on the reliability of the Life Events Checklist. *Psychological Reports, 50,* 1274.

Butcher, J. N. (1999). Research design in objective personality assessment. In P. C. Kendall, J. N. Butcher, & G. N. Holmbeck (Eds.), *Handbook of research methods in clinical psychology* (2nd ed., pp. 155–182). New York: Wiley.

Chaffin, M., & Valle, L. A. (2003). Dynamic prediction characteristics of the Child Abuse Potential Inventory, *Child Abuse & Neglect, 27,* 463–481.

Conners, C. K. (1997). *Conners' Rating Scales—Revised.* North Tonawanda, NY: Multi-Health Systems.

Danielson, C. K., Youngstrom, E. A., Findling, R. L., & Calabrese, J. R. (2003). Discriminative validity of the General Behavior Inventory using youth report. *Journal of Abnormal Child Psychology, 31,* 29–39.

Depue, R. A. (1987). *General Behavior Inventory (manual).* Minneapolis: University of Minnesota.

Dunn, L. M., & Dunn, L. M. (1997). *Peabody Picture Vocabulary Test—Third Edition: Manual.* Circle Pines, MN: American Guidance Services.

Endler, N. S., & Macrodimitris, S. D. (2003). Anxiety and depression: Congruent, separate, or both? *Journal of Applied Biobehavioral Research, 8,* 42–60.

Eyberg, S. M. (1985). Behavioral assessment: Advancing methodology in pediatric psychology. *Journal of Pediatric Psychology, 10,* 123–139.

Eyberg, S. M., McDiarmid, M. D., Duke, M., & Boggs, S. M. (2005). *Dyadic Parent–Child Interaction Coding System—Third Edition: A manual.* Manuscript in preparation.

Eyberg, S. M., & Pincus, D. (1999). *Eyberg Child Behavior Inventory and Sutter–Eyberg Student Behavior Inventory: Professional Manual.* Odessa, FL: Psychological Assessment Resources.

Eyberg, S. M., Schuhmann, E., & Rey, J. (1998). Psychosocial treatment research with children and adolescents: Developmental issues. *Journal of Abnormal Child Psychology, 26,* 71–82.

Fristad, M. A., Emery, B. L., & Beck, S. J. (1997). Use and abuse of the Child Depression Inventory. *Journal of Consulting & Clinical Psychology, 65,* 695–702.

Funderburk, B. W., Eyberg, S. M., Rich, B. A., & Behar, L. (2003). Further psychometric evaluation of the Eyberg and Behar rating scales for parents and teachers of preschoolers. *Early Education and Development, 14,* 67–81.

Hausknecht, J. P., Day, D. V., & Thomas, S. C. (2004). Applicant reactions to selection procedures: An updated model and meta-analysis. *Personnel Psychology, 57,* 639–683.

Haynes, S. N., & Lench, H. C. (2003). Incremental validity of new clinical assessment measures. *Psychological Assessment, 15,* 456–466.

Haynes, S. N., Nelson, K., & Blaine, D. D. (1999). Psychometric issues in assessment research. In P. C. Kendall, J. N. Butcher, & G. N. Holmbeck (Eds.), *Handbook of research methods in clinical psychology* (2nd ed., pp. 125–154). New York: Wiley.

Hops, H., Davis, B., Leve, C., & Sheeber, L. (2003). Cross-generational transmission of aggressive parent behavior: A perspective, mediational examination. *Journal of Abnormal Child Psychology, 31,* 161–169.

Hops, H., Davis, B., & Longoria, N. (1995). Methodological issues in direct observation: Illustrations with Living in Familial Environments (LIFE) coding system. *Journal of Clinical Child Psychology, 24,* 193–203.

Jacobs, J. R., Boggs, S. R., Eyberg, S. M., Edwards, D., Durning, P., Querido, J. G., McNeil, C. B., & Funderburk, B. W. (2000). Psychometric properties and reference point data for the revised edition of the school observation coding system. *Behavior Therapy, 31,* 695–712.

Johnson, J. H., & McCutcheon, S. M. (1980). Assessing life stress in older children and adolescents: Preliminary findings with the Life Events Checklist. In I. G. Sarason & C. D. Spielberger (Eds.), *Stress and anxiety* (Vol. 7, pp. 111–125). Washington, DC: Hemisphere.

Jones-Hiscock, C. (2004). Using depression inventories: Not a replacement for clinical judgment. *Canadian Journal of Psychiatry, 49,* 646–647.

Kamphaus, R. W. (2003). Psychometric properties of tests. In T. H. Ollendick & C. S. Schroeder (Eds.). *Encyclopedia of clinical child and pediatric psychology* (pp. 518–519). New York: Plenum Press.

Kamphaus, R. W., Dowdy, E., & Kroncke, A. P. (2003). Reliability. In T. H. Ollendick & C. S. Schroeder (Eds.). *Encyclopedia of clinical child and pediatric psychology* (pp. 545–546). New York: Plenum Press.

Kazdin, A. E. (1998). *Research design in clinical psychology* (3rd ed.). Boston: Allyn & Bacon.

Kovacs, M. (1992). *Children's Depression Inventory manual.* North Tonawanda, NY: Multi-Health Systems.

Lachenmeyer, C. M. (1974). Measurement and investigation: Five demands for social science measurement. *Journal of General Psychology, 93,* 173–182.

March, J. S., Parker, J. D. A., Sullivan, K., Stallings, P., & Conners, C. K. (1997). The Multidimensional Anxiety Scale for Children (MASC): Factor structure, reliability, and validity. *Journal of the American Academy of Child and Adolescent Psychiatry, 36,* 554–565.

Marcoulides, G. A., & Hershberger, S. L. (1997). *Multivariate statistical methods: A first course.* Mahwah, NJ: Erlbaum.

Mash, E. J., & Terdal, L. G. (1997). Assessment of child and family disturbance: A behavioral-systems approach. In E. J. Mash & L. G. Terdal (Eds.). *Assessment of childhood disorders* (3rd ed., pp. 3–68). New York: Guilford Press.

McDiarmid, M. D., Boggs, S. R., & Eyberg, S. M. (2004, November). *Development and Psychometric Properties of the Third Edition of the Dyadic Parent–Child Interaction Coding System.* Paper presented at the 38th annual Association for Advancement of Behavior Therapy Conference, New Orleans, LA.

Milner, J. S. (1986). *The Child Abuse Potential Inventory: Manual* (2nd ed.). Webster, NC: Psytec.

Molina, B. S. G., Pelham, W. E., Blumenthal, J., & Galiszewski, E. (1998). Agreement among teachers' behavior ratings of adolescents with a childhood history of Attention Deficit Hyperactivity Disorder. *Journal of Clinical Child Psychology, 27,* 330–339.

Ollendick, T. H., & Hersen, M. (1993). Child and adolescent behavioral assessment. In T. H. Ollendick & M. Hersen (Eds.). *Handbook of child and adolescent assessment* (pp. 3–14). Boston: Allyn & Bacon.

Popovic, M., Milne, D., & Barrett, P. (2003). The scale of perceived interpersonal closeness (PICS). *Clinical Psychology and Psychotherapy, 10,* 286–301.

Reynolds, C. R., & Kamphaus, R. W. (1992). *Manual for the BASC: Behavior Assessment System for Children.* Circle Pines, MN: American Guidance Service.

Reynolds, C. R., & Richmond, B. O. (1979). What I think and feel: A revised measure of children's manifest anxiety. *Journal of Abnormal Child Psychology, 6,* 271–280.

Rich, B. A., & Eyberg, S. M. (2001). Accuracy of assessment: The discriminative and predictive power of the Eyberg Child Behavior Inventory. *Ambulatory Child Health, 7,* 249–257.

Robins, P. M., Schoff, K. M., Glutting, J. J., & Abelkop, A. S. (2003). Discrimintative validity of the behavior assessment system for children–parent rating scales in children with recurrent abdominal pain and matched controls. *Psychology in the Schools, 40,* 145–154.

Saemundsen, E., Magnússon, P., Smári, J., & Sigurdardóttir, S. (2003). Autism diagnostic interview—revised and the Childhood Autism Rating Scale: Convergence and discrepancy in diagnosing autism. *Journal of Autism and Developmental Disorders, 33,* 319–328.

Sattler, J. M. (2001). *Assessment of children: Cognitive applications* (4th ed.). San Diego, CA: Sattler.

Schopler, E., Reichler, R. J., & Renner, B. R. (1990). *The Childhood Autism Rating Scale.* Los Angeles, CA: Western Psychological Services.

Shaffer, D., Fisher, P., Lucas, C. P., Dulcan, M. K., & Schwab-Stone, M. E. (2000). *NIMH diagnostic interview schedule for children, Version IV* (NIMH DISC-IV): Description, differences from previous versions, and reliability of some common diagnoses. *Journal of the American Academy of Child and Adolescent Psychiatry, 39,* 28–38.

Singleton, R. A., & Straits, B. C. (2005). *Approaches to Social Research* (4th ed.). New York: Oxford University Press.

Steele, R. G., Phipps, S., & Srivastava, D. K. (1999). Low-end specificity of childhood measures of emotional distress: Consistent effects for anxiety and depressive symptoms in a nonclinical population. *Journal of Personality Assessment, 73,* 276–289.

Smucker, M. R., Craighead, W. E., Craighead, L. W., & Green, B. J. (1986). Normative and reliability data for the Children's Depression Inventory. *Journal of Abnormal Child Psychology, 14,* 25–39.

Uchiyama, C. L., D'Elia, L. F., Dellinger, A. M., & Becker, J. T. (1995). Alternate forms of the Auditory-Verbal Learning Test: Issues of test comparability, longitudinal reliability, and moderating demographic variables. *Archives of Clinical Neuropsychology, 10,* 133–145.

Werba, B., & Eyberg, S. M. (2004). Introduction to Chapter VIII: Environment. In S. Naar-King, D. A. Ellis, and M. A. Frey (Eds.). *Assessing children's well-being: A handbook of measures* (pp. 147–150). New York: Erlbaum.

Wilder, L. K., & Sudweeks, R. R. (2003). Reliability of ratings across studies of the BASC. *Education and Treatment of Children, 26,* 382–399.

Yule, W. (1993). Developmental considerations in child assessment. In T. H. Ollendick & M. Hersen (Eds.), *Handbook of child and adolescent assessment* (pp. 15–25). Boston: Allyn & Bacon.

Zoltor, A. J., & Mayer, J. (2004). Does a short symptom checklist accurately diagnose ADHD? *Journal of Family Practice.* Retrieved February 14, 2005, from http://www.findarticles.com/p/articles/mi_m0689-is_5_53_ai_n6031048

4

Analogue and Virtual Reality Assessment

SARI D. GOLD
BRIAN P. MARX

Department of Psychology
Temple University
Philadelphia, Pennsylvania

INTRODUCTION

Behavioral assessment involves multimethod, multimodal, and multi-informant measurement of various independent and dependent variables and is derived from the assumption that environmental antecedent and consequent factors explain behavior (Haynes, 1998). The reason that behavioral assessment is so extensive is that behavior, behavioral problems, and causal relationships are assumed to vary across persons, time, and situations (Haynes). As such, flexibility and variability are essential features of a comprehensive and accurate behavioral assessment. Functional analysis, which emphasizes identification of stimuli and contingencies that elicit and maintain behaviors of interest, is one of the tenets of this method (Acierno, Hersen, & van Hasselt, 1998). In addition, behavioral assessment prioritizes the use of well-validated, psychometrically sound instruments that require minimal interpretation (Haynes). Behavioral assessment techniques allow for an empirical, hypothesis-based testing approach, with the goal of identifying causal relationships that can direct case conceptualization and treatment (Haynes).

Of the extant assessment protocols, behavioral assessment is likely to be the most dynamic (Haynes, 1998): Technological advancements are added to previously established methodologies in order to meet the varied and stringent requirements of this paradigm. This chapter will review the background information on analogue and virtual reality (VR) assessment, two relatively new developments in the childhood behavioral assessment field. It will begin with a broad and theoretical approach, by providing general background information on analogue and VR techniques and describing how they address the aforementioned goals of behavioral assessment, including functional assessment, case conceptualization, and treatment planning for children. An illustrative example will be provided to demonstrate how these techniques can be used to accomplish these goals. The chapter will then review and critique the empirical literature on the application of specific analogue and VR assessment techniques to diverse childhood problems. Finally, developmental considerations, which have been largely ignored by the literature, will be discussed.

BACKGROUND AND RELEVANCE TO CHILDHOOD BEHAVIORAL ASSESSMENT

Analogue assessment has been defined as "direct, systematic behavioral observations made of child behavior in a clinic or laboratory setting, especially where efforts are made to have the setting approximate in some ways more natural situations" (Barkley, 1991, p. 150). Analogue assessment takes on four different formats, including paper and pencil, audiotape, videotape, and enactment or role-play analogues (Nay, 1977). For the first three formats, children are asked to respond physically, verbally, or in writing to situations that are presented to them either in writing, on video, or on audiotape (Hintze, Stoner, & Bull, 2000a). Enactments involve the observation of a child's behavioral responses to circumscribed situations. Role-plays differ from enactments in that individuals are told ahead of time how to respond to a given scenario. For example, when assessing a child's social skills, an enactment would place her in a simulated classroom, and her responses to the other students would be observed. A role-play, on the other hand, would involve asking a child to behave as if she were meeting a new student for the first time (Hintze et al., 2000a). Analogue assessment relies on the assumption that an individual's behavior in a contrived environment approximates what would occur in a natural setting (Prout & Ferber, 1988).

Virtual reality technology is the most recent advance in the field of analogue assessment and falls into the enactment/role-play category. It has been defined as a "three-dimensional interface that puts the interacting subject in a condition of active exchange with a world re-created via the computer" (Vincelli & Molinari, 1998, p. 67). Such technology allows participants to feel fully present in this re-created environment by involving all of the sensorimotor channels and allowing for real-time navigation and interaction with the virtual environment (Vincelli & Molinari; Riva, 1997).

There are three types of VR systems: immersive VR, which utilizes head-mounted displays (HMDs), partially immersive VR, which involves a wide field-of-view display, such as a projection screen, and desktop VR, which uses a desktop monitor (McComas, Pivik, & Laflamme, 1998; Riva, 1998). Interaction occurs via joystick, keyboard, or a data glove, that is, a glove with sensors that transmit spatial and tactile information to a computer, thus allowing users to manipulate and explore VR environments (Ku et al., 2003). Although the full-immersion format may lead to an enhanced, all-encompassing experience for the user, this technology is much more expensive than the desktop version. In addition, some research on VR with adults has found that the use of HMDs causes symptoms of motion sickness in some subjects, resulting from a discrepancy between visual and vestibular inputs to the brain (Rose, Attree, & Johnson, 1996).

Virtual reality offers advantages over other analogue assessment techniques. First, it allows for increased confidentiality. The assessment procedure can be limited to the therapist's office and be devoid of human confederates while still immersing the subject in a simulated situation that involves others (North, North, & Coble, 1998). In addition, the technology allows the therapist to generate stimuli of greater perceived magnitude than may be possible with in vivo or imaginal techniques (North et al.). Furthermore, VR systems can simultaneously monitor diverse responses from the entire body and are sensitive to the properties of these responses, whereas other computer-based assessments can only accept one or two sources of input at a time (Riva, 1997). With respect to assessment, VR programs can alter what is presented auditorally, visually, olfactorially, etc., thus allowing for a flexible and multifaceted form of adaptive testing that is specifically tailored to the individual being tested (Riva, 1997). Finally, when compared with analogue assessments that involve contact with a feared stimulus, the VR methodology provides an added measure of safety by limiting contact to a computer-generated simulation within an office or clinic (North et al.). For example, if assessing a child with a dog phobia, the child's contact would be limited to a virtual animal rather than a real animal that could potentially harm the child. Because of its incipient status, the majority of systematic VR research has applied this technology to the assessment and treatment of adults, although some have commented on the potential application of VR to children (Muscott & Gifford, 1994; Rizzo, Wiederhold, & Buckwalter, 1998). The limited pilot data that have been generated thus far on the use of VR assessments with children have indicated that children find the technology usable and enjoyable (Rizzo et al., 2000).

Analogue assessment and VR assessment offer specific advantages over other assessment methods. First, they provide the therapist with the opportunity to observe behaviors that are difficult to assess via direct observation in natural settings, such as those that are highly situation-specific or occur infrequently (Hintze, Stoner, & Bull, 2000b). This may be particularly relevant for children whose behaviors of interest occur at recess or on the school bus, where gaining access is difficult and their behaviors are likely to be influenced by the obvious presence of an adult observer. Virtual reality assessment and analogue assessment differ from other techniques, such as retrospective self-report and naturalistic observation, in that they provide the therapist with environmental control, which is relevant to successful functional analysis. By manipulating external stimuli, the assessor can test ideographic hypotheses about the behavior of interest. Specific aspects of the behaviors can then be linked to environmental factors that explain their etiology and maintenance, thus clarifying and simplifying case conceptualization. In addition, this information can speak to treatment planning by finding ways to create an environment that fosters healthy behaviors and extinguishes those that are unhealthy (Hintze et al., 2000b).

A CASE EXAMPLE

Schill, Kratochwill, and Garner's (1996) case study of an 8-year-old girl with selective mutism provides an illustrative example of the use of analogue assessment. According to the American Psychiatric Association's *Diagnostic and Statistical Manual of Mental Disorders* (APA, 2000), children with selective mutism (SM) only speak to certain individuals or in specific situations, despite having intact language abilities. Most often, children with this disorder refuse to speak with nonfamily members, especially when they are outside of their home environments. Prior to devising the analogue, the researchers interviewed the girl's parents for two hours and received detailed information from them about their daughter's patterns of restricted speech. The interview was adapted from the Functional Diagnostic Protocol (FDP) (Cole & Gardner, 1993), a semistructured interview protocol that aids in the development of hypotheses about the factors that contribute to self-injurious behaviors. The protocol inquired about external factors, child characteristics, setting events, and behavioral consequences that may control the SM behaviors. In addition, the parents completed the Child Behavior Checklist (CBCL) (Achenbach & Edelbrock, 1983), a psychometrically sound paper-and-pencil measure. Using the information collected from the interview and checklist, the authors devised six hypotheses about the variables that initiated and maintained the concerning behavior. (1) The SM was negatively reinforced by the removal of aversive requests; (2) the child's perception of herself as incapable of performing certain tasks was related to the SM through negative reinforcement; (3) attention from others in response to speaking was aversive to the child and made it less likely that the child would repeat the behavior; (4) the child lacked coping skills to deal with aversive reactions such as teasing; (5) certain conditions and activities produced alternative behaviors to SM; (6) in certain settings, such as school, social feedback maintained the SM through positive reinforcement.

The analogue was used to test the first, second, and fifth hypotheses. Because of the child's history of refusing to speak in front of unfamiliar adults, all analogue tasks were performed both with an unfamiliar adult present (hard demand) and without (easy demand). The assessment procedure consisted of a baseline phase (a no-demand situation where the girl interacted freely with her family), an easy-demand task that allowed for a nonverbal response, a hard-demand task that allowed for a nonverbal response, an easy-demand task that did not allow for a nonverbal response, reading aloud in front of the parent, reading aloud in front of the parent and an unknown adult, playing an engaging board game with her family that required speech for participation (contingent play), playing the game without the required verbal participation (noncontingent play), and stimulus fading (the gradual introduction of an unknown adult to the contingent play situation).

Results indicated that hard-demand conditions produced significantly less speech than easy-demand situations. In addition, certain conditions, such as verbal interactions with family members, produced alternatives to SM (i.e., family members speaking for her). Within the easy-demand conditions, no behavioral differences were found between those that allowed for nonverbal responses and those that did not. When asked to read aloud, the child did so in front of her family but refused to do so in front of an adult stranger. Contingent play was found to increase speech in the hard-demand situation. The stimulus-fading technique was found to increase the amount of verbalization produced by the child in the presence of a stranger.

From these results, the investigators developed seven treatment recommendations for the parents and school professionals that would increase her use of language outside of the experimental setting. These recommendations included using the stimulus-fading technique with the reading-aloud task at school, keeping the child's brother and peers from speaking for her, ceasing the practice of rewording questions in such a way that they allowed a nonverbal response after her initial refusal to speak, providing the child with a longer response time rather than removing the request, the use of contingent play strategies that require verbalization in order for her to participate, avoiding enthusiastic feedback in response to her speech, and, finally, allowing the child some control over when and how she talks.

After three months elapsed, the child's behavior was again assessed. Multiple informant and method assessments indicated that the child's oral reading in front of a teacher, conversations with extended family members and other adults, talking on the phone, and ordering for herself in restaurants all increased.

Schill et al.'s (1996) analogue assessment technique accomplished several of the goals that underlie behavioral assessment. Specifically, they employed analogue assessment to identify the factors that supported the child's SM. Further, by breaking down this complicated behavioral repertoire into its antecedents and consequences, they were able to provide a clear conceptualization of her case and offer specific recommendations on how to effectively proceed with treatment.

A REVIEW AND CRITIQUE OF THE LITERATURE

Analogue and VR assessment have been used to investigate diverse childhood issues, including emotional problems, behavioral concerns, and academic problems (Hintze et al., 2000b; Mori & Armendariz, 2001). Within the emotional arena, these techniques have been employed to assess fears and phobias, depression, anxiety, and eating disorders. One of the most commonly used analogue assessments for investigating childhood fears and/or phobias is an enactment method known as the Behavioral Avoidance Test (BAT; Hamilton & King, 1991; Lang & Lazovik, 1963; Van Hasselt et al., 1981). In general, this test is administered in one of two ways. In the first variation, the child is placed in proximity to or contact with a feared stimulus and specific aspects of her behavior are observed, such as amount of time spent in the enactment or frequency of avoidance behaviors (Hintze et al., 2000a). Another iteration of this test involves placing the child in proximity to a feared stimulus but then requesting that she perform steps of a graded hierarchy of observable behaviors that continually bring her closer to the stimulus. Outcome measures of this task often include self-reported levels of distress and compliance with directions (Hintze et al., 2000a). The BAT has been used to investigate childhood fear of dogs (Bandura, Grusec, & Menlove, 1967; Hamilton & King, 1991), snakes (Kornhaber & Schroeder, 1975), water (Lewis, 1974), the dark (Kelley, 1976; Sheslow, Bondy, & Nelson, 1982), and spiders (Evans & Garfield, 1981). Butler, Miezitis, Friedman, and Cole (1980) applied this procedure to fifth and sixth grade children who evinced high levels of depression, wherein the children participated in enactments and role-plays involving depressogenic situations involving peer rejection.

Empirical support for the BAT's overall efficacy as an assessment and treatment instrument has been inconsistent (Mori & Armendariz, 2001). For example, both Kelley (1976) and Sheslow et al. (1982) used BATs that included gradual exposure to treat children's fear of the dark. Although Sheslow et al. (1982) found significant improvement, Kelley (1976) did not. These inconsistent findings could be due to the fact that the BAT procedures differed between the two studies (Mori & Armendariz). In fact, one of the most frequent criticisms leveled against this test has been its lack of standardization (Barrios & Hartmann, 1988; King, Ollendick, & Murphy, 1997). For example, the number of steps that made up the graded hierarchy has differed across various protocols (Mori & Armendariz). In addition, there was a lack of uniformity in the amount of calming statements that the children received and the extent of information that they were provided with regarding the feared statements. (Mori & Armendariz). These differences impede our ability to compare the findings across studies and interpret the results (Mori & Armendariz).

The Preschool Observation Scale of Anxiety (POSA; Glennon & Weisz, 1978), an analogue assessment method created for childhood separation anxiety, has also received attention in the literature. This 30-item scale delineates an observational rating system for specific anxious behaviors, such as gratuitous bodily movement and trembling voice. It has since been adapted for use with situational anxiety (Silverman & Serafini, 1998) and other childhood anxiety disorders (Kendall, 1994). Overall, the psychometric properties of the POSA have received support. Glennon and Weisz reported adequate interrater reliability (intraclass correlation = .77; correlation for the sum across items = .78). In addition, Kendall reported interrater reliability coefficient kappas that ranged from .79 to .93. The POSA has also been found to correlate with parent and teacher ratings of children's anxiety, thus supporting its convergent validity (Glennon & Weisz; Silverman & Serafini). These results allow for more cross-study comparison than has been afforded by the BAT.

Another area of psychopathology that has received attention from the analogue assessment literature is eating disorders. Specifically, VR technology is currently being developed for the assessment of eating disorders. The Body Image Virtual Reality Scale (BIVRS; Riva, 1997) assesses body image by presenting nine different-sized figures, varying from underweight to overweight, and asking individuals to identify the figures that concur with their current and desired body types. The discrepancy between these two selections translates into an index of dissatisfaction. Although similar techniques have previously been applied with sketches and other computer programs, the VR system will be an improvement because it adds a third dimension to the silhouettes (Riva). This is likely to improve participants' abilities to distinguish between figures and hone in on specific body areas, such as the stomach and thighs (Riva). This program has been designed to be inexpensive, compatible with personal computers, and run from the Internet, thus making it more accessible than many other VR techniques (Riva). Finally, this technique allows for increased standardization and cross-cultural comparisons (Riva).

In addition to emotional difficulties, analogue and VR assessment techniques have been applied to childhood behavioral difficulties, including Attention Deficit Hyperactivity Disorder (ADHD), noncompliance and aggression, social competence and cognition, and interpersonal problem solving. With regard to ADHD, researchers have used the analogue playroom as an assessment tool. In this procedure, children are observed while playing in a room with grids on the floor (e.g., Barkley & Ulman, 1975; Pope, 1970; Routh & Schroeder, 1976). Their locomotor activity level is assessed by counting the number of times they cross a grid line during a set period of time. In addition, attention is evaluated by observing the number of toys touched and the amount of time that children spend playing with them. Other researchers have adjusted this method to include an academic-like task in order to assess behaviors that are likely to occur in a classroom (Milich, 1984; Milich, Loney, & Roberts, 1986; M. A. Roberts, 1986, 1990). More specifically, children are asked to sit at a table, complete an academic task, remain seated, and avoid playing with any toys that are in the room. Investigators then assess the frequency of attentional shifts, off-task behaviors, leaving the seat, and touching of forbidden toys in order to quantify ADHD-type behavior (Mori & Armendariz, 2001). Like the BAT, both the free-play and academic-task ADHD analogue techniques have received criticism for lack of standardization. Specifically, researchers have varied their academic assignments, the types of toys present, and whether they include free play in isolation, an academic task in isolation, or both (Mori & Armendariz). This inconsistency hinders our ability to compare studies and interpret their results.

Rizzo et al. (2000) have piloted a VR ADHD assessment technique that speaks to these very criticisms. They have created a standardized virtual classroom that includes a teacher's desk, student desks, a virtual teacher, a chalkboard, a large window overlooking a playground and buildings, cars, and people, and a pair of doorways through which activity occurs. The technology provides a systematic, multisensory delivery that uses "typical" distracters, such as ambient classroom noise and a paper airplane flying around the room. During the procedure, the child sits at a virtual desk and is asked to perform specific tasks in the midst of the preprogrammed distractions, which can be varied based on the child's age or grade level. In addition to the reaction time and response variability on the task performance, the VR technology measures behavioral indicators associated with distractibility, such as head turning and gross motor movement. The task can be administered with and without distractions to allow for comparison and can also assess both audio and visual attention systems. The authors have piloted the technology on seven non-ADHD children and have found acceptable usability. The children expressed no hesitancy in using the equipment, none reported a sense of motion sickness, and all were able to read the virtual chalkboard. Although this technology holds the potential for increased standardization and control in the behavioral assessment of childhood ADHD, additional testing is needed to determine its reliability and validity.

In addition to ADHD, analogue assessment has been applied to childhood noncompliance and aggression, which, when severe, are strongly associated with the development of psychological problems in adulthood (Patterson, Reid, & Dishion, 1992). *Noncompliance* has been defined as the refusal to follow rules or comply with accepted standards of behavior (Forehand & McMahon, 1981). Several parent–child enactment procedures have been developed; their general format involves parents instructing their children to perform certain tasks. Both the child and parent behaviors are recorded and coded for items such as number of repeat commands, oppositional behaviors, and percent compliance (Forehand & McMahon; Barkley, 1987; M. W. Roberts & Powers, 1988; Robin & Foster, 1989). Of these methods, the Compliance Test (CT; Roberts & Powers) has received the most empirical evaluation (Hintze et al., 2000b). During the CT, parent–child dyads are placed in a playroom that contains distracter toys, instruction-designated toys, and instruction-designated containers. After a habituation period, the parent issues 30 standardized instructions to the child. These instructions are relayed to the parent by a clinician observing the two behind a one-way mirror via an earpiece worn by the parent. The observer notes whether or not the child initiates compliant behavior within five seconds of the instructions. The child's compliance ratio is quantified by dividing the number of compliant behaviors by 30.

Overall, the psychometric properties of the CT have been relatively strong. Roberts and Powers (1988) found interrater observer agreement to be greater than 97% and an internal consistency of .99. The CT's results have been shown to be significantly related to other measures of session behavior and other clinic-based analogues, thus supporting this method's criterion-related validity.

In general, analogue assessments typically used to evaluate noncompliance are similar to those used to assess aggression (Hintze et al., 2000b). Gable, Hendrickson, and Sasso (1995) outlined a specific and thorough assessment procedure based on the concept of data triangulation and involving three sources of information: record review and interviews, naturalistic observation, and analogue assessment. These varied methods are used to establish an operational definition of the child's aggression and also to determine the topographies, frequency, and severity of the behavior. Once this has been accomplished, the next step is to present five analogue situations that are based on the work of Iwata, Dorsey, Slifer, Bauman, and Richman (1982), Iwata, Pace, Kalsher, Cowdery, and Cataldo (1990), and Carr and Durand (1985) in order to identify the conditions maintaining the aggressive behavior. Specifically, the child is placed in five separate 10-minute situations that assess the relationship between her aggressive behavior and social attention, tangible reinforcement, escape, sensory reinforcement, and a control condition. Within the attention mode, the child plays in a room with multiple toys and an examiner present, who pretends to read or write. The examiner responds to the aggressive target behaviors with disapproving statements and ignores all other behaviors. During the tangible reinforcement condition, the child is directed to a specific task, with toys and edibles in plain view. The child is provided with the preferred items in response to her aggressive behavior. The escape analogue differs from the others in that the child is asked to perform a series of tasks, such as placing a block in a bucket, by the examiner. If the child refuses, the request is repeated and modeled by the examiner; if she continues to refuse, she is physically guided to complete the task. The examiner responds to aggressive behavior by removing the task and walking away and reintroducing the task when the aggression ends. Sensory reinforcement is assessed by having the examiner ignore the child, even in the face of the target behavior. The examiner also ignores aggression in the final control condition but provides her with social praise for appropriate behavior almost every 30 seconds. Out of concern for order effects, the authors suggest the replication of conditions. In addition, replication can allow for a more thorough assessment of whether certain forms of aggression are particular to specific conditions. The results of each condition are quantified using either frequency/event or interval recording and are then used to direct treatment recommendations. Two other sets of researchers have effectively utilized this approach to address aggressive behavior (Northup et al., 1991; Sasso et al., 1992).

In general, the few studies that have used Gable et al.'s (1995) technique have found support for its reliability, generalizability, and effectiveness. Their technique is consistent with the overall goals of behavioral assessment, including the use of multimethod, multimodal, and multi-informant measures and providing for an empirical, hypothesis-based testing approach. Importantly, their description of the procedure is specific enough to allow for sufficient standardization.

Although most of the assessment techniques described thus far are either enactments or role-plays, the most common analogue measures of children's social skills and competence used by researchers are sociometric measures of peer nominations and ratings that employ the pencil-and-paper method (Hintze et al., 2000a). Coie, Dodge, and Coppotelli (1982) developed a method that assesses the social composition of a classroom and establishes a method of comparing students against one another. According to the Coie et al. technique, each student in a classroom is asked to specify the three children in the class he likes the most and the least. Each student then receives a liked most (LM) and a liked least (LL) score based on the sums of the nominations that students receive in each category from the entire class. These scores are then used to calculate social preference (SP) scores, by subtracting the LL score from the LM score and a social impact (SI) score by adding the LL and LM scores together. The authors recommend interpreting the results by standardizing the scores for the entire class on each variable, thus allowing for comparison between students.

In addition, these standardized results can be used to classify children into sociometric status groups. Specifically, those children with a score above 1 on the SP category, a score above zero on the LM category, and an LL score of less than zero can be classified as *popular*. Children with SI scores greater than 1 and both LL and LM scores greater than zero can be considered *controversial*. *Neglected* children receive a SI score of less than –1 and an absolute LM score of zero. *Rejected* children receive a SP score less than –1, an LL score greater than zero, and an LM score less than zero. Finally, *average* children score close to the mean class score on both the SP and SI dimensions. By delineating a specific scoring method, Coie et al. (1982) allow for standardization and comparisons across studies. In addition, this technique relies on multi-informant sources, one of the priorities of behavioral assessment.

Children's social skills and competence have also been evaluated via role-plays. The Behavioral Assertiveness Test for Children (BAT-C; Bornstein, Bellack, & Hersen, 1977) consists of nine scenarios that a child is likely to encounter in daily interactions with other children. Children are introduced to the task by participating in a practice session. The format for each role-play involves a narrator introducing the scene, a role model delivering a prompt, and the child being asked to respond to the prompt as if the situation were happening in real life. For example, one of the scenes involves the narrator explaining that the child participant had lent her pencil to a classmate who then returned it with the point broken. The role model then states, "I broke the point." The child is then rated on the amount of eye contact she makes while speaking to the role model, loudness of speech, and whether or not she makes requests for new or alternate behaviors. In addition, two outside reviewers who are unfamiliar with the purposes of the vignettes rate the child's overall assertiveness on a scale of 1 to 5. The authors recommend that the scenarios be videotaped and coded. They also suggest carrying out the scenarios on three separate occasions per week for four weeks.

Several authors have examined the psychometric properties of the BAT-C. DiLorenzo and Michelsen (1982) evaluated the BAT-C by using observations of 46 role-playing situations in which 27 emotionally disturbed/learning-disabled children participated in four types of social interactions. Their results indicated that BAT-C possesses adequate internal reliability, as determined by split-half reliability and item-total correlations. In addition, Hobbs, Walle, and Hammersly (1984) found evidence for this test's convergent validity with fourth and fifth graders' peer nominations of the children they like and admire the most. At the same time, when compared to naturalistic observation, social skill role-plays have been found to have lower reliability and external validity (DuPaul & Eckert, 1994; Van Hasselt, Hersen, & Bellack, 1981).

Social cognition and interpersonal problem solving are often seen as contributors to the aforementioned social skills and competence abilities. Historically, the assessment of these constructs has relied on paper-and-pencil analogue measures rather than enactments or role-plays (Hintze et al., 2000b). One of the most popular paper-and-pencil methods utilized in the literature is the Assessment of Interpersonal Relations (AIR; Bracken, 1993a) (Hintze et al., 2000b). The AIR is a 35-item measure that evaluates children's perceptions of their social interactions with five different categories of people, including male and female peers, parents, and teachers. For each category, the children are asked to rate the degree to which they agree or disagree with statements such as "I am treated fairly." Bracken (1993a) normed this measure on 2501 children, who ranged from fifth to twelfth graders and whose demographic characteristics approximated those of the United States (Brooke, 1999). This effort allowed the authors to develop a system of translating a child's raw score to a standardized one based on her gender and age. The scoring system allows for the classification of child's relationships as very positive, moderately positive, average, moderately negative, or very negative. They provide guidelines for comparing the child's scores to those of her peers and also assessing her own relative strengths and weaknesses with respect to relationships.

Bracken (1993a) also evaluated the psychometric properties of this measure. The AIR's internal consistency coefficients ranged from .93 to .96, suggesting that this measure has strong internal consistency. In addition, correlations between pretest and post-test scores administered two weeks apart ranged from .94 to .98, providing further evidence of this measure's reliability. Unfortunately, interscorer reliability was not assessed (Brooke, 1999).

With respect to validity, Bracken (1993a) presented evidence of both age- and gender-based scoring differentials, which is consistent with the developmental literature on quality of interpersonal relationships. In addition, the test has been found to discriminate between "normal" adolescents and psychiatric inpatients (Bracken, 1993a; Brooke, 1999). Discriminant validity evidence was evaluated by comparing the AIR with the Multidimensional Self-Concept Scale (MSCS; Bracken, 1993b). Generally, correlations between the two scales were low, indicating that the tests were measuring different constructs. At the same time, the

AIR did correlate with the Social scale of the MSCS, as would be expected. These correlations ranged from .78 with female peers to .36 with male peers. The overall correlation between the two assessments was .55, suggesting a reasonable amount of overlap (Brooke). Factor analysis indicated seven meaningful items, five of which corresponded with the five AIR subscales (Bracken, 1993a). Bracken (1993a) cited the factor analysis results of another researcher, who found that each of the subscales measured a unique relationship (Brooke). However, factor validity coefficients were not reported (Brooke).

The AIR's normative data and clear scoring instructions allow for better standardization and cross-study and individual comparisons than most other analogue measures. At the same time, given that this instrument is billed as a diagnostic tool, more specific diagnostic research and interpretation instructions are warranted (Brooke, 1999). In addition, more attention needs to focus on how AIR's scores can translate into treatment recommendations (Hintze et al., 2000b).

In addition to emotional and behavioral assessment, analogue techniques have been used to measure children's academic abilities and learning behaviors. Within this context, analogue procedures typically involve interactions between the student and the examiner, and the goal is either to improve the skill being evaluated or to determine why the student is having difficulty and then to direct treatment accordingly (Gettinger & Seibert, 2000). In general, these assessment procedures occur under conditions similar to classroom instruction, so their results can be informed from and translated into that context (Gettinger & Seibert). Academic analogue procedures vary in format, technique, and purpose. The format can be one-to-one, can involve the whole class, or can be computer-based (Gettinger & Seibert). With respect to technique, analogue assessments differ in the way in which instruction occurs, such as the extent to which the child is instructed on how to complete tasks, how malleable that instruction is, and the types of materials used (Gettinger & Seibert). The purpose of the analogue may be to maximize test performance, to measure responsiveness to instruction, or to evaluate specific approaches or modifications (Gettinger & Seibert).

The literature has identified four different approaches to academic analogue assessment: dynamic assessment, curriculum-based assessment, think-aloud assessment, and computer-assisted assessment (Gettinger & Seibert, 2000). Dynamic assessment uses a pretest–teach–post-test procedure, with the goal of assessing children's potential for change and the type of instruction that will maximize on the students' abilities. Students respond to a brief set of specified instructions that then allow the examiner to make recommendations for intervention (Kirshenbaum, 1998). Some dynamic assessments relate to children's cognitive and learning abilities in general, while others focus on specific subject areas. Examples of analogue assessments of children's general abilities include Feurenstein's (1979) Learning Potential Assessment Device (LPAD), which measures cognitive abilities and growth, Jitendra and Kameenui's (1993) "testing the limits technique," which evaluates children's responses to different teaching methods, and Coleman's (1994) portfolio and dynamic assessment program, where children's behaviors during instruction are observed and then used to make recommendations for individual instruction. With respect to more specific applications of dynamic assessment, Campione and Brown (1987) developed a test–teach–test format that evaluates the amount of instruction necessary for the child to be able to master a mathematical skill and be able to generalize it to a related transfer task, such as independent mathematics problem solving. In addition, Carney and Cioffi (1990) developed a dynamic assessment tool for word-reading abilities.

Curriculum-based assessment (CBA) utilizes assessment materials and procedures that are taken from a student's current class curriculum and employs teaching methods that are consistent with those used by the teacher (Salvia & Ysseldyke, 1991). By identifying a student's strengths and weaknesses within the context of the classroom curriculum, this procedure can then be used to recommend specific curricular changes that will be beneficial to the child (Gettinger & Seibert, 2000). This assessment technique is used to monitor both current academic skills and progress toward a targeted outcome (Gettinger & Seibert). Although CBA has not received particularly stringent empirical evaluation, researchers have found positive reactions to this format. Both students and teachers have rated it as highly acceptable (Davis & Fuchs, 1995; Eckert & Shapiro, 1995). In addition, school psychologists reported that this method is more effective than norm-referenced protocols for identifying problems and communicating them to teachers and families. In addition, they reported feeling that these techniques are less biased than other formats in assessing children from diverse backgrounds (Shapiro & Eckert, 1993).

Think-aloud assessment focuses more on children's internal processes than the other scholastic assessment procedures described thus far (Gettinger & Seibert, 2000). During this procedure, children are asked to complete a task or learning situation and to report verbally and continuously what they are thinking while engaged with the activity. The examiner takes note of the cognitive processes and strategies employed by the child and her simultaneous performance. This information is then used to develop remedial methods to teach children new strategies or enhance the ones they already use to improve their classroom performance. The think-aloud method has been found to be effective for both reading comprehension and mathematics (Gettinger & Seibert).

Computer-assisted assessment programs—which provide instructional interventions, evaluate their effectiveness, determine children's skill level, analyze patterns of errors, and provide feedback and reinforcement—constitute the final method of analogue academic assessment (Gettinger & Seibert, 2000). One of the advantages of this method is the computer's ability to adapt the program to a student's current skill level, thus averting the frustration that accompanies tasks that are too difficult or the boredom of tasks that are too easy. In addition, when a child has not yet mastered a skill, the computer can present her with instructions that will help her to do so and then move her to an advanced level when appropriate. The highly interactive nature of this technology allows for immediate feedback for the student. Because computers have the ability to monitor, score, and preserve information about multiple students' individual abilities and changes, this technique is considered to be more efficient than other methods.

Two examples of computer-assisted programs that have been used in the academic assessment of children are Sherlock I and II (Lajoie & Lesgold, 1992). These programs ask children to solve problems that require the use of specific skills. As the students work through a problem, the computer provides individual tutoring and prompts in order to teach or improve on the skill in question. The children are then tested to see if they have mastered the skill and know when and where to apply it. If they have not completely mastered the skill or the ability to generalize it, the children are provided with additional instruction. The Sherlock programs focus on both academic skills and metacognitive abilities: Students are taught specific skills in addition to general approaches to effective problem solving.

Watkins and Kush (1988) examined the accuracy of computer-based assessment and compared it with paper-and-pencil measures. They found no difference between the two methods with respect to accuracy. In addition, students reported a preference for the computerized method over the others. Varnhagen and Gerber (1984), however, found that during a spelling exercise, children made more errors than they did with paper-and-pencil methods and took longer to complete the task. Future research should continue to examine the efficacy of computer techniques for academic assessment and evaluate the impact that children's comfort and experience with computers and knowledge of keyboard layout has on their performance.

The VR and analogue assessment techniques described thus far correspond with the variety of goals that accompany behavioral assessment. As part of a larger assessment package, these methods provide opportunities for multiple assessment methods, informants, and modes. In addition, the environmental control offered by these procedures makes them amenable to functional analysis and an empirical, hypothesis-based testing approach. The only behavioral assessment goal that is not addressed adequately, for the most part, by the analogue and virtual reality techniques is the use of well-validated, psychometrically sound instruments. Although many different researchers have employed these methods, their techniques vary from study to study, which makes it impossible to standardize and validate them. When conducting an extensive behavioral assessment that uses analogue techniques, it may be important to include well-validated measures in addition to these methods.

Some other areas of concern for these methodologies include their incremental utility, reliability, and ecological validity (Mori & Armendariz, 2001). Because analogue assessment techniques require significant time, space, equipment, and personnel, it is important to ensure their incremental utility. Their results need to provide accurate and unique information when compared with other, less cumbersome assessment methods in order to make them worthwhile endeavors. Research on the incremental utility of analogue and VR assessments is limited and contradictory. Although some researchers have found evidence for the accuracy of their analogue assessment results (e.g., M. W. Roberts & Powers, 1988), others have failed to do so (e.g., Routh & Schroeder, 1976). Future research should assess the amount of unique information provided by analogue and VR assessments when compared with other measures.

The reliability research on these measures is also contradictory and incomplete (Mori & Armendariz, 2001). The investigators who found evidence for temporal stability (e.g., Hamilton & King, 1991; Hinshaw, Simmel, & Heller, 1995) used brief intervals, with testings ranging from two consecutive days to one week apart. The preponderance of research, however, has found temporal stability for some but not all of the behavioral categories assessed (e.g., Millich, 1984; Rubin & Mills, 1988; Van Hasselt, Hersen, & Bellack, 1981). Kagan, Reznick, and Seidman (1988) found significant test–retest reliability only for the participants whose scores were most extreme. The timing intervals were broader for this latter research, ranging from one week to five years apart. The research on analogue assessment has been stronger, however, for interobserver reliability. Almost all of the researchers have assessed for this property and found satisfactory to high interobserver agreement (Mori & Armendariz, 2001).

Ecological validity, which refers to the extent to which children's behaviors in the analogue generalize to those outside of the experimental setting, is the final area of concern for analogue and VR assessment measures (Mori & Armendariz, 2001). The majority of research in this area has produced discouraging results. Sheridan, Dee, Morgan, McCormick, and Walker (1996) found that, although all of their participants' target behaviors improved from baseline to treatment and maintained at six-week follow-up, these improvements did not concur with naturalistic observations done at the school. Similarly, van Hasselt et al. (1981) found inconsistent to poor correlations between analogue and naturalistic observations. One the other hand, Hinshaw et al. (1995) found their analogue assessments of stealing and destruction in the lab did predict classroom observations of aggression. Researchers should continue to assess for the ecological validity of their measures. In addition, hypotheses as to why a particular analogue may or may not generalize should be developed and tested. Certain developmental, cognitive, or other variables may be able to shed light on this topic, thus improving the validity and treatment effectiveness of these techniques.

DEVELOPMENTAL CONSIDERATIONS

Although some have proposed that the inconsistent findings demonstrated by the analogue literature reflect a lack of standardization, it is possible that developmental factors have influenced these results as well. Most of the studies cited thus far place children in simulated environments within the confines of a laboratory or clinic that are supposed to mimic a classroom, playground, or other real-life situation. However, these studies have utilized children of various ages, and it is possible that their cognitive and developmental abilities affected their performance. Mental representation is a key component of most analogue assessments: Children are asked to interact with an experimenter or therapist as if she were someone else (e.g., teacher) within an environment that is supposed to represent an alternate location. At the same time, they are expected to do so in a way that represents reality rather than make-believe. In other words, they must use their imagination and "pretend" to be acting in reality. Children's capacities at mental representation and their understanding of and facility with pretence and imagination are likely to influence their immersion in the analogue and the generalizability of their behaviors.

Representational thinking is a multifaceted behavior that develops over time (Novak, 1996). An important milestone in this area, especially in relation to analogue assessment, develops around the age of 4, when children begin to grasp the distinction between appearance and reality (Flavell, 1999). For example, when shown a sponge that has been made to look like a rock, 4-year-olds are able to distinguish between the way the object looks and what it really is (Flavell). Three-year-olds, on the other hand, tend to see it as either a sponge or a rock and are not able to comprehend this duality (Flavell). This research suggests that behavioral responses to analogue procedures involving objects that approximate but are not identical to those in the child's world may not generalize to another setting until age 4. In addition, more advanced forms of mental representation do not develop until middle childhood. For example, research has indicated that children are unable to fully grasp the concept of interpretation until age 6 or 7. Pillow and Henrichon (1996) found that children who viewed a complete picture ascribed their own interpretation of the picture to an observer with a restricted view up until age 6. In addition, when interpreting an ambiguous event, children did not understand the influence that biases and expectations had on these interpretations until the same age (Pillow & Henrichon). As a result, children above and below the age of 6 may respond very differently to role-play techniques that involve either their own interpretations or assessing the interpretations of others.

There is disagreement within the literature about children's understanding of pretense and imagination, two additional developmental factors that may influence analogue assessment. Some researchers have found that children can distinguish between reality and fantasy by age 3; others suggest that this distinction solidifies in grade school (Woolley, 1995). Although children are able to engage in the action of pretending as young as age 18 months (Leslie, 1987, 1994) some research has indicated that they do not understand the activity as a mental process but rather an action until much later. For example, 18-month-olds are able to play with a banana and pretend that it is a telephone without confusion (Leslie, 1987, 1994). On the other hand, their understanding of what constitutes pretense is limited. Lillard (1993) found that when children as old as 5 were told that a doll who had never been exposed to a rabbit was hopping around, they claimed that the doll was pretending to be a rabbit, despite her lack of information about the animal. Lillard (1996) also found that children associated play with physical actions, such as clapping, rather than mental activities, such as thinking, until they reached age 7 or 8. Because there is so much dissension in the literature about children's cognitive development with respect to pretense and imagination (Woolley, 1995), it is difficult to predict the influence that age may have on the application of these behaviors to an analogue technique. However, the combination of pretense, imagination, and representational thinking toward reality that occurs in these techniques suggests that further attention to developmental characteristics is warranted. Behavioral psychologists view cognitive development as a hierarchical system that emerges and grows on the basis of contingencies (Novak, 1996). As skills emerge, they are reinforced, and the environment provides a context for the nascent skills to merge and further reinforces the emergence of more complex cognitive behavioral patterns (Novak). Because analogue assessment taps into a rich combination of various cognitive behaviors, young children, who are lower on this hierarchy of cognitive development and reinforcement, may respond differently to analogue techniques than those who are older. Perhaps children's developmental stages will impact how they respond to the analogue methods and the extent to which their behaviors translate out of session. In addition, differential cognitive capacities in the areas of representational thinking, pretense, imagination, and their coalescence may explain the contradictory findings in the extant literature.

SUMMARY

Analogue assessment techniques indirectly measure behaviors that are likely to occur in real life. In their most typical format, behaviors are observed in a simulated environment. The most recent advancements in analogue assessment methods have used virtual reality technology to immerse participants in an interactive environment that allows the computer to perform adaptive testing and precise measurement. Because analogue techniques allow for environmental control, these methods are particularly amenable to the multitudinous goals of behavioral assessment, including establishing functional analysis and hypothesis-testing approaches that direct treatment recommendations. Analogue and VR assessment techniques have been applied to a variety of childhood issues, including emotional concerns, behavioral problems, and academic assessment. Although these methods have great potential, they have received minimal empirical validation. The varied approaches and techniques have prohibited standardization, replication, and comparison. In addition, these methods have received inconsistent reviews with respect to their incremental utility, reliability, and ecological validity. The research has largely ignored developmental and cognitive factors that may influence their results. Future research should attempt to standardize these measures, allow for more systematic empirical evaluation, and, in the context of evaluating children, assess the interplay between cognitive and developmental abilities and resultant findings.

REFERENCES AND RESOURCES

Achenbach, T. M., & Edelbrock, C. (1983). *Manual for the Child Behavior Checklist and Revised Child Behavior Profile*. Burlington: University of Vermont Depatment of Psychiatry.

Acierno, R., Hersen, M., & van Hasselt, V. B. (1998). Prescriptive assessment and treatment. In A. S. Bellack & M. Hersen (Eds.), *Behavioral assessment: A practical handbook* (4th ed., pp. 47–62). Needham Heights, MA: Allyn & Bacon.

American Psychiatric Association. (2000). *Diagnostic and statistical manual of mental disorders* (4th ed., text revision). Washington, DC: Author.

Bandura, A., Grusec, J. E., & Menlove, F. L. (1967). Vicarious extinction of avoidance behavior. *Journal of Personality and Social Psychology, 5,* 16–23.

Barkley, R. A. (1987). *Defiant children: A clinician's manual for parent training*. New York: Guilford Press.

Barkley, R. A. (1991). The ecological validity of laboratory and analogue assessment methods of ADHD symptoms. *Journal of Abnormal Child Psychology, 19,* 149–178.

Barkley, R. A., & Ullmon, D. G. (1975). A comparison of objective measures of activity distractibility in hyperactive and nonhyperactive children. *Journal of Abnormal Child Psychology, 3,* 231–244.

Barrios, B. A., & Hartmann, D. (1988). Fears and anxieties. In E. J. Mash & L. G. Terdal (Eds.), *Behavioral assessment of childhood disorders* (pp. 259–304). New York: Guilford Press.

Bornstein, M. R., Bellack, A. S., & Hersen, M. (1977). Social skills training for unassertive children: A multiple baseline analysis. *Journal of Applied Behavior Analysis, 10,* 183–195.

Bracken, B. A. (1993a). *Assessment of Interpersonal Relations*. Austin, TX: Pro-Ed.

Bracken, B. A. (1993b). *Multidimensional Self-Concept Scale*. Austin, TX: Pro-Ed.

Brooke, S. L. (1999). Assessment of Interpersonal Relations: A test review. *Measurement and Evaluation in Counseling and Development, 32,* 105–111.

Butler, L., Miezitis, S., Friedman, R., & Cole, E. (1980). The effect of two school-based intervention programs on depressive symptoms in preadolescents. *American Educational Research Journal, 17,* 111–119.

Campione, J. C., & Brown, A. L. (1987). Linking dynamic assessment with school achievement. In C. S. Lidz (Ed.), *Dynamic assessment: An interactional approach to evaluating learning potential* (pp. 82–115). New York: Guilford Press.

Carney, J. J., & Cioffi, G. (1990). Extending traditional diagnosis: The dynamic assessment of reading abilities. *Reading Psychology, 11,* 177–192.

Carr, E. G., & Durand, V. M. (1985). Reducing behavior problems through functional communication training. *Journal of Applied Behavior Analysis, 18,* 111–126.

Coie, J. D., Dodge, K. A., & Coppotelli, H. (1982). Dimensions and types of social status: A cross-age perspective. *Developmental Psychology, 18,* 557–570.

Cole, C. L., & Gardner, W. I. (1993). Psychotherapy with developmentally delayed children. In T. R. Kratochwill & R. J. Morris (Eds.), *Handbook of psychotherapy with children and adolescents* (pp. 426–471). New York: Pergamon Press.

Coleman, L. J. (1994). Portfolio assessment: A key to identifying hidden talents and empowering teachers of young children. *Gifted Child Quarterly, 38,* 65–69.

Cone, J. D. (1978). The Behavioral Assessment Grid (BAG): A conceptual framework and taxonomy. *Behavior Therapy, 8,* 411–426.

Davis, L. B., & Fuchs, L. S. (1995). "Will CBM help me learn?" Students' perceptions of the benefits of curriculum-based measurement. *Education and Treatment of Children, 18,* 19–33.

DiLorenzo, T. M., & Michelson, L. (1982). Psychometric properties of the Behavioral Assertiveness Test for Children. *Child and Family Behavior Therapy, 4,* 71–76.

DuPaul, G. J., & Eckert, T. L. (1994). The effects of social skills curricula: Now you see them, now you don't. *School Psychology Quarterly, 9,* 113–132.

Durand, V. M., & Crimmins, D. B. (1988). Identifying the variables maintaining self-injurious behavior. *Journal of Autism and Developmental Disorders, 18,* 99–117.

Eckert, T. L., & Shapiro, E. S. (1995). Teachers' ratings of the acceptability of curriculum-based assessment methods. *School Psychology Review, 24,* 497–508.

Evans, P. D., & Garfield, H. (1981). Children's self-initiated approach to spiders. *Behavior, Research, and Therapy, 19,* 543–546.

Feurenstein, R. (1979). *The dynamic assessment of retarded performers: The Learning Potential Assessment Device, Theory, Instruments, and Techniques.* Baltimore: University Park Press.

Flavell, J. H. (1999). Cognitive development: Children's knowledge about the mind. *Annual Review of Psychology, 50,* 21–45.

Forehand, R. L., & McMahon, R. J. (1981). *Helping the noncompliant child: A clinician's guide to parent training.* New York: Guilford Press.

Gable, R. A., Hendrickson, J. M., & Sasso, G. M. (1995). Toward a more functional analysis of aggression. *Education and Treatment of Children, 18,* 226–242.

Gettinger, M., & Seibert, J. K. (2000). In E. S. Shapiro & T. R. Kratochwill (Eds.), *Behavioral assessment in schools: Ttheory, research, and clinical foundations* (2nd ed., pp. 139–167). New York: Guilford Press.

Glennon, B., & Weisz, J. R. (1978). An observational approach to the assessment of anxiety in young children. *Journal of Consulting and Clinical Psychology, 46,* 1246–1257.

Hamilton, D. I., & King, N. J. (1991). Reliability of a behavioral avoidance test for the assessment of dog phobic children. *Psychological Reports, 69,* 18.

Haynes, S. N. (1988). The changing nature of behavioral assessment. In A. S. Bellack & M. Hersen (Eds.), *Behavioral assessment: A practical handbook* (4th ed., pp. 1–21). Needham Heights, MA: Allyn & Bacon.

Hinshaw, S. P., Simmel, C., & Heller, T. L. (1995). Multimethod assessment of covert antisocial behavior in children: Laboratory observations, adult ratings, and child self-report. *Psychological Assessment, 7,* 209–219.

Hintze, J. M., Stoner, G., & Bull, M. H. (2000a). Analogue assessment: Emotional/behavioral problems. In E. S. Shapiro & T. R. Kratochwill (Eds.), *Conducting school-based assessments of child and adolescent behavior* (pp. 55–77). New York: Guilford Press.

Hintze, J. M., Stoner, G., & Bull, M. H. (2000b). Analogue assessment: Research and practice in evaluating emotional and behavioral problems. In E. S. Shapiro & T. R. Kratochwill (Eds.), *Behavioral assessment in schools: Theory, research, and clinical foundations* (2nd ed., pp. 104–138). New York: Guilford Press.

Hobbs, S. A., Walle, D. L., & Hammersly, G. A. (1984). Assessing children's social skills: Validation of the Behavioral Assertiveness Test for Children. *Journal of Behavioral Assessment, 6,* 29–35.

Iwata, B., Dorsey, M., Slifer, K., Bauman, K., & Richman, G. (1982). Toward a functional analysis of self-injury. *Analysis and Intervention in Developmental Disabilities, 2,* 3–20.

Iwata, B., Pace, G., Kalsher, M., Cowdery, G., & Cataldo, M. (1990). Experimental analysis and extinction of self-injurious escape behavior. *Journal of Applied Behavior Analysis, 23,* 11–27.

Jitendra, A. K., & Kameenui, E. J. (1993). Dynamic assessment as a compensatory assessment approach: A description and analysis. *Remedial and Special Education, 14,* 6–18.

Kagan, J., Reznick, J. S., & Seidman, N. (1988). Biological bases of childhood shyness. *Science, 240,* 167–171.

Kelley, C. K. (1976). Play desensitization of fear of darkness in preschool children. *Behavior Research and Therapy, 14,* 79–81.

Kendall, P. C. (1994). Treating anxiety disorders in children: Results of a randomized clinical trial. *Journal of Consulting and Clinical Psychology, 62,* 100–110.

King, N. J., Ollendick, T. H., & Murphy, G. C. (1997). Assessment of childhood phobias. *Clinical Psychology Review, 17,* 667–687.

Kirshenbaum, R. J. (1998). Dynamic assessment and its use with underserved gifted and talented populations. *Gifted Child Quarterly, 42,* 140–147.

Kornhaber, R. C., & Schroeder, H. F. (1975). Importance of model similarity on extinction of avoidance behavior in children. *Journal of Consulting and Clinical Psychology, 43,* 601–607.

Ku, J., Mraz, R., Baker, N., Zakzanis, K. K., Lee, J. H., Kim, I. Y., Kim, S. I., & Grahm, S. J. (2003). A data glove with tactile feedback for fMRI ofvirtual reality experiments. *Cyberpsychology and Behavior, 6,* 497–508.

Lajoie, S. P., & Lesgold, A. M. (1992). Dynamic assessment of proficiency for solving procedural knowledge tasks. *Educational Psychologist, 23,* 365–384.

Lang, P. J., & Lazovik, A. D. (1963). Experimental desensitization of a phobia. *Journal of Abnormal and Social Psychology, 66,* 519–525.

Leslie, A. (1987). Pretense and representation: Origins of "theory of mind." *Psychological Review, 94,* 412–426.

Leslie, A. (1994). ToMM, ToBY, and agency: Core architecture and domain specificity. In L. A. Hirschenfeld & S. A. Gellman (Eds.), *Mapping the mind: Domain specificity in cognition and culture* (pp. 119–148). Cambridge: Cambridge University Press.

Lewis, S. (1974). A comparison of behavior therapy techniques in the reduction of fearful avoidance behavior. *Behavior Therapy, 5,* 648–655.

Lillard, A. S. (1993). Young children's conceptualization of pretense: Action or mental representational state. *Child Development, 64,* 372–386.

Lillard, A. S. (1996). Body or mind: Children's categorization of pretense. *Child Development, 67,* 1717–1734.

McComas, J., Pivik, J., & LaFlamme, M. (1998). Current uses of virtual reality for children with disabilities. In G. Riva, B. K. Wiederhold, & E. Molinari (Eds.), *Virtual environments in clinical psychology and neuroscience: Methods and techniques in advanced patient–therapist interaction* (pp. 161–169). Amsterdam: IOS Press.

Milich, R. (1984). Cross-sectional and longitudinal observations of activity level and sustained attention in a normative sample. *Journal of Abnormal Child Psychology, 12,* 261–276.

Milich, R., Loney, J., & Roberts, S. 1986. Playroom observations of activity level and sustained attention. *Journal of Consulting and Clinical Psychology, 54,* 272–274.

Mori, L. T., & Armendariz, G. M. (2001). Analogue assessment of child behavior problems. *Psychological Assessment, 13,* 36–45.

Muscott, H. S., & Gifford, T. (1994). Virtual reality and social skills training for students with behavioral disorders: Applications, challenges, and promising practices. *Education and Treatment of Children, 17,* 417–434.

Nay, W. R. (1977). Analogue measures. In A. R. Ciminero, K. S. Calhoun, & H. E. Adams (Eds.), *Handbook of behavioral assessment* (pp. 233–277). New York: Wiley.

North, M., North, S., & Coble, J. (1988). Virtual reality therapy: An effective treatment for phobias. In G. Riva, B. K. Wiederhold, & E. Molinari (Eds.), *Virtual environments in clinical psychology and neuroscience: Methods and techniques in advanced patient–therapist interaction* (pp. 112–119). Amsterdam: IOS Press.

Northup, J., Wacker, D., Sasso, G. M., Steege, M., Cigrand, K., Cook, J., & DeRaad, A. (1991). A functional analysis of both aggressive and alternative behavior in an outclinic setting. *Journal of Applied Behavior Analysis, 24,* 509–522.

Novak, G. (1996). *Developmental psychology: Dynamical systems and behavior analysis.* Reno, NV: Context Press.

Patterson, G. R., Reid, J. B., & Dishion, T. B. (1992). *Antisocial boys: A social interactional approach.* Eugene, OR: Catalia.

Pillow, B. H., & Henrichon, A. J. (1996). There's more to the picture than meets the eye: Young children's difficulty understanding biased interpretation. *Child Development, 67,* 802–819.

Pope, L. (1970). Motor activity in brain-injured children. *American Journal of Orthopsychiatry, 40,* 783–794.

Prout, H. T., & Ferber, S. M. (1988). Analogue Assessment: Traditional personality assessment measures in behavioral assessment. In E. S. Shapiro & T. R. Kratochwill (Eds.), *Behavioral assessment in schools: Conceptual foundations and practical applications* (pp. 290–321). New York: Guilford Press.

Riva, G. (1997). Virtual reality as assessment tool in psychology. In G. Riva (Ed.), *Virtual reality in neuro-psycho-physiology* (pp. 71–80). Amsterdam: IOS Press.

Riva, G. (1998). Virtual reality in neuroscience: A survey. In G. Riva, B. K. Wiederhold, & E. Molinari (Eds.), *Virtual environments in clinical psychology and neuroscience: Methods and techniques in advanced patient–therapist interaction* (pp. 191–199). Amsterdam: IOS Press.

Rizzo, A. A., Buckwalter, J. G., Bowerly, T., Van Der Zag, C., Humphrey, L., Neumann, U., Chua, C., Kyriakakis, C., Van Rooyen, A., & Sisemore, D. (2000). The virtual classroom: A virtual reality environment for the assessment and rehabilitation of attention deficits. *CyberPsychology and Behavior, 3,* 483–499.

Rizzo, A. A., Wiederhold, M. D., & Buckwalter, J. G. (1998). Basic issues in the use of virtual environments for mental health applications. In G. Riva, B. K. Wiederhold, & E. Molinari (Eds.), *Virtual environments in clinical psychology and neuroscience: methods and techniques in advanced patient–therapist interaction* (pp. 21–42). Amsterdam: IOS Press.

Roberts, M. A. (1986). How is playroom behavior observation used in the diagnosis of attention deficit disorder? *Journal of Children in Contemporary Society, 19,* 65–74.

Roberts, M. A. (1990). A behavior observation method for differentiating hyperactive and aggressive boys. *Journal of Abnormal Child Psychology, 18,* 131–142.

Roberts, M. W., & Powers, S. W. (1988). The compliance test. *Behavioral Assessment, 10,* 375–397.

Robin, A. L., & Foster, S. L. (1989). *Negotiating parent–adolescent conflict: A behavioral–family systems approach.* New York: Guilford Press.

Rose, F. D., Attree, E. A., & Johnson, D. A. (1996). Virtual reality: An assistive technology on neurological rehabilitation. *Current Opinion in Neurology, 9,* 461–467.

Routh, D. K., & Schroeder, C. S. (1976). Standardized playroom measures as indices of hyperactivity. *Journal of Abnormal Child Psychology, 4,* 199–207.

Rubin, K. H., & Mills, R. S. L. (1988). The many faces of social isolation in childhood. *Journal of Consulting and Clinical Psychology, 56,* 916–924.

Salvia, J., & Ysseldyke, J. S. (1991). *Assessment* (5th ed.). Boston: Houghton Mifflin.

Sasso, G. M., Reimers, T. M., Cooper, L. J., Wacker, D., Berg, W., Steege, M., Kelly, L., & Allaire, A. (1992). Use of descriptive and experimental analysis to identify the functional properties of aberrant behavior in school settings. *Journal of Applied Behavior Analysis, 25,* 809–821.

Schill, M. T., Kratochwill, T. R., & Gardner, W. I. (1996). An assessment protocol for selective mutism: Analogue assessment using parents as facilitators. *Journal of School Psychology, 34,* 1–21.

Shapiro, E. S., & Eckert, T. L. (1993). Computer-based assessment among school psychologists: Knowledge, use, and attitudes. *Journal of School Psychology, 31,* 357–383.

Sheridan, S. M., Dee, C. C., Morgan, J. C., McCormick, M. E., & Walker, D. (1996). A multimethod intervention for social skills deficits in children with ADHD and their parents. *School Psychology Review, 25,* 57–76.

Sheslow, D. V., Bondy, A. S., & Nelson, R. O. (1982). A comparison of graduated exposure, verbal coping skills, and their combination in the treatment of children's fear of the dark. *Child and Family Behavior Therapy, 4,* 33–45.

Silverman, W. K., & Serafini, L. T. (1998). Assessment of child behavior problems: Internalizing disorders. In A. S. Bellack & M. Hersen (Eds.), *Behavioral assessment: A practical handbook* (4th ed., pp. 342–360). London: Jessica Kingsley.

Van Hasselt, V. B., Hersen, M., & Bellack, A. S. (1981). The validity of role play tests for assessing social skills in children. *Behavior Therapy, 12,* 202–216.

Varnhagen, S., & Gerber, M. M. (1984). Use of microcomputers for spelling assessment: Reasons to be cautious. *Learning Disability Quarterly, 7,* 266–270.

Vincelli, F., & Molinari, E. (1998). Virtual reality and imaginative techniques in clinical psychology. In G. Riva, B. K. Wiederhold, & E. Molinari (Eds.), *Virtual environments in clinical psychology and neuroscience: Methods and techniques in advanced patient–therapist interaction* (pp. 67–72). Amsterdam: IOS Press.

Watkins, M. W., & Kush, J. C. (1988). Assessment of academic skills of learning disabled students with classroom microcomputers. *School Psychology Review, 17,* 81–88.

Wellman, H. M., & Estes, D. (1986). Early understanding of mental entities: A reexamination of childhood realism. *Child Development, 57,* 910–923.

Whitehall, M. B., Hersen, M., & Bellack, A. S. (1980). A conversation skills training program for socially isolated children: An analysis of generalization. *Behavior Research and Therapy, 14,* 466–481.

Wolchik, S. A., Beals, J., & Sandler, I. N. (1989). Mapping children's support networks: Conceptual and methodological issues. In D. Belle (Ed.), *Children's social networks and social support* (pp. 191–220). New York: Wiley.

Woolley, J. D. (1995). The fictional mind: Young children's understanding of imagination, pretense, and dreams. *Developmental Review, 15,* 172–211.

5

BEHAVIORAL INTERVIEWING OF PARENTS

WILLIAM G. SHARP
CARA B. REEVES
ALAN M. GROSS

Department of Psychology
The University of Mississippi
University, Mississippi

INTRODUCTION

The behavioral interview is considered an essential component of the behavioral assessment process (Reitman, Hummel, Franz, & Gross, 1998). In addition to its function in facilitating communication, the interview provides an opportunity to make behavioral observations, to formulate a diagnosis, to identify environmental factors maintaining the problem behavior, to plan and evaluate treatment strategies, and to build rapport with the child and family. It also allows the interviewer to broach topics such as divorce, recent school change, and familial substance abuse that the interviewee may not have disclosed or considered relevant to the assessment process. Finally, it provides an opportunity for the interviewer to communicate to the client what therapy will be like and to articulate basic behavioral principles and assumptions through cues, probes, and summary statements (Sarwer & Sayers, 1998; Tombari & Bergan, 1978).

While perhaps the most essential and widely used tool in the assessment process, the interview has traditionally been viewed as an informal assessment method (Gresham, 1984). This lack of formal recognition was due, in part, to the generally unstructured format of traditional interviews as well as the paucity of information regarding the psychometric adequacy of behavioral interviews. Other contributing factors include the strong emphasis within the behavioral literature on direct observation as well as continued questions regarding the utility of subjective reports in behavioral assessment.

Although historically viewed as an informal method, the behavioral interview offers several advantages over other behavioral assessment strategies, such as behavioral checklists, direct observation, and self-monitoring. Most notably, the behavioral interview provides a flexible band of inquiry that can be broadened or narrowed as needed. This flexibility allows for the collection of general information regarding overall functioning as well as more detailed information about specific areas. The behavioral interview also provides the opportunity to collect information regarding the client's receptivity to certain intervention strategies, a variable not often captured by other assessment methods (Gresham & Davis, 1988). As noted by Sheridan, Krotochwill, and Bergan (1996), clients who find a treatment unacceptable due to the required investment of time and resources or who are unresponsive to a treatment strategy because of theoretical objections may be less likely to implement a treatment correctly, if at all. Therefore, the assessment of client receptivity to certain behavioral procedures during the interview process may aid in program design and implementation. Finally, the interview provides a setting in which the potential for greater confidentiality between patient and therapist exists. The patient may be more willing to divulge information verbally than to write it and provide a permanent record (A. A. Linehan, 1977). Information can also be obtained from people who, because of poor communication skills, are unable to provide it in other ways, such as questionnaires or behavioral checklists.

The goal of the present chapter is to review and clarify the major components involved in the behavioral interview. More specifically, the chapter focuses on the use of and issues involved with the behavioral interviewing of parents. The chapter begins with a discussion as to the distinction between child and adult assessment. We then define and provide a general overview of behavioral interviewing, which includes a review of the general assumptions and objectives of the behavioral interview. Next, we present examples of common interviewing formats, discuss the skills and strategies necessary in conducting a behavioral interview, and review the state of empirical research on the behavioral interview. The chapter concludes with a case illustration.

CHILD VERSUS ADULT ASSESSMENT

There are three aspects of child assessment that differentiate it from adult assessment (Boggs, Griffin, & Gross, 2003). First, while most adults who attend therapy identify themselves as having behavioral difficulties, children are typically referred for psychological services because an adult (e.g., parent, teacher) has determined that a behavioral problem exists. Based on this characteristic of child assessment, it is not uncommon for the child and adult to disagree about the actual existence of a problematic behavior as well as the exact specifics of the problem area. As such, it is important for the therapist to address any disparity in perceptions during initial stages of the treatment process in order to ensure efficient and effective data collection.

Child assessment is further distinguished from adult assessment by the critical role that developmental issues play in the assessment process. Given that childhood is a time marked by rapid growth and development, it is not uncommon for an adult to be concerned about developmentally appropriate behavior. Therefore, it is important for the therapist to consider a child's developmental context when determining whether a child's behavior is deviant. This entails having a clear understanding of normal developmental processes (i.e., typical age ranges by which children learn behaviors such as walking, talking, toileting, and reading) while recognizing that there will be some degree of variability within the normal range of meeting various milestones (Boggs et al., 2003). For example, most children become toilet-trained by approximately 3 years of age. Thus, children of this age are still within normal limits if they have not yet achieved bowel and bladder control. In contrast, toileting accidents are less common in children age 5 and up and, when present, should be addressed by appropriate health care professionals. Reviews of age-appropriate milestones in cognitive, emotional, and physical development have been provided in various psychological textbooks and may serve as a quick reference guide in identifying deviations along the developmental timeline (Sattler, 2002; Morrison & Anders, 1999).

Finally, child assessment can be differentiated from adult assessment by the common use of informant interviews (i.e., interviews conducted with individuals beyond the identified client, such as parents, teachers, or siblings) in the assessment process (Gresham & Davis, 1988). Several factors account for the ubiquity of informant interviews in child assessment. Most notably, many children are often unable, due to a limited verbal repertoire, or unwilling to report their own behaviors or symptoms (Beaver & Busse, 2000). Due to these communication difficulties, adults are often used as a primary source for information regarding a child's problem behavior. In addition, adults are typically powerful agents of behavior change in a child's environment, controlling many of the rewarding and aversive events that a child may experience. Therefore, the interview provides the therapist with the opportunity to assess an adult's current behavior management strategies as well as receptiveness to alternative behavioral procedures. For these reasons, the informant interview represents an important data collection method in child assessment, allowing the therapist to obtain detailed information regarding the problematic behavior and to develop treatment strategies that utilize the mediational potential of adults (Ciminero & Drabman, 1977).

In the outpatient setting, parents represent one of the most common sources of behavioral data (Beaver & Busse, 2000). As informants, parents have the potential to provide the therapist with a rich source of information, including a detailed description of the problem behavior and related environmental variables, as well as information regarding child discipline methods, marital status problems, and other home or community factors (Gresham & Davis, 1988). With this said, a child's behavioral difficulties often manifest themselves in multiple settings. Therefore, behavioral interviews typically extend beyond the child's primary caregiver, involving teachers and other significant adults. Although a variety of "traditional" interview formats are available for engaging parents and other informants in the interview process, the behavioral interview tends to provide the most relevant information for intervention planning and implementation.

GENERAL ASSUMPTIONS AND MAJOR OBJECTIVES IN BEHAVIORAL INTERVIEWING

BEHAVIORAL VERSUS TRADITIONAL INTERVIEWS

The *behavioral* interview is often distinguished from the traditional *psychological* interview in terms of the underlying assumptions and goals that guide its structure and format. In terms of theoretical assumptions, traditional psychological interviews tend to view current behavior problems as the product of remote environmental causes and/or internal states or traits (Gresham & Davis, 1988). Based on this assumption, traditional psychological interviews often inquire about the global concerns of the client and focus on gathering historical information (Gresham, 1984). In contrast, behavioral interviews tend to focus on the "here and now," emphasizing current environmental variables and minimizing inquiries regarding remote environmental events or personality traits (Sheridan et al., 1996). Based on this focus, the primary objective of a behavioral interview is to obtain descriptive information about problematic behavior and the environmental contingencies maintaining these behaviors.

The behavioral interview is further distinguished from the traditional psychological interview in terms of the emphasis placed on diagnostic concerns. More specifically, the primary goal of traditional psychological interviews is often equated with diagnostic assessment, while the overarching goal of the behavioral interview is typically associated with treatment planning (i.e., designing, implementing, and evaluating a treatment strategy). Consistent with this distinction, early behavior theorists tended to minimize the importance of formal diagnosis, shifting the focus of the assessment process to a more objective assessment of behavior (Beaver & Busse, 2000). While this initial distinction served to differentiate behavioral interviews from more dynamically oriented models, current behavioral theorists recognize that diagnostic assessment and treatment planning are interrelated processes (Hayes & Follette, 1992). More specifically, behavioral clinicians typically arrive at a diagnosis while gathering information regarding a problem or disorder during the assessment process. In turn, this diagnosis serves as the base on which a functional assessment is conducted and a treatment plan devised (Faul & Gross, in press).

FOUNDATION OF THE BEHAVIORAL INTERVIEW

The foundation of the behavioral interview rests on the general principles of conditioning and learning. Essential to this foundation is the assumption that behaviors are learned as a function of an individual's interaction with the environment (Sarwer & Sayers, 1998). Current behavior is conceptualized as a function of contingent reinforcement for a particular behavior as well as all other reinforcement operating in the environment at that point in time (Sheridan et al., 1996). In turn, patient difficulties are interpreted as maladaptive response tendencies both maintained and transformed by environmental contingencies (Beaver & Busse, 2000). Based on this perspective, problematic behavior may have multiple determinants, but the most important factors are typically viewed as occurring in close temporal proximity to the behavior of interest (Sarwer & Sayers).

Based on this foundation, the behavioral clinician attempts to elicit information necessary to perform a functional analysis of the problem throughout the interview process. This entails clearly defining (i.e., operationalizing) the problem behavior as well as developing an understanding of what environmental variables are functionally related to the client's behavior (Sarwer & Sayers, 1998). In doing so, the behavioral clinician is assessing a number of interrelated variables, including the antecedent (A) stimulus variables that set the stage for the maladaptive behavior, the problem behavior (B) of interest, and the environmental consequences (C) of behavior (Goldfried & Davison, 1994). Information regarding the "ABCs" of the problem is then used to formulate treatment strategies and evaluate treatment progress (O'Leary & Wilson, 1975). Approached in this manner, the behavioral interview is utilized throughout the assessment and treatment process, providing a vehicle to monitor progress in therapy and obtain feedback for making clinically sound adjustments in treatment.

MAJOR OBJECTIVES OF THE BEHAVIORAL INTERVIEW

Often cited as the most important aspect of behavioral interviewing, the first major objective of the behavioral interview is to obtain a complete and accurate description of the problem behavior (Morganstern, 1988). This should include information as to the frequency and duration of the behavior as well as behavioral excesses and deficits. Given the possible complexities of a presenting problem and its related environmental contingencies, it is often necessary to clarify the major components of a child's difficulties and then to prioritize these components into a manageable sequence (Sheridan et al., 1996). This enables a complex problem to be tackled in a more systematic fashion, allowing the therapist and parent to discuss immediate and long-term goals for behavior change. To aid in this process, several assessment strategies have been proposed (Goldfried & Pomeranz, 1968; Kanfer & Saslow, 1969; Mischel, 1973; Goldfried & Sprafkin, 1974; Kanfer & Grimm, 1977; Bergan, 1977; Bergan & Kratochwill,

1990). Although these guidelines differ in terms of specific areas of emphasis, all suggest gathering extensive information from clients or informants that describe the problem behavior in terms of affect, cognitions, and behavior (Morganstern). A number of these guidelines are discussed in more detail in the next section.

The second objective of the behavioral interview is to collect detailed and specific information regarding environmental variables potentially connected to the target behavior (Allen & Gross, 1994). These are factors that directly impact the child's experiences, including variables such as marital discord, divorce, parental psychopathology, and peer rejection. For example, parental depression has been consistently identified as a predictor of child behavior problems and peer rejection (Cicchetti & Toth, 1998). Findings such as these highlight the importance of environmental variables and their influence on child functioning. Furthermore, gathering information regarding the environmental contingencies will also provide a means for possible intervention. Specific questions regarding the details of the response and the situation in which it occurs will allow a thorough understanding of the associated antecedent and consequent stimuli maintaining the target behavior. Questions should address when the behavior started, in what context it occurs, and what consequences follow its occurrence: "What do you do when she does that?" "Does it only happen at school?"

Once the target behavior has been defined and environmental variables associated with the behavior have been identified, the third objective of the behavioral interview is to formulate a preliminary diagnosis. Although formal diagnosis is a multifaceted endeavor that continues throughout the assessment process, initial diagnostic impressions help steer the course of the functional analysis of the problem behavior (Boggs et al., 2003). More specifically, a preliminary diagnosis helps determine what, if any, additional assessments procedures (e.g., ability and achievement testing, structured interviews, behavioral checklists) are warranted. For example, after conducting unstructured interviews with the parents and teachers of a child who has difficulty completing classroom assignments, a clinician may decide that ability and achievement testing is warranted in order to rule out a possible learning disorder. In addition to aiding in the assessment process, diagnosis also facilitates communication between the clinician and other individuals involved in carrying out subsequent intervention strategies, allowing relevant parties to summarize complex problem behaviors with a diagnostic label (McClellan, 2000).

Based on information collected and synthesized during the first three objectives, the fourth objective of the behavioral interview is to design the most appropriate intervention (Allen & Gross, 1994). At this time, information pertaining to behavioral assets should be collected. Such data can help identify appropriate alternative behaviors to teach the child. Questions should address what new behaviors the parents would like to see and what current behaviors they like. Additionally, parents should be asked about the kinds of stimuli that are rewarding and aversive to the child. Asking "What does Joey like to do on the weekends?" and "Does he like to draw?" can prompt such information. It is also important for the clinician to consider the individual strengths and competencies of the child and how that may impact treatment efficacy. For example, if a child has strong communication skills, these abilities can be used to enhance other social skill deficits. Questions should also address current disciplinary strategies and their effectiveness in decreasing the behavior. Often parents are unwittingly reinforcing the problem, as in the case of a mother buying her child a toy to avoid the embarrassment of a tantrum. Such information can provide valuable insight into the nature of the problem as well as a mechanism for intervention.

The final major objective of the behavioral interview is to communicate basic behavioral principles to the client. This objective is accomplished throughout the interview process and may be done didactically or indirectly communicated through the use of cues, probes, and summary statements (Tombari & Bergan, 1978). Given that clients generally do not view the presenting problem as something influenced by their own behavior, it is important that clients understand how environmental factors may be maintaining the presenting problem (Sarwer & Sayers, 1998). This is especially true of parents, who often view the referral problem as something inherently wrong with the child. It is, therefore, the responsibility of the interviewer to correct these misconceptions and to educate parents on the general behavioral principles guiding the interview and subsequent interventions. An understanding of the relationship between the child's behavior and his or her environment is essential in helping parents provide the information needed. This information will then be used to connect the referral problem to malleable variables in the environment.

CONDUCTING THE INTERVIEW

SKILLS AND STRATEGIES

A primary purpose of the behavioral interview is to gather information about the presenting problem so that a behavior change strategy can be designed, implemented, and evaluated. Throughout this process, emphasis should be on obtaining valid and reliable information concerning the target behavior as well as the environmental contingencies associated with it. The collection and synthesis of this information will influence not only the direction of the interview itself, but also subsequent steps in the treatment process. Although the behavioral framework provides the structure for the interview process, a number of client–therapist relationship variables help determine a parent's continuation with the therapy process as well as compliance with treatment suggestions (Morganstern, 1988).

With this said, a common criticism of the behavioral approach is that it involves a cold, detached view of human behavior that has little regard for the therapeutic relationship (Morganstern, 1988; Goldfried & Davison, 1994). This image of behavior therapy can be attributed to (1) its use of a rather mechanistic language system when describing behavior (e.g., "antecedent," "response," "consequence") and (2) its adoption of an empirical stance when conceptualizing human functioning (Goldfried & Davison). Although these are common characteristics of the behavioral framework, the therapeutic alliance with the parent also plays a crucial role in determining effective treatment outcomes (Morganstern, 1988). More specifically, it is important that clinicians be prepared for the interview by considering not only *what* information they hope to obtain, but *how* they intend to obtain it. In this regard, there are a number of skills and strategies that should be incorporated throughout the interview process.

Rapport

The first skill necessary in conducting an interview is to establish a rapport with the parents. In doing so, it is important to create and maintain a warm and accepting environment, thus allowing the parents to feel safe and comfortable in discussing emotionally laden topics. This will help to establish a healthy working relationship with the parents and teachers. Parents often experience some uneasiness in discussing their children's problems and, to some extent, may feel responsible. For these difficulties, the clinician should provide reassurance that their child's problem is not beyond assistance and should refrain from insinuating blame or guilt (Boggs et al., 2003). Moreover, recognizing the parents' efforts and encouraging them to continue with effective strategies can serve to facilitate a collaborative relationship.

Effective Listening

In addition to establishing rapport, effective listening is important in conducting a successful interview (Sattler, 1998). To do so requires that the interviewer listen attentively and empathically to the client. Furthermore, it is important that the interviewer provide an environment free from distraction and interruption. The clinician should also be aware of the nonverbal communication of the parent. Tone of voice, body posture, facial expressions, and affect can provide useful information regarding intensity of experiences as well as prompt further questions if inconsistencies (between verbal and nonverbal communication) occur. For example, a parent may verbally report that the child's behavior at home is "fine" but present this information with a flat affect and sullen facial expression. Being aware of such inconsistencies can provide useful information into the nature of the problem.

Effective Communication

In addition to the development of listening skills, effective communication is essential for collecting information and establishing rapport. It is important that all communication be clear and precise and that clinicians refrain from technical jargon. Also important is that the interviewer communicate his/her understanding of what has been said. This can be accomplished by providing concise summary statements of shared information, which allow the parent to correct any miscommunication (Sattler, 2002). Furthermore, it is important for clinicians to be aware of their nonverbal communication. When engaging a client, the interviewer should be seated at eye level, facing the client. Warm facial expressions and eye contact communicate understanding and acceptance to the client and help in creating a trusting relationship.

COMMON INTERVIEWING FORMATS

Once the necessary skills are developed, the next step is to choose the interview format. Different techniques are available that vary along a dimension of structure or standardization. The most highly structured interviews ask a predetermined number of questions in a specific sequence (Sattler, 2002). In contrast, less structured interviews allow more latitude in terms of the question sequence or word use. The advantage in structured interviews is greater reliability, although it has been argued that this structure may restrict the flow of the interview and limit the ability to establish a rapport.

In the clinical setting, unstructured interviews with the child, parent(s), teacher(s), and others often precede more structured assessment procedures (Boggs et al., 2003). Through the unstructured interview, the clinician may gain a clear picture of what problematic behaviors are occurring and what personal or environmental variables seem to be contributing to or maintaining the behaviors. In addition, questions addressing duration, frequency, and intensity or severity of the behaviors as well as other key areas relevant to the referral question (e.g., developmental milestones, family history) can be asked. The clinician can then determine *if* and *which* one of several structured interview formats would be most appropriate. Throughout this process, a clinician may utilize a combination of unstructured and structured interview formats to assist with diagnosis and treatment planning.

Unstructured Interviews

As the name implies, the unstructured interview maintains an open format that allows clients to present their problem with minimal guidance. It is a versatile technique that allows clinicians to follow leads when and how they deem necessary. Typically, the interviewer will begin with general questions such as "What brings you here today?" and will then allow the client to discuss the problem situation. Eventually the questions will become more directed, as the clinician begins to formulate an understanding of the problem. Although their interviews were generally unstructured in nature, early behavioral theorists proposed a number of general guidelines for conducting a thorough behavioral assessment (Goldfried & Pomeranz, 1968; Kanfer & Saslow, 1969; Mischel, 1973; Goldfried & Sprafkin, 1974; Kanfer & Grimm, 1977). In general, these early models shared a common adherence to the ABC framework while varying on the emphasis placed on cognitive variables and the extent of historical data obtained.

Kanfer and Saslow (1969) describe one of the most comprehensive assessment guidelines. Their approach incorporates variables from the patient's current situation and past history, although historical data are considered relevant only if they contribute to the description of present problem responses or future interventions. According to Kanfer and Saslow's assessment schema, the following areas should be examined: (1) an analysis of the problem situation; (2) an elucidation of the factors maintaining the problem response; (3) a motivational analysis; (4) a developmental analysis; (5) an analysis of self-control; (6) an analysis of social relationships; and (7) an analysis of the sociocultural-physical environment. In addition to being extremely encompassing, Kanfer and Saslow's assessment approach represents one of the first systems that emphasized the importance of assessing the patient's behavior strengths along with the response deficits (Morganstern & Tevlin, 1981).

Mischel (1973) proposes a system of behavioral assessment that emphasizes the importance of evaluating cognitive variables when considering maladaptive behavior. In addition to environmental events, Michel suggests that cognitive social learning factors, or "person variables," play a role in shaping human behavior. From this perspective, cognitive social learning factors represent the product of an individual's social learning history and are theorized to influence the way in which environmental conditions affect human responding. Because these factors are unique to each individual, Michel asserts that it is imperative to study them if effective behavioral control is to be established. The person variables incorporated into this system include (1) cognitive and behavioral construction competence, (2) encoding strategies, (3) behavior-outcome and stimulus-outcome expectancies, (4) subjective stimulus values, and (5) self-regulatory systems and plans.

As with other interviewing techniques, the goal of these and other unstructured guidelines is to provide the clinician with a general framework for obtaining reliable data. Although sharing this common goal, these unstructured interview formats represent a less directive means of obtaining diagnostic and treatment information. With this said, the unstructured interview continues to play an intricate role in behavioral interviewing. As already noted, the unstructured interview typically precedes and determines the use of more structured assessment procedures. In addition, Sattler (2002) suggests that the unstructured interview is useful in identifying more general problem areas or when the interviewee is in crisis. For example, if a client were to present with suicidal ideation and needed an immediate risk assessment, an unstructured interview might be more useful than other techniques in determining the next course of action.

Semistructured and Structured Interviews

There is no clear delineation between semistructured interviews and structured interviews (Boggs et al., 2003; Hodges, 1993; Reich, 2000; Reitman et al., 1998; Sattler, 2002). Although both structured and semistructured interviews provide standardized procedures, they differ in the extent to which clinicians are allowed to deviate from the question order and wording as well as in their diagnostic reliability (Boggs et al., 2003). Thus, while semistructured interviews allow for deviations in protocol, structured interviews require more rigid sequencing of questions and verbatim instructions in an attempt to increase reliability. Unfortunately, there are no set criteria as to when an interview should be labeled as structured or semistructured, making the distinction somewhat difficult, even for the experienced clinician. Subsequently, there has been a great deal of inconsistency in categorizing interviews as structured or semistructured. Despite these difficulties, a brief review of semistructured and structured interviewing formats for use with parents is presented here. Although not exhaustive, an attempt was made to present a sample of psychometrically sound interviewing formats available to clinicians.

Intended for use with children ages 6–18 years, the Diagnostic Interview Schedule for Children—Fourth Edition (DISC-IV) and the DISC-P for parents (or knowledgeable caretakers) represent parallel forms of an instrument designed to assess over 30 psychological disorders (e.g., anxiety disorders, disruptive behavior disorders, mood disorders) over both the past four weeks and the past 12 months (Shaffer, Fisher, Lucas, Dulcan, & Schwab-Stone, 2000). Created by the National Institute of Mental Health (NIMH), the DISC-IV and DISC-P each contain nearly 3000 items assessing diagnostic classification corresponding with DSM-IV and the *International Classification of Diseases*, 10th edition (ICD-10; World Health Organization, 1993) criteria. However, it is unlikely that all questions will be administered, in that many are contingent on the endorsement of previous items (Shaffer et al., 2000). Questions addressing symptom duration, onset, and intensity are included as well as an introductory section covering demographic information. Its modular format allows for part or whole administration, and administration time typically ranges from 70 to 120 minutes. Test–retest reliabilities for the parent as well as for the combined parent/child have ranged from moderate to substantial across diagnostic categories. However, no formal validity data are available to date.

Appropriate for use with children age 9–17 years, the Child and Adolescent Psychiatric Assessment (CAPA; Angold et al., 1995) is a structured diagnostic interview, with versions available for use with children and their parents. Focusing on symptoms occurring during the preceding 3-month period, the CAPA provides the interviewer with a format for collecting data on the onset, duration, frequency, and intensity of symptoms in order to assign a diagnosis based on criteria from the DSM-IV (APA, 1994), the DSM-III-R (APA, 1987), and the ICD-10 (WHO, 1993). In addition to providing a diagnostic script, it includes questions regarding sociodemographic data, family structure and functioning, peer and adult relationships, and ratings of psychosocial impairment that may result from psychiatric symptomatology. Like the DISC-IV, the CAPA is modular in form and can be administered in part or in whole, at the interviewer's discretion. Thus, if an interviewer has ruled out the possibility of a mood disorder, those questions can be omitted, in the interest of time and rapport-building. Average administration time is approximately 1 hour for the parent version and an additional hour for the child report version. Although formal training is not required, the developers recommend that interviewers have at least a bachelor's degree. A unique feature of the CAPA is that it includes a glossary providing operational definitions of terminology, with the goal of minimizing subjectivity. Test–retest reliability is strong, ranging from .55 for Conduct Disorder to 1.0 for substance abuse (Angold & Costello, 1995, as cited in Angold & Costello, 2000).

The Schedule for Affective Disorders and Schizophrenia for School-Age Children (K-SADS; Puig-Antich & Chambers, 1978, as cited in Boggs et al., 2003), or "Kiddie SADS," is a semistructured interview for children ages 6–18 years, with both children and parents serving as informants. The primary purpose of the K-SADS is to generate DSM-IV diagnoses, including affective, psychotic, and behavioral disorders. Three versions are available: K-SADS-E (with an epidemiological focus), K-SADS-P IVR (with a present-state focus), and K-SADS-PL (with a present and lifetime focus). Each version has an average administration time of between 1 and 2 hours. The interview begins with an unstructured format, allowing the clinician to collect general information and establish rapport. The next section involves a *Screen Interview*, during which stem questions and probes are provided, with the aim of identifying a general problem area. Information collected in the *Screen Interview* will then determine which of five content modules (affective, psychotic, anxiety, behavioral, and substance abuse) will be subsequently administered. The K-SADS requires clinical judgment not only in determining content modules, but also in word use and item sequencing. The directions encourage administrators to tailor questions to the developmental level of the individual. Although this allows greater flexibility, it also requires a familiarity with child development and psychopathology. Because of this, administration should be limited to experienced professionals. Psychometric properties of the K-SADS have been reported to range from "acceptable" to "good" (Ambrosini, 2000).

Finally, Bergan and colleagues developed a semistructured interview system to be used within the context of behavioral consultation with parents and teachers (Bergan, 1977; Bergan & Tombari, 1975, 1976; Tombari & Bergan, 1978; Bergan & Kratochwill, 1990; Sheridan et al., 1996). Encompassing the major objectives of the behavioral interview, this model structures the interview process into four general stages: (1) Problem Identification, (2) Problem Analysis, (3) Plan Implementations, and (4) Problem Evaluation (Bergan, 1977). Procedurally, movement through the four stages of behavioral consultation is accomplished through a series of standardized behavioral interviews that correspond to the four stages of the consultative process (Sheridan et al.). During the problem identification interview (PII), the consultant and consultee define the target behavior, designate goals to be achieved through consultation, and determine the disparity between current and desired performance. Questions utilized during this interview stage include: "Which of the identified behaviors is most problematic?," "How often does the problem behavior occur?," and "What would be an easy method for you to track the problem behavior?" Following the PII, the problem analysis interview (PAI) is used to (1) identify the environmental variables that may contribute to the problem and (2) design a plan of behavior change that manipulates these variables. Occurring after baseline data have been collected, the PAI involves analyzing behavioral data and designing a plan of action. Examples of inquiries during this stage include: "Were you able to keep track of the problem?," "What typically occurred before the problem? After?," and "What are some things we could do to reach our behavior change goal?" Finally, the treatment evaluation interview (TEI) is used to analyze treatment data, evaluate the effectiveness of the treatment plan, and discuss future strategies for the maintenance of treatment gains. Sample interview questions used during the TEI include: "Were there any problems with implementing the plan?," "Should we continue to implement the plan over the next few weeks?," and "How could the plan be modified to make it more effective?" Bergan and Tombari (1975) have also developed a system for classifying the verbal behavior of both consultants and consultees during the interview process called the Consultation Analysis Record (CAR). As is discussed later, the CAR, used in conjunction with the behavioral consultative model, has contributed greatly to our understanding of the psychometric properties of behavioral interviews.

PSYCHOMETRIC CONSIDERATIONS

There is an abundance of research focusing on the psychometric properties of structured and semistructured interviews, with reliability and validity estimates accompanying most interviewing formats. The availability of psychometric data for these instruments can be attributed largely to the fact that their standardized nature makes them more amiable to traditional notions of reliability and validity. In general, this line of research indicates that structured interviews possess adequate reliability and validity, with estimates for most instruments ranging from moderate to substantial.

In contrast, there is a paucity of research focusing on the psychometric properties of unstructured behavioral interviews. This lack of research can be attributed to a number of interrelated factors. Most notable is a history of controversy regarding the application of traditional reliability and validity notions to behavioral assessment methods (Cone, 1977; Gresham, 1984; Nelson, Hay, & Hay, 1977). This debate has involved the argument that the subject matter of traditional assessment approaches (i.e., personality measures) and their associated measurement guidelines (i.e., reliability and validity) are incompatible with the subject matter of behavioral assessment (i.e., behavior that is situation and response specific; Cone, 1998). Conceptually, this contrasting view is due to the underlying assumption in behavioral assessment that observed behavior is the product of a dynamic interaction between environmental and individual factors, as opposed to the static underlying processes or hypothetical constructs often emphasized by traditional assessment approaches (Kratochwill & Shapiro, 2000).

Based on this assumption, the focus in behavioral assessment has been on determining what individual and environmental variables are responsible for inconsistencies in assessment data, rather than minimizing the error in the assessment method itself. As a result, behavioral researchers have tended not to establish the reliability of their assessment techniques with traditional psychometric criteria. In addition, many in the behavioral assessment framework failed to validate their assessment methods, due to the notion that the direct assessment of behavior is inherently valid, since the area of interest is being directly observed, removing the need for generalizing from a test score to a hypothetical construct (M. M. Linehan, 1980).

A rapprochement between behavioral assessment and psychometric concerns was reached during the 1970s when generalizability theory was proposed as a general framework for applying psychometric considerations to behavioral methods (Cone, 1977). In brief, generalizability theory represents a reinterpretation of traditional psychometric concepts that maintains that, at their core, the various forms of reliability and validity simply represent different ways in which data from one observation or measure can be generalized to other observations or measures (Gresham, 1984).[1] Based on this reinterpretation, it was argued that accuracy or correspondence between observations should be the primary method for establishing the psychometric properties of behavioral assessment strategies (Kratochwill & Shapiro, 2000).

Although behaviorists argued against the application of traditional notions of reliability to individual behavior (since behavior theory expects inconsistencies across environmental conditions), generalizability theory introduced the notion that reliability could be measured not only in terms of behavioral inconsistencies, but also as inconsistencies across observers. As noted by Gresham (1984), a major advantage of this view is that it conforms to many of the assumptions underlying behavioral assessment's theoretical framework, especially those assumptions that relate to estimating the extent to which scores obtained under one set of conditions (e.g., scorers, times, settings) correspond (i.e., are generalizable) to scores obtained under other sets of conditions. An additional value of applying generalizability theory to behavioral assessment is that its acceptance by many operating within the behavioral assessment framework helped to bolster the requirement that behavioral assessment methods be held to the same standards as more traditional assessment techniques (Gresham).

While a great deal of current research focusing on the psychometric adequacy of behavioral interviews no longer frames findings using the assumptions and/or language of generalizability theory, its application helped pave the way for the systematic evaluation of behavioral interviews. With this said, the initial rejection of traditional psychometric concerns by those operating within the behav-

[1] While a detailed review of generalizability theory and its application to behavioral assessment is beyond the scope of the current chapter, interested readers are referred to Cone (1977) and Nelson et al. (1977).

ioral framework impacted the quantity and scope of research in this area. More specifically, many of the psychometric features of behavioral assessment, such as norming, reliability, validity, and generalizability, have yet to be adequately addressed (Kratochwill & Shapiro, 2000). Given the strong emphasis on obtaining direct observations of behavior and an overall skepticism regarding the adequacy of subjective report of behavior by others, it is not surprising that the unstructured behavioral interview has received little attention when psychometric properties have been considered (Gresham, 1984). Such lack of investigation is problematic, given the frequent use and critical function of the behavioral interview in the assessment process. With this said, the few existing studies do suggest that it is both useful and feasible to study this important area of behavioral assessment (Sarwer & Sayers, 1998).

In terms of reliability, the majority of the research has focused on interobserver agreement, which measures the reliability or consistency between two or more interviewers. Based on this line of research, it appears that raters can reliably code interviewee verbalizations into the broad categories of *content*, *process*, and *control* in both analogue and actual case interviews using the CAR (Beaver & Busse, 2000). This finding has important implications for the training of psychologists involved in interviewing parents and teachers. For example, Bergan and Tombari (1975) suggest that the verbal-interaction categories described in their research be used to train psychologists to utter certain verbal statements that will facilitate effective behavioral interviews. Furthermore, reliable coding of interviews during training allows trainees to receive feedback regarding their verbal behavior and whether that behavior matches criteria specified for effective interviewing (Bergan & Tombari, 1975). Investigators have also focused on interobserver agreement in terms of problem identification and interview content (Helzer, Clayton, Pambakian, & Woodruff, 1978). This line of research suggests that interviewers can agree on the number of problem behaviors but that they may not always reach the same conclusions in terms of the specific nature of the problem. Reviewed evidence suggests that this lack of consensus may be due to differing interview content in terms of interviewer output and input. Given the growing body of evidence suggesting that training in behavioral interviewing skills can improve the integrity of behavioral interviews, it is likely that clinical training and manualization can improve the reliability of the behavioral interview (Sheridan, 1992; Kratochwill, Elliott, & Busse, 1995).

In terms of validity, an increasing body of evidence suggests that the behavioral interview generalizes to other domains of interest (Bergan & Tombari, 1975; Tombari & Bergan, 1978; Bergan & Neuman, 1980). A review of behavioral literature as well as research conducted with the CAR suggest that behavioral interviews possess content validity. It also appears that teacher verbalizations and expectations tend to converge with the underlying assumptions of the behavioral interview, providing evidence for the concurrent validity of behavioral interviews. Taken together, this line of evidence suggests that (1) behavioral interviews generalize to the larger domain of behavioral theory, and (2) the verbalizations uttered through the interview process communicate these underlying principles to the interviewee.

CASE ILLUSTRATION

To highlight the interviewing strategies presented previously in the chapter, consider the following case illustration. Allison B. is a 6-year-old Caucasian female referred by her pediatrician for possible ADHD. Allison was accompanied to the appointment by her 26-year-old single mother, Ms. B. Allison currently lives with her mother and her younger sister, Casey. Her parents divorced two years ago, and since then Allison has had no contact with her father.

During the initial stages of the interview, the clinician attempts to obtain a general description of the problematic behaviors and to formulate a diagnostic impression. Because a referral was made for ADHD, it is important to assess symptoms relevant to this diagnosis while at the same time not eliminating other possibilities. The following example is an excerpt from an unstructured interview with Ms. B.

Clinician: Ms. B., tell me what brings you here today.

Ms. B: Well, Dr. Smith thought I should get Allison checked for ADHD.

Clinician: Can you explain what has been going on?

Ms. B.: Allison will not mind me. I will tell her to do something and she simply will not do it. She always runs off from me when we are out together and when I tell her to come back, she just ignores me. It is embarrassing and I am worried that she will get lost or hurt.

Clinician: Do these behaviors occur at school as well?

Ms. B.: No—nothing has been brought to my attention.

Clinician: Does she do what the teacher asks of her?

Ms. B.: Yes. Her teachers rarely report having problems with Allison at school. She has a lot of friends and seems to be doing fine. It is only at home that I am seeing the problem.

Clinician: How is she with other adults? grandparents? babysitters?

Ms. B.: She does fine with her grandparents. She will often visit them for the weekend. They never have a problem with Allison or Casey.

Clinician: Have you observed Allison with other adults?

Ms. B.: Yes. I have seen her with her grandparents and her teacher. When they ask her to do something, she will do it without fussing. I guess it is just me (*Ms. B. becomes tearful*).

Clinician: It can be difficult having young children, especially when they are "willful." You are obviously a very dedicated parent to bring her here today.

Ms. B.: Thank you. I try. I love my daughters very much.

Clinician: Does Allison have a hard time attending to lessons at school or certain tasks at home?

Ms. B.: No. She loves to read books and always does well in school. Her teacher says that Allison always participates during lesson time and finishes all her work.

Clinician: Is she fidgety or does she move around excessively?

Ms. B.: I don't think so. I teach at Allison's school so I am exposed to a lot of children her age and I don't see Allison as more active than other children.

Clinician: Have her teachers mentioned anything to you about fidgety behavior?

Ms. B.: No.

Based on the present information, it does not appear that Allison has ADHD. To be diagnosed with this disorder requires the presence of six or more predefined behaviors (e.g., excessive talking, fidgetiness, excessive movement, disorganization, easily distracted) that fall in one of two categories: inattention or hyperactivity (American Psychiatric Association, 2000). Although more specific questions should be asked, Allison does not appear to meet the behavioral criteria. Moreover, the diagnosis requires that symptoms interfere with functioning across two or more settings. Based on Ms. B.'s report, Allison's problematic behavior occurs only at home. However, permission to speak with the teacher may provide additional information pertaining to the nature of the problem.

At this stage in the interview, having ruled out the ADHD diagnosis, it is important to collect more detailed information pertaining to the problem behavior and the environmental contingencies maintaining it.

Clinician: Can you tell me what you mean when you say that Allison does not mind you?

Ms. B.: Well, like last night—I told her to clean her room before we went to the store, and she refused.

Clinician: How did you respond to that?

Ms. B.: Well, it was getting so late that I just said that I would help her. I really needed to go to the grocery store for supper and couldn't wait all night for her to clean her room.

Clinician: Did Allison help you clean the room?

Ms. B.: No. Actually I am embarrassed to say that I ended up cleaning it by myself.

Clinician: Is this usually what happens when Allison disobeys?

Ms. B.: Well, I have tried everything and nothing works. I tried offering a dessert if she obeys, spanking her, and time out. Nothing works!

The interviewer is now collecting information relevant to the environmental contingencies maintaining the noncompliant behavior. More questions about the specific context and associated antecedents and consequences should be asked to provide a more thorough understanding of the problem. Additional questions regarding the intensity, frequency, and duration of the behavior are also necessary.

Clinician: You mentioned that Allison will frequently run off and leave you. Where does this occur?

Ms. B.: It usually happens when she is excited about going somewhere. Like when she is getting out of the car to go to a birthday party or even when crossing the street to get to school.

From the given information, the clinician has now identified the associated antecedent of the "running off" behavior. This information will be useful in designing treatment strategies. Other information that can be helpful for future interventions include Allison's behavioral attributes, things she enjoys doing, and favorite books and toys.

Clinician: What is Allison's favorite treat?

Ms. B.: She really likes to collect stickers. Her teachers give her stickers at school and she loves them. She also loves candy and cokes. But I try not to give her too many sweets.

Learning what activities and objects that Allison finds rewarding will assist the clinician in designing a successful treatment strategy. For example, stickers can be offered to Allison as a reward for walking with mom from the car to the school without running off.

Although unstructured interviews provide an opportunity to build rapport and speak freely with the client, structured clinical interviews can be useful in providing more organization in the interviewing process. In this example, the clinician used the Schedule for Affective Disorders and Schizophrenia for School-Age Children, Present Lifetime Version (K-SADS-PL; Kaufman, Birmaher, Brent, Rao, & Ryan, 1996). Because the referral question was to address possible ADHD, here is an excerpt from the ADHD module of the interview. In accordance to administration instructions, questions are only slightly modified to match the child's developmental level.

Clinician: Allison, do you get in trouble at school for talking too much in class?

Allison: No. I never get in trouble at school. I listen during math and reading.

Clinician: Do people tell you to be still often?

Allison: No. But my mom tells me to come back when I walk away from her.

Clinician: Do you have trouble staying still?

Allison: Sometimes. But usually I am ok. Except for when I have to go to the bathroom.

As can be seen, structured interviews provide a rigid format, while the unstructured interviews allow more time to establish rapport and follow the direction of the client. Some clinicians prefer to use an unstructured interview with young children to create a less intimidating atmosphere. However, there is no correct way to conduct the interview, and each strategy has its own associated advantages and disadvantages.

Speaking with other informants, such as the grandparents or teachers, can provide information about behavior across different environments. In this example, the teacher was contacted to assess Allison's behavior in the classroom setting. The unstructured interview with the teacher was quite similar to that with Ms. B., but it was adapted to fit the academic environment. Because the referral was made for ADHD, the clinician first assesses behaviors consistent with this diagnosis.

Clinician: How is Allison's behavior in the classroom?
Teacher: She is doing well and making good grades.
Clinician: Does she have a hard time paying attention to class lessons?
Teacher: No. Actually Allison is one of my best students. She asks good questions and always gets her work done on time.
Clinician: Does she have trouble remaining seated?
Teacher: No, not at all.
Clinician: Is she fidgety?
Teacher: No.

Although more specific questions should be asked for a full assessment, Allison does not appear to meet diagnostic criteria for ADHD according to teacher report. The clinician next decides to determine whether the noncompliant behavior occurs at school as well as at home.

Clinician: Does she follow through with instructions?
Teacher: Now she does. But when the school year started I was having some trouble with her. It's not that she didn't understand what I was asking of her, she just simply would refuse if it was something she didn't want to do. However, once she learned that behavior was unacceptable in my classroom, there has been no trouble.
Clinician: What did you do when she would disobey?
Teacher: If a student of mine does not mind, he or she will be punished. No exceptions.
Clinician: What form of punishment has Allison responded to?
Teacher: She really hates missing recess. Once she started missing recess time, she quickly began minding my instructions.

Allison's teacher has provided important information about the environmental contingencies maintaining the noncompliant behavior. It is apparent that Allison has learned to discriminate when there will be consequences for her noncompliant behavior. At school, consistent consequences are implemented for every occurrence of noncompliant behavior. As a result, Allison obeys her teacher. Conversely, there are no consequences for noncompliant behavior at home. Thus, she disobeys her mother.

The information provided by Ms. B. and the teacher served to lay the foundation for subsequent treatment strategies in this case. A contingency management program was implemented in the home, and Ms. B. was taught to issue simple and clear requests, to use appropriate punishment for every occurrence of noncompliant behavior, and to reinforce compliant behavior. Following 15 sessions of therapy, the frequency of noncompliant behavior diminished to near-zero levels.

SUMMARY

This chapter presented a broad overview of behavioral interviewing of parents, including a review of major goals and objectives of the behavioral interview, a presentation of common interviewing formats, and a discussion regarding the psychometric adequacy of the behavioral interview. Throughout, the chapter presented the crucial aspects and assumptions of the behavioral interview while emphasizing the underlying learning principles that frame the interview process. Given the ubiquity of the interview in behavioral assessment, an understanding of these assumptions, principles, and formats is considered crucial to the assessment and treatment of childhood behavior problems.

REFERENCES AND RESOURCES

Allen, J. B., & Gross, A. M. (1994). Children. In M. Hersen & S. M. Turner (Eds.), *Diagnostic interviewing* (2nd ed., pp. 305–326). New York: Plenum Press.

Ambrosini, P. J. (2000). Historical development and present status of the Schedule for Affective Disorders and Schizophrenia for school-age children (K-SADS). *Journal of the American Academy of Child and Adolescent Psychiatry, 39*(1), 49–58.

Angold, A., & Costello, E. J. (2000). The Child and Adolescent Psychiatric Assessment (CAPA). *Journal of the American Academy of Child and Adolescent Psychiatry, 39*(1), 39–48.

Angold, A., Prendergast, M., Cox, A., Harrington, R., Simonoff, E., & Rutter, M. (1995). The child and adolescent psychiatric assessment. *Psychological Medicine, 25,* 739–753.

American Psychiatric Association. (1987). *Diagnostic and statistical manual of mental disorders* (3rd ed.). Washington, DC: Author.

American Psychiatric Association. (1994). *Diagnostic and statistical manual of mental disorders* (4th ed.). Washington, DC: Author.

American Psychiatric Association. (2000). *Diagnostic and statistical manual of mental disorders* (4th ed., text revision). Washington, DC: Author.

Beaver, B. R., & Busse, R. T. (2000). Conceptual and research bases of interviews with parents and teachers. In E. S. Shapiro & M. T. R. Kratochwill (Eds.), *Behavioral assessment in schools: Theory, research, and clinical foundations* (2nd ed., pp. 257–286). New York: Guilford Press.

Bergan, J. R. (1977). *Behavioral consultation.* Columbus, OH: Merrill.

Bergan, J. R., & Kratochwill, T. R. (1990). *Behavioral consultation and therapy.* New York: Plenum Press.

Bergan, J. R., & Neumann, A. J. (1980). The identification of resources and constraint influencing plan design in consultation. *Journal of School Psychology, 17,* 307–316.

Bergan, J. R., & Tombari, M. L. (1975). The analysis of verbal interactions occurring during consultation. *Journal of School Psychology, 13,* 209–226.

Bergan, J. R., & Tombari, M. L. (1976). Consultant skill and efficiency and the implementation and outcomes in consultation. *Journal of School Psychology, 14,* 3–13.

Boggs, K. M., Griffin, R. S., & Gross, A. M. (2003). Diagnostic interviewing of children. In M. Hersen and S. Turner (Eds.), *Diagnostic interviewing.* (3rd ed., pp. 393–413) New York: Kluwer/Plenum Press.

Cicchetti, D., & Toth, S. L. (1998). The development of depression in children and adolescents. *American Psychologist,* 221–241.

Ciminero, A. R., & Drabman, R. S. (1977). Current developments in the behavior assessment of children. In B. B. Lahey & A. E. Kazden (Eds.), *Advances in clinical child psychology (Vol. 1).* New York: Plenum Press.

Cone, J. D. (1977). The relevance of reliability and validity for behavioral assessment. *Behavior Therapy, 8,* 411–426.

Cone, J. D. (1998). Psychometric considerations: Concepts, content, and methods. In A. S. Bellack & M. Hersen (Eds.), *Behavioral assessment: A practical handbook* (4th ed., pp. 22–46). Needham Heights, MA: Allyn & Bacon.

Faul, L. A., & Gross, A. M. (in press). Diagnoses and classification. In M. Hersen & J. C. Thomas (Eds.), *Comprehensive handbook of personality and psychopathology.* New York: John Wiley & Sons.

Goldfried, M. R., & Davison, G. C. (1994). *Clinical behavior therapy.* New York: John Wiley & Sons.

Goldfried, M. R., & Pomeranz, D. (1968). Role of assessment in behavior modification. *Psychological Reports, 23,* 75–87.

Goldfried, M. R., & Sprafkin, J. N. (1974). *Behavioral personality assessment.* Morristown, NJ: General Learning Press.

Gresham, F. M. (1984). Behavioral interviews in school psychology: Issues in psychometric adequacy and research. *School Psychology Review, 13*(1), 17–25.

Gresham, F. M., & Davis, C. J. (1988). Behavioral interviews with teachers and parents. In E. S. Shapiro & T. R. Kratochwill (Eds.), *Behavioral assessment in schools: Conceptual foundations and practical application* (pp. 455–493). New York: Guilford Press.

Hayes, S. C., & Follette, W. C. (1992). Can functional analysis provide a substitute for syndromal classification? *Behavioral Assessment, 14,* 345–355.

Helzer, J. E., Clayton, P. J., Pambakian, R., & Woodruff, R. A. (1978). Concurrent diagnostic validity of structured psychiatric interview. *Archives of General Psychiatry, 35,* 849–853.

Hodges, K. (1993). Structured interviews for assessing children. *Journal of Child Psychology and Psychiatry, 34,* 49–64.

Kanfer, F. H., & Grimm, L. G. (1977). Behavior analysis: Selecting target behaviors in the interview. *Behavior Modification, 1,* 7–28.

Kanfer, F. H., & Saslow, G. (1969). Behavioral diagnosis. In C. M. Franks (Ed.), *Behavior therapy: Appraisal and status.* New York: McGraw-Hill.

Kaufman, J., Birmaher, B., Brent, D., Rao, U., & Ryan, N. (1996). Kiddie-SADS-Present and Lifetime Version (K-SADS-PL). Retrieved April 3, 2004 from http://www.wpic.pitt.edu/ksads.

Kratochwill, T. R., Elliott, S. N., & Busse, R. T. (1995). Behavior consultation: A five-year evaluation of consultant and client outcomes. *School Psychology Quarterly, 10,* 87–117.

Kratochwill, T. R., & Shapiro, E. S. (2000). Conceptual foundations of behavioral assessment in schools. In E. S. Shapiro & T. R. Kratochwill (Eds.), *Behavioral assessment in schools: Theory, research, and clinical foundations* (2nd ed., pp. 3–15). New York: Guilford Press.

Linehan, A. A. (1977). Issues in behavioral interviewing. In J. D. Cone & R. P. Hawkins (Eds.), *Behavioral assessment: New directions in clinical psychology.* New York: Brunner/Mazel.

Linehan, M. M. (1980). Content validity: Its relevance to behavioral assessment. *Behavioral Assessment, 2,* 147–159.

McClellan, J. M. (2000). Special section: Research psychiatric diagnostic interviews for children and adolescents. *Journal of the American Academy of Child and Adolescent Psychiatry, 39*(1), 19–27.

Mischel, W. (1973). Toward a cognitive social learning reconceptualization of personality. *Psychological Review, 80,* 252–283.

Morganstern, K. P. (1988). Behavioral interviewing. In A. S. Bellack & M. Hersen (Eds.), *Behavioral assessment: A practical handbook* (4th ed., pp. 86–117). Needham Heights, MA: Allyn & Bacon.

Morganstern, K. P., & Tevlin, H. E. (1981). Behavioral interviewing. In M. Hersen & A. S. Bellack (Eds.), *Behavioral assessment: A practical handbook* (pp. 86–118). New York: Pergamon Press.

Morrison, J., & Anders, T. E. (1999). *Interviewing children and adolescents: Skills and strategies for effective DSM-IV diagnosis.* New York: Guilford Press.

Nelson, R. O., Hay, L. R., & Hay, W. L. (1977). Comments on Cone's "The relevance of reliability and validity for behavioral assessment." *Behavior Therapy, 8,* 427–430.

O'Leary, K. D., & Wilson, G. T. (1975). *Behavior therapy: Application and outcome.* Englewood Cliffs, NJ: Prentice Hall.

Reich, W. (2000). Diagnostic Interview for Children and Adolescents (DICA). *Journal of American Academy of Child and Adolescent Psychiatry, 39,* 59–66.

Reitman, D., Hummel, R., Franz, D. Z., & Gross, A. M. (1998). A review of methods and instruments for assessing externalizing disorders: Theoretical and practical considerations in rendering a diagnosis. *Clinical Psychology Review, 18,* 555–584.

Sarwer, D. B., & Sayers, S. L. (1998). Behavioral interviewing. In A. S. Bellack & M. Hersen (Eds.), *Behavioral assessment: A practical handbook* (4th ed., pp. 22–46). Needham Heights, MA: Allyn & Bacon.

Sattler, J. M. (1998). *Clinical and forensic interviewing of children and families.* San Diego, CA: Sattler.

Sattler, J. M. (2002). *Assessment of children: Behavioral and clinical applications* (4th ed.). San Diego, CA: Sattler.

Shaffer, D., Fisher, P., Lucas, C. P., Dulcan, M. K., & Schwab-Stone, M. E. (2000). NIMH Diagnostic Interview Schedule for Children Version IV (NIMH DISC-IV): Description, differences from previous versions, and reliability of some common diagnoses. *Journal of the American Academy of Child and Adolescent Psychiatry, 39*(1), 28–38.

Sheridan, S. M. (1992). Consulting and clients outcomes of competency-based behavioral consultation training. *School Psychology Quarterly, 30,* 117–139.

Sheridan, S. M., Krotochwill, T. R., & Bergan, J. R. (1996). *Conjoint behavioral interviewing: A procedural manual.* New York: Plenum Press.

Shriver, M. D., Anderson, C. M., & Proctor, B. (2001). Evaluating the validity of functional behavior assessment. *School Psychology Review, 30*(2), 180–192.

Tombari, M. L., & Bergan, J. R. (1978). Consultant cues and teacher verbalizations, judgments, and expectancies concerning children's adjustment problems. *Journal of School Psychology, 16,* 212–219.

World Health Organization. (1993). The ICD-10 classification of mental and behavioural disorders: Diagnostic criteria for research. Geneva, Switzerland: Author.

6

ACTIVITY MEASUREMENT

MARK D. RAPPORT
MICHAEL J. KOFLER
CARMEN HIMMERICH

Department of Psychology
University of Central Florida
Orlando, Florida

INTRODUCTION

Activity level is the first enduring trait or personality characteristic to develop in humans. Individual differences are apparent by the 28th week of gestation, and developmental trajectory studies suggest that activity level follows a curvilinear relationship between infancy and late adulthood. Its relationship with children's behavioral characteristics is intriguing. Heightened activity level following the neonatal period is associated with desirable behavioral attributes such as positive social interactions, motor and mental maturity, and inquisitiveness. This association rapidly reverses during preschool and early elementary school years. Pejorative characteristics such as aggression, distractibility, academic underachievement, learning disabilities, and strained peer and parent–child relationships are assigned to children exhibiting heightened activity after 5 years of age. These difficulties continue into middle childhood for many children, and they set the stage for a lifetime of disabilities, despite the diminution in activity level typically observed during adolescence.

Studies of activity level in children traditionally focus on understanding four interrelated areas: (a) the relative contribution of genetic, biological, and socialization developmental factors relevant to activity level; (b) the effects of activity level on physical growth and motor skill development; (c) age and gender trends in activity level across settings and situations; and (d) the role of activity level in understanding temperament or enduring personality differences. Collectively, this literature provides a strong foundation for understanding the origin, development, and expression of activity level in children (for a review, see Eaton, 1994). The next chapter section addresses the normal development and heritability of activity level in children as a reference for understanding abnormal activity—particularly age and gender effects.

Measurement of activity level in children is interesting in its own right, and it poses unique challenges to activity level research. It runs the gamut from subjective questionnaires to highly sophisticated and reliable actigraphs costing thousands of dollars. Sophistication and reliability alone, however, may be insufficient if our purpose is to understand the conditions under which activity level differs among children and how best to assess these differences. Consider the actigraph and its highly detailed output. Millisecond changes in activity level may be collected for several weeks at a time and downloaded to a computer to scrutinize differences between children with and without a particular clinical disorder. We determine that one group of children moves more frequently than another during the day. An interesting finding in its own right, but less than satisfactory if we wish to understand the underlying dynamics that contribute to the between-group differences. Combining the actigraph information with a daily activity log reveals that the first group of children is more active than the second group only when engaged in tasks or activities that require them to sit down and work on academic tasks. Our understanding of group differences gains further momentum as we add more information to the raw actigraph data, such as a videotape of the children's movements throughout the day. Video footage is analyzed using a computer scoring system. The analysis confirms between-group differences during academic assignment periods and reveals that activity level in the more active group of children constitutes two functionally distinct types of movement—one that appears to help them maintain alertness to the assignment, and the other, a form of escape behavior that removes them from the task. Our understanding of the phenomenon has increased exponentially from a simple statement of higher motor movement frequency in one group of children relative to another, to an inchoate appreciation of the dynamic interplay among activity level, cognitive function, and behavior. Other researchers may wish to explore the findings from a physiological perspective or use controlled laboratory investigations. The first group seeks to explain possible underlying differences in anatomical structure or processes serving these structures, whereas the second group is interested in determining whether particular cognitive variables or processes contribute to differences in activity level. The move from simple to complex and complementary measures of activity level in children is explored in the subsequent chapter section, which highlights the critical role assessment plays in scientific discovery.

EARLY DEVELOPMENT AND GENDER

A normative-developmental framework is adopted for examining activity level in developing children. This approach lays the groundwork for determining what is atypical and potentially pathological at other stages of development. For example, some instances of activity level may represent normal quantitative variations evident at other developmental periods or in less intense degree or form in same-age children. Other instances may represent qualitative variations that are not normal for any developmental period.

ACTIVITY LEVEL IN INFANCY

Differences in human activity level are evident by the 28th week of gestation and predict several aspects of infant behavior. For example, fetal movement recorded during the last three months of pregnancy is significantly correlated with infants' motor, language, and personal-social skills at 12 weeks of age (Walters, 1965). Children with higher activity levels in utero evidence more advanced motor development at 8–12 weeks, including lifting their head for a prolonged period of time when lying on their stomach, recognizing familiar voices, using variations of cry tones to signify different needs, and smiling responsively to their parents. The cephalocaudal developmental sequence of activity level—beginning with the head and proceeding to the arms and finally to the legs—suggests a strong genetic influence.

Increases in activity level following the neonatal period are readily noticeable in infants and include rhythmical stereotypic movements involving the extremities, such as repetitive hand movements and leg kicks. Desirable behavioral characteristics begin to develop at this stage. Infants become interested in social interactions, recognize pleasant objects such as a bottle, and react with excitement and increased activity to a wide range of environmental stimuli. The corresponding development of locomotor behavior is easily observed in maturing infants. Movement becomes increasingly more coordinated, purposeful, and functional during the first 18 months of life. These rapid changes are evident in the progression of developmental milestones, such as lifting the head (approximately 2–3 months of age), rolling over (4–6 months), sitting unassisted and crawling (7–9 months), standing (10–12 months), and eventually walking unassisted (12–18 months). The sequence of these milestones is typically the same in children, with occasional variations. Activity level peaks at approximately 8 years of age (based on a review of 12 studies involving 840 children between 1 and 24.6 years of age), and these findings are relatively consistent across different cultures (Eaton, McKeen, & Campbell, 2001).

ACTIVITY LEVEL AND HERITABILITY

Heritability plays an important role in determining activity level. Twin studies reveal that a significant degree of infant activity is genetically determined. Monozygotic (identical) twins are significantly more similar in activity level than dizygotic (fraternal) twins at 30 weeks, based on actometer and parent ratings (Saudino & Eaton, 1991). This finding has been confirmed by every published twin study of activity level to date, but it is weakened somewhat because twin study methodology cannot completely control for or rule out third-factor influences. Selective breeding experiments, however, are designed to directly address the degree to which activity level is inheritable. A compelling example is derived from a study involving 30 generations of selective breeding (DeFries, Gervais, & Thomas, 1978). Ten random litters were randomly chosen from 40 possible litters of mice, and the most active and inactive females were selected to become progenitors of a high- and low-activity breeding line. Replicate (high- and low-activity) and control lines were also established. High-active, low-active, and control (intermediate activity) mice were subsequently mated at random within their respective line (e.g., high active with high active, low active with low active) to produce first-generation offspring. The most active male and female were selected from each subsequent litter in the high-active line, and these same procedures were followed for the low-active and control lines for 30 generations of selective breeding. The authors report a tenfold difference in activity level in open field activity between the two highly inbred stains (high and low active), with the control group falling intermediate between the two groups. High-active mice became significantly more active, low-active mice became less active, and intermediate-active mice remained about the same after 30 generations of breeding. These results provide compelling evidence that activity level is significantly influenced by genetic factors.

ACTIVITY LEVEL IN EARLY CHILDHOOD

Motor behavior continues to show an upward trajectory in toddlers and early preschoolers, but the changes are less pronounced and slower relative to those observed during infancy. Development of gross and fine motor behavior dominates this period as children explore and interact with their environment and acquire myriad skills, ranging from using scissors and crayons to riding a tricycle. Environmental and particularly setting effects may significantly influence children's activity level during this time. Some children attend nursery schools and day-care facilities, whereas others have limited access to playgroups and other children. The stability of children's activity level over this time period is remarkable, despite differences in context and environment. For example, the test–retest correlation for a sample of 129 boys and girls assessed at age 3 and again at age 4 was .44 and .43, respectively. This finding indicates strong continuity in children's activity level at a time when development is proceeding rapidly.

The relationship between age and activity level again changes rapidly in late preschool and elementary school (age 5–10), but for the first time it shows a *decline*, due in part to setting effects and societal demands. Children are expected to sit and engage in academic tasks and other cognitive activities for increasingly longer periods of time. Those able to do so are praised for their concentration abilities and tenacity, with accompanying high grades and test scores. Pejorative characteristics are conferred on those less able to regulate their activity level after entering elementary school—they are described as distractible, aggressive, restless, hyperactive, and impulsive. A significant majority of these children develop serious learning problems, make marginal or failing grades, exhibit a wide range of externalizing behavior problems, and experience impaired social relationships.

ACTIVITY LEVEL AND GENDER

Anecdotal evidence has proliferated for years concerning gender differences in activity level, viz., that boys are more active than girls. The topic has undergone considerable empirical scrutiny by investigative teams throughout the world and was recently summarized in a meta-analytic review (Campbell & Eaton, 1999). Results of 46 studies comparing boys' and girls' activity level revealed that male infants are more active than female infants when measured by parent ratings, direct observations, and actometers. Gender differences in activity level become more noticeable during toddlerhood and early preschool, with boys being more active than girls regardless of whether they play with male or female friends (Tryon, 1991). The higher activity level is readily visible through the physical vigor and roughness in boys' play and may contribute to the preference of young children to play with same-gender children. These differences continue through senior high school, with boys engaging daily in vigorous activity for significantly longer periods of time relative to girls. Overall activity level, however, declines exponentially with increasing age and grade—males and females show a decline in total activity level of 69% and 36%, respectively, during school days from childhood through adolescence (Gavarry, Giacomoni, Bernard, Seymat, & Falgairette, 2003).

TECHNIQUES AND MEASUREMENT OF ACTIVITY LEVEL IN CHILDREN

Myriad approaches and techniques are available for measuring activity level in children. Some are developed specifically for clinical settings, others are better suited for educational settings, and some can be used across settings. The type of information and precision required by the clinician or investigator dictates the selection of measures. For example, several rating scales provide teacher, parent, or clinician judgments concerning a child's overall activity level in a particular setting. These same scales may be useful for monitoring changes in activity level associated with behavioral or pharmacological treatment. Their greatest attribute—cost effectiveness—is also their most significant shortcoming. Rating scales are subject to numerous influences, and at best reflect judgments about, rather than being actual measures of, activity level. Moreover, surprisingly few child rating scales have established convergent validity with objective measures such as actigraphs. Conversely, actigraphs provide highly accurate information concerning activity level and can document even minor movement differences between different body parts 24 hours a day for several weeks. Software scoring programs facilitate data analysis and interpretation. The actigraph's greatest attribute—precision of measurement—is also its most significant shortcoming. Moment-to-moment changes in activity level provide no context for understanding the functional nature of children's behavior, and most commercially available systems are prohibitively expensive. Child activity level measures and techniques reviewed next highlight these issues, and an evidence-based approach for practice is recommended.

SUBJECTIVE MEASURES OF ACTIVITY LEVEL: PARENT, TEACHER, AND CLINICIAN RATING SCALES

Practice

Rating scales are the most commonly used measures of children's activity level. Some are subscales of broadband rating instruments (e.g., the Nervous-Overactive subscale of the Teacher Report Form), whereas others are stand-alone measures of children's activity level (e.g., Werry–Weiss–Peters Activity Rating Scale) or contain the DSM-IV (American Psychiatric Association, 1994) hyperactivity items in rating scale format. Commonly used scales for measuring children's activity level are shown in Table 6.1, coupled with their psychometric properties and other characteristics.

Clinicians use activity rating scales primarily for diagnosis and treatment monitoring. The considerable weight assigned rating scale scores for determining a child's diagnostic standing is associated with several factors: (a) the unrealistic time parameters permitted by health maintenance organizations (HMOs) for assessment purposes; (b) a need to obtain information from multiple informants to assess the breadth, severity, and situational or pervasive nature of problems relative to established norms; (c) the limited insight of children concerning their behavioral and emotional problems; (d) their cost effectiveness; and (e) recognition that a child's activity level in an assessment setting fails to augur their activity level in naturalistic settings. A past study illustrates this latter point—approximately 80% percent of children meeting ADHD diagnostic criteria were misdiagnosed by their primary pediatrician because they failed to exhibit a higher-than-normal level of motor activity during the office examination. At 3-year follow-up, these children were no different from obviously hyperactive children with respect to their continuing behavior problems, poor grades, and medication status (Sleator & Ullmann, 1981).

Using activity rating scales for diagnostic purposes requires age and gender norms. Published normative data are available for some rating scales. Others, however, fail to include sex and age norms, which limit their usefulness (see Table 6.1). Most scales can be completed quickly and reflect observer judgments over time periods ranging from days to months. Test–retest reliability varies considerably and reflects scale integrity, situational variability, and the assessment time interval. Most scales demonstrate adequate short-term test–retest reliability, although there is substantial variability between the subscales of some forms. For example, the 2-week CBCL-TRF retest reliabilities range from .60 for the Withdrawn/Depressed subscale to .96 for the Total Problems measure and .93 for the Hyperactivity-Impulsivity scale. High test–retest reliability increases the likelihood that differences found during frequent administration (e.g., when monitoring changes during treatment) are due to clinical factors and not measurement error.

Internal consistency, a measure of the extent to which items on a scale measure the same underlying construct, range from an alpha of .58 to .99 for these scales. The former value may be too low, whereas the latter is also problematic, because it suggests redundancy within the item pool. Support for the validity of most available scales comes from comparisons with existing scales or demonstrations of the scale's ability to differentiate between clinical and nonclinical samples (e.g., significant group differences between ADHD and non-ADHD children). The only scales correlated significantly with objective measures are the WWPARS (with actometer ratings) and the CRS-R (with the computerized Continuous Performance Test of vigilance/sustained attention).

Age and gender norms are available for several of the rating scales. Some scales, such as the CRS-R series, provide norms for multiple age groups within their reported age range (e.g., the CRS-R provides separate norms for each gender at ages 3–5, 6–8, 9–11, 12–14, and 15–17). Others dichotomize children into larger age groupings (e.g., ages 6–11 and 12–18 for the CBCL) or provide only overall norms (e.g., WWPARS). Due to rapid changes in children's activity level, a scale that provides incremental norms is recommended for children between the ages of 5 and 10. Although some scales report the time interval rated (e.g., the CBCL asks informants to consider the child's behavior during the last 6 months), many fail to specify a rating period, an important limitation when interpreting available norms. The cost of rating scales is as variable as their psychometric properties, with starter kits ranging from $98 (CSI-4) to $425 (CRS-R) for broadband scales, and $42 (ADHD-IV) to $206 (ADDES-2) for narrow-band DSM-IV scales. The cost of reordering forms ranges from free (ADHD-IV) to more than $2 per form (RBPC). As revealed in Table 6.1, psychometric properties are not necessarily correlated with cost. Most scales can be administered quickly (range: 2–20 minutes), and some have software available for quick scoring.

Activity rating scale scores complement conventional diagnostic practice. They provide an important but limited piece of information that is juxtaposed with extensive history taking, record review, parent and child semistructured clinical interview, psychoeducational assessment results, and broad- and narrow-band scale scores. This information is coupled with details concerning the onset, course, and duration of presenting problems and serves as the basis for case conceptualization.

TABLE 6.1 Broadband, Stand-alone, and DSM-IV-Oriented Rating Scales Used to Measure Activity Level in Children

Scale		Psychometric Properties											
		No. of Items	Item Type	Completion Time (min)	Test–Retest	Internal Consistency (alpha)	Convergent/ Divergent	Validity Evidence: Criterion	Validity Evidence: ROM	Norms: Age	Norms: Sex	Rating Period	Publisher/Cost
BROADBAND SCALES													
BASC Reynolds & Kamphaus, 1992 Hyperactivity Scale Note: BASC-2 available soon	P T	126–138	0–3 freq.	10–20	.85–.95	mid. –70s .80s–.90s	CBCL (.71–.84) CPRS Hyperactivity scale = .56	BGD: With and without CD, behavior disorder, Depression, emotional disturbance, ADHD, LD, Mild MR, and Autism	*NR*	4–18	Y	*NR*	American Guidance Services, Inc. Complete kit: $330/$450 (with or without software; manual, 25 of each form type, 25 DO forms) Forms: 25 @ $39
CBCL Achenbach & Rescorla, 2001 Nervous-Overactive scale Rater: Parent		118	0–2 freq.	15–20	(1 wk) .80–.94 (3 mo) M = .84	.63–.97	93 items identical between CBCL & TRF See manual for detailed validity information	Discriminant analysis (referred v. nonreferred: 80– 88% correctly identified BGD: ADHD v. non-ADHD, LD	NS correlation with actometer (Aronen et al., 2002)	2–18	Y	Past 6 mo.	ASEBA Complete computer scoring kit: $325 (manual, software, 50 CBCL, TRF, & YSR forms) Forms: 50 @ $25 (any type)
CBCL-TRF Achenbach & Rescorla, 2001		118	0–2 freq.	15–20	(2 wk) .60–.96	.72–.95	Factor scores "correlate well" with equiv. CTRS scales	Discriminant analysis (referred v. nonreferred	*NR*	5–18	Y	Past 2 mo.	see CBCL

Nervous-Overactive scale Rater: Teacher						(2 mo) .63–.88		Significant correlation between scores and DO	74–80% correctly identified BGD: ADHD v. non-ADHD, LD					
CBRF-A Van Egeren, Frank, & Paul, 1999 Overactivity (OA) Scale Inpatient only			65	0–3 sev.	*NR*	(2 wk) .63–.76 (3 wk) .38 (OA)	*NR*	Overactivity scale with: CBCL: .23–.28 (Externalizing, Aggressive Behavior) –.21 (Internalizing)	Overactivity scale did not predict length of hospital stay	*NR*	3–17	N	8-hour shift	Author Cost: *NR*
CBRSC Neeper, Lahey, & Frick, 1990 Motor Hyperactivity scale (4 items) Rater: Teacher			70	0–5 freq.	10–15	Published norms based on earlier 81-item of test—*NR* for available scale					6–14	Y	*NR*	Harcourt Assessment, Inc. Complete kit: $133 (contents unspecified) Forms: $29 (number unspecified)
CRS-R Conners, 1997	Long	P	80	0–3 freq.	15–20	(6–8 wk) . .47–.85	.73–.94	Long: Short: .95–1.00 P:T: .12–.55 CDI:	BGD: ADHD v. non-ADHD, *emotional problems*	CPT: $r =$ .33–.44	3–17	Y	Last month	Multi-Health systems, Inc. Complete kit: $425 (manual, 25 of each form type, etc.)

(*continues*)

TABLE 6.1 (*continued*)

Scale		No. of Items	Item Type	Completion Time (min)	Test–Retest	Internal Consistency (alpha)	Convergent/ Divergent	Validity Evidence: Criterion	Validity Evidence: ROM	Norms: Age	Norms: Sex	Rating Period	Publisher/Cost
							Psychometric Properties						
Hyperactivity Scale		T 59			.47–.88	.77–.96							
Rater: Parent, Teacher		P 28					.40–.82 (teacher)						Forms: 25 @ $26 (any version)
Self-report and							.36–.79 (parent)						
ADHD DSM-IV	Short			5–10	.89–.96	.86–.94							
Scales also available		T 27		.72–.92	.88–.95								
CSI-4		P 77	0–3 freq.	10–20	(2 wk)	.74–.94	ADHD-HI & (C) vs:	ADHD category (6 studies):		5–12	Y	"Overal 1 bx"	Checkmate Plus, Inc.
Gadow & Sprafkin, 1994, 2002		T 99			.66–.88 (P & T)	(both)	TRF-Externalizing: .69 (.53)	Mean sensitivity: .64 (.87 if using either teacher or parent)					Complete kit:
Screens for DSM disorders, including ADHD							IOWA-Conners-IO: .70 (.83)	Mean specificity: .77 (.62 if using either teacher or parent)					$98/$358 (with or without software; manuals, 25 each form, plus scoring sheets, profiles) Forms: 50 @ $32
MCBC		P 77	T-F	10–15	(unknown)	.58–.83	*NR*	*NR*	*NR*	9–14	Y	*NR*	Author
Sines, 1986, 1988					.49–.78								Cost: *NR*
Activity Level Scale													
		T 68			*NR*	*NR*							

PBQ Behar & Stringfield, 1974 Hyperactive-distractible factor		30	0–2 freq.	5–10	(3–4 mo) .60–.94	*NR*	Significantly correlated with DO of classroom bx and interactions	BGD: Normal v. hyperactive, emotionally disturbed preschool children	*NR*	3–6	*NR*	*NR*	Author Cost: *NR*
RBPC Quay & Peterson, 1993 Motor Excess (ME) Scale (5 items)		89	0–3 sev.	15–20	(2 mo) .49–.83	.73–.94	Original BPS: .63–.97 CBCL: .43–.92 among alike scales ME not significantly correlated with DO of gross motor activity (r = .00; N = 34)	Discriminate clinical from nonclinical groups of children	*NR*	5–18	N	*NR*	Psychological Assessment Resources, Inc. Complete kit: $172 (manual, 50 forms & profile sheets) Forms: 25 @ $55
STAND-ALONE SCALES													
WWPARS Werry, 1968 Rater: Parent		22	0–2 freq.	5	*NR*	*NR*	WWPARS rating at age 4.5 significantly related to CPRS rating at 6.5 years (Campbell et al., 1978)	Predicted some improvements in mother–child interactions in response to stimulant meds in hyperactive children (Barkley & Cunningham, 1980)	Actometer M = .65 Range: .24 (classroom) to .77 (woodshop); .67 during gym	2–9	*NR*	*NR*	Free online:
DSM-IV SCALES													
ACTeRS	P	25	1–5 freq.	5–15	(2 wk)	.78–.96	CBCL (.80–.81)	Hyperactivity scores medication sensitive in ADHD students; BGD: ADHD/non-ADHD	*NR*	5–14	N	*NR*	MetriTech, Inc. Complete kit: $54 (manual + 50 forms; parent OR teacher)

(*continues*)

TABLE 6.1 *(continued)*

Scale		No. of Items	Item Type	Completion Time (min)	Test–Retest	Internal Consistency (alpha)	Convergent/ Divergent	Validity Evidence: Criterion	Validity Evidence: ROM	Norms: Age	Norms: Sex	Rating Period	Publisher/Cost
Ullmann et al., 1997					.68–.78								
Hyperactivity scale	T	24				.92–.97	CPRS (.78–.90)						Forms: 50 @ $37
ADDES-2	P	46	0–4 freq.	15–20	(1 mo)	.96–.98	TRF (.79–.87)	BGD: ADHD v. non-ADHD	*NR*	3–20	Y	*NR*	Hawthorne Educational Services, Inc.
McCarney, 1995a, 1995b					.88–.93								
Hyperactive/impulsive subscale Note: ADDES-3 available soon	T	60			.88–.97	.98–.99	CTRS: –2: (.51–.83) -S: (.42–.80) -S: ADHDT (.76–.93) -S: TRF (.51–.87)			4–19			Complete kit: $206 Forms: 50 @ $31 (either version) $20 per 50 ADDES/DSM-IV forms
ADHD-SC-4	P	50	0–4 freq.	*NR*	(6 wk)	.93–.95	CBCL (.48–.81)	Sensitivity	*NR*	3–18	Y	*NR*	Slosson Educational Publications, Inc.
Gadow & Sprafkin, 1997a, 1997b					.75–.82		TRF (.45–.88)	.81–.85 Specificity .57–.94					Complete kit: $78 Forms: 50 @ $28
	T				.70–.89	.92–.95		Sensitivity .61–.89 Specificity .57–.94					

ADHD-IV	P	18	0–3 freq.	10	(4 wk)	.86–.92	CPRS-R: .10–.80	65–84% (teacher); 60–68% (parent) of		5–18	Y	Last 6 mo.	Guilford Publications, Inc.
DuPaul, Power, Anastopoulos, & Reid, 1998					.78–.86		CRTS-R: .12–.41 ADHD Bx Code: .25–.26	ADHD children correctly classified via logistic regression					Complete kit: $42 (book, manual, scale)
Hyperactivity/ Impulsivity scale	T				.88–.90	.88–.96	AES: –.36	BGD: ADHD-I, ADHD-C, and controls (parent and teacher)					Forms: Photocopiable
ADHD-SRS		56	0–4 freq.	10–15	(2 wk)	.92–.99	ADDES: .80–.95	BGD: ADHD v. non-ADHD	*NR*	5–18	Y	*NR*	Wide Range, Inc.
Holland, Gimpel, & Merrell, 1998 Hyperactive-Impulsive Scale Rater: Parent, teacher (same form; separate norms provided)					.93–.98		CTRS: .64–.97 (like scales) ADHD-IV: .89–.93						Complete kit: $85 (manual, 25 forms) Forms: 25 @ $38
ADHDT		36	0–2 sev.	5–10	(1 wk)	.91–.97	Compared to seven other tests used to diagnose ADHD or bx concerns: "satisfactory"	BGD: ADHD v. non-ADHD	*NR*	3–23	Y	*NR*	Pro-Ed, Inc.
Gilliam, 1995					.85–.94			True positives/ negatives: 92%					Complete kit: $95 (manual, 50 summary/response forms)
Hyperactivity scale					(2 wk)			False positives: 7.7%					
Rater: Parent or Teacher					.85–.92		CTRS: .53–.72 ADDES-S: –.81 to –.88 ACTeRS: –.71 to –.78						Forms: 50 @ $42

(*continues*)

TABLE 6.1 *(continued)*

Scale		Psychometric Properties											
								Validity Evidence		Norms			
Scale		No. of Items	Item Type	Completion Time (min)	Test–Retest	Internal Consistency (alpha)	Convergent/ Divergent	Criterion	ROM	Age	Sex	Rating Period	Publisher/Cost
BASC-M	P	47	0–3 freq.	5–10	(2–8 wk)	.64–.83	CBCL: –.68 to .79	BGD: ADHD v. non-ADHD &	*NR*	4–18	Y	*NR*	American Guidance Services, Inc.
Reynolds, & Kamphaus 1992					.57–.90			ADHD-I v. ADHD-C (both versions)					Complete kit: $129 (manual, 25 each form, scoring template)
Hyperactivity Scale	T				.72–.93	.78–.93	CTRS-R (–.36–.62)						Forms: 25 @ $32
CAAS	P	31	1–4 freq.	2–5	(3 yr)	.75–.81	*NR*	*NR*	*NR*	5–13	*NR*	*NR*	American Guidance Services, Inc.
Lambert, Hartsough, & Sandoval, 1990					.32–.44								Complete kit: $150 (manual, 25 each form, scoring profile)
Hyperactivity scale	T				.40–.82	.78–.94							
Rater: Teacher or parent													Forms: 25 @ $48
ECADDES	P	50	0–4 freq.	12–15	(1 mo)	.87–.97	CPRS-R: .41–.71	BGD: ADHD v. non-ADHD	*NR*	2–6	Y	*NR*	Hawthorne Educational Services, Inc.
McCarney & Johnson, 1995					.82–.89		ADHDT: .46–.81						Complete kit: $162 (technical and intervention manuals, parent's guide, 50 school, home, & DSM-IV forms)
Hyperactive-Impulsive Index	T	56			.90–.98								Forms: $35 per 50 forms (home or school); $22 per 50 DSM-IV

S-ADHD-RS Spadafore & Spadafore, 1997 Impulsivity/ Hyperactivity scale (20 items) Rater: Teacher	50	0–4 freq.	10	(2 wk to 1 mo) .88–.90	*NR*	*NR*	Correctly identified: 50/50 ADHD Incorrectly identified 2/50 non-ADHD as ADHD	*NR*	5–19	Y		Complete Kit: $80 (manual, 25 Scoring Protocols, 25 Observation Forms, 25 Med Tracking Forms) Forms: 25 @ $25
SNAP-IV Swanson, 1992 Hyperactivity/ Impulsivity scale (9 items) Rater: Teacher or parent (same form)	90	0–3 freq.	10–15	(2 wk) .70–.90	.90+	*NR*	*NR*	*NR*	*NR*	Y	*NR*	Form and scoring guidelines are free online: http://www.adhd.net

Abbreviations: ACTeRS, ADD-H: Comprehensive Teacher's Rating Scale; ADDES-2, Attention Deficit Disorders Evaluation Scale—2nd edition; ADDES-S, Attention Deficit Disorders Evaluation Scale—Secondary-Age Student; ADHD-IV, ADHD Rating Scale-IV; ADHD-SC-4, ADHD Symptom Checklist—DSM-IV edition; ADHD-SRS, ADHD Symptoms Rating Scale; ADHDT, ADHD Test; BASC, Behavior Assessment System for Children; BASC-M, Behavior Assessment System for Children—Monitor for ADHD; BGD, Between-group differences; CADS, Conners' ADHD/DSM-IV Scales; CAAS, Children's Attention and Adjustment Survey; CBCL, Child Behavior Checklist; CBRF-A, Child Behavior Rating Form—Abbreviated; CBRSC, Comprehensive Behavior Rating Scale for Children; CDI, Children's Depression Inventory; Con., Convergent; CPRS-R, Conners' Parent Rating Scale—Revised; CPT, Continuous Performance Test; CRS-R, Conners' Rating Scales—Revised; CSI-4, Child Symptom Inventory—4th edition; CTRS, Conners' Teacher Rating Scale—Revised; ECADDES, Early Childhood Attention Deficit Disorders Evaluation Scale; freq., frequency; M, mean; MCBC, Missouri Children's Behavior Checklist; *NR*, P, Parent; PBQ, Preschool Behavior Questionnaire; RBPC, Revised Behavior Problem Checklist; ROM, relation to objective measures; S-ADHD-RS, Spadafore ADHD Rating Scale; sev., severity; SNAP-IV, Swanson, Nolan, & Pelham Rating Scale—Version IV; T, Teacher; TRF, Teacher Report Form; WWPARS, Werry–Weiss–Peters Activity Rating Scale.

Pricing information obtained from publishers' Web sites, retrieved January 2005.

Another common use of children's activity rating scales is for monitoring treatment effectiveness. Teachers and parents frequently complete short-form activity scales during the initial titration period to inform physicians of pharmacological treatment effectiveness. Instruments such as the Conners' Teacher Rating Scale (CTRS; Conners, Sitarenios, Parker, & Epstein, 1998), SNAP-IV (Swanson, 1992), ACTeRS (Ullman et al., 1997), and ADHD-IV (DuPaul, Powers, Anastopoulos, & Reid, 1998) are useful for this purpose because of their proven sensitivity to overall and between-dose psychostimulant effects (Rapport, 1990). These and other scales are also useful for monitoring changes in activity level that accompany behavioral interventions (e.g., Rapport, Murphy, & Bailey, 1982; Multimodal Treatment Study of Children with ADHD Cooperative Group, 1999).

Research

Activity rating scales are commonly used in research studies for a variety of purposes. Some studies use a particular score (e.g., ≥2 SD above the mean) as one of several selection criteria for identifying sample participants. Scales with published norms (age, gender) and reasonably high sensitivity and specificity are best suited for this purpose (see Table 6.1).

Other researchers obtain rating scale scores to investigate relationships between children's activity level and other characteristics, such as aggression, as potential marker variables of particular outcomes, or as mediators and moderators of other variables under study. Examples of these studies are common in the developmental psychopathology literature, whose central question addresses frequently the identification of early child characteristics and their continuity with later adverse outcomes. Fergusson, Lnyskey, and Horword (1997), for example, found that early ratings of hyperactivity predict adverse scholastic achievement during adolescence, even after controlling for IQ and other family background factors. These findings were replicated by an independent investigative team and were expanded to show that a dual-developmental model involving cognitive as well as behavioral pathways accounted more fully for the relationship between early attention deficit and long-term scholastic achievement (Rapport, Scanlan, & Denney, 1999). Scales that can be readministered over extended time intervals and have strong test–retest reliability and internal consistency are preferred in these types of studies.

Gauging treatment success by obtaining measures before and after behavioral or psychopharmacological treatment is a third common use of activity rating scales in child research. Rating scales used for assessing treatment outcome need to have high test–retest reliability over brief periods of time and with repeated administration (>.70), demonstrated sensitivity to treatment-related activity level change, and scale construction that minimizes floor and ceiling effects. Several scales possess these characteristics (see Table 6.1), and some are exquisitely sensitive in detecting overall and between-dose effects (see Rapport, 1990).

Limitations

Inadequate measurement units, insufficient psychometric properties, and the lack of age and sex norms limit the usefulness of many child activity rating scales. None of the available child activity level rating scales has a standard unit of measurement—that is, a meaningful unit of activity or movement that is equivalent within and across measures and raters. This lack of a basic measurement unit renders it impossible to accurately define activity level and leaves us in the uncomfortable position of referring to differences and changes in children's activity level by referring back to the scales used initially to quantify the behavior. The fact that many available scales are moderately or even strongly correlated with one another partially mitigates this concern. Correlations between activity rating scales and objective activity measures, however, are generally much weaker and in the .32–.58 range. These values indicate that 66% to 91% of the variability in activity rating scale scores is not linearly related to variability in actigraph scores in the same children measured at the same time. This finding probably reflects the fact that children's activity rating scales tend to reflect other aspects of behavior and not just activity level—an expected circumstance, given the wording of most scale items and reliance on factor analytic scale construction methodology (i.e., descriptions of activity level may correlate highly but tend to reflect a broader range of behavior than just movement).

Psychometric limitations of rating scales include imprecise measurement, inadequate construct validity, and a lack of established research documenting their diagnostic utility. Most scales use a Likert-type rating format, and comparisons within and between scales assume that a specific interval reflects the same unit of behavior (i.e., that the unit of measure between a 2 and 4 is identical to the difference between a 1 and 3 and that these behavioral units are consistent across scales). This is a speculative assumption at best. Moreover, the psychometric properties of most child activity rating scales are wanting. Activity scale validity is usually accomplished by demonstrating that scores derived from one instrument correlate with those derived from an already established scale of activity level or by demonstrating that children known to be highly active (e.g., ADHD) score significantly higher than normal peers on the scale. Most activity rating scales meet at least one of these two criteria. Extant research, however, reveals that even when activity scale scores are correlated, they may be unrelated to objective measures of activity level (Rapoport, Abramson, Alexander, & Lott, 1971; Stevens, Kupst, Suran, & Schulman, 1978). Other studies demonstrate that children receiving higher teacher activity ratings than other children in the same classroom may actually be less motorically active, according to precision counters used concurrently to measure motor movement. For example, when measured by step counter, nearly 64% of children rated as clinically hyperactive were less active than the most active child rated as being normal by the teacher (Tryon & Pinto, 1994). Collectively, these shortcomings limit the interpretability and usefulness of activity rating scales.

The diagnostic utility of most activity rating scales is unknown. Four metrics address this concern: sensitivity, specificity, positive predictive power (PPP), and negative predictive power (NPP). Sensitivity and specificity indicate the proportion of the group with a target diagnosis who test positive and negative on a measure, respectively. These two indices are useful for examining the overall classification accuracy of rating scales and other instruments but are not particularly valuable to clinicians unaware of a child's diagnostic standing prior to referral. PPP and NPP are the statistics most relevant for this purpose. PPP, as it applies to rating scale utility, indicates the conditional probability that a child exceeding a rating scale cutoff score meets criteria for a particular diagnosis such as ADHD (i.e., the ratio of true positive cases to all test positives). NPP, in contrast, indicates the conditional probability that a child who doesn't exceed an established cutoff score will not meet criteria for a particular clinical diagnosis (i.e., the ratio of true negative cases to all test negatives). High values (e.g., >.80) for all four indices are desirable.

Sensitivity, specificity, PPP, and NPP are also used to examine individual scale items and specific clinical diagnostic criteria. For example, the diagnostic utility of DSM-III (1980) activity level descriptions was investigated in a study of 76 6- to 12-year-old boys referred to a child psychiatry outpatient clinic (Milich, Widiger, & Landau, 1987). Children met diagnostic criteria for ADHD, Conduct Disorder (CD), both diagnoses, some other diagnosis, or an unspecified deferred diagnosis based on a comprehensive clinical assessment. Base rates for DSM-III items "shifts activities," "runs/climbs," "can't sit still," "runs around," and "on the go" ranged from .25 to .51 in the children with ADHD. As such, these descriptions occurred with relatively low frequency, and only two (shifts activities, on the go) identified a reasonably large proportion of the children (i.e., sensitivity rates of .70, .40, .38, .38, .68, respectively). The items were fairly specific to the disorder (specificity rates of .69, .78, .89, .86, .67, respectively) and served as moderately strong inclusion criteria (PPP rates of .72, .67, .79, .75, .69, respectively). NPP rates ranged from .54 to .68 and indicate that none of the items are particularly useful as exclusion criteria—that is, the absence of the symptoms do not necessarily mean that ADHD can be ruled out. Collectively, these findings support current clinical practice parameters that recommend conducting a comprehensive clinical assessment as opposed to relying on activity rating cutoff scores.

A final limitation of many child activity rating scales is their failure to include information concerning temporal changes in activity level relative to age, gender, and cultural norms. This is important because children exhibit differences or changes in activity level for myriad reasons, and some patterns are associated with particular psychological disorders, diseases, and situational demands. Complementary information is always needed, such as whether the change is abrupt or gradual, situational or pervasive, acute or chronic, and stable or waxing and waning.

Recommendation

Activity rating scales play a vital role in clinical diagnosis and treatment monitoring. Astute clinicians and researchers recognize that scales with established psychometric properties provide important information concerning children's activity level if they include age and gender norms and are culturally appropriate. Reviewing a scale's psychometric properties is particularly important when assessing low rates of activity level such as those observed in some cases of childhood depression—reliability (and hence, validity) tends to be lower in these cases. Monitoring treatment effects with activity rating scales requires prudence. Diminished activity level in children may or may not correspond with positive change in other aspects of their behavior. Scales such as the Academic Performance Rating Scale (APRS: DuPaul, Rapport, & Periello, 1991) are recommended to obtain complementary information concerning corresponding changes in adaptive functioning.

OBJECTIVE MEASURES OF ACTIVITY LEVEL: ANALOGUE, ACTOMETER, ACTIGRAPH, AND BEHAVIOR OBSERVATION SYSTEMS

Practice

Objective measures of children's activity level have been available for decades, but few make their way into everyday clinical practice. The primary reasons for their infrequent adoption are cost, time demands, and the widely held belief that they provide diminutive incremental benefit in diagnostic accuracy relative to information derived from parent and teacher activity rating scales. Several of the newer measures are less expensive and require minimal time to download collected data, and recent empirical evidence suggests that some instruments and observational systems hold excellent promise for improving diagnostic sensitivity and specificity. Objective measures of children's activity level include analogue measures, behavioral observation systems, actometers and actigraphs, and other measures used exclusively in research settings, such as stabilometers, photoelectric cells, ultrasound, and infrared motion analysis (see Table 6.2).

Analogue measures of children's activity level are occasionally used in research-oriented clinical outpatient facilities. An area within the clinic is established that approximates some aspect of children's natural environment, with the expectation that evoked activity level will resemble behavior observed typically in *esse situ*. This setting can take many different forms, depending on the information desired. Clinicians measuring children's movement associated with avoidance of or escape from a feared stimulus, such as a spider, will frequently utilize an elongated *approach* corridor and record steps taken or grid lines crossed as an indicator of fearfulness. Other common applications involve the use of analogue classrooms or activity rooms to assess motor movement in children referred for

ADHD, and topographical movement idiosyncrasies in children with pervasive developmental disorder. Activity level in these settings is usually assessed by trained observers *in vivo* or afterwards by tape review. Measurement may be as simple as counting floor marked grid changes over a preestablished time interval (e.g., Partington, Lang, & Campbell, 1971) or as sophisticated as using a computer-based, behavioral observation system to review taped sessions and code multiple behavior categories.

Direct observation has several advantages over other methods for measuring children's activity level. Some observational coding schemas are highly correlated with mechanical measures such as actometers, motion sensors, and calorimetry (Tryon, 1991). They do not hinder a child's movement as do some mechanical devices. In addition, they can be used to reflect specific types of movement in a variety of settings and over defined time periods. This latter information is particularly important if the goal is to understand the functional nature of children's movement rather than simply measuring quantitative differences. Most observation coding schemas, however, require that one or more trained individuals observe a child for a designated time interval (e.g., 20–30 minutes) on several occasions within or across weeks to render a valid sampling of behavior. For this reason, they are impractical for most clinicians.

An interesting alternative to *in vivo* observations is to digitally record the child's behavior in the setting and situation of interest and to transfer this information to a computer mpeg file for later viewing and analysis via the Noldus Observer (Noldus Information Technology, Inc.). This sophisticated software program permits continuous recording of any behavior while time-locking the observation with noted changes in the environment. Additional features include the ability to view, stop, and reverse the observation at any time at significantly reduced speeds, to enhance accuracy, and to modify behavioral codes for additional analyses. Newer versions and complementary software facilitate the exploration of sequential behavioral events that may not be immediately apparent to a trained observer—for example, to determine whether particular behaviors systematically precede other behaviors. A screen shot of the Noldus Observer is depicted in Figure 6.1.

Pedometers are inexpensive instruments used occasionally to measure one aspect of children's activity level—steps taken. Past studies, however, indicate that actometers are much more sensitive than pedometers for both detecting overall activity level and discriminating between children with and without ADHD (Barkley & Ullman, 1975; Rapoport et al., 1971).

Actometers are modified wristwatches capable of recording the frequency of movement occurring along the horizontal plane crossing through 3 and 9 o'clock on the watch (Bell, 1968). Removing the balance and hairspring assemblies and adding a small weight to the lever causes the second hand to move incrementally each time the device is moved. Frequency of movement, or how many distinct movements occur (i.e., changes in direction), is estimated by comparing the starting and ending times shown on the watch face. These instruments, however, are

TABLE 6.2 Objective Measures of Activity Level in Children: Mechanical and Direct Observational Approaches

Instrument/ Distributor	Age Range	Recording Length	Norms	Software Available	Cost
MECHANICAL					
Actigraphs Ambulatory Monitoring MiniMitter MTI, Inc.	Any	22 days per 32 KB of memory	No	Yes	Starter: $1000+ (with necessary software and reader interface); $500–$2000 for each additional actigraph
Actometers[a] Model 108 Engineering Department Times Industries, Waterbury, CT 06720	Any	Variable	No	Yes[b]	*NR*
Pedometers (available at sporting goods stores)	Any	Range: 99,999 steps (~5.25 miles) to 1000 miles	No		
Stand-Alone				No	$10–$40
With data downloadable to PC				Yes	$125–$400+
DIRECT OBSERVATIONS					
ADHD BCS Barkley, 1990	*NR*	15 min.	No	No	*NR*
ADHD-SOC Checkmate Plus, Ltd.	School age	16 min.			Kit: $25
BASC SOS AGS, Inc.	School age	15 min.	No	Yes	25 forms @ $33
COC Abikoff, 1977/1980	School age	32 min.	No	No	*NR*
DOF ASEBA	5–14	10 min.	Yes	Yes	*NR*
Noldus Observer Noldus Information Technology	Any	Variable	No	Yes	Observer Basic 5.0 $1795; Observer Video Pro 5.0 $5850

Abbreviations: BCS, Behavior Coding System; COC, Classroom Observation Code; DOF, Direct Observation Form; SOC, School Observation Code; SOS, Student Observation System;

[a]Many studies report either using the Kaulins and Willis actometers (no longer manufactured) or enlisting a jeweler to modify a self-winding wristwatch, as described by Schulman and Reisman (1959).

[b]Eaton, McKeen, & Saudino (1996) provide SAS syntax for performing group-level data analysis based on actometer readings.

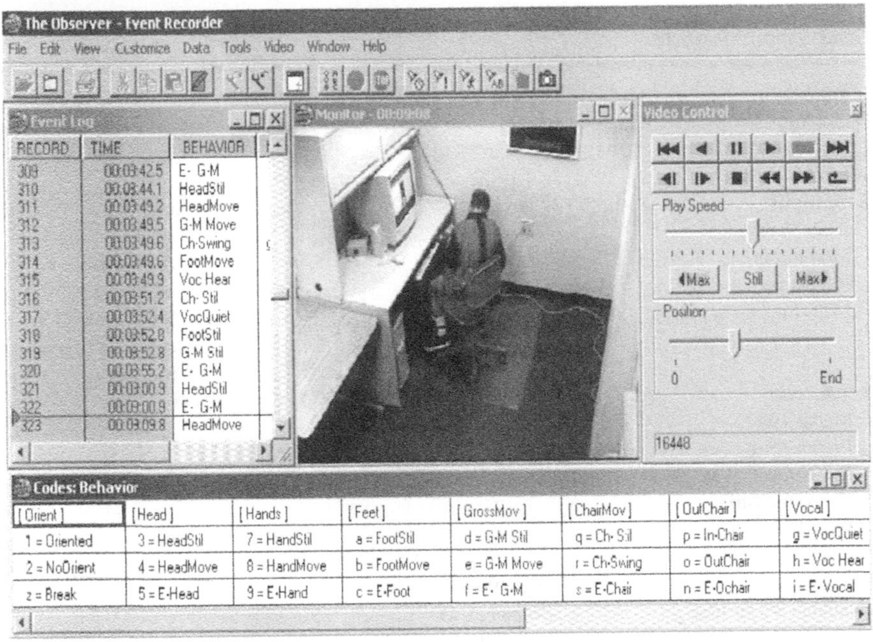

FIGURE 6.1 A screenshot of the Noldus Observer. Trained observers watch the video file (center) and code behavior (top left) according to prespecified behavior codes (bottom left).

incapable of measuring the duration or intensity of movement, which may be important for clinical diagnosis.

Newer *actigraphs* generate a current (voltage) each time the instrument is moved in a direction vertical to the instrument face. The current is passed through an amplifier and filtered based on factory and user settings. The result of this process is an analogue waveform—a histogram of measured voltage over time—from which movement frequency, intensity, and duration is extracted (for a detailed review, see Tyron, 1991). These devices allow for more precise recording of activity or movement, with excellent test–retest stability. An oft-cited actigraphy study examined movement differences in 12 children with ADHD and 12 age-matched classmates based on 24-hour waist activity for 7 days (Porrino et al., 1983). Children with ADHD were found to be approximately 25% to 30% more active than normal controls, particularly in school and at home when completing in-seat academic assignments. Deciding on where to place the actigraph (e.g., waist, arm, leg) and which recording modes to utilize are critical elements that must be considered prior to clinical assessment. These and other relevant parameters are reviewed below.

Settings and Recording Modes

Actometers do not have programmable settings, and they report only an average frequency of movement. In contrast, actigraphs provide many options for data collection, and the settings and mode of an actigraph determine the type of data recorded. Different modes return significantly different data points, and careful consideration of the purpose of data collection may prove critical when selecting among possible settings. The primary distinction is between actigraph placement and variable sampling intervals and among frequency, duration, and intensity of movement selections—these and other dimensions are reviewed next.

Placement of the actigraph influences the amount and type of movement it records. Common placement locations are the wrist, trunk, and ankles. Actigraphs placed on a belt or in a pouch around the waist are more likely to detect gross body movements, due to the motion and energy expenditure necessary to move this area. In contrast, arm recordings detect lower-intensity, more subtle movements and result in higher activity recordings, regardless of the time of day. Precise placement on the arm is also worth noting because even small variations may yield differences in activity level. Some research on the older, less precise actometer suggests that larger readings are typically obtained as a function of how far the recording site is from the axis of rotation (Johnson, 1971). Other researchers, however, have found that forearm length is not significantly related to obtained movement counts (Eaton, 1983). Thus, wrist recordings may detect higher activity than will forearm recordings, highlighting the importance of consistent placement across subjects or patients. Either wrist may be used for recording (i.e., handedness does not appear to affect differentially recorded activity levels in children). As a general rule of thumb, integrated generalized movements like postural shifts are detected by all sites, whereas small movements associated with distal extremities are best detected by wrist-worn monitors.

Filters involve measurement parameters such as sampling rate and epoch length. Sampling rate, measured in hertz (Hz), determines how many samples per second are taken by the actigraph. This rate is factory set at 10 Hz (i.e., 10 samples per second) for many actigraphs, although some models are programmable. In the most general sense, more precise data are garnered as a function of higher sampling rates (i.e., more data sampled per time unit). An *epoch* is the unit of time that the actigraph combines into one data point. Some models have factory-set epochs (e.g., Ambulatory Monitoring's MicroMini is preset at 1-minute epochs), whereas others are customizable. Epoch length represents a trade-off between specificity and duration of continuous monitoring—the shorter the epoch, the more specific the data. For example, a 1-minute epoch at a 10-Hz sampling rate over 60 contiguous minutes will produce 60 distinct data points, with each point based on 60 samples. Changing the epoch length to 10 minutes yields only six data points for the same length of observation (each based on 600 samples). Most modern actigraphs have at least 32K of memory, which translates into approximately 22 days of continuous data using 1-minute epochs. This memory is reused once data have been downloaded from the actigraph, indicating that short epochs are feasible for all but the longest continuous measurements. The nature of the data recorded for each point, however, varies considerably based on the actigraph's mode.

Mode is set depending on whether the user is interested in frequency, duration, and/or intensity of movement. Common available modes include full-waveform, zero-crossing, time above threshold, and proportional integrating measure modes. A visual heuristic of data characteristics associated with different settings is depicted in Figure 6.2. Full-waveform mode collects the entire analogue waveform for analysis, whereas the other options record only certain characteristics of this wave. This mode is typically available only on high-end actigraphs. Zero-crossing mode (ZCM) records the number of times the waveform voltage crosses a set reference voltage—as the voltage changes in response to movement, ZCM counts each instance the waveform crosses a preset threshold. Consider a swing on a child's swingset held at a determined height and released. ZCM counts the number of times the swing crosses a height just above its resting point. As the swing slows, it continues to cross this threshold, and each pass is counted until it stops. Zero-crossing mode is thus a measure of movement frequency.

Time above threshold (TAT) measures the *duration* of movement, or time spent in movement. Once the set threshold is reached, the actigraph counts each sampling period (e.g., every tenth of a second at 10 Hz) until the movement-generated voltage falls below this level. This mode determines that movement is above a threshold, but it does not measure *how much* above threshold. Consider the child's swing again—as it slows, less and less time is spent above any given height, and the number of counts will be considerably less than would be the case if the same swing were measured using ZCM. For this reason, zero-crossing is often considered a more sensitive measure than TAT.

Proportional integrating measure (PIM) mode measures the absolute value of the area under the waveform curve or, stated differently, the *intensity* of movement or activity level. To illustrate the difference between frequency and intensity of movement, consider the *test of strength* machines at state fairs. Two individuals may swing the hammer in a nearly identical manner, however, the intensity or force can vary considerably—PIM mode detects these differences. PIM mode measures gross activity level instead of counting time above threshold or merely changes in movement. Two subgroups, low PIM and high PIM, are available. The difference is that high PIM applies an extra filter, which further amplifies the analogue waveform signal and allows comparison of more minute movements. Unless one is measuring premature infants or individuals with movement-related disabilities, the standard low-PIM mode is preferred. Using high PIM with normal or hyperactive populations may result in a ceiling effect because much of the activity may be amplified to the maximum value possible for the actigraph. Hypothetical differences in data counts across the three modes are depicted in Figure 6.2.

Mode Comparisons

Zero-crossing and time-above-threshold options quantify how often movement occurs—in contrast, PIM mode examines how *much* movement occurs. PIM mode may also be the most sensitive measure, especially when examining

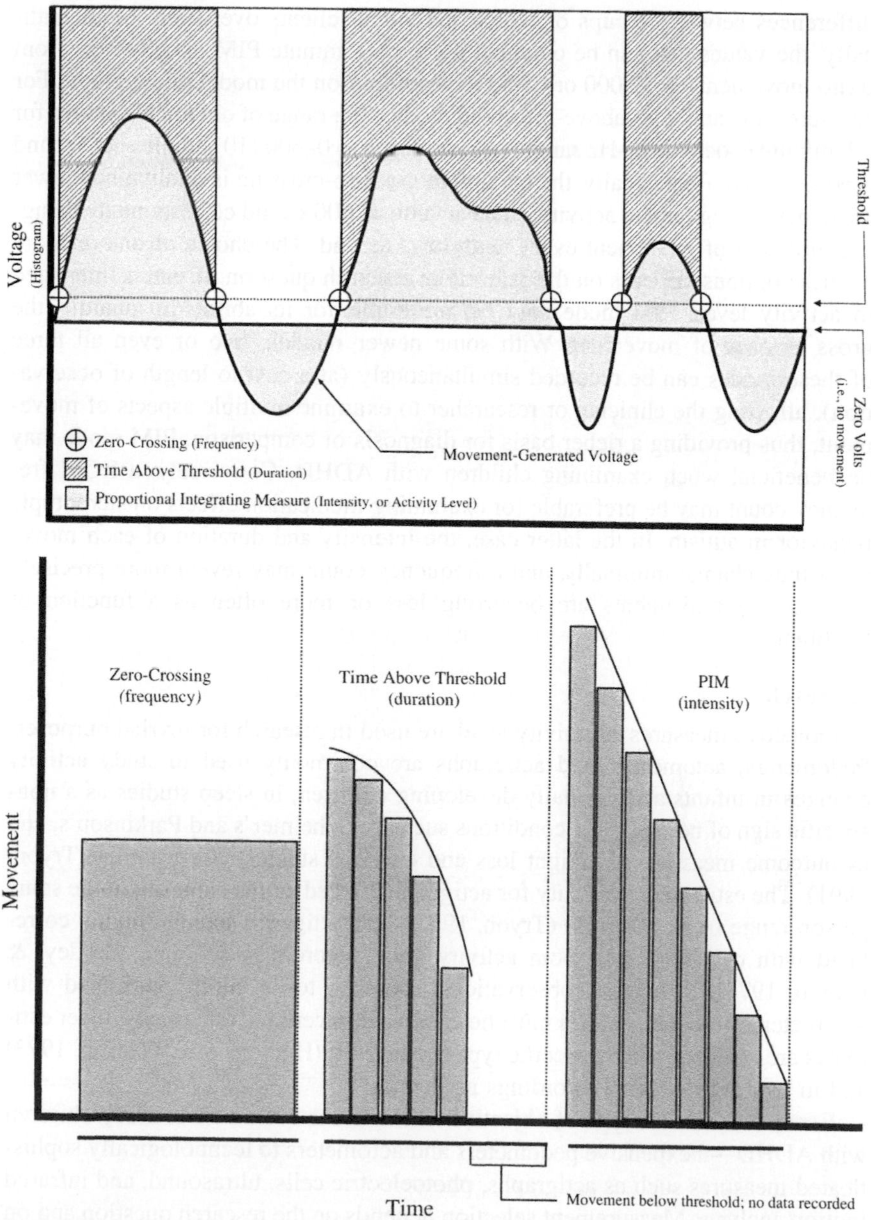

FIGURE 6.2 A visual heuristic depicting the movement-generated waveform characteristics associated with different modes (top), and hypothetical data for three actigraph modes measuring the same swing from start to stop (bottom).

differences between groups or within individual clients over time. Mathematically, the values that can be obtained for each 1-minute PIM epoch range from 0 (no movement) to 32,000 or 65,535, depending on the model of actigraph. For zero-crossing and time-above-threshold modes, the range of obtainable values for a 1-minute epoch (at 10-Hz sampling rate) drops to 0–600 (10 samples per second × 60 seconds). Realistically, the maximum for zero-crossing is likely much lower when measuring human activity, since a value of 600 would correspond to changing direction of movement every tenth of a second. The choice of one or more of these options depends on the referral or research question. If one is interested in activity level, PIM mode may be preferable for its ability to quantify the gross amount of movement. With some newer models, two or even all three of these modes can be recorded simultaneously (at a cost to length of observation), allowing the clinician or researcher to examine multiple aspects of movement, thus providing a richer basis for diagnosis or comparison. PIM mode may be beneficial when examining children with ADHD. Conversely, a ZCM frequency count may be preferable for examining medication effects on stereotypic behavior in autism. In the latter case, the intensity and duration of each movement may change minimally, and a frequency count may reveal more precisely whether the movements are occurring less or more often as a function of treatment.

Research

Objective measures of activity level are used in research for myriad purposes. Pedometers, actometers, and actigraphs are commonly used to study activity changes in infants and normally developing children, in sleep studies as a nonspecific sign of neurological conditions such as Alzheimer's and Parkinson's, and as outcome measures in weight loss and exercise studies (for a review, Tryon, 1991). The estimated reliability for actigraphs placed at the same site in the same person range from .90 to .99 (Tryon, 1985), and actigraph data are highly correlated with children's playroom activity level recordings (Ullman, Barkley, & Brown, 1978). Behavioral observations also tend to be highly correlated with actometers; however, caution must be exercised in certain situations—lower estimates are obtained during specific types of activity (Halverson & Waldrop, 1973) and in low activity level recordings in general.

Every conceivable type of objective measure has been used to study children with ADHD—inexpensive pedometers and actometers to technologically sophisticated measures such as actigraphs, photoelectric cells, ultrasound, and infrared motion analysis. Measurement selection depends on the research question and on the level of precision required by the investigator. Studies of ADHD illustrate this point adeptly. Simple actometers placed on ankles and wrists and in waist belt pockets consistently reveal overall activity level differences between children with ADHD and control children. More sophisticated actigraphs are required to determine whether these children move more than their peers throughout the day and during different activities (e.g., Porrino et al., 1983). These devices, however, are unable to address questions concerning the type, site, and complexity of movement. For example, Teicher et al. (1996) used infrared motion analysis to track the precise two-dimensional location of four reflective markers taped to a cap and clothing worn by children with ADHD and normal controls. Children with ADHD exhibited two to three times more movement during a vigilance task at every body location, and covered a fourfold-wider area in their movements relative to control children. Motion analysis also revealed that children with ADHD moved their entire body to a greater degree, kept their extremities still 66% less and their trunk still 74% less, and exhibited less complex movement overall (i.e., more linear side-to-side movement) relative to control children. Information gleaned from this investigation confirms that children with ADHD emit significantly more movement relative to age-matched controls, regardless of body location monitored. It also reveals that the excessive movement is less complex relative to same-age peers. But why do children with ADHD display a higher rate of movement? And are these excesses merely random movement, or do they serve some functional purpose? Complementary studies suggest that their excessive movement may be related to particular task demands and, in some cases, serve to compensate for an inability to maintain sufficient arousal (Zentall & Leib, 1985). These and related questions must be addressed by behavioral observation and complex coding schemas.

Research has also sought to determine whether actigraphs are diagnostically useful given their exceptional reliability and established validity. Studies have not been designed to address definitively whether they can serve this function, but some have examined pieces of the puzzle. For example, a belt-worn activity monitor showed exceptionally high positive predictive power (.91) for discriminating between children with ADHD and normal controls undergoing psychometric evaluation (Matier-Sharma, Perachio, Newcorn, Sharma, & Halperin, 1995). Sensitivity, however, was unacceptably low (.25). Collectively these findings indicate a very strong likelihood that children will meet ADHD diagnostic criteria if they exhibit higher-than-normal activity during psychometric evaluation, whereas nearly 75% of children with a diagnosis of ADHD fail to show this behavioral pattern. Conclusions derived from this and similar studies are complicated by methodological factors. The aforementioned cited study, as an example, relied on the least sensitive placement for detecting activity level changes—the waist, which primarily detects major postural shifts.

Limitations

Even objective measures of children's activity level have relative strengths and shortcomings. It is unclear whether analogue test settings elicit a representative sample of children's behavior shown at school and home. This limitation raises questions about the validity and generalization of findings. The relatively brief behavioral samples of 10–30 minutes in analogue settings are particularly suspect. Children most likely to be assessed for excessive movement in analogue settings are those suspected of ADHD. These children are known to be highly variable, which decreases the likelihood that brief behavior samples will serve as adequate behavioral samples for either diagnostic or treatment purposes.

Direct observation bypasses many of the shortcomings inherent in analogue assessment but tends to be quite costly, even when volunteers are recruited and trained. Required training time is proportional to the complexity of the coding scheme and behavior being observed. Periodic retraining is required to minimize *observer drift*—a well-documented phenomenon that refers to the likelihood that observers will alter their definitions of the behaviors they are observing over even short time periods. Taping observations can dramatically improve reliability by creating a permanent record of behavior, but observers must still be trained to review and code the data reliably. Sophisticated observational and data-handling programs represent a clear improvement over existing observation instruments and procedures, but they remain too costly for most practice settings. High-tech instruments are procured to conduct investigative studies of children's activity level and usually represent a trade-off between measurement precision and transportability. The stabilometer lies on the simpler end of the spectrum and provides highly defined measurement of a child's buttocks movement while seated. The very nature of the apparatus, however, places serious limits on a child's mobility and may offer a limited behavioral sample. Pedometers are limited to providing somewhat crude measures of steps taken, whereas actigraphs allow for more precise recording of activity or movement over extended time periods, with excellent test–retest stability. Their most significant limitations are that they are limited to detecting movement of particular extremities, due to the attachment locale or site; they remain too costly for widespread clinical adoption; and age, gender, and cultural norms are unavailable. Instruments at the upper end of the measurement spectrum, such as ultrasonic, are somewhat unreliable in detecting gross and fine motor movements—others, such as infrared motion analysis, are prohibitively expensive and must be supplemented by observation to judge the functional nature and contextual variables associated with movement.

Recommendations

Behavioral observation is an expensive and time-consuming practice unlikely to enjoy widespread adoption among practicing clinicians. This said, it remains one of the truly valid means by which to gain an appreciable understanding of children in their natural environment and remains a cornerstone for school psychologists and empirical investigations. A practical alternative is to video record children's behavior for later coding and analysis; however, this raises thorny ethical concerns and is unlikely to be permitted in most educational settings. Actometers represent a reasonable compromise between the rather limited and somewhat unreliable pedometer and highly precise but costly actigraph until the latter becomes more affordable for clinical practices. Either leg or wrist placement is preferred, coupled with a supplementary daily activity log to facilitate interpretation. Due to the limitations of the actometers, such a log must include the starting and ending "times" shown on the actometer for each activity listed in order to be useful. Multiday samples of behavior are recommended, particularly for children suspected of ADHD, owing to their high within- and across-day variability. Combining activity level data with information gleaned from extensive histories, semistructured clinical interview, and appropriate rating scales is required for effective case conceptualization, consistent with evidence-based practice.

FUTURE DIRECTIONS

Little is known about the activity level in children with clinical disorders relative to the burgeoning literature on normal development. Extant literature suggests that activity level differences associated with most clinical disorders of childhood represent quantitative deviations. For example, heightened activity level is frequently observed in children with attention-deficit/hyperactivity disorder (ADHD) and some forms of anxiety, whereas lower-than-normal levels of activity are often related to childhood depression. Differences in activity level topography—activity level's unique form and expression in a particular situation or setting—may also have special meaning for understanding the movement of some children. Topographical differences are frequently observed in children with autism (e.g., stereotypic, ritualistic behavior), who display self-injurious behavior, and as a result of untoward side effects associated with short-term (e.g., akathesia) and chronic (e.g., tardive dyskinesia) neuroleptic administration. Measuring activity level in children with particular clinical disorders using the measures reviewed must be supplemented by behavioral observation to understand the subtleties, contextual factors, and possible functional nature of children's motor activity. Actigraphs may play an increasingly larger role in clinical assessments, but they are functionally limited until standardized age and gender norms are developed.

REFERENCES AND RESOURCES

Achenbach, T. M., & Rescorla, L. A. (2001). *Manual for the ASEBA School-Age Forms & Profiles.* Burlington, VT: University of Vermont Research Center for Children, Youth, & Families.

Aman, M. G., & Werry, J. S. (1984). The revised behavior problem checklist in clinic attenders and nonattenders: Age and sex effects. *Journal of Clinical Child Psychology, 13,* 237–242.

Ambulatory Monitoring. (2004). The micromini motionlogger actigraph and family of single-sensor recorders [User's manual to accompany Act Millennium version 3.5.0.0 and higher (3rd ed.)]. New York: Author. Retrieved from http://www.ambulatory-monitoring.com/, 7 October 2004.

American Psychiatric Association. (1980). *Diagnostic and statistical manual of mental disorders, 3rd edition (DSM-III).* Washington, DC: Author.

American Psychiatric Association. (1994). *Diagnostic and statistical manual of mental disorders* (4th ed.). Washington, DC: Author.

Angello, L. M., Volpe, R. J., DiPerna, J. C., Gureasko-Moore, S. P., Gureasko-Moore, D. P., Nebrig, M. R., & Ota, K. (2003). Assessment of attention-deficit/hyperactivity disorder: An evaluation of six published rating scales. *School Psychology Review, 32,* 241–262.

Aronen, E. T., Fjällberg, M., Paavonen, E. J., & Soininen, M. (2002). Day-length associates with activity level in children living at 60 degrees north. *Child Psychiatry and Human Development, 32,* 217–226.

Barkley, R. A. (1988). Child behavior rating scales and checklists. In M. Rutter, A. H. Tuma, & I. S. Lann (Eds.), *Assessment and diagnosis in child psychopathology* (pp. 113–155). New York: Guilford Press.

Barkley, R. A., & Ullman, D. G. (1975). A comparison of objective measures of activity and distractibility in hyperactive and nonhyperactive children. *Journal of Abnormal Child Psychology, 3,* 231–244.

Behar, L., & Stringfield, S. (1974). A behavior rating scale for the preschool child. *Developmental Psychology, 10,* 601–610.

Bell, R. Q. (1968). Adaptation of small wristwatches for mechanical recording of activity in infants and children. *Journal of Experimental Child Psychology, 6,* 302–305.

Butcher, J. E., & Eaton, W. O. (1989). Gross and fine motor proficiency in preschoolers: Relationships with free play behavior and activity level. *Journal of Human Movement Studies, 16,* 27–36.

Campbell, D. W., & Eaton, W. O. (1999). Sex differences in the activity level of infants. *Infant and Child Development, 8,* 1–17.

Conners, C. K., Parker, J. D. A., Sitarenios, G., & Epstein, J. N. (1998). The Revised Conners' Parent Rating Scale (CPRS-R): Factor structure, reliability, and criterion validity. *Journal of Abnormal Child Psychology, 26,* 257–268.

Conners, C. K., Sitarenios, G., Parker, J. D. A., & Epstein, J. N. (1998). Revision and restandardization of the Conners' Teacher Rating Scale (CTRS-R): Factor structure, reliability, and criterion validity. *Journal of Abnormal Child Psychology, 26,* 279–291.

Conoley, J. C., & Impara, J. C. (1995). *The twelfth mental measurements yearbook.* Lincoln, NE: Buros Institute of Mental Measurements.

DeFries, J. C., Gervais, M. C., & Thomas, E. A. (1978). Response to 30 generations of selection for open-field activity in laboratory mice. *Behavior Genetics, 8,* 3–13.

Demaray, M. K., Elting, J., & Schaefer, K. (2003). Assessment of attention-deficit/hyperactivity disorder (ADHD): A comparative evaluation of five, commonly used, published rating scales. *Psychology in the Schools, 40,* 341–361.

DuPaul, G. J., Power, T. J., Anastopoulos, A. D., & Reid, R. (1998). *ADHD rating scale—IV: Checklists, norms, and clinical interpretation.* New York: Guilford Press.

DuPaul, G. J., Rapport, M. D., & Perriello, L. M. (1991). Teacher ratings of academic skills: The development of the Academic Performance Rating Scale. *School Psychology Review, 20,* 284–300.

Eaton, W. O. (1983). Measuring activity level with actometers: Reliability, validity, and arm length. *Child Development, 54,* 720–726.

Eaton, W. O. (1994). Temperament, development, and the five-factor model: Lessons from activity level. In G. F. Habversow, G. A. Kohastamm, & R. P. Mecten (Eds.), *The developing structure of temperament and personality from infancy to adulthood* (pp. 173–187). Hillsdale, NJ: Erlbaum.

Eaton, W. O., McKeen, N. A., & Campbell, D. W. (2001). The waxing and waning of movement: Implications for psychological development. *Developmental Review, 21,* 205–223.

Eaton, W. O., McKeen, N. A., & Saudino, K. J. (1996). Measuring human individual differences in general motor activity with actometers. In K. P. Ossenkopp, M. Kavaliers, & P. R. Sanberg (Eds.), *Measuring movement and locomotion: From invertebrates to humans* (pp. 79–92). Austin, TX: R. G. Landes.

Emerson, E. N., Crowley, S. L., & Merrell (1994). Convergent validity of the school social behavior scales with the Child Behavior Checklist and teacher's report form. *Journal of Psychoeducational Assessment, 12,* 372–380.

Fergusson, D. M., Lynskey, M. T., & Horwood, L. J. (1997). Attentional difficulties in middle childhood and psychosocial outcomes in young adulthood. *Journal of Child Psychology and Psychiatry, 38,* 633–644.

Gadow, K. D., & Sprafkin, J. (1997a). *ADHD Symptom Checklist—4 manual*. Stony Brook, NY: Checkmate Plus.

Gadow, K. D., & Sprafkin, J. (1997b). *Child symptom inventories norms manual*. Stony Brook, NY: Checkmate Plus.

Gadow, K. D., & Sprafkin, J. (2002). *Child Symptom Inventory 4: Screening and norms manual*. Stony Brook, NY: Checkmate Plus.

Gadow, K. D., Sprafkin, J., & Nolan, E. E. (1996). *Attention Deficit Hyperactivity Disorder School Observation Code*. Stony Brook, NY: Checkmate Plus Ltd.

Gadow, K. D., Sprafkin, J., Salisbury, H., Schneider, J., & Loney, J. (2004). Further validity evidence for the teacher version of the Child Symptom Inventory—4. *School Psychology Quarterly, 19*, 50–71.

Gavarry, O., Giacomoni, M., Bernard, T., Seymat, M., & Falgairette, G. (2003). Habitual physical activity in children and adolescents during school and free days. *Medicine & Science in Sports & Exercise, 35*(3), 525–531.

Gilliam, J. E. (1995). *Examiners manual for the Attention-Deficit/Hyperactivity Disorder Test: A method for identifying individuals with ADHD*. Austin, TX: Pro-Ed.

Halverson Jr., C. F., & Waldrop, M. F. (1973). The relations of mechanically recorded activity level to varieties of preschool play behavior. *Child Development, 44*, 678–681.

Hogan, A. E., Quay, H. C., Vaughn, S., & Shapiro, S. K. (1989). Revised Behavior Problem Checklist: Stability, prevalence, and incidence of behavior problems in kindergarten and first-grade children. *Psychological Assessment: A Journal of Consulting and Clinical Psychology, 1*, 103–111.

Holland, M. L., Gimpel, G. A., & Merrell, K. W. (1998). Innovations in assessing ADHD: Development, psychometric properties, and factor structure of the ADHD Symptoms Rating Scale (ADHD-SRS). *Journal of Psychopathology & Behavioral Assessment, 20*, 307–332.

Impara, J. C., & Plake, B. S. (1998). *The thirteenth mental measurements yearbook*. Lincoln, NE: Buros Institute of Mental Measurements.

Johnson, C. F. (1971). Hyperactivity and the machine, the actometer. *Child Development, 42*, 2105–2110.

Kramer, J. J., & Conoley, J. C. (1992). *The eleventh mental measurements yearbook*. Lincoln, NE: Buros Institute of Mental Measurements.

Lahey, B. B., & Piacentini, J. C. (1985). An evaluation of the Quay–Peterson Revised Behavior Problem Checklist. *Journal of School Psychology, 23*, 285–289.

Lambert, N., Hartsough, C., & Sandoval, J. (1990). *Manual for the Children's Attention and Adjustment Survey*. Circle Pines, MN: American Guidance Service.

Matier-Sharma, K., Perachio, N., Newcorn, J. H., Sharma, V., & Halperin, J. M. (1995). Differential diagnosis of ADHD: Are objective measures of attention, impulsivity, and activity level helpful? *Child Neuropsychology, 1*, 118–127.

McCarney, S. B. (1995a). *Attention deficit disorders evaluation scale* (2nd ed.). Columbia, MO: Hawthorne Educational Services.

McCarney, S. B. (1995b). *The Early Childhood Attention Deficit Disorders Evaluation Scale (ECADDES)*. Columbia, MO: Hawthorne Educational Services.

Milich, R., Widiger, T. A., & Landau, S. (1987). Differential diagnosis of attention deficit and conduct disorders using conditional probabilities. *Journal of Consulting and Clinical Psychology, 55*, 762–767.

Mitchell, J. V. (1985). *The ninth mental measurements yearbook—Volume II*. Lincoln, NE: Buros Institute of Mental Measurements.

Multimodal Treatment Study of Children with ADHD Cooperative Group (US). (1999). A 14-month randomized clinical trial of treatment strategies for attention-deficit/hyperactivity disorder. *Archives of General Psychiatry, 56*, 1073–1086.

Neeper, R., Lahey, B. B., & Frick, P. J. (1990). *Manual for the Comprehensive Behavior Rating Scale for Children (CBRSC)*. San Antonio, TX: Psychological Corporation.

Partington, M. W., Lang, E., & Campbell, D. (1971). Motor activity in early life. I. Fries' congenital activity types. *Biology of the Neonate, 18,* 94–107.

Peach, W. J., & Cobb, S. E. (1990). Student ratings vs. teacher ratings on the Revised Behavior Problem Checklist. *Journal of Instructional Psychology, 17,* 194–196.

Plake, B. S., & Impara, J. C. (2001). *The fourteenth mental measurements yearbook.* Lincoln, NE: Buros Institute of Mental Measurements.

Plake, B. S., Impara, J. C., & Spies, R. A. (2003). *The fifteenth mental measurements yearbook.* Lincoln, NE: Buros Institute of Mental Measurements.

Porrino, L. J., Rapoport, J. L., Behar, D., Sceery, W., Ismond, D. R., & Bunney, W. E. (1983). A naturalistic assessment of the motor activity of hyperactive boys: I. Comparison with normal controls. *Archives of General Psychiatry, 40,* 681–687.

Quay, H. C. (1983). A dimensional approach to behavior disorder: The Revised Behavior Problem Checklist. *School Psychology Review, 12,* 244–249.

Quay, H. C., & Peterson, D. R. (1993). *The Revised Behavior Problem Checklist: Manual.* Odessa, FL: Psychological Assessment Resources.

Rapoport, J., Abramson, A., Alexander, D., & Lott, I. (1971). Playroom observations of hyperactive children on medication. *Journal of the American Academy of Child Psychiatry, 10,* 524–534.

Rapport, M. D. (1990). Controlled studies of the effects of psychostimulants on children's functioning in clinic and classroom settings. In C. K. Conners & M. Kinsbourne (Eds.), *Attention Deficit Hyperactivity Disorder* (pp. 77–111). Munich, Germany: Medizin Verlag Munchen.

Rapport, M. D., Murphy, H. A., & Bailey, J. S. (1982). Ritalin vs. response cost in the control of hyperactive children: A within-subject comparison. *Journal of Applied Behavior Analysis, 15,* 205–216.

Rapport, M. D., Scanlan, S. W., & Denney, C. B. (1999). Attention-deficit/hyperactivity disorder and scholastic achievement: A model of dual developmental pathways. *Journal of Child Psychology and Psychiatry, 40,* 1169–1183.

Reynolds, C. R., & Kamphaus, R. W. (1992). *Behavior Assessment System for Children: Manual.* Circle Pines, MN: American Guidance Service.

Routh, D. K., Schroeder, C. S., & O'Tuama, L. A. (1974). Development of activity level in children. *Developmenal Psychology, 10,* 163–168.

Saudino, K. J., & Eaton W. O. (1991). Infant temperament and genetics: An objective twin study of motor activity level. *Child Development, 62,* 1167–1174.

Schulman, J. L., & Reisman, J. M. (1959). An objective measure of hyperactivity. *American Journal of Mental Deficiency, 64,* 455–456.

Shelton, T. L., & Barkley, R. A. (1993). Assessment of attention-deficit/hyperactivity disorder in young children. In J. L. Culbertson & D. J. Willis (Eds.), *Testing young children: A reference guide for developmental, psychoeducational, and psychosocial assessments* (pp. 290–318). Austin, TX: Pro-Ed.

Sines, J. O. (1986). Normative data for the revised Missouri Children's Behavior Checklist—Parent form (MCBC-P). *Journal of Abnormal Child Psychology, 14,* 89–94.

Sleator, E. K., & Ullmann, R. K. (1981). Can the physician diagnose hyperactivity in the office? *Pediatrics, 67,* 13–17.

Spadafore, G. L., & Spadafore, S. J. (1997). *Spadafore attention deficit hyperactivity disorder rating scale.* Novato, CA: Academic Therapy Publications.

Sprafkin, J., Gadow, K. D., & Nolan, E. E. (2001). The utility of a DSM-IV-referenced screening instrument for attention-deficit/hyperactivity disorder. *Journal of Emotional and Behavioral Disorders, 1,* 182–191.

Stevens, T. M., Kupst, M. J., Suran, B. G., & Schulman, J. L. (1978). Activity level: A comparison between actometer scores and observer ratings. *Journal of Abnormal Child Psychology, 6,* 163–173.

Swanson, J. M. (1992). *School-based assessments and interventions for ADD students.* Irvine, CA: K. C. Publications.

Teicher, M. H., Ito, Y., Glod, C. A., & Barber, N. I. (1996). Objective measurement of hyperactivity and attentional problems in ADHD. *Journal of the American Academy of Child and Adolescent Psychiatry, 35,* 334–342.

Tryon, W. W. (1985). Human activity: A review of quantitative findings. In W. W. Tryon (Ed.), *Behavioral assessment in behavioral medicine* (pp. 257–299). New York: Springer.

Tryon, W. W. (1991). *Activity measurement in psychology and medicine.* New York: Plenum Press.

Tryon, W. W. (1993). Activity level and DSM-IV. In M. Hersen & S. M. Turner (Eds.), *Adult psychopathology and diagnosis* (4th ed., pp. 104–150). New York: Wiley.

Tryon, W. W., & Pinto, L. P. (1994). Comparing activity measurements and ratings. *Behavior Modification, 18,* 251–261.

Ullman, D. G., Barkley, R. A., & Brown, H. W. (1978). The behavioral symptoms of hyperkinetic children who successfully respond to stimulant drug treatment. *American Journal of Orthopsychiatry, 48,* 425–437.

Ullmann, R. K., Sleator, E. K., & Sprague, R. L. (1984). A new rating scale for diagnosing and monitoring of ADD children. *Psychopharmacology Bulletin, 20,* 160–164.

Ullmann, R. K., Sleator, E. K., & Sprague, R. L. (1997). *ACTeRS teacher and parent forms manual.* Champaign, IL: MetriTech, Inc.

van Egeren, L. A., Frank, S. J., & Paul, J. S. (1999). Daily behavior ratings among children and adolescent inpatients: The abbreviated child behavior rating form. *Journal of the American Academy of Child and Adolescent Psychiatry, 38,* 1417–1425.

Walters, C. E. (1965). Prediction of postnatal development from fetal activity. *Child Development, 36,* 801–808.

Werry, J. S. (1968). Developmental hyperactivity. *Pediatric Clinics of North America, 15,* 581–599.

Wilson, M. J., & Bullock, L. M. (1989). Psychometric characteristics of behavior rating scales: Definitions, problems, and solutions. *Behavioral Disorders, 14,* 186–200.

Zentall, S. S., & Leib, S. L. (1985). Structured tasks: Effects on activity and performance of hyperactive and comparison children. *Journal of Educational Research, 79,* 91–95.

7

Structured and Semistructured Interviews

HELEN ORVASCHEL

Center for Psychological Studies
Nova Southeastern University
Fort Lauderdale, Florida

INTRODUCTION

The purpose of this chapter is to provide an overview of the current state of the art of structured and semistructured interviews for use with children and adolescents. This author was involved in the first centralized review of instruments designed to assess psychopathology in youth (Orvaschel, Sholomskas, & Weissman, 1980a), as part of an NIMH initiative to determine the availability of instruments suitable for large-scale epidemiologic research in the child and adolescent psychopathology arena. In that monograph we challenged the field by stating, "Relatively few adequate, well-developed, and widely used instruments are available to assess psychiatric disorders in children. . . . It is hoped that this report will be viewed as an initial effort to centralize and disseminate information relevant to investigators of child psychopathology and that individuals are stimulated to improve the techniques of evaluation that are currently lacking" (p. 1).

The resulting monograph provided an impetus for ongoing development and progress in the field of diagnostic assessment procedures in youth and also served as a starting point for an NIMH initiative on assessment of child and adolescent psychopathology (the NIMH DISC; Costello, Edelbrock, Dulcan, Kalas, & Klaric, 1984). During the succeeding 25 years, many reviews on these assessments have been published (Edelbrock & Costello, 1988; Hodges & Zeman, 1993; Orvaschel, 1986, 1988, 1989; Orvaschel, Sholomskas, & Weissman, 1980b), in an ongoing effort to keep the field apprised of changes and progress in the availability of diagnostic interviewing measures. Given the maturity of the field, it is appropriate that this effort to update the subject be undertaken at this time.

This overview is intended to inform readers on the issues in diagnostic interviewing methods by discussing their commonalities as well as differences, such as developmental issues, distinctions between structured and semistructured, computerization, handling of multiple informants, and the utility and context of psychometrics. It should be noted, however, that this work is not intended to be an exhaustive examination of available instruments, for such reviews can be found in a variety of texts. On the contrary, the emphasis will be to provide a historical context on the subject, an update on the K-SADS-E, for which this author is best known (Orvaschel, 1995; Orvaschel & Puig-Antich, 1987), and an overview of established interviews.

HISTORICAL PERSPECTIVE

The use of structured and semistructured interviews with children has its history routed in the efforts of Rutter and Graham (1968) in the United Kingdom, who introduced semistructured diagnostic interviews with children as well as the inclusion of the child as informant, and Robins and Guze (1970), who pioneered diagnostic interviews with adults in the United States in order to establish diagnostic reliability. In the adult arena, the development of such assessments in the United States followed the establishment of specified diagnostic criteria. For example, the Research Diagnostic Criteria (RDC) (Spitzer, Endicott, & Robins, 1978) led to the development of the Schedule for Affective Disorders and Schizophrenia (SADS) (Spitzer & Endicott, 1978). The RDC was a precursor to the DSM-III (APA, 1980), which then led to the Diagnostic Interview Schedule (DIS; Robins, Helzer, Croughan, & Ratcliff, 1981) and subsequently to the Structured Clinical Interview for DSM-III-R (SCID; Spitzer & Williams, 1985). All this led to improved reliability in diagnosis by reducing both criteria and information variance (Spitzer et al., 1978). The move toward some degree of standardization of diagnostic assessment strategies for younger populations followed similar efforts successfully used with adults, but at a lagging pace. While those in the United Kingdom were innovating child assessments in the 1960s, the United States did not progress in this arena until the 1980s (Costello et al., 1984; Hodges, McKnew, Cytryn, Stern, & Kline, 1982; Kovacs, 1985; Orvaschel, Puig-Antich, Chambers, Tabrizi, & Johnson, 1982; Reich, Herjanic, Welner, & Grandhy, 1982; Schaffer, Fisher, Piacentini, Schwab-Stone, & Wicks, 1989).

The early efforts of Herjanic with the DICA (Herjanic, Herjanic, Brown, & Wheatt, 1975), Kovacs with the ISC (Kovacs, 1985), and Puig-Antich with the K-SADS (Puig-Antich & Chambers, 1978), as well as others mentioned in the original review (Orvaschel et al., 1980a), were largely motivated by their specific research interests and the need for systematic and replicable diagnostic procedures that could achieve appropriate levels of reliability and validity. The three interviews specifically just mentioned are still in use, despite many changes and revisions. Those in the original review that are not noted have largely disappeared from the field, while others have emerged. In all, seven structured and semistructured interviews appropriate for children and adolescents will be examined in this review. The three oldest interviews will be reviewed first, beginning with a more extensive review of the K-SADS/KSADS-E, which is the most widely used semistructured interview, followed by a review of the DICA and ISC/ISCA. The newer instruments will then be presented, beginning with the DISC, which is the most widely used structured interview, followed by the ADIS, CAPA, and CHIPS. Before discussing any specific interviews, some discussion on general issues about these assessment procedures is warranted.

ELEMENTS OF THE DIAGNOSTIC INTERVIEW

The diagnostic interviews currently available have several commonalities as well as significant differences. The selection process for a user should be based on how and why the evaluations are needed. When examining the commonalities, it should be noted that the interviews differ, even on features that they share. For example, virtually all interviews included here assess according to the *DSM-IV criteria*. However, several also include items for DSM-III, DSM-III-R, RDC, and even the ICD. Also, all assessments provide for broad *coverage of Axis I disorders*; only one or two attempt to include some elements of Axis II diagnosis. Nevertheless, some interviews clearly place greater emphasis on one or two categories of disorder (e.g., anxiety, mood), because the authors developed their interview with particular research interests in mind.

All the assessment procedures provide for evaluations of both children and adolescents, with some recommended *age ranges* from about 5 or 6 to 17 or 18. Such a large age range raises developmental issues regarding the wording of questions, length of interview, appropriate areas of assessment, and the like. The issues are not handled in a uniform manner across interviews, but they are always addressed. Some interviews have different questions for particular ages, some write questions primarily for the younger age group, and some include specific areas only for some ages (e.g., dating behavior for adolescents).

Another similarity across interviews is that all assess some aspects of *functioning* to determine if impairment is present. Nevertheless, they differ in how the assessment is made. Some ask about functioning in a global context, some cover specific areas of functioning, and some ask about functioning within particular episodes of psychopathology.

Finally, all interviews reviewed here include *parallel forms* for an adult informant (parent, caretaker) and a child/adolescent informant. Some have separate forms for the different informants, while some use the same form and simply provide a separate place for coding responses. Procedures also differ on whether the same or a different interviewer interviews both informants, as well as which informant goes first and how or if the information derived will be combined or kept separate.

Differences between interviews should also be noted. One such difference is the issue of *structured vs. semistructured format.* An interview that is presented as "structured" generally means that the questions written should be posed precisely and that the interviewer is given no discretion on what is asked or how it is asked. The procedures are more strictly adhered to, discouraging or precluding clinical judgment, because the interview is intended for use by lay interviewers, who should not be making decisions that have clinical implications. This is contrary to semistructured interview designs, which are intended to be used by professionals, individuals expected to make clinical judgments throughout the interview process. The semistructured arrangement provides latitude on wording of questions and flexibility in determining the clinical significance of responses.

Another factor that differentiates interviews is whether they are *symptom vs. syndrome oriented.* Some interviews cluster questions that are connected, such as all items related to sleep in one section and those related to school behavior in another section. Interview developers believe this format makes more logical sense to the informant, makes the interview flow more smoothly, and avoids redundancy. On the other hand, a syndrome-oriented interview clusters questions according to the disorder of inquiry. For example, sleep questions on a syndrome-oriented interview would be included in the depression section and would be asked about again, albeit somewhat differently, in the mania section. This allows the symptom to be evaluated in the time frame related to the disorder in question and follows the pattern of the psychopathology. The authors of these interviews argue that such groupings aid the informants in recall, help the respondents feel more understood in relation to their psychopathology (because symptom placement acknowledges that these behaviors are how the problem is often experienced), and follow more closely how clinicians make diagnostic determinations.

The *time frame* for the psychopathology assessed also differs from one interview to another and is somewhat related to the previous distinction on symptom vs. syndrome orientation. Some assessments target "current" behavior, in whatever format that term is applied (i.e., past month, past 3 months, past year), and some make "lifetime" assessments, which include "current" and "past" psychopathology. It is difficult for an interview to go beyond a current-psychopathology format if questions are grouped according to behaviors rather than syndromes, because symptoms must be clustered in time to determine if a diagnosable disorder is present. Therefore, while syndrome-oriented interviews may assess current or lifetime psychopathology, symptom-oriented interviews are more likely to be current only. Additionally, some interviews or parts of interviews assess behaviors as present (and clinically significant) or absent, while others assess behaviors according to *gradations of severity*, and the levels of severity also vary considerably across and within interviews.

Another important area of variability between evaluation procedures is how they are intended to derive a diagnosis. When more than one individual is interviewed, *informant variance* is the rule and not the exception (Kashani, Orvaschel, Burk, & Reid, 1985). Some assessments are designed to have different individuals interview informants and to then add together symptoms endorsed by either informant to derive a diagnosis. Other procedures include the use of separate diagnoses based on each informant or the use of another party to review some or all assessment material and provide a diagnosis; others use a summary procedure (clinically combining information from all informants) to determine diagnosis.

Finally, the issue of *computerization* also distinguishes interviews. While all the instruments included in this review allow for symptoms and disorders to be entered onto computer, some provide for computer administration and even computer-generated diagnoses. This feature is advantageous for many running research programs, reducing personnel needs and even diminishing errors. However, this attribute is best reserved for those interviews with a structured format. Efforts to "computerize" semistructured interviews ultimately lead to a reduction in the use of clinical judgment and turn the process into a far more structured effort than was originally intended.

PSYCHOMETRICS

Psychometric data are available for all diagnostic interviews generally recognized in the field, as well as those included in this review. These data generally refer to the validity and reliability of the interview in question. However, there is considerable disagreement as to what constitutes an appropriate test of validity or reliability for a diagnostic instrument. With respect to validity, the controversy is due, in part, to the relationship between the validity of the measure and the validity of the underlying construct. More specifically, an evaluation of this type cannot reflect the accurate measurement of a disorder if the fundamental paradigm on which the disorder is based is invalid. Therefore, the validity of an interview is dependent on the nosologic system it represents.

With the foregoing caveat in mind, it is clear that all the interviews included here have achieved face and content validity. That is to say, they have all been constructed by experts in the field who are knowledgeable about and understand psychopathology contained in their respective instruments and who complied with current criteria systems when devising the interviews. Correspondingly, all available interviews have demonstrated some discriminate validity by distinguishing disorder rates in patient and nonpatient populations, or high- and low-risk samples, or similarly appropriate differentials. Most have also shown some level of concurrent validity, in that they have been compared favorably to another available interview or have shown comparability with a purported benchmark, such as a professional assessment, chart diagnosis, and the like. The difficulty here is that the field has been unable to agree on a "gold standard" with which to compare interview-derived diagnoses, so the benchmark varies for each.

Reliability has also been established for all available instruments. This has been primarily in the form of test–retest and interrater procedures. The test–retest paradigm is useful but may be compromised by informants' tendency to underreport on a second interview. In addition, symptoms and disorders may indeed change from one time period to another as the result of actual decline or improvement in functioning, again reducing reliability coefficients. These difficulties are avoided when examining interrater agreement, necessary to demonstrate the instruments' consistency in the hands of different examiners. Nevertheless, rater agreement can be affected by the nature of the population studied, the severity of the psychopathology, and the age and communication skills of the informant.

Irrespective of the psychometric data available, those who use a structured or semistructured diagnostic interview must establish its reliability at the site in which it will be used and with the personnel who are responsible for its administration. Given the nature of these instruments, they may be highly reliable in a particular site, but this reliability does not automatically transfer to new users. Rater agreement and comparability of administration cannot be assumed unless established and tested; even then, ongoing maintenance and monitoring is needed to avoid the gradual introduction of error and interviewer drift. Therefore, researchers and clinicians alike must ensure appropriate training and supervision of staff responsible for the ascertainment of data from diagnostic interviews.

Finally, structured and semistructured interviews are expected to provide comprehensive and systematic data relevant to making a diagnosis, but they were never intended to rule out or replace other evaluations. Their employment does not preclude the use of supplementary measures to assess additional domains that may be relevant to understanding the subject or patient. These include assessments such as I.Q. tests, life events, family functioning or family psychiatric history, and paper-and-pencil measures of severity for particular areas of symptomatology (e.g., anxiety, depression, ADHD). The latter would be particularly helpful additions for quantifying treatment progress or outcome or more closely examining particular domains of psychopathology.

SPECIFIC DIAGNOSTIC INTERVIEWS

SCHEDULE FOR AFFECTIVE DISORDERS FOR SCHOOL-AGED CHILDREN—PRESENT STATE OR EPIDEMIOLOGIC VERSION (K-SADS-P OR K-SADS-E)

The history of the K-SADS, in all its incarnations, is intricately intertwined with overall efforts in child diagnostic assessment since around 1980 and should be viewed in that context. The K-SADS is a semistructured diagnostic interview designed to ascertain and record the signs and symptoms of Axis I child and adolescent psychopathology. It was developed initially by Joaquim Puig-Antich and William Chambers (working at the Psychiatric Institute, Columbia University School of Medicine) in the late 1970s to provide a systematic method for assessing children who participated in a psychobiology of prepubertal depression research program (Puig-Antich & Chambers, 1978). They used the adult version of the Schedule for Affective Disorders and Schizophrenia (SADS) (Endicott & Spitzer, 1978) as a point of departure, hence the name, KIDDIE-SADS, coined by Kim Puig-Antich. At that time in its use, the interview was referred to simply as the K-SADS. The 1978 version assessed Research Diagnostic Criteria (RDC) (Spitzer et al., 1978) for affective disorders, schizophrenia, some of the anxiety disorders (separation anxiety, generalized anxiety, phobias, obsessions, compulsions, and depersonalization/derealization), and many of the symptoms of Conduct Disorder.

It was in 1978 that this author first met with Drs. Puig-Antich and Chambers and discussed using the K-SADS in a pilot study to assess psychopathology in children of depressed parents (Orvaschel, Weissman, Padian, & Lowe, 1981). However, because the proposed study population was not of identified patients but of "at-risk" children, the interview needed to be modified to assess past as well as current symptoms and disorders. As a result, the first version of a "lifetime" K-SADS was born, although no name had as yet been assigned. The interview was constructed on a typewriter and was virtually identical to the existing (version 2) K-SADS, except that rather than a rating for "current episode" and for "last week" as in the original, ratings were made for "current episode" and "past episode." In addition, space was allocated to record some aspects of chronology (i.e., ages at first and last episode, durations of current and longest episode) for each of the disorders covered.

While conducting that study, this author began working with Drs. Puig-Antich and Chambers and another member of their research team (Mary Ann Tabrizi) on the refinement of an alternative version of the K-SADS that would assess past and current psychopathology. The second working draft, completed in June 1979, was the product of that collaboration and was the first time the term *Epidemiologic Version* (K-SADS-E; Orvaschel, Puig-Antich, Tabrizi, & Chambers, 1979) was used. The interview form contained columns for coding current and most severe past episodes of disorder, screen questions that allowed the interviewer to skip sections, and additional categories, such as attention deficit, conduct, alcohol abuse, and drug abuse disorders. Reference to the K-SADS as the Present State (P) version did not begin with any consistency until the 1980s, when data were presented on its test–retest reliability (Chambers, Puig-Antich, Hirsch, Paez, Ambrosini, Tabrizi, & Davies, 1985). Revisions of the P version through at least the fourth working draft were motivated primarily by changes in diagnostic criteria systems, but the interview's primary format and most of the original wording to questions were retained (Puig-Antich & Ryan, 1986).

While some of us preferred calling the modified interview the "lifetime" version, again Dr. Puig-Antich prevailed, and the cover page of this version stated, "It is designed to ascertain both past and current episodes of psychopathology in epidemiologic research. Issues concerned with levels of symptom severity and treatment effects are best addressed by use of the K-SADS-P. For clinical studies of past psychopathology the K-SADS-L is recommended." Dr. Puig-Antich intended for the lifetime version, or "L-version," to assess only past episodes of disorder; in fact, a draft of the K-SADS-L was completed in December 1979 (Puig-Antich, Chambers, Orvaschel, & Tabrizi, 1979). It contained screen questions that assessed whether the child "ever" suffered from a particular problem (e.g., depressed mood). Notes were recorded for chronology, and symptom ratings were recorded only for worst past episode. If an ongoing disorder was noted, the interviewer was instructed to switch to the present episode version of the K-SADS. Because of the cumbersome nature of this procedure, the L-version was eventually dropped from the K-SADS repertoire in the early 1980s and only the P and E versions were retained to assess present episode and lifetime psychopathology. Nevertheless, the name "epidemiologic version" had already been established and was therefore retained.

The third version of the K-SADS-E (Puig-Antich, Orvaschel, Tabrizi, & Chambers, 1980), written to follow DSM-III criteria (APA, 1980), was used to test the reliability of retrospective assessment (Orvaschel, Puig-Antich, Chambers, Tabrizi, & Johnson, 1982). Although very similar to version 2 in all respects except for criteria changes from RDC to DSM-III, this version added a separate Scoring Form, anorexia nervosa, and diagnostic decision trees for the mood and psychosis sections. The decision to move from severity ratings to a presence-or-absence coding system for individual symptoms was predicated on previous experience demonstrating difficulty in obtaining information on past behaviors that would yield adequate reliability at that level of specificity. Therefore, from version 2 through version 4, items on the K-SADS-E were rated as present (2) or absent (1), with a code 2 affirming that the item was present at a clinically significant level, generally corresponding to a code 3 or higher on the K-SADS-P.

Version 3 remained in use until DSM-III-R (APA, 1987) was introduced, necessitating the move to version 4 of the K-SAD-E (Orvaschel & Puig-Antich, 1987). This revision resulted in far more dramatic changes to the interview in both content and structure. In addition to accommodating to new or different criteria, content changes included the addition of depression and mania not otherwise specified (NOS), sections for bulimia nervosa, oppositional disorder, cigarette use, and, later, post-traumatic stress disorder (PTSD). Structural changes were, at times, necessitated by changes in DSM criteria. For example, because of the increased clarity in the conceptualization of phobias, this disorder was divided into three distinct subsections in place of one global phobia category.

However, some criteria changes in the nosologic system appeared to be less conceptually or empirically based. This resulted in a section added to many of the disorder categories called "other characteristics," or OC. These sections of the interview often incorporated items that had been part of a previous criteria system but were excluded from the DSM revision of the time (i.e., alcohol-use items from RDC) or were considered of clinical interest but were not required in the DSM (i.e., ADD items). It was hoped that the addition of this material would allow users and investigators to record information that could be reconstituted at a later date, if needed, because of subsequent changes in the DSM system and even the potential return to previous criteria. It was also hoped that the material in the OC section might be useful to those who wished to further describe and elucidate characteristics of some forms of child psychopathology beyond the criteria provided in the DSM system of the day.

Additional structural changes included extensive alterations in the substance use sections and the recording of chronology for all disorders covered. Changes in the drug abuse category were inspired by the format used in the Diagnostic Interview Schedule (DIS) (Robins, Helzer, Ratcliff, & Seyfried, 1982). In addition to ascertainment of symptoms that were present, this innovative procedure allowed for recording of specific drug classes involved in each criterion.

K-SADS-E VERSION 5

The decision to again revise the K-SADS-E was based on the publication of DSM-IV diagnostic criteria, with which version 5 is compatible. However, more than criterion-based questions were changed. During the eight years of use of version 4, many suggestions for revision were provided by users from around the world, and some of these suggestions were incorporated in the most recent interview. The most frequent requests concerned the provision of severity ratings for specific symptom items rather than just for overall categories of disorder. This was especially important to those who wished to use the E rather than the P version of the K-SADS with patient populations and for treatment outcome studies.

Because concerns regarding poor reliability for past symptom-severity ratings did not hold true for ratings of current behaviors, a compromise decision was made. This compromise resulted in the most salient change in this latest version of the K-SADS-E, the availability of severity ratings for current symptoms, while retaining the previous format of ratings of present (clinically significant = code 2) or absent (code 1) for past symptoms. Not all current behaviors have a severity-rating choice attached. The presence of psychotic symptoms is considered severe by definition, and they are therefore rated as absent, suspected, or definite (as in version 4). Additional changes include the permanent addition of a PTSD section, the inclusion of criteria items for a proposed alternate version of dysthymia contained in the DSM-IV appendix, and myriad changes needed to accommodate disorder criteria changes in the DSM.

Of course, much was retained and sometimes expanded from previous versions, such as the "Other Characteristics" sections (non-DSM-IV criteria items carried over from previous systems or items of potential clinical interest), systematized chronology sections, overall disorder severity ratings, and especially the interview format. The order of interview sections, informants, and flow has remained stable, as has the use of summary ratings, the inquiry and notation of chronology before specific coding of items, and the need for use of interviewer discretion and clinical judgment in questioning. In fact, the omission of a computer-administered version of the K-SADS-E as well as a computerized scoring system is intentional and predicated on the assumption that such a development would undermine the semistructured nature of the interview intended by the authors and ultimately lead to its use in a structured format by lay interviewers.

Administration of the K-SADS-E, a syndrome-oriented instrument, requires a brief unstructured time (about 5 minutes) during which rapport is established and the interviewer inquires about the child's interests, school functioning, family relationships, and physical health. This information is intended for use later, in the more structured portion, when the previously acquired details may be used to determine functional impairment in these areas. Inquiry proceeds to sections on history of treatment and medication for emotional/behavioral problems, also intended for use later in the interview. The discussion then moves to specific topics of psychopathology, beginning with mood disorders, psychosis, anxiety disorders, and so on. Questions are written in wording most appropriate for younger children. Interviewers are instructed to alter wording as needed for adolescents and to use third person when speaking with the parent. The mother (parent, caretaker) is always interviewed first, followed by an interview with the child/adolescent. Responses of each informant are recorded, and summary ratings for each symptom are made during the interview with the child. Attempts to resolve discrepancies in information are made during the course of the interview with the child so that the summary rating reflects the best estimate of information provided by all sources. Diagnoses are based on the summary ratings. These are not intended to be additive versions of the mother's and child's responses, but the clinician's best judgment of that which approximates "truth." The interview takes between 30 and 60 minutes per informant to administer, depending on the nature and extent of psychopathology present.

Psychometric data on the K-SADS have been examined from its earliest adaptations (Chambers et al., 1985; Orvaschel et al., 1982) to its most recent edition. Interrater reliability for version 5 of the K-SADS-E has yielded a mean kappa coefficient of .66. Kappa coefficients for specific disorders are as follows: MDD .73; Dysthymia .72; Other Depression (i.e., Adjustment Disorder with depressed mood and Depression NOS) .49; Separation Anxiety .65; Any Phobia/Panic .75; Other Anxiety Disorder (i.e., GAD/OAD, OCD, PTSD) .63; ADHD .77; Conduct Disorder .68; and Oppositional Disorder .51. Mean correlation coefficients for past symptoms of major depression were .81, .72, and .69 for mother, child, and summary ratings, respectively; for current symptoms of major depression the mean correlations were .81, .79, and .70 for mother, child, and summary ratings, respectively. Mean correlations for mother, child, and summary ratings for current dysthymia were .65, .59, and .66, respectively, and for current mania, .75, .72, and .45, respectively (sample size was insufficient to calculate correlations for past symptoms for these disorders).

Evolution of the interview has always been guided by the intent to provide a vehicle for the systematic ascertainment of signs and symptoms of psychopathology in school-age children, appropriate for use by clinicians and clinical researchers. The point of departure was the diagnostic system available at the time, beginning with the RDC (Spitzer & Endicott, 1978), through the DSM-III, III-R (in varying stages of draft form), and culminating in the DSM-IV. But beyond this framework was the hope of providing a bridge between the current epistemology and the data needed to bring us to the next phase of diagnostic clarity. The K-SADS-E version 5 is the most recent stage of the process described. It was copyrighted so that efforts to present altered versions under its name are prevented. It is widely used in clinical and epidemiologic research in the United States and worldwide, including countries in Europe, Asia, Africa, South America, and the Middle East.

DIAGNOSTIC INTERVIEW FOR CHILDREN AND ADOLESCENTS (DICA)

The DICA was initially developed by Herjanic and her colleagues at Washington University in St. Louis as a semistructured interview for research purposes (Herjanic et al., 1975). While many report that the DICA was modeled after the adult Diagnostic Interview Schedule (DIS) by Robins (Robins et al., 1981), the first version predated the DIS by almost a decade. Following the introduction of the DIS in epidemiologic research, Herjanic joined with others to revise the DICA to make it more structured and to improve reliability (Herjanic & Reich, 1982). Its most recent incarnations assess symptoms for most Axis I disorders according to DSM-IV criteria, assess "lifetime" disorders, have separate interviews for children (6–12) and adolescents (13–18), and fall somewhere between structured and semistructured in organization, requiring what is referred to as "highly trained" lay interviewers (Reich, 2000). There is also a computerized version, although reliability rates have been reportedly lower than for the interviewer-administered version (Reich, Cottler, McCallum, Corwin, & VanEerdwegh, 1995).

The DICA is syndrome oriented and, although the format allows the interviewer to probe responses, the probes are predefined in the interview process. Requests for explanations or clarification are also handled by material already written and provided in the interview manual. Despite the authors' claim that the DICA is semistructured, its reliance on lay interviewers and the formulaic responses to questions have it fall more closely in the structured-interview camp. It is unclear how a composite diagnosis is derived; but, similar to the DISC, the DICA appears to derive diagnoses in separate or additive formats. The interview is reported to take between 1 and 3 hours to administer by an interviewer, depending on the extent of psychopathology present. Reliability and validity have been studied over the years for various versions of the interview (Herjanic & Reich, 1982; Reich et al., 1982; Welner, Reich, Herjanic, Jung, & Amado, 1987).

Test–retest reliability for a recent version reports kappas ranging from .32 for ADHD in children to .92 for Conduct Disorder in adolescents (Reich, 2000). Most of the kappas reported for the diagnostic categories were in the moderate-to-high range. The report did not indicate if these data were for current or lifetime disorders or whether the diagnoses were based on one informant or were derived from composite information.

The DICA has a lengthy history and has been available and used since the 1970s. It has evolved over the years to address changes in criteria and has attempted to deal with developmental considerations in the assessment process. Although Dr. Herjanic retired many years ago, the interview's current authors have continued efforts to improve the diagnostic process, and modifications have resulted in specialized offshoots that examine specific areas of assessment appropriate for studies on the genetics of alcoholism, ADHD, and the like. The DICA is widely used in the United States and other countries, particularly targeting genetic and smaller-scale epidemiologic studies, and remains an interesting and viable diagnostic assessment choice.

INTERVIEW SCHEDULE FOR CHILDREN AND ADOLESCENTS (ISCA)

The ISCA, originally named the Interview Schedule for Children (ISC), was developed in the mid- to late 1970s (Kovacs, 1985) for use with Kovacs' longitudinal study of depression in children. Like the other diagnostic interviews that are still in use and were part of that first review (Orvaschel et al., 1980a), this instrument has undergone many revisions and alterations. Nevertheless, its initial focus and underlying structure have remained intact. The ISCA is a semistructured diagnostic interview for school-aged children (8–17). It is symptom oriented, has parallel versions for parent and child, and asks information on signs and symptoms that cover a range of diagnostic categories. In addition to symptoms of psychopathology, the interview contains items to assess mental status, dating and sexual behavior, and some interviewer observations.

It was designed to be administered by experienced clinicians who undergo extensive training on the instrument. Interviews are conducted separately with each informant, by the same interviewer. Composite diagnoses are derived from summary ratings that reflect the best estimate of the information obtained. Initial evaluations with this interview are estimated to range between 2 and 4 hours (2–2½ for parent; 45 minutes to 1½ hours for child). Ratings of symptom severity are made, although the range may vary from 0 to 8 points to 0 to 3 points. Timelines are used to chart onsets and offsets of symptoms and disorders, and the interview's time frame is current psychopathology (past 2 weeks to past 6 months, depending on the disorder). However, a revision is available that provides instruction for obtaining information that reportedly assesses "lifetime" diagnoses (ISCA-C & L). There are also versions that focus on follow-up for both children and adults and some that are appropriate for collateral informants (ISCA-

Current and Interim version, ISCA-C & I; Follow-up Interview Schedule for Adults, FISA) (Sherrill & Kovacs, 2000). The development of these alternative or supplemental evaluations has been motivated by the needs of the longitudinal research conducted by its author.

The ISCA allows diagnoses to be derived from most nosologic systems (e.g., DSM-IV, ICD) and covers a comprehensive range, including all mood categories (i.e., MDD, dysthymia, mania, hypomania), anxiety (i.e., phobias, OCD, GAD, SAD), elimination (i.e., enuresis, encopresis), disruptive (i.e., ADHD, CD, ODD), eating, and substance disorders. Reliability and validity have been studied over the years for various versions of the interview. Current reports on intraclass correlations for rater agreement are generally high, with correlation coefficients ranging mostly in the .80s and .90s; far fewer kappas were reported and they ranged from .22 to 1.0. Intraclass correlations for depression items, mania items, conduct items, and anxiety items are .96, .85, .93, and .95, respectively (Sherrill & Kovacs, 2000). Users should note that many of these interrater reliability correlations are based on ratings from interviewers who may have been trained for weeks or even months. Additional categories covered in the ISCA include some Axis II categories (i.e., antisocial, borderline, histrionic, schizotypal, compulsive) and groupings such as bereavement, sleep disorder, somatization, and psychosis, but the reliabilities of these clusters are unclear.

The ISCA/ISC has a lengthy history and has been available and used since the late 1970s. It has evolved over the years, primarily to address the needs of its developer, and has been a valuable research tool for diagnostic determination and the measurement of severity in research. Despite these assets, several disadvantages have limited its use. The ISCA is time consuming to administer and requires a more extensive training period than any of the other diagnostic interviews available, even when used by experienced clinicians. As a result, this interview has rarely been used by investigators other than its author. There have been exceptions, such as occasional use by researchers of anxiety (Last, Francis, Hersen, Kazdin, & Strauss, 1987) and suicidal behavior (Goldston et al., 1996), but even in these circumstances alternative assessments were sometimes utilized by these investigators (i.e., ADIS). The ISCA remains a more cumbersome diagnostic tool than its contemporaries, with idiosyncrasies that continue to limit more widespread appeal.

NATIONAL INSTITUTE OF MENTAL HEALTH DIAGNOSTIC INTERVIEW SCHEDULE FOR CHILDREN—VERSION IV (NIMH DISC-IV)

The NIMH DISC-IV was developed originally between 1979 and 1984 (Edelbrock, Costello, Dulcan, Conover, & Kala, 1986) as a result of an initiative intended to launch a multisite study of children and adolescents. This endeavor was similar to the Epidemiologic Catchment Area (ECA) study of adults (Myers et al., 1984) and resulted in the multisite Methods for the Epidemiology of Child and Adolescent Mental Disoders (MECA) study (Lahey et al., 1996), using the DISC available at the time. Version IV of this instrument, made available in 1997, follows criteria of the DSM-IV and the ICD-10. Adaptations have also been (or are in the process of being) developed and include telephone, teacher, and brief versions. While initial development of the DISC was motivated by the needs of large-scale epidemiologic research, it has since been, and continues to be, used in other types of research and sometimes in clinical settings.

The history of the DISC is lengthy, and changes from the first version to its current state are so extensive that its likeness to the original is largely in principal only. From its onset, the DISC has been a fully structured diagnostic interview designed for administration by lay interviewers. As with most such interviews, there are parallel versions administered to children (DISC-Y) and their parents or caretakers (DISC-P). It is symptom oriented in design, and composite diagnoses are derived by adding information from parent and child interviews. The DISC-IV allows for the assessment of approximately 30 Axis I diagnoses and is available in both English and Spanish translation (Shaffer, Fisher, Lucas, Dulcan, & Schwab-Stone, 2000). Psychometric testing of all versions was conducted, and data on the most recent version indicates kappa test–retest reliability ranging from .05 to .96, depending on the disorder, informant, and sample tested (Shaffer, Fisher, Lucas et al., 2000). For example, the kappa for panic disorder with child informants in a community sample is reported to be .05, while the kappa for specific phobia with parent informants in a clinical sample is reported to be .96. In light of the original purpose of the DISC, use in large-scale epidemiologic research, the more relevant data may be its reliability from combined (parent and child) informants in community samples. Kappa statistics for diagnostic categories include ADHD .48, ODD .59, CD .66, OAD .52, SAD .49, social phobia .44, and MDD .45, suggesting moderate test–retest reliability in many disorders of interest. Validity studies have largely not been conducted. Administration of the interview in its entirety takes between approximately $2\frac{1}{2}$ and 4 hours, the shorter range for community samples and the latter for clinical samples.

Considerable NIMH resources, financial and otherwise, have been expended to develop and refine the DISC and to encourage its use. In this respect, it has a number of advantages, such as more variety of parallel versions and translations than any other child and adolescent diagnostic interview. It is widely used in the United States and in many other countries, allowing for some cross-national and international comparisons in prevalence and incidence data. Its structured format allows for lay interviewer or computer administration and for computer-derived diagnoses. Efforts at modularization and the development of shorter versions may enhance its attractiveness to users. Interestingly, the characteristics that make it attractive to some consumers make it unattractive to others. Specifically, its highly structured format, administration by lay interviewers, and computer compatibility are viewed by many researchers and clinicians as undesirable, and the exercise of clinical judgment is considered an asset, particularly for those who place a strong premium on questions linked to diagnostic validity.

ANXIETY DISORDERS INTERVIEW SCHEDULE FOR CHILDREN (ADIS)

The ADIS was developed by Silverman and Nelles (1988) in order to overcome noted shortcomings of existing child and adolescent interviews. The authors correctly observed that other assessments had reported unacceptably low reliability scores for anxiety disorders, making them particularly less suitable for research in this category of psychopathology. The ADIS is a semistructured, syndrome-oriented diagnostic interview targeting children between the ages of 6 and 18. It is intended to be administered by trained clinicians, has parallel versions administered directly to children (ADIS-C) and to their parents/mothers (ADIS-P), and takes approximately 1 hour per informant to administer.

Coverage of anxiety disorders on the ADIS includes separation anxiety (SAD), generalized anxiety/overanxious (GAD/OAD), post-traumatic stress (PTSD), obsessive-compulsive (OCD), all the phobias (agora-, social, specific, and school), panic, and avoidant disorders. In addition, the interview assesses such additional categories of psychopathology as mood and disruptive behavior (ADHD, ODD, and CD) disorders, schizophrenia, enuresis, and sleep terrors. Interrater and test–retest reliability and validity data have yielded promising results, particularly when compared with other interviews, and established the ADIS as an important competitor when selecting an evaluation tool for child anxiety. In one report, test–retest reliability coefficients were lowest for agoraphobia and OCD in children aged 6–11, but were generally moderate to high for most other categories of anxiety (i.e., .51–.75 for SAD; .67–.73 for GAD; .44–.61 for social phobia) (Silverman & Eisen, 1992). Results were less promising for mood disorders. In a subsequent report, kappas for the anxiety disorders were excellent, yielding composite scores of .84 for SAD, .92 for social phobias, .81 for specific phobia, and .80 for GAD, as well as high coefficients for symptom scales and severity ratings (Silverman, Saavedra, & Pina, 2001). Interrater agreement is also reportedly excellent, with kappas of .84 for child interviews, .83 for parent interviews, and .78 for composite interviews.

Similar to other instruments, impetus for development of the ADIS was spearheaded by the research interests of its authors. Existing measures were not providing sufficiently reliable assessments of anxiety disorders in childhood and a need arose for a more satisfactory procedure. The authors expanded questioning in the anxiety categories to achieve their objective of a more thorough evaluation of child anxiety disorders. Administration is achieved by trained clinicians, and most questions require elaboration. The interview obtains quantifiable data on symptoms and assesses course and severity of pathology. The ADIS may be a later addition to the diagnostic interview arsenal, but it has acquired many adherents with interests in child and adolescent anxiety. However, its attention to other categories (than anxiety) of disorder is primarily for the purposes of differential diagnosis, making it less advantageous for general clinical use or research targeting nonanxiety categories of psychopathology.

CHILD AND ADOLESCENT PSYCHIATRIC ASSESSMENT (CAPA)

The CAPA is a structured diagnostic interview for children between the ages of 9 and 17 years (Angold & Costello, 2000). It was designed in "modular form" so that individual sections can be administered independent of the rest of the interview. The authors also provide a glossary that defines each symptom in very specific detail as well as how to code different levels of symptom severity. The manual for the interview provides strict rules for how to ask questions, including when questions are mandatory and when they are considered discretionary. Most symptoms are assessed for the 3-month period prior to interview, although exceptions are noted for infrequently occurring behaviors.

The CAPA covers symptoms of psychopathology for most Axis I disorders, including the disruptive (e.g., ADHD, CD, ODD), mood, anxiety, substance use, eating, elimination, sleep, and tic disorders. There are also sections on observable behavior, social functioning (i.e., school, home, etc.), the family, life events, sociodemographics, and the like. It can be administered by professionals or lay interviewers, although extensive training is required irrespective of qualifications. There is a parallel version for parents, and there are versions for young adults (YAPA) age 18+, preschoolers (PAPA) ages 3–6, which is administered to their parents, a Spanish translation, and a shortened version of the interview with more skip-outs. Administration of the regular interview is estimated to take approximately an hour per informant.

The psychometric properties of the CAPA have been examined, and kappa coefficients for test–retest reliability have been reported to range from .55 for CD to 1.0 for substance use disorders (Angold & Costello, 1995). Various measures of concurrent validity have also yielded promising results (Angold & Costello, 2000). Despite these assets, the CAPA has not been widely used by researchers other than the authors and their colleagues and collaborators. This may be due to its unwieldy design and burdensomely expensive training, estimated by its authors as costing approximately $600 per trainee and $2000 in fixed costs (Angold & Costello, 200).

CHILDREN'S INTERVIEW FOR PSYCHIATRIC SYNDROMES (ChIPS)

The ChIPS was developed by Elizabeth Weller and colleagues (Weller, Weller, Fristad, Rooney, & Schecter, 2000) to target diagnostic assessment in young children and to stick more closely to symptoms in the available nosologic system.

More specifically, the authors stated that they reviewed the most frequently used diagnostic interviews at the time (e.g., CAS, DISA-R, DISC, ISC, and K-SADS) and decided that existing questions were too complex for younger children and that better adherence to the DSM-III criteria was needed. The resulting tool was believed to provide a structured psychiatric interview with shorter, more easily understood questions that could be comprehended by children ages 6–11 years with I.Q.s of 70 and over.

Development of the specific interview format and questions is somewhat different than most available assessments of its type. In this syndrome-oriented interview, the authors designed the interview so that syndromes were assessed in the order of their estimated prevalence in the general population. Therefore, disruptive behavior disorders (e.g., ODD, CD, substance disorders) are assessed first, followed by anxiety disorders (e.g., phobias, SAD, GAD), eating disorders, mood disorders, elimination disorders, and psychosis, and ending with two sections on stressors, viewed as potentially sensitive and requiring rapport. The questions within each disorder are also ordered as they appear in the DSM, which is assumed to be in decreasing order of frequency. This interview is highly structured, provides frequent skips out of sections for which initial (screen) questions are not endorsed, and is intended for administration by trained lay interviewers. A parent version (P-ChIPS) parallels the child version, and revised additions extend the interview into adolescence, so the age range of the ChIPS is now 6–18 years. Administration time is reportedly estimated to range from about 20 minutes to a little less than an hour, depending on subject's age and extent of psychopathology, and it is assumed that this estimate is per informant.

Several studies have examined the psychometric properties of the ChIPS, particularly how it compares with similar assessments of psychopathology (Fristad et al., 1988b). Concurrent validity was examined by comparing the ChIPS to the DICA on child inpatients. Kappa coefficicents between .31 and .73 were reported for 13 of the disorders covered (Teare, Fristad, Weller, Weller, & Salmon, 1998a). Similar studies on subsequent (DSM-IIIR and DSM-IV) versions of the interviews, with both inpatient and outpatient children and adolescents, reported kappas ranging from .28 to .75, with reported mean kappas between .4 and .5. (Fristad et al., 1988a, 1988b). It should be noted that some agreement rates may have been inflated, because some of the samples assessed included inpatients.

Motivation for development of this instrument again appears to be the research interests of its authors, who describe it as a structured, diagnostic screening instrument. It is briefer than its "competitors" and is purportedly appropriate for trained lay interviewer administration. However, "lay" interviewers used in the studies reported would be viewed by many as clinicians (e.g., psychology graduate students, medical students). Therefore, it is unclear whether the interview's reliability would fare as well if it were in the hands of truly lay interviewers.

As to the interview's structure, the authors designed the order of syndromes assessed according to their estimated prevalence in the general population. Problems with this pattern may occur because diagnostic decision making sometimes requires the clustering of syndromes so that issues relevant to differential questions can be addressed. For example, the prevalence of psychosis is low in the child population, but its presence requires differentials of mood disorder with psychotic features or schizophrenia or schizo-affective disorder, questions that may be difficult to resolve when their assessment lacks temporal proximity. Similarly, assessing for CD precludes the need to assess for ODD, despite the fact that the latter occurs with greater prevalence. Concerns about the ordering of questions within each disorder, in decreasing order of frequency according to the DSM, should also be noted. For many of the disorders, the DSM-assumed frequency of symptoms is the rate reported for adults and not for children (i.e., mood disorders). Finally, there is some lack of clarity on how or whether a consensus diagnosis is derived. The use of this instrument by clinical and epidemiologic researchers other than the authors is not yet widespread.

SUMMARY

Structured and semistructured diagnostic interviews appropriate for use with school-age children are reviewed. Emphasis is placed on the historical context of the subject and on updating readers on the K-SADS-E. A discussion of issues relevant to diagnostic interviewing is also provided, particularly with respect to developmental issues, distinctions between structured and semistructured, computerization, handling of multiple informants, and the utility and context of psychometrics. While the review is not intended as an exhaustive look at all available child diagnostic interviews, it is intended to provide an overview of established interviews, their advantages and disadvantages, and the direction of the field.

REFERENCES AND RESOURCES

American Psychiatric Association. (1980). *Diagnostic and statistical manual of mental disorders, 3rd edition (DSM-III)*. Washington, DC: Author.

American Psychiatric Association. (1987). *Diagnostic and statistical manual of mental disorders, 3rd edition revised (DSM-III-R)*. Washington, DC: Author.

Angold, A., & Costello, E. J. (1995). A test–retest reliability study of child-reported psychiatric symptoms and diagnoses using the Child and Adolescent Psychiatric Assessment (CAPA-C). *Psychological Medicine, 25,* 755–762.

Angold, A., & Costello, E. J. (2000). The Child and Adolescent Psychiatric Assessment. *Journal of the American Academy of Child Psychiatry, 39,* 39–48.

Chambers, W. J., Puig-Antich, J., Hirsch, M., Paez, P., Ambrosini, P., Tabrizi, M. A., & Davies, M. (1985). The assessment of affective disorders in children and adolescents by semistructured interview. *Archives of General Psychiatry, 42,* 696–702.

Costello, A. J., Edelbrock, C. S., Dulcan, M. D., Kalas, R., & Klaric, S. H. (1984). Report of the NIMH Diagnostic Interview Schedule for Children (DISC). Washington, DC: National Institute of Mental Health.

Edelbrock C., & Costello, A. J. (1988). A review of structured psychiatric interviews for children. In M. Rutter, A. H. Tuma, & I. Lann (eds.), *Assessment and diagnosis in child and adolescent psychopathology*. New York: Guilford.

Edelbrock, C., Costello, A. J., Dulcan, M. K., Conover, N. C., & Kala, R. (1986). Parent–child agreement on child psychiatric symptoms assessed via structured interview. *Journal of Child Psychology Psychiatry, 27,* 181–190.

Endicott, J., & Spitzer, R. L. (1978). A diagnostic interview: The SADS. *Archives of General Psychiatry, 35,* 837–853.

Fristad, M. A., Cummins, J., Verducci, J. S., Teare, M., Weller, E. B., & Weller, R. A. (1988a). Study IV: Concurrent validity of the DSM-IV revised Children's Interview for Psychiatric Syndromes (ChIPS). *Journal of Child and Adolescent Psychopharmacology, 8,* 227–236.

Fristad, M. A., Glickman, A. R., Verducci, J. S., Teare, M., Weller, E. B., & Weller, R. A. (1988b). Study V: Children's Interview for Psychiatric Syndromes (ChIPS): psychometrics in two community samples. *Journal of Child and Adolescent Psychopharmacology, 8,* 237–245.

Goldston, D. B., Daniel, S. S., Reboussin, D. M., Kelley, A., Ievers, C., & Brunstetter, R. (1996). First-time suicide attempters, repeat attempters, and previous attempters on an adolescent inpatient psychiatry unit. *Journal of the American Academy of Child Psychiatry, 35,* 631–639.

Herjanic, B., Herjanic, M., Brown, F., & Wheatt, T. (1975). Are children reliable reporters? *Journal of Abnormal Child Psychology, 3,* 41–48.

Herjanic, B., & Reich, W. (1982). Development of a structured psychiatric interview for children: Agreement between child and parent on individual symptoms. *Journal of Abnormal Child Psychology, 10,* 307–324.

Hodges, K., McKnew, D., Cytryn, L., Stern, L., & Kline, J. (1982). The Child Assessment Schedule (CAS) diagnostic interview: A report on reliability and validity. *Journal of the American Academy of Child Psychiatry, 21,* 468–473.

Kashani, J. H., Orvaschel, H., Burk, J. P., & Reid, J. C. (1985). Informant variance: The issue of parent–child disagreement. *Journal of the American Academy of Child Psychiatry, 24,* 437–446.

Kovacs, M. (1985). The Interview Schedule for Children. *Psychopharmacology Bulletin, 21,* 991–994.

Lahey, B. B., et al. (1996). The NIMH Methods for the Epidemiology of Child and Adolescent Mental Disorders (MECA) Study: background and methodology. *Journal of the American Academy of Child and Adolescent Psychiatry, 35,* 855–864.

Last, C. G., Francis, G., Hersen, M., Kazdin, A. E., & Strauss, C. C. (1987). Separation anxiety and school phobia: A comparison using DSM-III criteria. *American Journal of Psychiatry, 144,* 653–657.

Myers, J. K., et al. (1984). Six-month prevalence of psychiatric disorders in three communities: 1980–1982. *Archives of General Psychiatry, 41,* 959–967.

Orvaschel, H. (1986). Psychiatric interviews suitable for use in research with children and adolescents. *Psychopharmacology Bulletin, Special Issue, 21,* 737–745.

Orvaschel, H. (1988). Structured and semistructured psychiatric interviews for children. In C. J. Kestenbaum & D. T. Williams (Eds.), *Handbook of clinical assessment of children and adolescents (Vol. I)* (pp. 31–42). New York: New York University Press.

Orvaschel, H. (1989). Diagnostic interviews for children and adolescents. In C. G. Last & M. Hersen (Eds.), *Handbook of child psychiatric diagnosis* (pp. 483–495). New York: John Wiley & Sons.

Orvaschel, H. (1995). *Schedule for Affective Disorders and Schizophrenia for School-Age Children—Epidemiologic Version 5 (K-SADS-E-5).* Ft. Lauderdale, FL: Nova Southeastern University.

Orvaschel, H., & Puig-Antich, J. (1987). *Schedule for Affective Disorders and Schizophrenia for School-Age Children—Epidemiologic Version 4 (K-SADS-E).* Philadelphia: Medical College of Pennsylvania.

Orvaschel, H., Puig-Antich, J., Chambers, W., Tabrizi, M. A., & Johnson, R. (1982). Retrospective assessment of child psychopathology with the Kiddie-SADS-E. *Journal of the American Academy of Child Psychiatry, 21,* 392–397.

Orvaschel, H., Puig-Antich, J., Tabrizi, M. A., & Chambers, W. (1979). *The Schedule for Affective Disorders and Schizophrenia for School-Age Children-Epidemiologic Version 1 (K-SADS-E)*. New York: New York Psychiatric Institute.

Orvaschel, H., Sholomskas, D., & Weissman, M. M. (1980a). *The assessment of psychopathology and behavioral problems in children: A review of scales suitable for epidemiological and clinical research (1967–79)*. Monograph for NIMH Series AN No. 1, DDHS Publication No. (ADM) 80–1037. Washington, DC: U.S. Government Printing Office.

Orvaschel, H., Sholomskas, D., & Weissman, M. M. (1980b). Assessing children in epidemiologic studies: A review of interview techniques. In F. Earls (Ed.), *Monographs in psychosocial epidemiology I. Studies of children*. New York: Prodist.

Orvaschel, H., Weissman, M. M., Padian, N., & Lowe, T. (1981). Assessing psychopathology in children of psychiatrically disturbed parents: A pilot study. *Journal of the American Academy of Child Psychiatry, 20,* 112–122.

Puig-Antich, J., & Chambers, W. (1978). The Schedule for Affective Disorders and Schizophrenia for School-Age Children (KIDDIE-SADS). New York: New York State Psychiatric Institute.

Puig-Antich, J., Chambers, W., Orvaschel, H., & Tabrizi, M. A. (1979). *The Schedule for Affective Disorders and Schizophrenia for School-Age Children—Lifetime Version (K-SADS-L)*. New York: New York State Psychiatric Institute.

Puig-Antich, P., Orvaschel, H., Tabrizi, M. A., & Chambers, W. (1980). *The Schedule for Affective Disorders and Schizophrenia for School-Age Children—Epidemiologic Version (K-SADS-E)*. New York: New York State Psychiatric Institute.

Puig-Antich, J., & Ryan, N. (1986). *The Schedule for Affective Disorders and Schizophrenia for School-Age Children (K-SADS-P)*. Pittsburgh, PA: Western Psychiatric Institute and Clinic.

Reich, W. (2000). Diagnostic Interview for Children and Adolescents (DICA). *Journal of the American Academy of Child and Adolescent Psychiatry, 39,* 59–66.

Reich, W., Cottler, L. B., McCallum, K., Corwin, D., & VanEerdwegh, M. (1995). Computerized interviews as a method of assessing psychopathology in children. *Comprehensive Psychiatry, 36,* 40–45.

Reich, W., Herjanic, B., Welner, Z., & Grandhy, P. R. (1982). Development of a structured interview for children: Agreement on diagnosis comparing child and parent interviews. *Journal of Abnormal Child Psychology, 10,* 325–336.

Robins, E., & Guze, S. B. (1970). Establishment of diagnostic validity in psychiatric illness: Its application to schizophrenia. *American Journal of Psychiatry, 44,* 854–861.

Robins, L., N., Helzer, J. E., Croughan, J., & Ratcliff, K. S. (1981). National Institute of Mental Health diagnostic interview schedule: Its history, characteristics, and validity. *Archives of General Psychiatry, 38,* 381–389.

Robins, L. N., Helzer, J. E., Ratcliff, K. S., & Seyfried, W. (1982). Validity of the Diagnostic Interview Schedule, Version II: DSM-III diagnoses. *Psychological Medicine, 12,* 855–870.

Rutter, M., & Graham, P. (1968). The reliability and validity of the psychiatric assessment of the child: I. Interview with the child. *British Journal of Psychiatry, 114,* 563–579.

Shaffer, D., Fisher, P., Piacentini, J., Schwab-Stone, M., & Wicks, J. (1989). *Diagnostic Interview Schedule for Children (DISC 2.1)*. Rockville, Md: National Institute of Mental Health.

Shaffer, D. M., Fisher, P. W., Dulcan, M. K., et al. (1996). The NIMH *Diagnostic Interview Schedule for Children (DISC-2.3)*: Description, acceptability, prevalences, and performance in the MECA study. *Journal of the American Academy of Child and Adolescent Psychiatry, 35,* 865–877.

Shaffer, D. M., Fisher, P. W., Lucas, C., Dulcan, M. K., & Schwab-Stone, M. E. (2000). NIMH Diagnostic Interview Schedule for Children—Version IV (NIMH DISC-IV): Description, differences from previous versions, and reliability of some common diagnoses. *Journal of the American Academy of Child and Adolescent Psychiatry, 39,* 28–38.

Sherrill, J. T., & Kovacs, M. (2000). Interview Schedule for Children and Adolescents (ISCA). *Journal of the American Academy of Child Psychiatry, 39,* 67–75.

Silverman, W. K., & Eisen, A. R. (1992). Age differences in the reliability of parent and child reports of child anxious symptomatology using a structured inverview. *Journal of the American Academy of Child Psychiatry, 31,* 117–124.

Silverman, W. K., & Nelles, M. A. (1988). The Anxiety Disorders Interview Schedule for Children. *Journal of the American Academy of Child Psychiatry, 27,* 772–778.

Silverman, W. K., Saavedra, L. M., & Pina, A. A. (2001). Test–retest reliability of anxiety symptoms and diagnoses with the Anxiety Disorders Interview Schedule for DSM-IV: Child and Parent Versions. *Journal of the American Academy of Child Psychiatry, 40,* 937–944.

Spitzer, R. L., & Endicott, J. (1978). *Schedule for Affective Disorders and Schizophrenia.* New York: Biometrics Research, Evaluation Section, N.Y. State Psychiatric Institute.

Spitzer, R. L., Endicott, J., & Robins, E. (1978). Research diagnostic criteria: Rationale and reliability. *Archives of General Psychiatry, 35,* 773–782.

Spitzer, R. L., & Williams, J. B. W. (1985). Structured clinical interview for DSM-III-R 9SCID). New York: Biometrics Research Department, New York Psychiatric Institute.

Teare, M., Fristad, M. A., Weller, E. B., Weller, R. A., & Salmon, P. (1998a). Study I: Development and criterion validity of the Children's Interview for Psychiatric Syndromes (ChIPS). *Journal of Child and Adolescent Psychopharmacology, 8,* 205–211.

Teare, M., Fristad, M. A., Weller, E. B., Weller, R. A., & Salmon, P. (1998b). Study II: Concurrent validity of the DSM-III-R Children's Interview for Psychiatric Syndromes (ChIPS). *Journal of Child and Adolescent Psychopharmacology, 8,* 213–219.

Weller, E. B., Weller, R. A., Fristad, M. A., Rooney, M. T., & Schecter, J. (2000). Children's Interview for Psychiatric Syndromes (ChIPS). *Journal of the American Academy of Child and Adolescent Psychiatry, 39,* 76–84.

Welner, Z., Reich, W., Herjanic, B., Jung, K. G., & Amado, H. (1987). Reliability, validity, and parent–child agreement studies of the diagnostic interview for children and adolescents. *Journal of the American Academy of Child and Adolescent Psychiatry, 5,* 649–653.

8

CHILD SELF-REGULATION

MARTIN AGRAN

Department of Special Education
University of Wyoming
Laramie, Wyoming

MICHAEL L. WEHMEYER

Beach Center
University of Kansas
Lawrence, Kansas

INTRODUCTION

A dramatic shift has occurred in special education practice since the mid-1990s. The traditional instructional model used in special education was clearly a teacher-directed model, in which the teacher was responsible for all executive decisions relating to curriculum development, instructional delivery, and evaluation; that is, the teacher determined what students learned and under what conditions, as well as the consequence of management system operative in the classroom (Agran, 1997). In contrast, the students' roles were correspondingly passive and involved responding to the cues and consequences delivered by the teacher. This approach has been challenged by a number of researchers (Agran & Wehmeyer, 1999; King-Sears & Carpenter, 1997; Mithaug, Mithaug, Agran, Martin, & Wehmeyer, 2003; Wehmeyer, Agran, & Hughes, 1998) who suggested that such a teacher-directed approach promotes dependency, minimizes motivation, and restricts student engagement and transfer of learning. Instead, to enhance learning and skill development, it is critical that we maximize involvement of students with disabilities in self-directed decision making and actions in school that directly impact their learning, that is, enable students to become more self-determined and more self-regulated (Agran, King-Sears, Wehmeyer, & Copeland, 2003; Wehmeyer, Agran, & Hughes, 1998). This involves teaching students to use learning strategies that allow them to modify and regulate their own behavior (Agran, 1997). These strategies are referred to as *student-directed learning* or *self-regulation strategies.* Such strategies enable students to regulate their own behavior, independent of external control, and allow students to become active participants in their own learning and to enhance self-determination. In all, student-directed learning strategies have demonstrated educational efficacy across a wide age range of learning and adaptive skills and students with a variety of disabilities and have been well validated and supported in the literature. Specifically, they aim to teach students how to set their own learning goals, monitor their own performance, identify problems and solutions to present or future problems, verbally direct their behavior, administer reinforcement, or evaluate their own performance.

The purpose of this chapter is to discuss the value of utilizing a student- or child-directed learning approach. First, the benefits of this approach are discussed. Following, the characteristics of student-directed learning strategies are described. Next, recommended assessment approaches are presented. In particular, a self-regulated problem-solving model is presented. Last, recommendations to promote self-regulation are discussed.

PASSIVE STUDENT ENGAGEMENT

Historically, instruction in special education practice has relied on a mechanistic, environmentally determined model of behavioral development (Kanfer, 1977). That is, skill development or learning was thought of as the "continuous, quantitative accumulation of behavior," and learning, as such, was derived from a conditioning model (Langer, 1969, p. 55). Accordingly, learning was based on stimulus–consequence relationships, which were contingent on the strength of the reinforcing properties of the consequences available and the student's history of experiences with these or similar consequences. Given the student's history and saliency of environmental stimuli and the established strength of consequences, the student was perceived accordingly as having a relatively passive role, in which development was subject to the overarching power of the laws of stimulus–response relationships. Learning could be advanced via environmental manipulations or modifications that systematically altered environmental cues and consequences and increased the probability that a desired response will occur in the future. Management of the learning environment was the teacher's responsibility and involved a thorough understanding of behavior analysis. As a result, teachers were given full responsibility for selecting student goals, developing actions and activities, conducting evaluations, and later determining adjustments to improve desired results or learning outcomes for their students (Agran, 1997). In this respect, they had full control over the learning experience.

Special education has relied on such a model since the mid-1970s. To its credit, it has allowed students with disabilities, regardless of their instructional needs, to achieve unexpectedly high performance levels. But it has resulted in a situation in which many students with disabilities have been denied the opportunity to participate in their educational program in an active and self-directed way (Sands & Wehmeyer, 1996; Wehmeyer & Sands, 1998). Making choices, taking risks, having control over outcomes, and assuming responsibility for personal action are highly valued societal goals (Wehmeyer, 1992). However, instructional activities to promote and support self-regulation and student-directed learning have largely been left out of educational programs for students with disabilities, particularly for students with more significant disabilities (Agran & Hughes, 1997; Mithaug, Martin, & Agran, 1987). Consequently, as mentioned previously, many students become dependent on external supports provided by teachers and associates, exhibit only a passive level of engagement in school, and show little motivation or self-initiative in responding to new learning challenges. Eisenberger, Conti-D'Antonio, and Bertrando (2000) described this situation as follows:

> Students with learning disabilities may not approach tasks with a plan of action or be able to estimate accurately how much time a task will require. Some of these students may exhibit disorganized thinking and have problems in planning, organizing, and controlling their lives in academic and social settings. Their school performance, when compared with their ability, may be poor. This issue may be evidenced on report cards that are rife with Ds and Fs. The work that they do may be incomplete or of poor quality. They may attribute their lack of work to personal feelings, request adult intervention and "help" before making an attempt, or avoid tasks completely by treating teachers and other adults as enemies to fight. They often have no strategies for comprehending, retrieving, or using information. They may have a tendency to complete only work that is effortless, and they openly complain if work requires effort. They behave as though they have no influence over how they live their lives. These are students who have not developed self-efficacy, the belief that they have the abilities needed to produce quality work through sustained effort. Because these students approach difficult tasks without self-efficacy, they make very poor use of their capabilities (pp. 3–4).

All too often, students with disabilities experience the same difficulties. They enter learning situations with little initiative, motivation, or a sense of self-efficacy. Unfortunately, our reliance on a teacher-directed instructional model has only exacerbated the situation. As mentioned before, such a model has only helped to reinforce student dependency and left motivation, engagement, and learning as the responsibility of the teacher, not the student.

A FUNCTIONAL MODEL OF SELF-DETERMINED BEHAVIOR

Self-determination is a complex construct involving the interplay of several components. Most definitions of self-determination focus on the specific behaviors or actions in which people engage that, in turn, enable them to exert increased control over their lives (Wehmeyer & Agran, 2004; Sands & Wehmeyer, 1996; Wehmeyer, 1996a, 1998). However, we have suggested that one cannot define self-determination as a set of skills or behaviors, but must look at the function of

TABLE 8.1 Components of Self-Determination

Choice-making skills
Decision-making skills
Problem-solving skills
Goal-setting and -attainment skills
Self-monitoring, -evaluation, and -reinforcement skills
Self-instruction skills
Self-awareness
Self-efficacy
Internal locus of control

that behavior in the person's life. People who are self-determined act in ways that enable them to achieve desired goals and enhance their quality of life. Reflecting this emphasis, Wehmeyer (1996b) defined self-determined behavior as "acting as the primary causal agent in one's life and making choices and decisions regarding one's quality of life free from undue external influence or interference" (p. 24). In this context, *causal agency* implies that it is the individual who makes or causes things to happen in his or her life. An agent is a person or thing through which power is exerted or an end is achieved. Thus, a *causal agent* is someone who makes or causes things to happen in his or her life. Self-determined people act as the causal agent in their lives.

Self-determination emerges across the life span as children and adolescents learn skills and develop attitudes that enable them to become causal agents in their own lives. These attitudes and abilities are the *component elements* of self-determination, and it is this level of the theoretical framework that drives instructional activities. As they acquire these component elements, individuals become increasingly self-determined. Table 8.1 lists these elements.

A complete discussion of each of these component elements is not feasible within the context of this chapter (see Agran, 1997; Wehmeyer, Agran, & Hughes, 1998; Wehmeyer, 2001). However, two issues relating to these components are important to consider. First, it is this level at which assessment can be conducted and instruction occurs. That is, there are instructional strategies and methods that can be implemented and evaluated to enhance student capacity in each of these component areas. Wehmeyer, Agran, and Hughes identified numerous methods, materials, and supports to promote these component elements. Second, each of these component elements can be acquired through specific learning experiences. Development and acquisition of these component elements is lifelong and begins when children are very young. Some elements have greater applicability for secondary education and transition; others will focus more on elementary years. As such, promoting self-determination as an educational outcome involves systematic student-directed learning experiences across the span of a student's educational experience.

ASSESSING INSTRUCTIONAL NEEDS IN SELF-DETERMINATION

Because self-determination is a complex construct, it defies easy definition and topography. Likewise, it is a phenomenon that cannot be assessed via pencil-and-paper standardized assessments. As a multidimensional construct, measurement in self-determination must involve multiple indicators that include participant observation, personal interviews, subjective and objective indicators, and standardized instruments. Only when there are ample sources of data generated from these multiple methods and perspectives can we begin to adequately measure self-determination. Determining instructional and curricular needs in the area of self-determination will involve a combination of standardized and informal procedures incorporating input from multiple sources, including the student, his or her family, teachers, and other stakeholders (e.g., peers, related service professionals).

A key distinction in efforts to promote self-determination is the role of the student. In traditional assessments, the student's performance is evaluated via permanent products (e.g., written examination) or via third-party observation. Because self-determination is focused on the student's empowerment and self-advocacy, students can and should play an active role in the assessment process (Field, Martin, Miller, Ward, & Wehmeyer, 1998). As they noted, students can provide insight on evidence of self-regulated behavior and environmental stimuli that either facilitated or hindered their self-determination.

There are a few standardized measures of self-determination and its component elements that could be used to identify instructional and curricular needs. The *Arc's Self-Determination Scale* (Wehmeyer & Kelchner, 1995a) is a 72-item self-report measure that provides data on each of the four essential characteristics of self-determination identified by Wehmeyer and colleagues (Wehmeyer, Kelchner, & Richards, 1996). The scale measures (a) student autonomy, including the student's independence and the extent to which he or she acts on the basis of personal beliefs, values, interests, and abilities; (b) student self-regulation, which includes interpersonal cognitive problem solving and goal setting and task performance; (c) psychological empowerment, which involves assessing the student's sense of self-efficacy or perception that he or she has some degree of control over his or her circumstances; and (d) student self-realization, or knowledge of his or her strengths and limitations. The *Arc's Self-Determination Scale* was normed with 500 students with and without intellectual disabilities in rural, urban, and suburban school districts across five states. Its primary purpose is to enable students with cognitive disabilities to self-assess strengths and limitations in the area of self-determination and to provide students and teachers a tool with which they can jointly determine goals and instructional programming to promote self-determination.

Another measure of self-determination is the *AIR Self-Determination Scale* (Wolman, Campeau, DuBois, Mithaug, & Stolarski, 1994), which measures individual student capacity for and opportunity to practice self-determination. There are three forms of the scale (i.e., educator, student, and parent), and the results of each can be used to develop a profile of a student's level of self-determination, areas of strength and areas needing improvement, educational goals and objectives, and recommended strategies to build student capacity and increase opportunities to become self-determined.

The *Choice Maker Self-Determination Assessment* (Martin & Huber Marshall, 1996) is a curriculum-based assessment that provides teachers an opportunity to rate both student self-determination skills and the opportunity in school for students to perform these skills. It measures students' skills across three areas: choosing goals, expressing goals, and taking action. Skills are rated from 0 to 4. There is also a profile that allows teachers to visually analyze the relationship of student skills relative to school opportunity. Last, the assessment includes a list of goals and objectives relating to teaching priorities.

The *Self-Determination Assessment Battery* (Hoffman, Field, & Sawilowsky, 1995) measures a variety of cognitive, behavioral, and affective factors relating to self-determination. The battery includes five instruments. First is a multiple-choice assessment of the students' knowledge of self-determination skills. Second, a 38-item behavioral checklist allows teachers to observe student performance of these skills in classroom settings. Third, a 92-item self-report scale is included to measure the students' perceptions about self-determination. Fourth, a scale in which teachers can rate their students across a variety of skills and behaviors associated with self-determination is provided. Last, a scale for parents to rate their children across a variety of skills associated with self-determination is included.

In summary, although self-determination represents a complex construct, open to interpretation, several instruments are available to provide evaluative measures of skills, behavior, and knowledge associated with it. It would, however, be imprudent to suggest that any such instrument can yield a definitive assessment as to whether a student is self-determined, since there are any of a number of setting- and person-specific variables that can impact a child's execution of self-determined behavior. However, these instruments can be helpful in identifying teaching priorities and the student's overall skills in this area.

SELF-REGULATION STRATEGIES

Mithaug, Martin, and Agran (1987) conducted a comprehensive literature review on "success" behaviors—behaviors associated with successful outcomes, as reported by a sample of notable individuals, and identified over 40 skills and four major activities or skill clusters. Although the language differed across the papers, strong similarities were noted across the works reviewed. First, successful individuals set goals for themselves. They identified and set goals that were clearly defined, identified a specific purpose, and were feasible to achieve.

Second, successful individuals engaged in independent performance; that is, they used a variety of self-directed strategies (e.g., self-monitoring) to achieve their aims. Third, successful people were able to evaluate their performance in terms of how well they had achieved a specified level of performance. Last, successful individuals appeared to have the capacity to learn from their mistakes and to change or adjust their goals or the actions as needed. Based on these findings, Mithaug et al. (1987) developed the A*daptability Instructional Model*, which seeks to teach students with disabilities how to regulate their own behavior using the four activities described earlier. This model represented one of the first comprehensive models to promote the self-determination of students with mental retardation and developmental disabilities and provided the template for self-determination programs that followed, including the *Self-Determined Learning Model of Instruction* (Wehmeyer, Palmer, Agran, Mithaug, & Martin, 2000) to be described later in the chapter.

Critical to an individual's success in learning and task performance is the ability to self-regulate his or her performance (Watson & Tharp, 1989). To achieve goals (self- or other-selected), standards or desired levels of performance (self- or other-selected) must be present. With these standards, the individual can determine if a discrepancy exists between the existing level of performance and the desired level of performance. With this information, an appropriate action can be made to modify the situation.

Typically, the following strategies are associated with self-regulation: goal setting, self-monitoring, self-evaluation, and self-reinforcement (Smith & Nelson, 1997). *Goal setting* refers to setting a performance goal to achieve for oneself, *self-monitoring* refers to observing and recording one's performance, *self-evaluation* involves comparing these recordings to a known performance standard, and *self-reinforcement* involves the selection and administration of reinforcement to oneself. Each of these may be used alone or in combination. Clearly, all humans self-regulate, but not with equal success (Mithaug, 1993). The reasons for this are several. Standards may be lacking; if they are present, the students may not be aware of them. Also, students may not know how to observe their own behavior or how to compare their behavior to these standards (Watson & Tharp, 1989). Further, they may lack the strategies needed to achieve their goals, even if they have been able to compare their performance to known standards.

It is not surprising that the success behaviors discussed previously function as self-regulation strategies. These strategies allow individuals to pursue self-selected goals, initiate and follow through on a course of action, and adjust their performance as needed. Without self-regulated performance, the likelihood that a student will achieve success is minimized. A description of each of these strategies follows.

Self-monitoring, or *self-recording*, involves teaching students to observe whether they have performed a desired behavior. These procedures have been shown to improve the motivation and performance of students with disabilities (Agran, 1998; Wehmeyer, 1998). For example, McCarl, Svobodny, and Beare

(1991) found that teaching three students with intellectual disabilities to record progress on classroom assignments improved on-task behavior for all students and increased productivity for two of the three. Agran, Sinclair, Alper, Cavin, and Hughes (in press) taught students with intellectual disabilities to monitor their own behavior so as to increase their following-direction skills. Kapadia and Fantuzzo (1988) used self-monitoring procedures to increase attention to academic tasks for students with developmental disabilities and behavior problems. Lovett and Haring (1989) demonstrated that self-recording activities enabled adults with intellectual disabilities to improve task completion of daily living activities. Last, Chiron, and Gerken (1983) reported that students with intellectual disabilities who charted their progress on school reading activities achieved improvements in their reading levels.

Self-evaluation involves teaching the student to compare his or her performance, based on self-monitored records, to a desired goal, standard, or outcome. Schunk (1981) reported that students who verbalized cognitive strategies related to evaluating their study and work skills increased their math achievement scores. Brownell, Colletti, Ersner-Hershfield, Hershfield, and Wilson (1977) indicated that students who determined their performance standards demonstrated increased time on-task when compared with students operating under externally imposed standards.

Last, *self-reinforcement* involves teaching students to select and administer consequences to themselves (e.g., verbally telling themselves they did a good job). Self-reinforcement allows students to provide themselves with reinforcers that are accessible and immediate. Lagomarcino and Rusch (1989) used a combination of self-reinforcement and self-monitoring procedures to improve the work performance of a student with mental retardation in a community setting. Moore, Agran, and Fodor-Davis (1989) used a combination of student-directed activities, including self-instructions, goal setting, and self-reinforcement, to improve the production rate of workers with mental retardation. Self-reinforcement has also been used to improve academic performance (Stevenson & Fantuzzo, 1984), work productivity (Moore et al.) and leisure/recreational skills (Coleman & Whitman, 1984).

SELF-MONITORING

It is widely accepted that learning to monitor one's behavior is the key or prerequisite to self-regulation (Kanfer, 1970). Students who monitor their own behavior are better able to identify a discrepancy between an actual or existing performance level and a future or desired level. As noted previously, self-monitoring involves a student's observation of his or her own behavior and recording whether the behavior had occurred or not. The strategy requires that a student discriminate whether the desired or goal behavior was or was not performed and then accurately record the occurrence on a monitoring card or recording device. Essentially any discrete behavior that can be operationally defined can be self-monitored.

Self-monitoring usually focuses on tasks, behaviors, or processes a student already performs. It is the most basic form of student-directed learning, and it involves having a student respond to simple self-prompts or questions about what he or she has done.

Target behaviors may include practically any behavior the student (or teacher) wishes to modify. For example, Agran, Blanchard, Wehmeyer, and Hughes (2001) taught six secondary-level students with varying disabilities to employ and monitor their use of several classroom study and organizational skills (e.g., recording and completing assignments, using day planner). The students were instructed to place a tally mark on a card after they performed a target behavior. Dramatic improvements were reported for all students. Gilbert, Agran, Hughes, and Wehmeyer (2001) taught five middle school students with severe cognitive disabilities to monitor a set of classroom "survival" skills. These skills included being in class and in seat when the bell rings, having appropriate materials, greeting the teacher and other students, asking and answering questions, sitting up straight and looking at teacher when addressed, acknowledging teacher and student comments, and using a planner. Positive changes were reported for all students, and the behaviors were maintained at 100%.

Students' self-monitoring should be evident in any setting, but it is especially important in inclusive settings. Agran and Alper (2000) surveyed a sample of general and special educators, and a majority of respondents indicated that self-regulation/student-directed learning is one of the most important skill areas needed for successful inclusion.

A question often asked is the importance of accuracy relative to the student who is self-monitoring. Interestingly, students who may not be accurate or honest in monitoring their behaviors can still exhibit desirable behavior changes (Reinecke, Newman, & Meinberg, 1999). Ample research suggests that self-monitoring will produce a desired effect even if the student's recordings are inaccurate. That is, self-monitoring produces a reactive effect in which the student attends more to his or her behavior and, by doing so, provides stimuli to cue the response (Smith & Nelson, 1997). Consequently, the self-monitoring procedure may produce a desired effect without any other intervention (Agran & Martin, 1987; Wehmeyer, 1998). Nevertheless, it is helpful to build into the self-monitoring process occasional teacher checks for accuracy; these external checks may occur less frequently as the student becomes more proficient with self-monitoring.

Self-monitoring produces behavior change because it may serve as a discriminative stimulus to the student and, thus, cue the desired response. Self-monitoring allows the student to recognize that the specific target behavior has occurred and reminds the student of present and future contingencies (i.e., "If I perform this response, this will happen"). The target behavior is more likely to occur when this information is available to the student. As Mithaug (1993) noted, the more often the student has the opportunity to monitor his or her behavior, the more competent he or she will be and the more likely he or she is to appreciate the value and utility of self-monitoring.

SELF-EVALUATION

Self-evaluation involves the comparison of the behavior monitored to the student's desired goal or a teacher-determined standard. It is a critical self-regulation skill because it allows the student to be aware of whether she or he is meeting a desired goal and may potentially serve as a reinforcing event (Agran & Hughes, 1997). Self-evaluation extends self-monitoring methods from a frequency tally to an informed judgment. Self-evaluation provides the student with a standard against which to assess his or her behavioral performance (Agran, 1997). If the standard is met, the strategy may assume a reinforcing property, which will promote the likelihood that the behavior will occur in the future. If the standard is not met, the student is alerted to the apparent discrepancy between the desired performance level and the observed performance level. Of critical importance is the fact that the student provides him- or herself with the feedback and is not dependent on a teacher or other individual to evaluate his or her behavior. In a study conducted by Agran, Blanchard, and Wehmeyer (2000), a student was taught to evaluate whether she had sufficient insulin to give herself the correct amount of insulin at lunchtime. This responsibility was based on the consequences of making an error. The goal was for the student to become 100% proficient in following the procedures outlined since anything less could have life-threatening consequences. The strategy proved to be successful. In this self-evaluation application, the student was literally given control over her own health and well-being.

In another application, three adolescents with developmental disabilities were taught to evaluate their classroom behavior relative to goals they had initially set for themselves (Wehmeyer, Yeager, Bolding, Agran, & Hughes, 2003). The target behaviors included improving their listening skills, not touching other students, increasing on-task behavior, decreasing inappropriate verbalizations, and decreasing disruptive behavior. The students compared their self-monitored recordings to those of a second observer to determine if they met the self-selected goal. Improvements in behavior were reported for all students.

Finally, Hoff and DuPaul (1998) taught students with attention deficit and oppositional defiant disorders to self-evaluate their compliance with classroom rules. Initially, the teacher rated the students' compliance behaviors; then the students were instructed to use the same rating system so that they could self-evaluate every 5 minutes. The students' disruptive behaviors decreased during math, recess, and social studies. Compliance with rules increased and was maintained even when the teacher was absent. All students indicated that they appreciated the self-evaluation procedure.

The advantages of self-evaluation are obvious. Needless to say, teachers spend considerable time providing feedback to students. When students learn how to self-evaluate their own behavior, teachers can shift their attention to other responsibilities. Most importantly, students are not dependent on teachers to judge how well they are doing but, instead, learn how to self-evaluate their behaviors and make changes toward improvements. The gains in doing this are well supported in the self-regulation literature (see Mithaug, Mithaug, Agran, Martin, & Wehmeyer, 2003).

Self-evaluation can be taught independently or as part of a total self-regulation package, which typically involves goal setting, self-monitoring, and self-reinforcement. Also, and most importantly, it serves as a critical step in problem solving (Wehmeyer, 1998). Prior to determining if an action was successful or not and warranted reinforcement, the student must evaluate (or compare) the self-monitored records to the goal standard (either self- or teacher-determined). Inherent in the self-regulation process is the role of the student in evaluating his or her progress in meeting goals and then making a data-based decision on what needs to be done so that progress can be facilitated. The obvious advantage of self-evaluation is it allows the student to engage in an evaluative activity that traditionally has only been done by teachers and, in doing so, provides the student with increased ownership of and motivation to change.

Self-evaluation can be combined with other procedures to promote efficacy. For example, middle school students with learning disabilities learned how to both self-monitor their behaviors during class and then self-evaluate their classroom behavior at the end of class to increase their on-task behaviors (Dalton, Martella, & Marchand-Martella, 1999). The students used the classroom clock as their cueing system to monitor their work performance ("Are you working?") every 5 minutes. Also, they used a checklist noting specific classroom tasks (e.g., "Did you get your homework done?"), which also required a "yes" or "no" response. The checklist contained a series of questions for selected classroom behaviors required at the beginning of class ("Did you get started on time?"), during class ("Did you self-monitor to stay on-task?"), and at the end of class ("Did you follow the teacher's directions?"). After completing the checklist throughout each class session, the students evaluated their behavior. The intervention increased the student's on-task behaviors and resulted in increasing the teachers' ratings of the students' classroom behavior.

SELF-REINFORCEMENT

Self-reinforcement represents a major component of most conceptualizations of self-regulation or self-determination. There is evidence to suggest that self-reinforcement is as effective as, if not more effective than, teacher-delivered reinforcement. Since the aim of self-regulation is to promote students' independence and control over their learning and development, it is a critical self-regulation strategy. Bandura and Perloff (1973) indicated that humans routinely compare themselves to self-prescribed standards and administer self-rewarding or self-punishing consequences accordingly. Skinner (1953) explained in early research on self-control that when discussing the capacity of individuals to control or direct their own behavior, two responses are involved. The first refers to a controlling response, which affects the probability that the target response will occur, and the second is the controlled or desired behavior. Self-reinforcement clearly serves the function of a controlling response and increases the likelihood the target behavior will occur again.

Self-reinforcement involves a procedure in which students are taught to reinforce themselves immediately after a desired behavior has occurred (Wehmeyer, 1998). Students are always present to administer their own consequences or feedback, so the possibility of lost reinforcement is greatly minimized. Also, students may have difficulty acquiring desired outcomes because the available consequences are too delayed, too small, or not achievable. Self-reinforcement solves this potential problem in providing an opportunity for the student to reinforce him- or herself immediately (Malott, 1984). Traditionally, teachers have always been in control of the consequences in a learning situation. Self-reinforcement shifts that control the student, and it is this shift that provides considerable potency to self-regulation.

Two activities are involved in self-reinforcement: discrimination and delivery. A student must discriminate that the target behavior has occurred before he or she can deliver a reinforcer to him- or herself. In this sense, self-reinforcement is functionally linked to self-monitoring. Similar to self-monitoring, self-reinforcement has stimulus properties that may cue appropriate responding.

It is safe to say that many individuals, with or without disabilities, are not experienced in overtly reinforcing themselves. However, students with varying support needs can be taught systematically to reinforce themselves. For example, Lagomarcino and Rusch (1989) taught a student with profound mental retardation to reinforce himself by placing a coin into an empty slot in a board after completing a work task.

As mentioned previously, the learning experiences of most students with disabilities have been controlled by others (Agran, 1998). Traditionally, students have only had a passive role, in which they have responded to the cues and consequences delivered by teachers or paraprofessionals. Students had little or no active involvement in the determination, delivery, or evaluation of their educational experiences. Consequently, although providing opportunities to students to evaluate and reinforce their own behavior appear to be appealing to students, students may initially perceive opportunities to evaluate and reinforce their own behavior as beyond their capacity. As with self-monitoring or self-evaluation, concentrated efforts must be made to ensure that self-regulatory experiences produce positive outcomes. That is, students need to select behaviors they can easily perform, monitor, and evaluate and that occur frequently enough so that students can reinforce themselves. Based on a history of past negative experiences at school, many students may not believe they have the capacity to produce a desired learning outcome or do not believe they know how to modify or adjust their behavior to achieve desired goals. Once students can understand the dynamic connectivity of the self-regulation strategies described in this chapter, they will increasingly realize how much control over the learning process they really have.

THE SELF-DETERMINED LEARNING MODEL OF INSTRUCTION

Wehmeyer and colleagues (Mithaug, Wehmeyer, Agran, Martin, & Palmer, 1998; Wehmeyer, Palmer, Agran, Mithaug, & Martin, 2000) developed a model of teaching that enables teachers to teach students to problem solve. This model, called the *Self-Determined Learning Model of Instruction*, was derived from the *Adaptability Instruction Model* developed by Mithaug, Martin, and Agran (1987) and Mithaug, Martin, Agran, and Rusch (1988), described previously, and incorporates principles of self-regulated learning.

The model consists of a three-phase instructional process depicted in Figures 8.1, 8.2, and 8.3. Each instructional phase presents a problem to be solved by the

Problem for Student to Solve: What is my goal?

Student Questions	Teacher Objectives	Supports
SQ 1: What do I want to learn?	• Enable students to identify specific strengths and instructional needs • Enable students to communicate preferences, interests, beliefs, and values	Student self-assessment of interests, abilities, and instructional needs Awareness training
SQ 2: What do I know about it now?	• Teach students to prioritize needs • Enable students to identify their current status in relation to the instructional need	Choice making Problem-solving instruction
SQ 3: What must change for me to learn what I don't know?	• Assist students gather information about opportunities/barriers in their environments • Enable students to decide if action will be focused toward capacity building, modifying the environment or both	Decision-making instruction Goal-setting instruction
SQ 4: What can I do to make this happen?	• Support students to choose a need to address from prioritized list • Teach students to state a goal and identify criteria for achieving goal	

FIGURE 8.1 Self-Determined Learning Model of Instruction: What is my goal?

Problem for Student to Solve: What is my plan?

Student Questions	Teacher Objectives	Supports
SQ 5: What can I do to learn what I don't know?	• Enable student to self-evaluate current status and self-identified goal status	Self-scheduling Self-instruction
SQ 6: What could keep me from taking action?	• Enable student to determine plan of action to bridge gap between self-evaluated current status and self-identified goal status	Antecedent cue regulation Choice-making instruction
SQ 7: What can I do to remove these barriers?	• Collaborate with student to identify most appropriate instructional strategies • Teach student and support needed student-directed learning strategies • Provide mutually agreed upon teacher-directed instruction	Goal-attainment strategies Problem-solving instruction Decision-making instruction Self-advocacy instruction
SQ 8: When will I take action?	• Enable student to determine schedule for action plan • Enable student to implement action plan • Enable student to self-monitor progress	Assertiveness training Communication skills training Self-monitoring

FIGURE 8.2 Self-Determined Learning Model of Instruction: What is my plan?

Problem for Student to Solve: What have I learned?

Student Questions	Teacher Objectives	Supports
SQ 9: What actions have I taken?	• Enable student to self-evaluate progress toward goal achievement	Self-evaluation strategies Choice-making instruction
SQ 10: What barriers have been removed?	• Collaborate with student to compare progress with desired outcomes • Support student to reevaluate goal if progress is insufficient	Problem-solving instruction Decision-making instruction
SQ 11: What has changed about what I don't know?	• Assist student to decide if goal remains the same or changes • Collaborate with student to identify if action plan is adequate or inadequate, given revised or retained goal • Assist student to change action plan if necessary	Goal-setting instruction Self-reinforcement strategies Self-monitoring strategies Self-recording strategies
SQ 12: Do I know what I want to know?	• Enable student to decide if progress is adequate or inadequate or if goal has been achieved	

FIGURE 8.3 Self-Determined Learning Model of Instruction: What have I learned?

student. The student solves each problem by responding to a sequence of questions in each phase. Additionally, each question is linked to a set of *Teacher Objectives* and a list of *Educational Supports* teachers can use to enable students to self-direct their learning. In each phase, the student is the primary agent for choices, decisions, and actions, even when actions are teacher directed.

The *Student Questions* in the model are constructed to direct the student through a problem-solving sequence in each phase. The solutions to the problems in each phase lead to the problem-solving sequence in the next phase. Their construction was based on theory in the problem-solving and self-regulation literature that suggests that there is a *sequence* of thoughts and actions, a means–ends problem-solving sequence, that must be followed for any person's actions to produce results that satisfy their needs and interests. Following the model, students learn to solve a sequence of problems to construct a means–ends chain—a causal sequence—that moves them from an *actual state* (i.e., not having their needs and interests satisfied) to a *goal state* (i.e., having those needs and interests satisfied by connecting their needs and interests to their actions and results via goals and plans).

To answer the questions in this sequence, students regulate their own problem solving by setting goals to meet needs, constructing plans to meet goals, and adjusting actions to complete plans. Each instructional phase poses a problem the student must solve (What is my goal? What is my plan? What have I learned?). The four questions differ from phase to phase, but they represent identical steps in the problem-solving sequence. These include: (1) identify the problem, (2) identify potential solutions to the problem, (3) identify barriers to solving the problem, and (4) identify consequences of each solution. These steps represent the fundamental steps in any problem-solving process and form the means–end problem-solving sequence represented by the *Student Questions* in each phase.

Teaching students to use the *Student Questions* will teach them a self-regulated problem-solving strategy. Concurrently, teaching students to use various self-regulated learning strategies provides students with additional means to become the causal agent in their lives.

Wehmeyer, Palmer, Agran, Mithaug, and Martin (2000) conducted a field test of the model, with teachers responsible for the instruction of adolescents receiving special education services. The sample involved a total of 40 students with mental retardation, learning disabilities, or emotional or behavioral disorders. Students identified a total of 43 goals they wanted to address (three students chose two goals). Of the 43 goals, 10 focused on acquiring or modifying social skills or knowledge, 13 focused on behavioral issues (compliance with school procedures, controlling behavior in specific circumstances, learning more adaptive behavior), and 20 addressed academic needs. The field test indicated that the model was effective in enabling students to attain educationally valued goals. Also, Agran, Blanchard, and Wehmeyer (2000) taught 19 students with severe disabilities to use the model to promote transition-related outcomes in classroom settings. The target behaviors included following directions, improving job task performance, improve budgeting skills, independently making transportation arrangements, and improving personal hygiene skills. Positive increases in targeted behaviors were observed for 17 of the students. The model permitted students to identify meaningful goals for themselves and actions to achieve self-set goals. Last, four transition-age youth with mental retardation or developmental disabilities were taught to use the model to increase direction following, contributions to classroom discussion, and appropriate touching (Agran, Blanchard, Wehmeyer, & Hughes, 2002). All students increased their performance levels to 100% and maintained that level for the duration of the study. Also, social validation data indicated that all students had positive feelings about the strategy and their improvements in problem solving.

In summary, the *Self-Determined Learning Model of Instruction* allows students to assume more control over the learning process by allowing them to understand the connectivity of self-directed goals, actions, and outcomes. As such, self-regulated problem solving provides them a logical and systematic way to facilitate goal attainment.

SUMMARY

The strategies described in this chapter serve to expand and enhance a student's capacity but also to change his or her place and order in the learning configuration. These strategies provide students with increased opportunities to literally regulate their own learning and development. Once students can understand the dynamic connectivity of the self-regulation strategies, they will increasingly realize how much control over the learning process they have. Many students with disabilities experience little control over their own learning. They have a restricted sense of self-efficacy and do not believe they have control over learning outcomes (Wehmeyer, 1998). Based on a history of negative experiences at school, they do not believe they have the capacity to consistently produce a desired learning outcome. Most importantly, they do not know how to modify or adjust their behavior to achieve these goals. As Mithaug (1993) noted, success involves the interaction of opportunity and capacity. Self-regulation provides students with the tools to maximize their capacity to assess existing opportunity and to determine if and how gain can be derived. Self-regulation seeks in part to teach this relationship and, in doing so, will allow the student to achieve a level of engagement and motivation infrequently experienced.

REFERENCES AND RESOURCES

Agran, M. (1997). *Student-directed learning: Teaching self-determination skills.* Pacific Grove, CA: Brooks/Cole.

Agran, M. (1998). Student self-evaluation techniques: Students as decision makers in program evaluation. In M. Wehmeyer & D. J. Sands (Eds.), *Making it happen: Student involvement in educational planning* (pp. 355–379). Baltimore: Paul H. Brookes.

Agran, M., & Alper, S. (2000). Curriculum and instruction in general education: Implications for service delivery and teacher preparation. *Journal of the Association for Persons with Severe Handicaps, 25,* 167–174.

Agran, M., Blanchard, C., & Wehmeyer, M. L. (2000). Promoting transition goals and self-determination through student-directed learning: The self-determined learning model of instruction. *Education and Training in Mental Retardation and Developmental Disabilities, 35,* 351–364.

Agran, M., Blanchard, C., Wehmeyer, M. L., & Hughes, C. (2001). Teaching students to self-regulate their behavior: The differential effects of student- versus teacher-delivered reinforcement. *Research in Developmental Disabilities, 22,* 319–332.

Agran, M., Blanchard, C., Wehmeyer, M., & Hughes, C. (2002). Increasing the problem-solving skills of students with developmental disabilities participating in general education. *Remedial and Special Education, 23,* 279–288.

Agran, M., & Hughes, C. (1997). Problem solving. In M. Agran (Ed.), *Student-directed learning: Teaching self-determination skills* (pp. 171–198). Pacific Grove, CA: Brookes-Cole.

Agran, M., King-Sears, M. E., Wehmeyer, M. L., & Copeland, S. R. (2003). *Teachers' guide to inclusive practices: Student-directed learning.* Baltimore: Paul H. Brookes.

Agran, M., & Martin, J. E. (1987). Applying a technology of self-control in community environments for individuals who are mentally retarded. In M. Hersen, R. M. Eisler, & P. M. Miller (Eds.), *Progress in behavior modification* (pp. 108–151). Newbury Park, CA: Sage Publications.

Agran, M., Sinclair, T., Sitlington, P., Cavin, M., & Wehmeyer, M. L. (in press). Using self-monitoring to increase following-direction skills of students with moderate to severe disabilities in general education. *Education and Training in Developmental Disabilities.*

Agran, M., & Wehmeyer, M. (1999). *Teaching problem solving to students with mental retardation.* Washington, DC: American Association on Mental Retardation.

Bandura, A., & Perloff, B. (1973). Relative efficacy of self-monitored and externally imposed reinforcement systems. In M. R. Goldfried & M. Merbaum (Eds.), *Behavior change through self-control* (pp. 152–161). New York: Holt, Rinehart and Winston.

Brownell, K. D., Colletti, G., Ersner-Hershfield, R., Hershfield, S. M., & Wilson, G. T. (1977). Self-control in school children: Stringency and leniency in self-determined and externally imposed performance standards. *Behavior Therapy, 8,* 442–455.

Chiron, R., & Gerken, K. (1983). The effects of a self-monitoring technique on the locus of control orientation of educable mentally retarded children. *School Psychology Review, 3,* 87–92.

Coleman, R. S., & Whitman, T. L. (1984). Developing, generalizing, and maintaining physical fitness in mentally retarded adults: Toward a self-directed program. *Analysis and Intervention in Developmental Disabilities, 4,* 109–127.

Dalton, T., Martella, R. C., & Marchand-Martella, N. E. (1999). The effects of a self-management program in reducing off-task behavior. *Journal of Behavioral Education, 9,* 157–176.

Eisenberger, J., Conti-D'Antonio, M., & Bertrando, R. (2000). *Self-efficacy: Raising the bar for students with learning needs.* Larchmont, NY: Eye on Education.

Field, S. S., Martin, J. E., Miller, R. J., Ward, M., & Wehmeyer, M. L. (1998). Student self-determination guide. Reston, VA: Council for Exceptional Children.

Gilberts, G. H., Agran, M., Hughes, C., & Wehmeyer, M. (2001). The effects of peer-delivered self-monitoring strategies on the participation of students with severe disabilities in general education classrooms. *Journal of the Association for Persons with Severe Handicaps, 26,* 25–26.

Hoff, K. E., & DuPaul, G. J. (1998). Reducing disruptive behavior in general education classrooms: The use of self-management strategies. *School Psychology Review, 27,* 290–303.

Hoffman, A., Field, S., & Sawilowsky, S. (1995). *Self-Determination Assessment Battery User's Guide.* Detroit, MI: Wayne State University Press.

Hughes, C., & Agran, M. (1998). Introduction to the special issue on self-determination. *Journal of the Association for Persons with Severe Handicaps, 23,* 1–4.

Kanfer, F. H. (1970). Self-regulation: Research, issues, and speculations. In C. Neuringer & J. L. Michael (Eds.), *Behavior modification in clinical psychology* (pp. 178–220). New York: Appleton-Century-Crofts.

Kanfer, F. H. (1977). The many faces of self-control, or behavior modification changes its focus. In R. B. Stuart (Ed.), *Behavioral self-management: Strategies, techniques and outcomes* (pp. 1–48). New York: Brunner/Mazel.

Kapadia, S., & Fantuzzo, J. W. (1988). Training children with developmental disabilities and severe behavior problems to use self-management procedures to sustain attention to preacademic/academic tasks. *Education and Training in Mental Retardation, 23,* 59–69.

King-Sears, M. E., & Carpenter, S. L. (1997). *Teaching self-management to elementary students with developmental disabilities.* Washington, DC: American Association on Mental Retardation.

Lagomarcino, T. R., & Rusch, F. R. (1989). Utilizing self-management procedures to teach independent performance. *Education and Training in Mental Retardation, 24,* 297–305.

Langer, J. (1969). *Theories of development.* New York: Holt, Rinehart & Winston.

Lovett, D. L., & Haring, K. A. (1989). The effects of self-management training on the daily living of adults with mental retardation. *Education and Training in Mental Retardation, 24,* 306–307.

Malott, R. W. (1984). Rule-governed behavior, self-management, and the developmentally disabled: A theoretical analysis. *Analysis and Intervention in Developmental Disabilities, 4,* 199–209.

Martin, J. E., & Huber Marshall, L. (1996). ChoiceMaker: A comprehensive self-determination transition program. *Intervention in School and Clinic, 30*(3), 147–156.

McCarl, J. J., Svobodny, L., & Beare, P. L. (1991). Self-recording in a classroom for students with mild to moderate mental handicaps: Effects on productivity and on-task behavior. *Education and Training in Mental Retardation, 26,* 79–88.

Mithaug, D. E. (1993). Self-regulation theory: How optimal adjustment maximizes gain. Westport, CT: Praeger.

Mithaug, D. E., Martin, J. E., & Agran, M. (1987). Adaptability instruction: The goal of transition programming. *Exceptional Children, 53,* 500–505.

Mithaug, D. E., Martin, J. E., Agran, M., & Rusch, R. F. (1988). *Why special education graduates fail.* Colorado Springs, CO: Ascent Publications.

Mithaug, D. E., Mithaug, D. K., Agran, M., Martin, J. E., & Wehmeyer, M. L. (2003). *Self-determined learning theory: Predictions, prescriptions, and practice.* Mahwah, NJ: Erlbaum.

Mithaug, D., Wehmeyer, M. L., Agran, M., Martin, J., & Palmer, S. (1998). The self-determined learning model of instruction: Engaging students to solve their learning problems. In M. L. Wehmeyer & D. J. Sands (Eds.), *Making it happen: Student involvement in educational planning, decision-making and instruction* (pp. 299–328). Baltimore: Brookes.

Moore, S. C., Agran, M., & Fodor-Davis, J. (1989). Using self-management strategies to increase the production rates of workers with severe handicaps. *Education and Training in Mental Retardation, 24,* 324–332.

Reinecke, D. R., Newman, B., & Meinberg, D. L. (1999). Self-management of sharing in three preschoolers with autism. *Education and Training in Mental Retardation and Developmental Disabilities, 34,* 312–317.

Sands, D. J., & Wehmeyer, M. L. (1996). *Self-determination across the life span: Independence and choice for people with disabilities.* Baltimore: Brookes.

Schunk, D. H. (1981). Modeling and attributional effects on children's achievement: A self-efficacy analysis. *Journal of Educational Psychology, 73,* 93–105.

Skinner, B. F. (1953). *Science and human behavior.* New York: Free Press.

Smith, D. J., & Nelson, J. R. (1997). In M. Agran (Ed.), *Student-directed learning: Teaching self-determination skills* (pp. 80–110). Pacific Grove, CA: Brooks/Cole.

Stevenson, H. D., & Fantuzzo, J. W. (1984). Application of the "generalization map" to a self-control intervention with school-aged children. *Journal of Applied Behavior Analysis, 17,* 203–212.

Watson, D. L., & Tharp, R. G. (1989). *Self-directed behavior: Self-modification for personal adjustment.* Pacific Grove, CA: Brooks/Cole.

Wehmeyer, M. L. (1992). Self-determination and the education of students with mental retardation. *Education and Training in Mental Retardation, 27,* 302–314.

Wehmeyer, M. L. (1996a). Self-determination as an educational outcome: Why is it important to children, youth, and adults with disabilities? In D. J. Sands & M. L. Wehmeyer (Eds.), *Self-determination across the life span: Independence and choice for people with disabilities* (pp. 17–36). Baltimore: Brookes.

Wehmeyer, M. L. (1996b). A self-report measure of self-determination for adolescents with cognitive disabilities. *Education and Training in Mental Retardation and Developmental Disabilities, 31,* 282–293.

Wehmeyer, M. L. (1998). Self-determination and individuals with significant disabilities: Examining meanings and misinterpretations. *Journal of the Association for Persons with Severe Handicaps, 23,* 5–16.

Wehmeyer, M. L. (2001). Self-determination and mental retardation. In L. M. Glidden (Ed.), *International review of research in mental retardation* (Vol. 24, pp. 1–48). San Diego, CA: Academic Press.

Wehmeyer, M. L., & Agran, M. (2004). Promoting access to the general curriculum for students with significant cognitive disabilities. In F. Spooner & D. Browder (Eds.), *Teaching reading, math, and science to students with significant cognitive disabilities.* Baltimore: Paul H. Brookes.

Wehmeyer, M. L., Agran, M., & Hughes, C. (1998). *Teaching self-determination to students with disabilities: Basic skills for successful transition.* Baltimore: Paul H. Brookes.

Wehmeyer, M. L., & Kelchner, K. (1995a). Measuring the autonomy of adolescents and adults with mental retardation: A self-report form of the Autonomous Functioning Checklist. *Career Development for Exceptional Individuals, 18,* 3–20.

Wehmeyer, M. L., Kelchner, K., & Richards, S. (1996). Essential characteristics of self-determined behaviors of adults with mental retardation and developmental disabilities. *American Journal on Mental Retardation, 100,* 632–642.

Wehmeyer, M. L., Palmer, S. B., Agran, M., Mithaug, D. E., & Martin, J. E. (2000). Promoting causal agency: The Self-Determined Learning Model of Instruction. *Exceptional Children, 66,* 430–453.

Wehmeyer, M. L., & Sands, D. J. (1998). *Making it happen: Student involvement in education planning, decision making, and instruction.* Baltimore: Paul H. Brooks.

Wehmeyer, M. L., Yeager, D., Bolding, N., Agran, M., & Hughes, C. (2003). The effects of self-regulation strategies on goal attainment for students with developmental disabilities in general education. *Journal of Physical and Developmental Disabilities, 15,* 79–91.

Wolman, J. M., Campeau, P. L., DuBois, P. A., Mithaug, D. E., & Stolarski, V. S. (1994). *AIR self-determination scale and users guide.* Palo Alto, CA: American Institutes for Research.

9

Psychophysiological Assessment*

Frank H. Wilhelm

Department of Clinical Psychology and Psychotherapy
Institute for Psychology
University of Basel
Basel, Switzerland

Silvia Schneider

Department of Clinical Child and Adolescent Psychology
Institute for Psychology
University of Basel
Basel, Switzerland

Bruce H. Friedman

Department of Psychology
Virginia Polytechnic Institute and State University
Blacksburg, Virginia

Conceptual Framework and Practical Considerations

Considerable progress has been made in systematically exploring psychophysiological functioning in infants, children, and adolescents. Assessment of psychophysiological reactions opens unique ways of understanding cognitive and emotional processes and provides insights that cannot be obtained by behavioral

*Preparation of this chapter was supported by Grants 105311-105850 (FHW) and PP001-68701 (SS) from the Swiss National Science Foundation.

Correspondence concerning this article should be addressed to Frank Wilhelm, Health Psychophysiology Laboratory, Institute for Psychology, University of Basel, CH-4055 Basel, Switzerland. Electronic mail may be sent to frank.wilhelm@unibas.ch.

observation, interview, or questionnaire. The increasing availability of easy-to-use high-technology tools for psychophysiological assessment brings this domain into the reach of child psychologists and clinicians who do not intend to spend years becoming technical experts. Nevertheless, psychophysiology is a matured scientific field, with its own nomenclature, concepts, and methodological approaches, that requires careful study. While attempting not to replicate what is covered regarding adult psychophysiolgy in Chapter 8 (Kevin T. Larkin) of the book *Clinician's Handbook of Adult Behavioral Assessment*, we will outline methodological considerations specifically germane to assessment in children and review part of the relevant literature to provide a concise introduction into this exciting field. Research examples are offered to illustrate the utility of psychophysiology in child clinical assessment. The interested reader is referred to more specialized chapters in the *Handbook of Psychophysiology* (Cacioppo, Tassinary, & Berntson, 2000), which is particularly thorough in outlining concepts and reviewing the literature and provides a chapter on developmental psychophysiology (Fox, Schmidt, & Henderson, 2000), and *Psychophysiological Recording* (Stern, Ray, & Quigley, 2000), which excels in providing details on psychophysiological data acquisition and interpretation. In addition, a series of papers on methods and guidelines is made available to the public on the Web site of the Society for Psychophysiological Research (SPR) (http://www.sprweb.org). Lists with measurement device manufacturers and software for psychophysiological signal recording and analysis have been collected by SPR members and been made available through their associated Web site (www.psychophys.com).

UTILITY OF PSYCHOPHYSIOLOGICAL ASSESSMENT IN CHILDREN

Psychophysiological assessment is language free and thus transcends cultural, ethnic, and age boundaries in a unique way. Depending on their age, children may not be well aware of their emotional or cognitive processes and/or may lack the language to describe them. Such obstacles may be amplified in children with clinical disorders that involve communication impairment. Thus, questionnaire or interview methods might be biased or inappropriate to infer such information. Psychophysiological science tries to understand interactions of physiological and psychological processes. An important context for understanding complex psychophysiological responses may be provided by self-report and behavioral measures that are often obtained in conjunction with psychophysiological responses. The three-systems approach to emotion assessment, as first formulated by Lang (1968, 1978), stipulates a comprehensive measurement of physiological function, overt behavior, and self-report since no single mode fully captures emotional response. Behavioral observation and interviews have been weighted heavily in child assessment practice. However, conceptually and statistically, by adding psychophysiological variables with sources of measurement error and biases independent of the other assessment modes, the overall validity and reliability of assessment of attention, emotion, and cognition may be improved (see, for example, Wilhelm & Roth, 2001).

Furthermore, psychophysiology methods can add insights into how basic physiological mechanisms may be involved in shaping child behavior. For example, since autonomic nervous system (ANS) regulation can dispatch or withdraw resources to muscles and organs, children with generally high sympathetic reactivity to stressors are likely predisposed to overreact behaviorally to challenging situations. Moreover, since ANS regulation changes during the course of development due to structural and functional changes in the central and peripheral nervous systems, the perspective for understanding developmental changes in child behavior may be widened considerably by examining physiological data. There are few extant cross-sectional or longitudinal studies that examine such important intersections between child behavior and physiology.

ASPECTS OF PSYCHOPHYSIOLOGICAL ASSESSMENT UNIQUE TO CHILDREN

Many concepts and methods from the adult psychophysiology literature referred to in Chapter 8 of the book *Clinician's Handbook of Adult Behavioral Assessment* are in principle applicable to children. Children have an orienting response, habituate to stimuli, exhibit a startle reflex that is attenuated when in a positive emotional state, show spontaneous electrodermal responses, accelerate their heartbeat when anxious, show evidence of heart rate variability locked to autonomic rhythms, and demonstrate almost all basic psychophysiological processes extensively studied in adults. Thus, most of the measurement methods developed for adults can be productively applied in children and even in infants, although they may require modification. For example, at the most mundane level, to accommodate a smaller body, the electrocardiogram (ECG) in infants and children is best measured with smaller electrodes. For many measurement devices, special sensors can be obtained from the manufacturer; for example, a smaller upper arm cuff for blood pressure or a special child head garment for obtaining multilead electroencephalogram (EEG) activity at the scalp. Gain settings of amplifiers might need to be adjusted to compensate for the smaller electrical potentials of child bioelectrical activity. Furthermore, for the analysis of these biosignals, the analysis software settings might need to be adjusted to accommodate the typically higher frequency in cardiovascular and respiratory rhythmic activity.

On the other hand, children differ from adults in certain aspects of psychophysiological response, with implications for assessment. This point is particularly relevant to perceptual, cognitive, and emotional functioning in early life when the central and peripheral nervous systems are still developing. Interpreting what a specific measure taken in a certain context from a particular child actually means may be difficult, since it may deviate considerably from the adult literature. For example, event-related brain potentials (ERPs) change through the course of child development (Cycowicz, 2000; Ridderinkhof & van der Stelt, 2000), and simply comparing a child's reactions to adult studies may lead to erroneous conclusions. Currently, few data exist on age-related norms for psychophysiological reactions to child-relevant testing paradigms, so diagnostically meaningful assessment in individual children is typically not practical. Psychophysiological assessments need to be obtained within the context of an age-matched group—in either a clinical practice, hospital, or research setting—to allow drawing any conclusions regarding the normality or abnormality of perceptual, cognitive, or emotional functions in individual children. In this respect, child psychophysiology research is still in its infancy, which is understandable, given the cost and complexity of obtaining normative data.

Ethical Issues

Children need, and are granted by law, special protections when participating in clinical exams or research studies. Thus, any invasive or unpleasant assessment method requires even more justification in children than in adults. Most psychophysiological measurement methods, such as electrocardiography (ECG) and electrodermal activity, are noninvasive and have minimal potential for harm when applied correctly (Putnam, Johnson, & Roth, 1992). Some newer and diagnostically very strong assessment techniques, such as functional magnetic resonance imaging (fMRI) and positron emission tomography (PET), are used increasingly in psychophysiological studies and can be disagreeable to some children because of their potentially frightening nature. Also, certain paradigms for assessment of conditionability utilize rather unpleasant stimuli, for example, loud noise bursts. Ethical principles imply that such techniques require special justification before being applied in children by carefully weighing potential risks and benefits.

Sensor overload might be a problem when attempting to measure responses in every possible physiological system at the same time. Here again, the incremental utility of adding a sensor should be examined carefully to minimize the burden to the child, both during setup and removal of the sensors and during the assessment. Often, similar information can be obtained by using another, less invasive sensor type; for example, a pulse plethysmograph that is easily attached to the finger can measure heart rate almost as reliably as ECG, which requires putting three sticky patches and cables on the chest.

Task overload is another problem to be aware of—children generally have a much smaller attention span than adults and might easily get distracted and eventually fail to follow the stimuli presented on a computer screen. Safeguards against this possibility should be part of the assessment procedure to avoid unreliable data. Much can be gained by redesigning assessment paradigms in a child-friendly way. For example, instead of using squares and circles as conditioned stimuli in a discriminatory conditioning paradigm, one may consider using frogs and birds. Reaction-time tasks can be reappraised as a game where the child competes against other children. Standard psychological stressors such as mental arithmetic can be introduced as an exercise known from school and of course need to be carefully adjusted to the age of the child.

Creating Child Friendly Assessment

Even if the assessment paradigm is optimized, many children may not comply with instructions to sit still for extended periods of time. In particular, assessments of children with Attention-Deficit Hyperactivity Disorder (ADHD) have to consider this issue carefully. If an assessment is longer than 20–30 minutes, it should be designed so that the child can have breaks to interact with a parent or other children, get something to drink, or play with a toy. Of course, taking off sensors or unplugging cables might be so much effort that other solutions, e.g., several shorter experimental sessions instead of a single long session, may need to be found. During the preparatory phase when sensors are attached and when they are removed it is often a good idea to have the child watch an age-appropriate movie. There are creative ways to make the assessment more child friendly and to optimize child compliance, including how the assessment room is equipped, task design, and how the child is treated by the examiner. For example, tasks can be made appealing to children by using stimuli depicting animals or scenes that children can relate to. The task may be introduced in an interactive way by asking the child a question such as "Do you think you can keep your eyes open and watch the pictures on the screen?" Many children like to have their imagination involved: The room can be set up to reflect a theme from a popular children's TV series or movie and assessment can be put into this context. However, care must be taken to keep the assessment standardized and not to induce distortions or even bias measurements.

Compliance of children with the instructions is crucial for the success of most assessments. An important first step is to ensure that instructions are optimized for children of the examined age group by doing some piloting and adjustments as necessary. One can make sure that the instructions have been understood by asking children to repeat what is asked from them. To keep children engaged even with monotonous tasks, it has proven beneficial in our research to use a systematic operant conditioning approach. For example, the child receives a stamp on a prepared sheet for completion of each part of a lengthy assessment session (see, for example, Figure 9.1). The child is told that after the assessment, the size of the box with presents he or she will receive depends on how many stamps were collected. One can even make special medals or stickers that certify the child's participation in the study. As a beneficial side effect, his or her friends may tell their parents that they want to participate in the study as well, which may help with recruitment efforts.

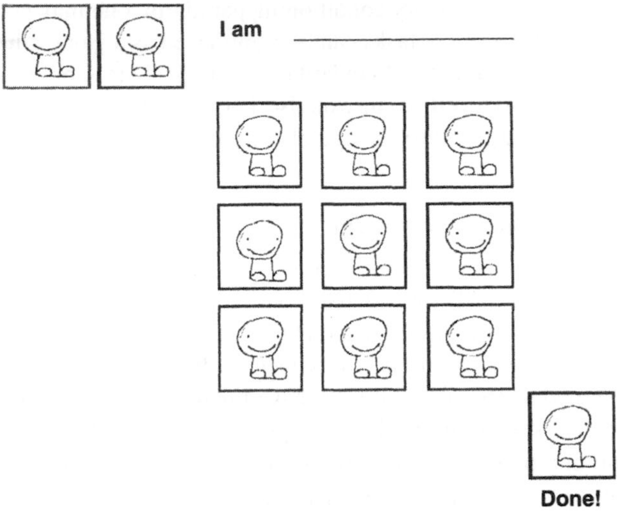

FIGURE 9.1 Chart used for enhancing compliance of children during a lengthy assessment session (90 min) for a psychophysiological study at the Institute for Psychology, University of Basel. For completion of each part of the assessment, the child receives a stamp and later a reward (toy) that depends on the number of stamps received. The first two stamps are given before the start of the session; stamp 12 is a bonus if all parts are finished.

Even the attachment of electrodes, which can take 20 minutes or more in some paradigms (especially when using an array of EEG or EMG electrodes), can be made more conducive to children. Having a boy or girl imagine that he/she is a space flight commander and that his/her vital signs will be monitored during takeoff can be rather engaging. Some setups allow the child to watch the physiological signals on the computer monitor. In this case, it is good to provide some insights to the child as to what the signal means. By showing that just by clapping her hand the examiner can make the child's EDA signal go up is highly interesting for most children. Some laboratory setups have an assessment room connected by one-way mirror or monitor and intercom to the control room. The intercom can of course be playfully woven into the space commander theme.

Many psychophysiological studies also collect subjective data on moods and symptoms. With adequate introduction, in our experience, most children will be able to use rating scales with text as descriptors and anchors starting at the age of 8. In younger children, iconing anchors, such as the Self-Assessment Manikin (Bradley & Lang, 1994), might be employed starting at the age of 4 years. We have developed iconic self-assessment scales covering a range of moods and symptoms related to anxiety and successfully used them in children at age 6 years onward (for examples, see Figure 9.2) (Schneider, Wilhelm, & Martin, 2005). To ensure that children understand the concept of gradual increase in symptoms (as opposed to on/off), it is recommended to initially review the questions to be used during the assessment and have the children describe and then rate their current

My strongest anxiety **during fast breathing:**

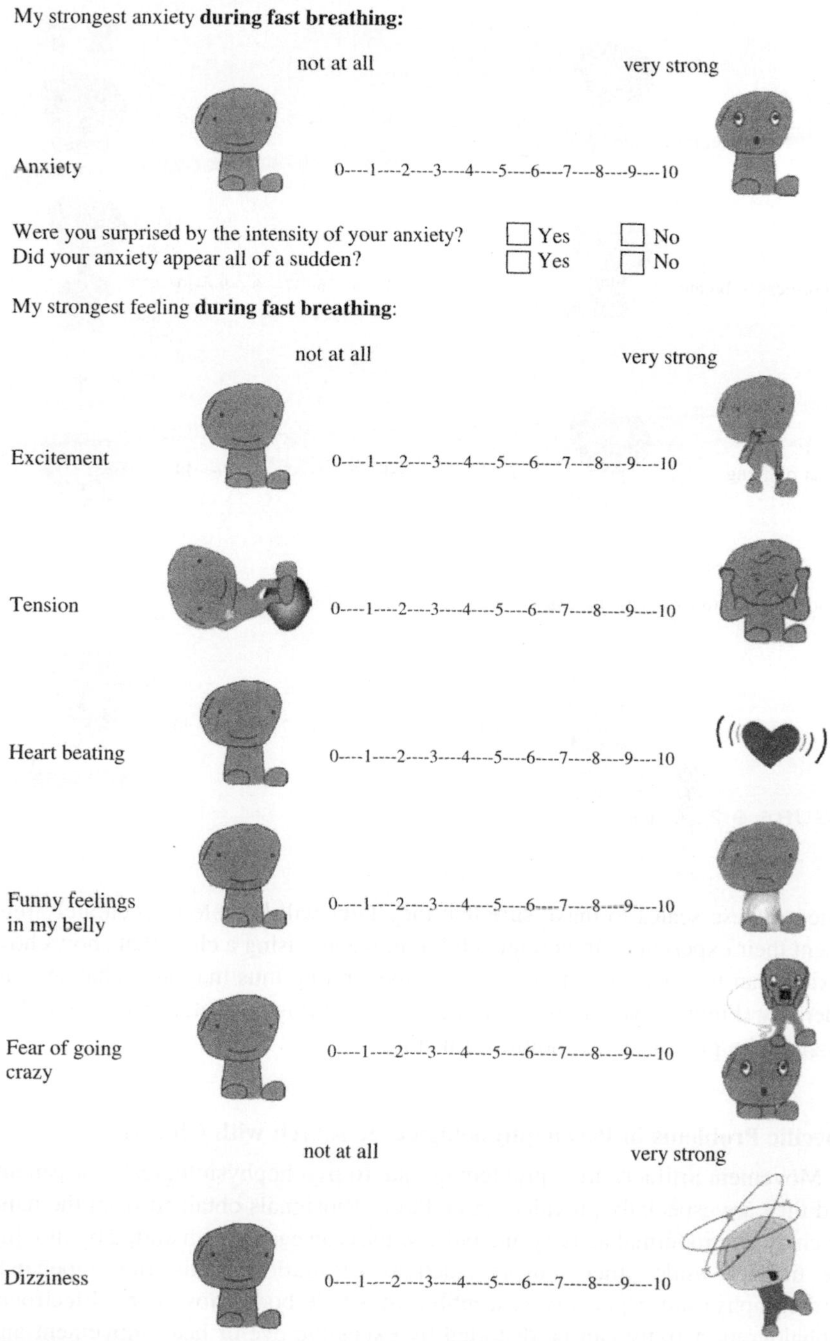

not at all   very strong

Anxiety   0----1----2----3----4----5----6----7----8----9----10

Were you surprised by the intensity of your anxiety?   ☐ Yes   ☐ No
Did your anxiety appear all of a sudden?   ☐ Yes   ☐ No

My strongest feeling **during fast breathing**:

not at all   very strong

Excitement   0----1----2----3----4----5----6----7----8----9----10

Tension   0----1----2----3----4----5----6----7----8----9----10

Heart beating   0----1----2----3----4----5----6----7----8----9----10

Funny feelings
in my belly   0----1----2----3----4----5----6----7----8----9----10

Fear of going
crazy   0----1----2----3----4----5----6----7----8----9----10

not at all   very strong

Dizziness   0----1----2----3----4----5----6----7----8----9----10

FIGURE 9.2 Child self-assessment questionnaire enhanced with iconic representations of symptoms and emotions, as developed for a child research program at the Institute for Psychology, University of Basel.

(continues)

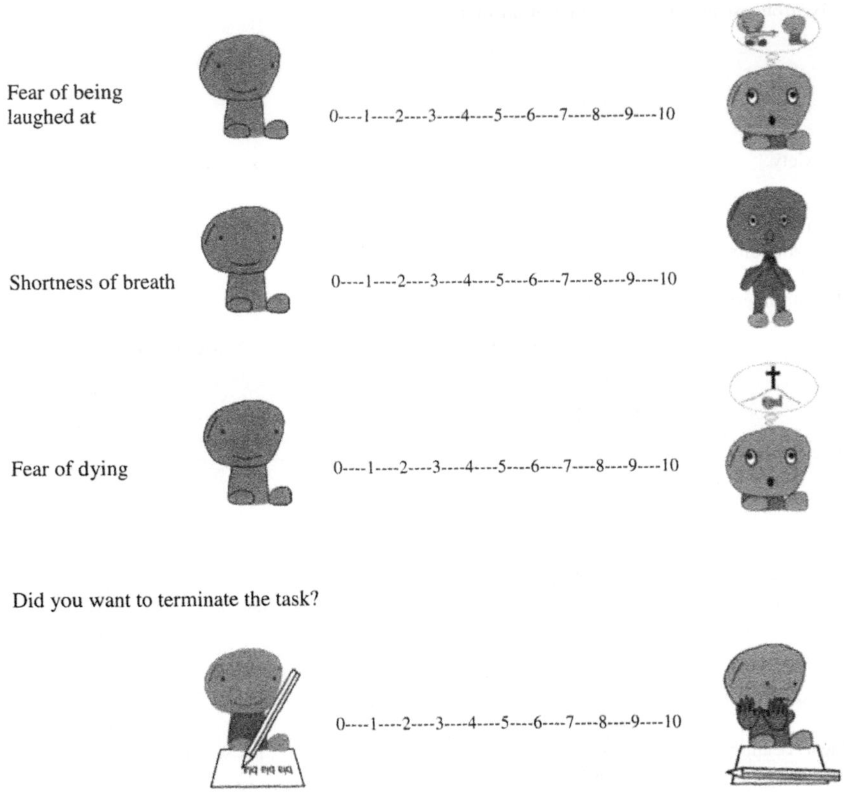

Fear of being laughed at
0----1----2----3----4----5----6----7----8----9----10
Shortness of breath
0----1----2----3----4----5----6----7----8----9----10
Fear of dying
0----1----2----3----4----5----6----7----8----9----10
Did you want to terminate the task?
0----1----2----3----4----5----6----7----8----9----10

FIGURE 9.2 *Continued*

state on these scales to make sure that they later will be able to accurately represent their experience. In younger children, we are using a chart that shows how anxiety can fluctuate over time and how their rating thus may also change considerably (Figure 9.3). Of course, if a child is marking a sheet, sensors should, if possible, be put on the nondominant hand.

Specific Problems in Psychophysiological Research with Children

Movement artifacts are a problem unique to psychophysiological assessment, and they are especially prevalent in children. Biosignals obtained from the hand (such as electrodermal activity and pulse wave) can easily be distorted by moving the fingers, while other sensors (such as respiration bands and impedance cardiography) are especially susceptible to whole-body movement. Electroencephalogram activity can be distorted by excessive eye or head movement and clenching of the jaw. fMRI and PET brain scans can get blurred with even subtle head movement. Thus, as an aid in detection of these problematic movement

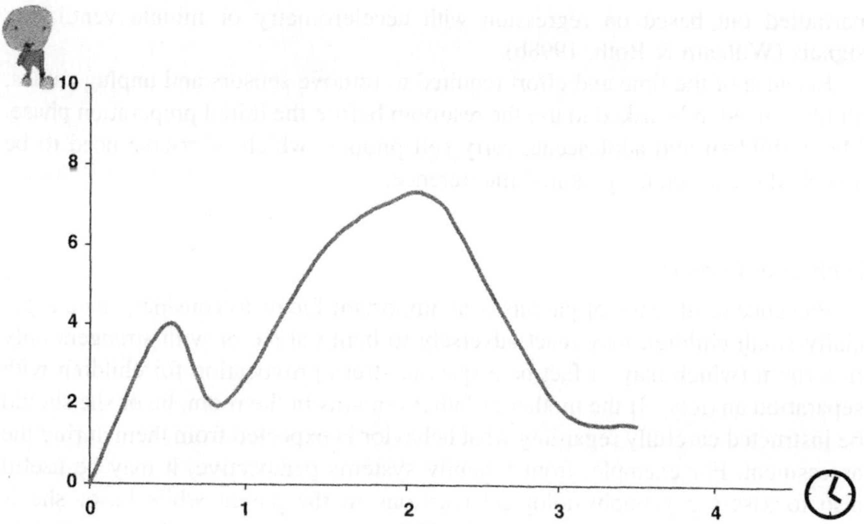

FIGURE 9.3 Chart showing how anxiety can fluctuate over time, to instruct children about the use of self-assessment scales.

intervals it is highly advisable to record physical activity with an accelerometer attached to the child or chair. These intervals need to be carefully screened during the signal analysis, and affected signals need to be edited, interpolated, or excluded.

Physical activity not only induces biosignal artifacts but also might make the results of certain measurements ambiguous or inconclusive; most psychophysiological measures of emotional activation, including heart rate, electrodermal activity, blood pressure, respiratory sinus arrhythmia, and salivary cortisol, also react strongly to muscular activity. This problem is further complicated by the fact that emotions not only influence autonomic function but also often induce restlessness (for example, as part of the fight-or-flight response). One can somewhat guard against ambiguities in the results with careful instructions to the child, age-appropriate duration of assessment, and continuous recording of physical activity as described earlier. In a research context, any conclusions as to underlying autonomic mechanisms for a specific state or trait (for example, Attention-Deficit Hyperactivity Disorder) are most convincing when it can be demonstrated that it is not related to differences in physical activity (for example, by analysis of covariance). Otherwise, the results from the physiological measurements are rather trivial, and psychophysiological assessment may not really add anything to a much simpler accelerometry or behavioral observation approach. Special procedures have been developed to account for the confounding effects of physical activity on autonomic function measures, e.g., estimation of the "additional heart rate" component in the heart rate signal, after the physical component has been partialled out based on regression with accelerometry or minute ventilation signals (Wilhelm & Roth, 1998b).

Because of the time and effort required to remove sensors and unplug cables, children need to be asked to use the restroom before the initial preparation phase. Many children and adolescents carry cell phones, which of course need to be switched off to reduce potential interference.

Including Parents

Presence or absence of parents is an important factor to consider, since especially small children may react adversely to being alone or with strangers only in a room (which may in fact be a specific stress provocation for children with separation anxiety). If the mother or father remains in the room, he or she should be instructed carefully regarding what behavior is expected from them during the assessment. For example, from a family systems perspective, it may be useful also to assess psychophysiological reactions in the parent while he or she is observing or interacting with the child. If the assessment room does not accommodate parent–child dyadic examinations, at the very least one may consider measuring heart rate responses in the parent using an inexpensive wristwatch heart rate monitor, which can later be synchronized with data obtained from the child (for details, see the upcoming section on ambulatory monitoring).

A parent in the room will typically increase considerably a child's compliance with the assessment procedures (although there are exceptions where the opposite is true). Some child maladjustment problems change the style of dyadic interaction with parents and how parents react to their child, or the maladjustment might even be triggered or maintained by parental style. For instance, an overprotective and worried mother may be a risk factor for a child developing an anxiety disorder. Understanding the physiological reactions and communication style of the mother while the child undergoes anxiety challenges may reveal important insights. One way to quantify this is by analysis of cross-correlations or coherence between mother and child in physiological, self-report, and behavioral responses (Gottman & Roy, 1990). Behavioral data can best be gathered by digital video, using a second camera focusing on the parent and mixing this signal onto one-half of a split screen, with the other half showing the child.

Another important factor is the compliance of parents. They need to be well informed and understand the importance of the assessment procedures to help the child develop a positive attitude toward the assessment. Often, a child arrives for the examination with one parent (usually the mother) and is later alone in the assessment room. The parent may stay in the adjacent room, together with the assessor, to see the child's reactions and ask questions. After the procedures, it is important to offer a debriefing with child and parent, which ideally includes having them look at a few parts of the physiological recordings and give some interpretation of what they mean.

Medication and Timing of Assessment

Many psychophysiological measures are affected by medications that are commonly prescribed to children, such as Ritalin and antihistamines, which have moderate to strong side effects on autonomic nervous system function. If possible and approved by the pediatrician or child and adolescent psychiatrist, these drugs may be discontinued during the assessment day. Beverages containing caffeine should be taken in the usual amount for the child and the amounts taken during the day before the assessment noted on a sheet as a control variable.

Timing of assessment should be scrutinized because circadian rhythms can influence wakefulness and psychophysiological responding. For many children and parents, assessment will only fit to their schedule conveniently at the end of a school- and workday, when they are already tired and have diminished capacity for attention. The wakefulness state during the assessment needs to be monitored carefully and, if necessary, modulated by instructions or breaks. This is especially important in infants, who frequently change their state. Assessments will work best if the sleeping–waking–eating cycle of the infant or child is taken into account.

PARADIGMS FOR PSYCHOPHYSIOLOGICAL ASSESSMENT IN CHILDREN

FROM LABORATORY TO AMBULATORY ASSESSMENT

Most psychophysiological assessment will take place in a laboratory, clinic, or private practice under controlled conditions, where children are supervised and the context of physiological recording is well known. Measurement systems and analysis software are well developed, documented, user friendly, and reliable (for a register of manufacturers and devices, see, for example, www.psychophys.com). Movement artifacts can be minimized, and analysis and statistical procedures are well established. However, the laboratory can be an intimidating environment to children. By constraining children to perform certain tasks, their reactions may not be representative of normal function. For example, children with anxiety disorders will likely not show real "baseline" values when assessed in the laboratory, and any acute anxiety episode elicited there may or may not represent what is going on in real life. Growing concern about low external validity and the increasing availability of alternative high-tech solutions makes ambulatory monitoring a desirable option for a variety of assessment questions (Maheu et al., 2005; Wilhelm & Roth, 1996). For some clinical problems, only "real-life" assessment can establish the validity of laboratory results and help disentangle the effects of trait or temperament from state–trait interaction unique to the laboratory.

Modern multichannel ambulatory monitoring devices such as the LifeShirt system (Vivometrics, Inc., Ventura, CA) are available specifically for children and allow a comprehensive assessment of various physiological systems during day and night (Wilhelm & Grossman, in press; Wilhelm, Roth, & Sackner, 2003). Understanding sleep processes and nocturnal autonomic function may help better explain behavioral problems in children. By extending the observation window, some rare episodes that are unlikely to happen spontaneously in the laboratory (e.g., seizures, temper tantrums, and panic attacks) may be captured. Frequency and distribution of motoric tics across the day can be measured with an accelerometry sensor attached to the affected area. Simple wristwatch heart rate monitors (e.g., from Polar, Inc., and Timex, Inc.) or actigraphs (e.g., from Ambulatory Monitoring, Inc., and Mini Mitter, Inc.) are basic tools that can estimate sleep–wake cycles, sleep efficiency, daytime physical activity level, and circadian rhythm (Teicher, 1995). There are very few studies that have examined the evolution of sleep parameters with age in school-aged children and adolescents. In these studies, total sleep time has been found to decrease with age only on school days (Ohayon, Carskadon, Guilleminault, & Vitiello, 2004).

Data on physical activity, autonomic function, and subjective experience (when using an integrated or separate electronic diary) may be supplemented by endocrine measures. Special saliva collection swabs that children can chew on and store in a small plastic container (Salivettes) can later be analyzed for concentration of the stress hormone cortisol and other compounds (see also the upcoming section on neuroendocrine function). There are also ambulatory monitors that offer measures of impedance cardiography and heart rate variability (described later) as well as electrodermal activity (e.g., Ambulatory Monitoring System, Vrije Universiteit Amsterdam, the Netherlands; Varioport, Becker Meditec, Germany).

However, ambulatory monitoring has its unique challenges: The amount of data collected can be staggering, and without contextual information the physiological information may be uninterpretable. Modern devices have advanced analysis capabilities for efficient data reduction and built-in sensors that help provide contextual information (for example, level of physical activity, posture, speaking). More specific information can be entered into an electronic diary by the parent or child. Electronic momentary assessment with e-diaries has been used in adults and recently has been shown to be feasible in children ages 8 years and older and even superior to paper-and-pencil measures in terms of compliance and accuracy when assessing pain (Palermo, Valenzuela, & Stork, 2004). Ambulatory recording may in some instances require a semistandardized protocol, for example, by having the child sit quietly at various times during the day for establishing baselines of autonomic activation and then estimating circadian variation without any physical activity confound. This procedure can be quite efficient and eliminate the need for more burdensome long-term laboratory assessments.

Ambulatory monitors may be beneficially applied as an adjunct to observational studies in the laboratory since the children are able to move freely. With some systems (e.g., LifeShirt, Vivometric, Inc., Ventura, CA), data are not only stored internally for later download but can be wirelessly transmitted in real time to a computer for display and analysis. Such telemetric capacity may be useful not only for assessment but also for targeted treatment. For example, when monitoring physical activity in children with impulsivity problems, an operant intervention might be triggered when the activity exceeds a certain level. A similar kind of biofeedback application is built into some wrist actigraphs intended, for example, for operant treatment of children with Attention-Deficit Hyperactivity Disorder. These devices beep when activity level surpasses defined thresholds of intensity and duration to remind the child to calm down (see also the upcoming section on pediatric biofeedback applications).

FROM BEHAVIORAL CHALLENGES TO COMPUTERIZED STIMULUS PRESENTATION

Even the most sophisticated physiological measures lack meaning without relating them to the condition(s) under which they were collected. The most basic paradigm is the resting baseline, and any abnormality seen there usually indicates a pervasive trait feature. Most medical measurements (e.g., blood pressure and blood draws) are taken under supposed baseline conditions. However, as discussed earlier, laboratory baselines may not well represent real-world functioning, especially in children, because of reactivity to the setting. An example of this effect in the adult medical literature is "white-coat hypertension": high blood pressure in the clinic but not at home.

Psychophysiology is mostly used in reactivity paradigms in which a psychologically meaningful situation or stimulus is presented and reactions to it are quantified, typically in reference to a prechallenge or prestimulus baseline. A multitude of behavioral challenge and stimulus presentation paradigms has been developed and are well standardized. Some of the procedures have been utilized for child assessment.

Among behavioral challenges, mental stress inductions such as the Trier Social Stress Test (Kirschbaum, Pirke, & Hellhammer, 1993), consisting of a preparatory period, simulated speech, and mental arithmetic, each with a duration of 5 minutes, have been adapted to children (Kudielka, Buske-Kirschbaum, Hellhammer, & Kirschbaum, 2004). Next to the assessment of behavioral responses, potency and timing of this test allow quantifying the course of salivary cortisol and autonomic response to stress (and over a 30- to 60-minute period following the stress). For anxiety assessment, child-relevant paradigms that have been used for social fears include, for example, reading aloud and singing a children's song (Martel et al., 1999). Stimuli such as animals or needles can be used to induce anxiety in children with specific phobias. For children with separation anxiety, a provocation might involve having the mother leave the room. Some data exist on physiological reactions to the Strange Situation test (Ainsworth, Blehar, Waters, & Wall, 1978), a putative measure of attachment style applied in children as early as 12 months of age (Donovan & Leavitt, 1989). The test consists of a baseline with the parents and short periods of 3–6 minutes of separation. For example, it has been shown that, despite less overt distress in insecure-avoidant infants after short separations from the mother, overall cardiac measures indicate physiological activation patterns similar to those of the secure infants during separation (Spangler & Grossmann, 1993). Behavioral and physiological reactions to novel situations (e.g., a stranger entering the room) are taken as indication of the extent of behavioral inhibition in children (Kagan, Reznick, & Snidman, 1987), which has been shown to be related to adult anxiety disorders (Rosenbaum et al., 1993). Depending on the assessment goals, relevant situations may also be interactions with other children in standardized or unstandardized situations, playing with toys or a computer game, and induction of frustration or anger.

Physical stressors are sometimes used to quantify general autonomic response patterns. These responses can easily be probed by a change of posture (standing up from sitting or by using a tilt table), cold pressor (holding the hand into a bucket with 4°C cold water), or physical exercise (handgrip dynamometer, bicyle ergometer). Measurements taken during these tests allow calibration of each child's psychophysiological response to the more general autonomic response tendencies to aversive or physical stimuli. For example, a child that is physically not very fit may react with large heart rate increase to a standardized ergometer load, and it might be useful to know this when interpreting the heart rate responses to mental stressors. Physical stress reactivity may then be used as a covariate in the mental stress analyses.

Respiratory challenge procedures have been used for questions related to panic disorder or the propensity for it, for example, in children diagnosed with anxiety disorders (Pine et al., 1998) or in offspring of parents with panic disorder (Pine et al., 2005), because respiratory regulation seems to be particularly unstable in this clinical condition (Gorman et al., 1988; Papp et al., 1989; Wilhelm, Trabert, & Roth, 2001a, 2001b). A respiratory challenge may consist of having the child breathe 5% concentrations of carbon dioxide (CO_2) for several minutes or 20% for a single breath repeatedly with pauses. A less threatening procedure that may provide similar information is the hyperventilation test with a following extended recovery period (Wilhelm, Gerlach, & Roth, 2001), but its validity for child assessment has not yet been established. Interest in physiological recovery has also emerged as an important factor, since the speed of recovery may be as telling in regard to emotion regulation processes as the extent of reactivity (Fredrickson, Mancuso, Branigan, & Tugade, 2000; Roth, Wilhelm, & Trabert, 1998).

General style and capacity for emotion regulation have been probed using video film clips of 2–5 minutes' duration (Gross & Levenson, 1995). Film clips can be taken from children's movies after securing permission to use them in studies. Sequences from commercial movies can be excellent emotional provocations. Basic emotions that can be evoked with films include anxiety or fear, anger, sadness, disgust, contempt, joy, and surprise. Despite different forms of emotional expression across cultures and age ranges, there are common elements, or prototype patterns, that can be identified (Plutchik, 1980). Physiologically, many emotions are similar, in that they produce generalized activation or arousal, which allows an objective quantification of emotion intensity, especially when aggregating across several measures. Differences in the pattern of physiological responses to several emotional provocations ("situational response specificity") can be small in comparison to differences between individuals in their preferred physiological response pattern ("individual response stereotypy"). Thus, inferring the kind of emotion a child experiences solely from the physiological signature is typically not possible and requires additional context information, for example, about the task or situation, facial expression, and verbalizations. However, efforts are currently being made to apply modern pattern recognition procedures to classification of affective state solely on the basis of physiological signals (Christie & Friedman, 2004; Picard, Vyzas, & Healey, 2001).

Interpretation of psychophysiological responses in infants and young children benefits from synchronized coding of overt behavior, including facial expression and social interaction. Behavioral responses can act as an anchor and validate that the child responded to a task in the intended way. Commercial software commonly used for this purpose is the Observer® (Noldus Information Techology, The Netherlands), which also has a mobile version for field studies that can be installed on a Palm-type pocket computer. A relevant coding scheme for a specific assessment question can be programmed rather easily. Certain keys, mouse clicks, or input fields on the touch screen are assigned to a certain behavior and record the time of each instance when they are activated and deactivated. A software solution that is experienced as more intuitive to handle by some users is INTERACT (Mangold, Germany). As an important feature, such a behavioral coding tool allows importing physiological data to graph them together with behavioral responses and do advanced statistical analyses that relate these different measurement domains to each other (e.g., cross-correlation, sequential analysis, pattern identification). Such analyses allow inferences to be made about conditional probabilities and causal attributions (e.g., What comes first, physiological activation or impulsive behavior?).

Much basic work in psychophysiology has been devoted to understanding the short-term reactions (within 5 seconds or so) to specific stimuli, which may be used as objective index of attention and perception and help elucidate early emotional and cognitive processes. Instead of conceiving physiological measures as convergent indicators of a construct (such as a specific emotion), it has proven fruitful to embed the psychological construct within a biological framework, e.g., the orienting reflex, defense response, voluntary attention, affective space, sensory intake-rejection dichotomy, and conditioning. With the advent of commercial software for scripting computerized stimulus presentation (e.g., Presentation, SuperLab, E-Prime; MacWhinney, St. James, Schunn, Li, & Schneider, 2001) classical paradigms from emotion research, cognitive psychology, and neuroscience can be implemented rather easily and modified for specific assessment needs. The basic principle of such paradigms is to compare physiological reactions to different categories of stimuli (typically two or three) by averaging across several examples for each category (at least two or three to allow generalization), often with several repetitions to increase measurement reliability. The interstimulus interval has a length sufficient for physiological responses to return to baseline (e.g., 25 seconds, with some variability to reduce expectation effects).

At the most basic level, human and animal action tendencies are determined by appetitive vs. defensive emotional systems on the one hand and the intensity of the response tendency on the other. Thus, one of the primary psychophysiological assessment paradigms allowing inferences about emotion and motivation processes records a small set of physiological responses during the presentation of pictorial stimuli varying on the independent dimensions of valence (related to approach/withdrawal) and arousal (related to intensity), thus each picture referring to a specific coordinate in "affective space." To promote standardized assessment, a large set of pictures has been developed, with norms for adults and children specifying their level of valence and arousal (International Affective Picture System, IAPS; Lang, Bradley, & Cuthbert, 1995). Similarly, sounds of about 6 seconds' duration have been assembled for the same purpose (International Affective Digital Sounds, IADS; Bradley & Lang, 2000). Both stimulus sets are available from the NIMH Center for the Study of Emotion and Attention (CSEA), University of Florida, Gainesville.

These stimuli have been widely used in adults (Lang, Bradley, & Cuthbert, 1990) and to a lesser extent in children (McManis, Bradley, Berg, Cuthbert, & Lang, 2001) to probe basic affective response tendencies. The magnitude of the skin conductance response (SCR) to the stimulus is typically the index of general physiological activation or arousal provoked. The magnitude of the eye-blink startle reflex to a 95-dB noise burst (50 ms) measured with two small EMG electrodes below the eye (orbicularis oculi muscle) is typically used as the best index of valence appraisal. This reflex is potentiated when the valence of a stimulus is appraised as negative (e.g., spider, injury, weapon). It is attenuated when the valence is positive (e.g., baby, flower, chocolate).

Other stimuli for specific purposes have been developed. To probe children's reactions to faces displaying basic emotions, the NimStim faces set has been developed and is available for download (http://www.macbrain.org/faces). Individual research teams have developed their own stimuli for specific assessment purposes, including stimulus material for measuring event-related brain potentials (e.g., Benasich, Thomas, Choudhury, & Leppanen, 2002). Basic paradigms measure the speed of habituation in ERP components to sinusoidal tones of different pitch presented with different probabilities or ask subjects to attend to tones of a certain pitch and ignore the others to assess the attentional P300.

Conditioning studies also profit from computerized stimulus presentation. After repeatedly coupling a neutral stimulus (e.g., a geometrical shape) with a strong appetitive (e.g., food) or aversive (e.g., loud noise) stimulus that provokes unconditioned responses (UCRs), the neutral stimulus can elicit a similar physiological reaction (conditioned response, CR). The most commonly used physiological measure for conditioned response is the skin conductance response magnitude (see later section for more detail). Using this basic paradigm, the speed of acquisition, general appetitive or aversive conditionability, and speed of extinction can be modeled to assess basic emotional learning processes.

FROM THE CENTER TO THE PERIPHERY: MEASUREMENT METHODS IN CHILDREN

We have already referred to several commonly used psychophysiological measures when describing methodological issues and paradigms relevant in psychophysiological assessment. Here we will give a more systematic account of commonly used measures and their relevance and specific issues in child assessment. We will largely stay within and build on the framework used in the adult psychophysiology chapter (Chapter 8) in *Clinician's Handbook of Adult Behavioral Assessment.*

Central Nervous System Functioning

Electroencephalographic (EEG) measures, including evoked response potentials (ERPs), offer a noninvasive method for monitoring physiological activity with excellent temporal resolution. However, spatial resolution is limited, even when using high-density electrode head gowns. Magnetoencephalographic (MEG) measures have excellent temporal and good spatial resolution, but they are very expensive to implement, and not many facilities exist. Some medical centers have positron emission tomography (PET) to measure localized activation in the brain. However, this method requires injecting a radioactive tracer and as such is not typically a measure of choice for psychophysiological assessment, especially in children. Functional magnetic resonance imaging (fMRI) facilities are becoming available at many universities and hospitals. Similar to PET, the fMRI signal relies on the hemodynamic changes associated with brain cell activity (blood flow, blood oxygenation, etc.), and, because of delays in hemodynamic responses to local brain activity changes, the measurements are more indirect and have a time resolution only on the order of seconds. What is recorded is the so-called BOLD signal. fMRI allows mapping areas in the brain that are involved in attention, perception, emotion, and cognition. Good primers and lectures about these methods have been made available on the Internet in visual and audio format (e.g., http://www.cis.rit.edu/htbooks/mri/inside.htm, http://www.umich.edu/~fmri/course, and http://biac.stanford.edu).

Although fMRI is an exciting tool for psychophysiological assessment, it has distinct disadvantages, especially when applied to children. The strong magnet in a scanning room requires special supervision to prevent ferrous parts from entering the room and potentially causing damage or injury. The scanner is a large machine that can be frightening to some children, and having to lie down on a table that is moved into a narrow tube can be a claustrophobic experience for many. For scanning sequences, strong radio waves are used that react with the magnetic field lines and produce a very loud noise. There are likely no side effects, but because of the relative novelty of the technology, long-term data on the effects of accumulated MRI brain scanning time during infancy or childhood are missing. Even when an fMRI center is close by, scanning time is typically limited and expensive. Thus, a compelling alternative for certain research questions in children is to use peripheral measures. Many map well into certain brain processes. For example, SCR is a good index of amygdala activation, is inexpensive and very unobtrusive, and has no potential for side effects; depending on the site location, components of the ERP morphology are good indices of a large variety of central processes. In child research, before submitting children to fMRI assessment it is generally a good idea to establish the relevance of a novel or adapted adult paradigm by using peripheral psychophysiological measures.

Advanced EEG measurement systems with many electrodes incorporated in a head cap that can be applied with children are now commercially available. These systems contain sophisticated software for screening out artifacts (which is especially important in child assessment) and provide analysis tools for addressing specific questions, such as power within specific frequency bands at certain scalp locations, source localization, timing, and pattern of activation spread in response to a stimulus, ensemble averaged ERP curves, and wave coherence between different loci. Because these tools have not yet been widely applied to the study of infants and children, especially in longitudinal designs, there is much need and opportunity for making important scientific contributions to the understanding of human brain development.

The relatively modest amount of research on biology–behavior relations during development using EEG and ERP measures has already provided important insights into the emergence and reorganization of brain processes during infancy and childhood. Dramatic changes in the power and center frequencies of the resting EEG (e.g., an upward shift in alpha rhythm recorded over the occipital cortex indicative of visual attention; changes in sleep EEG) are likely primarily a function of structural changes, including myelination of axons, changes in dendritic branching, and reorganization of neural networks. On the other hand, these modifications also correspond to functional changes as cognitive and emotional regulation becomes more sophisticated and as experience shapes the child's thinking. For example, patterns of frontal EEG alpha asymmetry have been examined in relation to emotional and cognitive development in early childhood and have been related to social maladaptation later (e.g., Henderson, Fox, & Rubin, 2001). Early severe abuse may have a deleterious effect on brain development, as indicated by an increased left EEG coherence in abused patients, pointing to a deficit in left cortical differentiation (Ito, Teicher, Glod, & Ackerman, 1998). Perceptual deficits have been related to functional changes. For example, the typical left-hemisphere distribution of the ERP in response to language stimuli was relocated to the other hemisphere in deaf children, indicating a greater focus on visual-spatial information during processing (Neville, Kutas, & Schmidt, 1982).

Somatic Nervous System Functioning

Muscular responses are at the direct intersection between physiology and overt behavior. They can easily be measured with small surface electromyographic (EMG) electrodes placed at appropriate locations. For example, tension in the forearm or neck that may accompany stress or anxiety states can be quantified reliably this way. More specialized applications are the measurement of changes in facial expression by placing the electrodes over specific muscles involved in emotional expression. The most commonly assessed are probably the corrugator muscle, involved in frowning, and the zygomaticus muscle, involved in smiling. Both have been established to be good measures of valence appraisals of stimuli. Eye-blink startle EMG amplitude was described earlier in the context of measuring responses using IAPS pictures to characterize responses within affective space. This measurement requires applying a secondary stimulus that is potent enough to trigger a defensive startle reflex. Commonly used startle probes are 95-dB white noise (50 ms in duration) delivered through headphones, air puffs applied to the eye, and flashing lights. A variant of the startle measurement method is prepulse inhibition. Here, a weaker tone (e.g., 1000 Hz, 70 dB) precedes the startling noise burst and inhibits the reflex from being fully triggered. The relative difference between the full reflex and the inhibited reflex is taken as a measure of prepulse inhibition magnitude. This measure has been linked to dopaminergic brain activity and temperament in adults (e.g., Alessi, Greenwald, & Johanson, 2003) and has been explored in infants (Blumenthal, Avendano, & Berg, 1987) and children (Castellanos et al., 1996), where it was related to hyperactivity and tics.

An easy way to measure direction of gaze without an often obtrusive and expensive eye-tracking device is by electrooculography (EOG). The eyes act as a dipole, and their direction can be inferred from the changes in voltage, measured with four electrodes positioned above and below one eye (at the forehead and cheekbone) and on the left and right temples. It is, of course, important for the child to keep the head in a stable position, which can be ensured by using an easy chair that is tilted backward slightly and a special headrest. The gaze direction initially needs to be calibrated individually by having each child look at stimuli presented in each corner of the computer monitor. The time course of gaze direction can serve as a more direct measure of attention allocation than reaction time paradigms like the dot-probe test (MacLeod, Mathews, & Tata, 1986). EOG signals can also be analyzed for the frequency of spontaneous eye blinks, which has been related to anxiety (increased; Kojima et al., 2002) and Attention-Deficit/Hyperactivity Disorder (decreased; Konrad, Gauggel, & Schurek, 2003).

An accelerometer attached to the chair, chest, or shoulder can measure gross body movement. This device can be used for detecting movement artifacts when scoring other biosignals or as an index of restlessness in conditions like anxiety, depression, and hyperactivity. Mobile, wristwatch devices are especially appropriate for children and can be worn for days or weeks for charting activity and sleep patterns (Teicher, 1995).

Autonomic Nervous System Functioning

The autonomic nervous system is relatively well developed at birth and consists of a sympathetic and a parasympathetic branch that innervates a variety of target organs, including the heart, lungs, skin, intestines, and vasculature. Many commonly used psychophysiological measures are an index of sympathetic or parasympathetic function or both. Until recently, researchers typically assumed that autonomic control of dually innervated target organs was best viewed as a continuum extending from parasympathetic to sympathetic dominance. It is now apparent that these two systems may operate rather independently ("autonomic space"; Berntson, Cacioppo, & Quigley, 1991). Even within autonomic branches, activation patterns can be organ specific. This arrangement ensures efficient coordination between systems when different demands are imposed on each, but it also raises caution not to overgeneralize from a specific measure. Thus, although measures have been established to characterize certain physiological responses with psychological importance, no single measure can characterize the multiple modes of autonomic control within the entire body.

Prenatal recording of fetal heart rate by sonographic methods is standard obstetric diagnostic practice (Pardey, Moulden, & Redman, 2002). Reliable recording of heart rate using ECG is relatively easy shortly after birth. Heart rate is dually innervated by the sympathetic (increase) and parasympathetic (decrease) branches of the autonomic nervous system and is probably the strongest peripheral indicator of anxiety when physical activity is controlled (Wilhelm & Roth, 1998a). Heart rate has been extensively used as a tool for assessment of perceptual and cognitive development in infants because the decelerative response to stimuli can be used as an objective index of basic sensory capacities (e.g., Berg & Berg, 1979). For example, the habituation–dishabituation paradigm repeatedly presents a stimulus until the decelerative response has habituated, and then it presents a different stimulus that restores decelerative responding only if it is perceived as novel, which, depending on the stimuli used, may indicate attentional, perceptual, and cognitive development (Graham & Clifton, 1966).

In order to characterize sympathetic and parasympathetic innvervation of the heart independently, pre-ejection period (PEP) and respiratory sinus arrhythmia (RSA) are commonly used measures (Berntson et al., 1991). PEP, which is measured by combining ECG and impedance cardiography (ICG) signals, refers to the period between the onset of left ventricular depolarization (indicated by the ECG) and the start of ejection of blood during systolic contraction (indicated by the ICG). Increased β-adrenergic sympathetic activation of the cardiac muscle accelerates this process. At least four electrodes (at the neck and chest) need to be attached, and movement needs to be minimized for reliable assessment. Best results in infants and children are obtained by averaging across at least 10 beats to overcome movement artifacts.

RSA can be measured from the variations in heart period (interval between consecutive ECG R-waves) occurring synchronous with respiratory phase. During inspiration the RR interval is shorter (heart rate is faster) than during expiration, an effect mediated primarily by the cardiac parasympathetic nerve. A straightforward method calculates the difference between minimum and maximum heart periods associated with respiration ("peak–valley method"; Grossman, van Beek, & Wientjes, 1990). In the child literature, estimation of the variance of the heart rate signal after moving polynomial filtering has been used frequently (Porges & Byrne, 1992; Porges, Doussard-Roosevelt, Portales, & Greenspan, 1996). However, equating this measure with "vagal tone," as is often done, is an unwarranted oversimplification. An alternative parasympathetic index sometimes seen in the literature, mean successive differences (MSD), can be derived by statistical filtering of the cardiac interbeat interval time series. Computationally simple, MSD tends to correlate highly with other RSA indices (Friedman, Allen, Christie, & Santucci, 2002; Hayano et al., 1991), but its validity as a parasympathetic index has been questioned (e.g., Berntson et al., 1997; Task Force of the European Society of Cardiology and the North American Society of Pacing and Electrophysiology, 1996).

More complex methods use spectral analytic, autoregressive, or complex demodulation calculations (Wilhelm, Grossman, & Roth, 2005) and typically rely on the definition of a fixed respiratory frequency band (high frequency, or HF, 0.15–0.50 Hz). However, these need to be carefully monitored and adjusted for a particular age group because of changes in respiratory regulation during infancy and childhood. Furthermore, the predictive relations of RSA and parasympathetic cardiac control can be diminished with acute changes in respiratory frequency and depth often associated with emotional state changes since both have been demonstrated to be confounds. Methods for adjusting for these confounds have been developed (e.g., Grossman, Wilhelm, & Spoerle, 2004; Wilhelm, Grossman, & Coyle, 2004). Thus, one may argue that by concurrent measurement of respiratory pattern one can optimize estimation of parasympathetic control by RSA during development. However, many studies in infants and children have not measured respiration concurrently, and findings indicate that this can be a productive approach (e.g., Porges et al., 1996).

RSA is only one component of heart rate variability (also sometimes termed *heart period variability*). Another source of systematic fluctuation in heart rate is the occurrence of slower waves about every 10 seconds (low frequency, or LF, 0.04–0.15 Hz), which reflect both sympathetic and parasympathetic influences on the cardiovascular system and are associated with efficient blood pressure regulation. The LF/HF ratio has been used as an index of sympathovagal balance, but its validity has been criticized widely and it is not recommended as a primary measure (Berntson et al., 1997). Of course, another important source of heart rate variability is physical activity. Because waking infants and young children can be quite restless, their LF heart rate variability can be spuriously inflated. Valid measurement is best attempted during periods of 1 minute or more with little movement (as indicated, e.g., by accelerometry). A third established source of heart rate variability is occurring with even slower waves about every 25–300 seconds (very low frequency, or VLF, 0.0033–0.04 Hz), which, in addition to sympathetic and parasympathetic inputs, may be influenced by the thermoregulatory, peripheral vasomotor, and renin-angiotensin systems. This measure, of course, may also be spuriously inflated by repeated changes in physical activation about every 25–300 seconds. In general, one needs to caution against an uncritical use of these measures in children. At the very least, manual editing of misdetected beats in the often-noisy child ECG signal is important, as is concurrent monitoring of physical activity and respiration.

RSA and other measures of cardiac parasympathetic and sympathetic control have been used in diverse contexts relevant to child and adolescent clinical psychology. Such indices have figured prominently in developmental theories of conduct disorder and antisocial behavior (Beauchaine, 2001; Mezzacappa et al., 1997). In general, these models are consistent with the view that low parasympathetic heart rate control marks maladaptive and inflexible responsiveness (see Friedman, in press). For example, in 12-week-old infants, high RSA was associated with less negative behaviors and less tendency to be disrupted by the experimental procedures; in 9-month-old infants, high RSA was prospectively related to reduced behavioral problems at 3 years of age, as assessed by maternal report (Porges et al., 1996; Porges, Doussard-Roosevelt, Portales, & Suess, 1994); in very-low-birth-weight infants, high RSA was associated with better behavior regulation at 3 years (Doussard-Roosevelt, Porges, Scanlon, Alemi, & Scanlon, 1997) and was predictive of social competence in school (Doussard-Roosevelt, McClenny, & Porges, 2001); in 2-year-old children, a high-risk group with low RSA displayed more negative affect and dysregulated emotion-regulation behaviors than did the low-risk group (Calkins & Dedmon, 2000). In addition, heart rate variability measures have yielded fresh insights into the development of information-processing deficits in autism spectrum disorders (Althaus et al., 2004). Cardiac autonomic indices may also be sensitive to clinically relevant personality and psychosocial variables in children and adolescents, such as hostility and family conflict (Salomon, Matthews, & Allen, 2000). Preliminary data from an ongoing study of one-session treatment of childhood-specific phobias suggest that parasympathetic control of heart rate may be an informative treatment outcome variable (Hurley, Friedman, Scarpa, & Ollendick, 2002).

A number of other cardiovascular activity measures has been meaningfully applied in infants and children to study emotional reactions, e.g., blood pressure (using an inflatable cuff around the upper arm), finger pulse wave (using a sensor clipped to the finger), and finger temperature (using a small thermistor attached to the fingertip). Finger pulse amplitude and finger temperature are good measures of peripheral vascoconstriction, often associated with enduring anxiety or stress. Electrodermal activity is an important and often-used measure of sympathetic response and arousal in adults that can be measured relatively easily in children by attaching two small electrodes to the palm of the hand or fingers. The measured skin conductance level is a result of sympathetically activated sweat gland activity. Skin conductance responses (SCRs) are phasic fluctuations of about 5–10 seconds on top of the more tonic level changes and can be observed during behavioral tasks to derive the number of nonspecific fluctuations per minute or to quantify the magnitude of the SCR to specific stimuli.

Although both heart rate and electrodermal activity are influenced by sympathetic efferents they are not redundant. Gray's (1975) theory distinguishes between two motivational systems, which he refers to as the behavioral activation system (BAS) and the behavioral inhibition system (BIS). Fowles (1980, 1987, 1988) has shown that heart rate responses primarily reflect activity of the BAS, and electrodermal responses primarily reflect activity of the BIS. Thus it would appear that in infant and child studies, both heart rate and skin conductance level would complement each other for probing the underlying mechanisms for problems with impulse control or anxiety.

Respiratory activity is influenced by the autonomic nervous system. But because it is also tightly linked with regulation of arterial CO_2 levels, it has a great deal of independence and may yield additional information. Respiration is typically measured by attaching a stretchable belt around the thorax, and respiratory rate can be easily computed from this. To also reliably measure changes in the amount of air inhaled with each breath, a second belt around the abdomen is required. Both signals then need to be added, since breathing can shift between these two compartments. In infant care, often the transcutaneous CO_2 is measured using a small sensor attached to the forearm to monitor blood gases. An alternative is to measure end-tidal CO_2 with small plastic cannulas in front of the nostrils. Both are good measures of hyperventilation, which is associated with anxiety in general (Alpers, Wilhelm, & Roth, 2005) and specifically with a diagnosis of panic disorder in adults (Klein, 1993; Wilhelm, Gevirtz, & Roth, 2001). Recent reports have extended findings of respiratory dysregulation to children and adolescents with anxiety disorders (Pine et al., 1998, 2005).

Neuroendocrine System Functioning

Assessment of psychophysiological functioning in infants and children would not be complete without an appreciation of neuroendocrine measures. Salivary cortisol is the measure most commonly used because of its outstanding cost–benefit ratio: On the one hand, it can be collected rather easily and noninvasively (i.e., without blood draws) in children with modern methods (Schmidt, 1998), and assays have gone down in cost tremendously in recent years. On the other hand, it is a reliable marker of hypothalamic-pituitary-adrenocortical axis function and can yield a better understanding of a child's stress response. For example, salivary cortisol can be used to assess children's stress responses to phobic stimuli in treatment-outcome studies (Hurley, Scarpa, Friedman, & Ollendick, 2003). Children comply well with instructions to chew on a cotton swab for about a minute, so repeated sampling during a stressful procedure is feasible. Unfortunately, certain hormones specifically important for understanding adolescent development during puberty, e.g., growth or sex hormones, cannot reliably be obtained from saliva samples but, rather, need to be collected by 24-hr urine sampling or blood draws. Paediatric endocrine abnormalities can have particularly detrimental effects on the developing brain (Northam, 2004).

PSYCHOPHYSIOLOGICAL ASSESSMENT IN PEDIATRIC BIOFEEDBACK APPLICATIONS

Biofeedback involves electronically measuring a physiological value and immediately communicating any change to train the child to function better. Subtle body changes can be "amplified" and presented to the child to change cognitive, emotional, physiological, or overt behavior (Schwartz & Andrasik, 2003). A well-known example is the urine alarm device that immediately rings and wakes the child with sleep enuresis whenever bedwetting occurs (Schwartz, 2003). Biofeedback applications often use heart rate or skin conductance to capture the most basic of emotion-relevant factors, calm versus aroused. The "fight-or-flight" response of acutely anxious or stressed individuals is also characterized by increases in blood pressure and breathing rate and by vasoconstriction. Children are often unaware of subtle bodily changes, but through biofeedback-mediated training they can learn to reduce physiological overreaction, which can also diminish the cognitive and affective experience of anxiety and stress.

Progress in microelectronics and interfaces with personal computers have filled the marketplace with devices that are simple to operate, compact, and affordable. Biofeedback methods were researched heavily in the 1980s for treating such disorders as headaches, incontinence, temporomandibular syndrome, and irritable bowel syndrome. Particularly for treatment of psychophysiological disorders and pain, biofeedback has been shown to be a cost-effective option as a component of an integrated behavioral medicine treatment program (Schneider, 1987). Although the results were quite positive, the cost, size, and intricacy of the equipment and the shortage of trained professionals kept biofeedback from widespread adoption. Relatively inexpensive devices and efficient biofeedback protocols are now available (http://www.aapb.org). Biofeedback has been made attractive to children via specially designed interfaces that allow exploration of their own bodily functions in a playful way.

Mental health care professionals sometimes treat children with incapacitating physical symptoms for which no organic cause can be medically determined (Binder & Campbell, 2004). An influential article published in 1998 in *the Journal of the American Medical Association* reported an astounding 629 million total visits (primarily adults) to alternative medicine professionals in 1997 in the United States, a 47% increase from 1990, thereby exceeding total visits to all U.S. primary care physicians (Eisenberg et al., 1998). Alternative therapies were used most frequently for chronic conditions, including headaches, insomnia, anxiety, and depression. Biofeedback, which clearly has specific indications for many of these disorders, was used rarely (1%), although it had better insurance coverage than most other alternative treatments (30% of visits were fully covered and 44% were partially covered). Figures for children do not exist, but one may expect that many concerned parents seek alternative treatment modalities for their child when they do not agree with standard medical treatment options, such as psychopharmacology.

Biofeedback is highly compatible with standard cognitive-behavioral treatment, which emphasizes self-regulation and focuses on behavior change. This suggests that biofeedback may be helpful, as a secondary modality, in treating psychological problems and disorders (Futterman & Shapiro, 1986). There are some important stand-alone or adjunctive biofeedback applications tested in adults with emotional, behavioral, or psychosomatic problems that might be productively applied in children, such as EMG biofeedback-assisted progressive relaxation (Lehrer, Carr, Sargunaraj, & Woolfolk, 1994), biofeedback of specific symptomatic organ systems (Schwartz & Andrasik, 2003), CO_2 biofeedback training for hyperventilation (Meuret, Wilhelm, & Roth, 2001; Wilhelm, Gevirtz, & Roth, 2001), heart rate variability biofeedback training (Lehrer, Vaschillo, & Vaschillo, 2000), frontal EEG asymmetry biofeedback training to enhance mood (Allen, Harmon-Jones, & Cavender, 2001), and neurofeedback for the management of Attention-Deficit/Hyperactivity Disorder (Lubar, 2003).

SUMMARY

Psychophysiological science is an exciting field with great potential for researchers and practitioners interested in exploring the microcosmos relating to the intricate interactions between human experience, behavior, and physiology. Psychophysiological methods provide a window for understanding the biological bases of cognition, emotion, and behavior in infants and children. In clinical applications, these methods may be useful for objectifying diagnoses relating to emotional disturbance and track progress with treatment or as an adjunctive treatment modality in itself. Psychophysiological research has largely been occupied with basic questions, such as identifying pathways in the brain and peripheral nervous system involved in specific emotional responses. Although this research has greatly enhanced our understanding of mind–body connections, the impact of the field on clinical practice has been small except in the assessment of sleep disturbance and pain management (Roth, 1998). The increasing availability of inexpensive yet sophisticated noninvasive measurement devices and information on their use and interpretation may change this picture.

What is perhaps most unique to psychophysiological assessment in infants and children is the developmental perspective. Interestingly, most developmental research has been conducted cross-sectionally; i.e., it compared groups of children at different ages. However, it has been convincingly argued that the limitations of this approach are often seriously underestimated (Kraemer, Yesavage, Taylor, & Kupfer, 2000). Under many circumstances, only a longitudinal design can provide reliable delineation of the course of development and provide answers to etiological questions such as "Which processes during development constitute risk or mediating factors for subsequent maladjustment?" (Kraemer et al., 1997; Kraemer, Stice, Kazdin, Offord, & Kupfer, 2001). Developmental psychophysiology has important connections to the emerging field of genetic psychophysiology (de Geus, 2002). Because basic psychophysiological processes related to attention and emotion regulation can be assumed to act as intermediaries between gene expression and complex psychosocial behaviors, cognitive abilities, and mental health, much can be gained in our understanding of genetic factors by an assessment of psychophysiology in infancy, childhood, and adolescence.

REFERENCES AND RESOURCES

Ainsworth, M. D. S., Blehar, M. C., Waters, E., & Wall, S. (1978). *Patterns of attachment: A psychological study of the strange situation.* Hillsdale, N.J.: Erlbaum.

Alessi, S. M., Greenwald, M., & Johanson, C. E. (2003). The prediction of individual differences in response to D-amphetamine in healthy adults. *Behavioral Pharmacology, 14*(1), 19–32.

Allen, J., Harmon-Jones, E., & Cavender, J. (2001). Manipulation of frontal EEG asymmetry through biofeedback alters self-reported emotional responses and facial EMG. *Psychophysiology, 38*(4), 685–693.

Alpers, G. W., Wilhelm, F. H., & Roth, W. T. (2005). Psychophysiological assessment during exposure in driving phobic patients. *Journal of Abnormal Psychology, 114*(1), 126–139.

Althaus, M., Van Roon, A. M., Mulder, L. J., Mulder, G., Aarnoudse, C. C., & Minderaa, R. B. (2004). Autonomic response patterns observed during the performance of an attention-demanding task in two groups of children with autistic-type difficulties in social adjustment. *Psychophysiology, 41*(6), 893–904.

Beauchaine, T. P. (2001). Vagal tone, development, and Gray's motivational theory: Toward an integrated model of autonomic nervous system functioning in psychopathology. *Developmental Psychopathology, 13*(2), 183–214.

Benasich, A. A., Thomas, J. J., Choudhury, N., & Leppanen, P. H. (2002). The importance of rapid auditory processing abilities to early language development: Evidence from converging methodologies. *Developmental Psychobiology, 40*(3), 278–292.

Berg, W. K., & Berg, K. M. (1979). Psychophysiological development in infancy: State, sensory function and attention. In J. D. Osofsky (Ed.), *Handbook of infant development* (pp. 283–343). New York: Wiley.

Berntson, G. G., Cacioppo, J. T., & Quigley, K. S. (1991). Autonomic determinism: The modes of autonomic control, the doctrine of autonomic space, and the laws of autonomic constraint. *Psychological Review, 98,* 459–487.

Berntson, G. G., Bigger, J. T., Jr., Eckberg, D. L., Grossman, P., Kaufmann, P. G., Malik, M., et al. (1997). Heart rate variability: Origins, methods, and interpretive caveats. *Psychophysiology, 34*(6), 623–648.

Binder, L. M., & Campbell, K. A. (2004). Medically unexplained symptoms and neuropsychological assessment. *Journal of Clinical Experimental Neuropsychology, 26*(3), 369–392.

Blumenthal, T. D., Avendano, A., & Berg, W. K. (1987). The startle response and auditory temporal summation in neonates. *Journal of Experimental & Child Psychology, 44*(1), 64–79.

Bradley, M. M., & Lang, P. J. (1994). Measuring emotion: The Self-Assessment Manikin and the Semantic Differential. *Journal of Behav Ther Exp Psychiatry, 25*(1), 49–59.

Bradley, M. M., & Lang, P. J. (2000). Affective reactions to acoustic stimuli. *Psychophysiology, 37*(2), 204–215.

Cacioppo, J. T., Tassinary, L. G., & Berntson, G. G. (2000). *Handbook of psychophysiology* (2nd ed.). Cambridge, UK: Cambridge University Press.

Calkins, S. D., & Dedmon, S. E. (2000). Physiological and behavioral regulation in two-year-old children with aggressive/destructive behavior problems. *Journal of Abnormal & Child Psychology, 28*(2), 103–118.

Castellanos, F. X., Fine, E. J., Kaysen, D., Marsh, W. L., Rapoport, J. L., & Hallett, M. (1996). Sensorimotor gating in boys with Tourette's syndrome and ADHD: Preliminary results. *Biological Psychiatry, 39*(1), 33–41.

Christie, I. C., & Friedman, B. H. (2004). Autonomic specificity of discrete emotion and dimensions of affective space: A multivariate approach. *International Journal of Psychophysiology, 51*(2), 143–153.

Cycowicz, Y. M. (2000). Memory development and event-related brain potentials in children. *Biol Psychol, 54*(1–3), 145–174.

de Geus, E. J. (2002). Introducing genetic psychophysiology. *Biol Psychol, 61*(1–2), 1–10.

Donovan, W. L., & Leavitt, L. A. (1989). Maternal self-efficacy and infant attachment: Integrating physiology, perceptions, and behavior. *Child Development, 60*(2), 460–472.

Doussard-Roosevelt, J. A., McClenny, B. D., & Porges, S. W. (2001). Neonatal cardiac vagal tone and school-age developmental outcome in very low-birth-weight infants. *Developmental Psychobiology, 38*(1), 56–66.

Doussard-Roosevelt, J. A., Porges, S. W., Scanlon, J. W., Alemi, B., & Scanlon, K. B. (1997). Vagal regulation of heart rate in the prediction of developmental outcome for very low-birth-weight preterm infants. *Child Development, 68*(2), 173–186.

Eisenberg, D. M., Davis, R. B., Ettner, S. L., Appel, S., Wilkey, S., Van Rompay, M., et al. (1998). Trends in alternative medicine use in the United States, 1990–1997: Results of a follow-up national survey. *Journal of the American Medical Association, 280*(18), 1569–1575.

Fowles, D. C. (1980). The three arousal model: Implications of Gray's two-factor learning theory for heart rate, electrodermal activity, and psychopathy. *Psychophysiology, 17*(2), 87–104.

Fowles, D. C. (1987). Application of a behavioral theory of motivation to the concepts of anxiety and impulsivity. *Journal of Research in Personality, 21*(4), 417–435.

Fowles, D. C. (1988). Psychophysiology and psychopathology: A motivational approach. *Psychophysiology, 25*(4), 373–391.

Fox, N. A., Schmidt, L. A., & Henderson, H. A. (2000). Developmental psychophysiology: Conceptual and methodological perspectives. In J. T. Cacioppo, L. G. Tassinary, & G. G. Berntson (Eds.), *Handbook of psychophysiology* (2nd ed., pp. 665–686). Cambridge, UK: Cambridge University Press.

Fredrickson, B. L., Mancuso, R. A., Branigan, C., & Tugade, M. M. (2000). The undoing effect of positive emotions. *Motivation and Emotion, 24,* 237–258.

Friedman, B. H. (in press). Anxiety and cardiac vagal tone: Central and peripheral processes. *Biological Psychology.*

Friedman, B. H., Allen, M. T., Christie, I. C., & Santucci, A. K. (2002). Validity concerns of common heart-rate variability indices. *IEEE Eng Med Biol Mag, 21*(4), 35–40.

Futterman, A., & Shapiro, D. (1986). A review of biofeedback for mental disorders. *Hospital Community Psychiatry, 37*(1), 27–33.

Gorman, J. M., Fyer, M. R., Goetz, R., Askanazi, J., Liebowitz, M. R., & Fyer, A. J. (1988). Ventilatory physiology of patients with panic disorder. *Archives of General Psychiatry, 45,* 31–39.

Gottman, J. M., & Roy, A. K. (1990). *Sequential analysis. A guide for behavioral researchers.* Cambridge, UK: Cambridge University Press.

Graham, F. K., & Clifton, R. K. (1966). Heart-rate change as a component of the orienting response. *Psychol Bull, 65*(5), 305–320.

Gray, J. A. (1975). *Elements of a two-process theory of learning*. New York: Academic Press.

Gross, J. J., & Levenson, R. W. (1995). Emotion elicitation using films. *Cognition & Emotion, 9*(1), 87–108.

Grossman, P., van Beek, J., & Wientjes, C. (1990). A comparison of three quantification methods for estimation of respiratory sinus arrhythmia. *Psychophysiology, 27*(6), 702–714.

Grossman, P., Wilhelm, F. H., & Spoerle, M. (2004). Respiratory sinus arrhythmia, cardiac vagal control and daily activity. *American Journal of Physiology, 287*(2), H728–734.

Hayano, J., Sakakibara, Y., Yamada, A., Yamada, M., Mukai, S., Fujinami, T., et al. (1991). Accuracy of assessment of cardiac vagal tone by heart rate variability in normal subjects. *Am J Cardiol, 67*(2), 199–204.

Henderson, H. A., Fox, N. A., & Rubin, K. H. (2001). Temperamental contributions to social behavior: The moderating roles of frontal EEG asymmetry and gender. *J Am Acad Child Adolesc Psychiatry, 40*(1), 68–74.

Hurley, J. D., Friedman, B. H., Scarpa, A., & Ollendick, T. H. (2002). The utility of psychophysiological assessment in one-session treatment of specific phobias in children. *Psychophysiology, 39,* S12.

Hurley, J. D., Scarpa, A., Friedman, B. H., & Ollendick, T. H. (2003). Treatment of specific phobias in children: Effect on salivary cortisol. *Psychophysiology, 39,* S49.

Ito, Y., Teicher, M. H., Glod, C. A., & Ackerman, E. (1998). Preliminary evidence for aberrant cortical development in abused children: a quantitative EEG study. *Journal of Neuropsychiatry Clin Neurosci, 10*(3), 298–307.

Kagan, J., Reznick, J. S., & Snidman, N. (1987). The physiology and psychology of behavioral inhibition in children. *Child Dev, 58*(6), 1459–1473.

Kirschbaum, C., Pirke, K., & Hellhammer, D. (1993). The "Trier Social Stress Test"—a tool for investigating psychobiological stress responses in a laboratory setting. *Neuropsychobiology, 28*(1–2), 76–81.

Klein, D. F. (1993). False suffocation alarms, spontaneous panics, and related conditions. An integrative hypothesis. *Archives of General Psychiatry, 50,* 306–317.

Kojima, M., Shioiri, T., Hosoki, T., Sakai, M., Bando, T., & Someya, T. (2002). Blink rate variability in patients with panic disorder: New trial using audiovisual stimulation. *Psychiatry Clin Neurosci, 56*(5), 545–549.

Konrad, K., Gauggel, S., & Schurek, J. (2003). Catecholamine functioning in children with traumatic brain injuries and children with attention-deficit/hyperactivity disorder. *Brain Res Cogn Brain Res, 16*(3), 425–433.

Kraemer, H., Kazdin, A., Offord, D., Kessler, R., Jensen, P., & Kupfer, D. (1997). Coming to terms with the terms of risk. *Arch Gen Psychiatry, 54*(4), 337–343.

Kraemer, H., Stice, E., Kazdin, A., Offord, D., & Kupfer, D. (2001). How do risk factors work together? Mediators, moderators, and independent, overlapping, and proxy risk factors. *Am J Psychiatry, 158*(6), 848–856.

Kraemer, H., Yesavage, J., Taylor, J., & Kupfer, D. (2000). How can we learn about developmental processes from cross-sectional studies, or can we? *Am J Psychiatry, 157*(2), 163–171.

Kudielka, B. M., Buske-Kirschbaum, A., Hellhammer, D. H., & Kirschbaum, C. (2004). HPA axis responses to laboratory psychosocial stress in healthy elderly adults, younger adults, and children: Impact of age and gender. *Psychoneuroendocrinology, 29*(1), 83–98.

Lang, P. J. (1968). Fear reduction and fear behavior: Problems in treating a construct. In J. M. Shlien (Ed.), *Research in psychotherapy* (Vol. 3, pp. 90–103). Washington, DC: American Psychological Association.

Lang, P. J. (1978). Anxiety: Toward a psychophysiological definition. In H. S. Akiskal & W. L. Webb (Eds.), *Psychiatric diagnosis: Exploration of biological criteria* (pp. 265–389). New York: Spectrum.

Lang, P. J., Bradley, M. M., & Cuthbert, B. N. (1990). Emotion, attention, and the startle reflex. *Psychological Review, 97*(3), 377–395.

Lang, P. J., Bradley, M. M., & Cuthbert, B. N. (1995). *International Affective Picture System (IAPS): Technical manual and affective ratings*. Gainesville, FL: University of Florida, Department of Psychology, Center of Research in Psychophysiology.

Lehrer, P., Carr, R., Sargunaraj, D., & Woolfolk, R. (1994). Stress management techniques: Are they all equivalent, or do they have specific effects? *Biofeedback Self Regul, 19*(4), 353–401.

Lehrer, P., Vaschillo, E., & Vaschillo, B. (2000). Resonant frequency biofeedback training to increase cardiac variability: Rationale and manual for training. *Appl Psychophysiol Biofeedback, 25*(3), 177–191.

Lubar, J. F. (2003). Neurofeedback for the management of attention-deficit/hyperactivity disorder. In M. S. Schwartz & F. Andrasik (Eds.), *Biofeedback: A practitioner's guide* (3rd ed.). New York: Guilford Press.

MacLeod, C., Mathews, A., & Tata, P. (1986). Attentional bias in emotional disorders. *Journal of Abnormal Psychology, 95*(1), 15–20.

MacWhinney, B., St. James, J., Schunn, C., Li, P., & Schneider, W. (2001). STEP—A system for teaching experimental psychology using E-Prime. *Behavior Research Methods, Instruments, & Computers, 33*(2), 287–296.

Maheu, M. M., Pulier, M. L., Wilhelm, F. H., McMenamin, J. P., & Brown-Connolly, N. E. (2005). *The mental health professional and the new technologies*. Mahwah, NJ: Erlbaum.

Martel, F. L., Hayward, C., Lyons, D. M., Sanborn, K., Varady, S., & Schatzberg, A. F. (1999). Salivary cortisol levels in socially phobic adolescent girls. *Depress Anxiety, 10*(1), 25–27.

McManis, M. H., Bradley, M. M., Berg, W. K., Cuthbert, B. N., & Lang, P. J. (2001). Emotional reactions in children: Verbal, physiological, and behavioral responses to affective pictures. *Psychophysiology, 38*(2), 222–231.

Meuret, A. E., Wilhelm, F. H., & Roth, W. T. (2001). Respiratory biofeedback-assisted therapy for panic disorder. *Behavior Modification, 25*, 584–605.

Mezzacappa, E., Tremblay, R. E., Kindlon, D., Saul, J. P., Arseneault, L., Seguin, J., et al. (1997). Anxiety, antisocial behavior, and heart rate regulation in adolescent males. *Journal of Child Psychol Psychiatry, 38*(4), 457–469.

Neville, H. J., Kutas, M., & Schmidt, A. (1982). Event-related potential studies of cerebral specialization during reading. II. Studies of congenitally deaf adults. *Brain Lang, 16*(2), 316–337.

Northam, E. A. (2004). Neuropsychological and psychosocial correlates of endocrine and metabolic disorders—a review. *J Pediatr Endocrinol Metab, 17*(1), 5–15.

Ohayon, M. M., Carskadon, M. A., Guilleminault, C., & Vitiello, M. V. (2004). Meta-analysis of quantitative sleep parameters from childhood to old age in healthy individuals: Developing normative sleep values across the human lifespan. *Sleep, 27*(7), 1255–1273.

Palermo, T. M., Valenzuela, D., & Stork, P. P. (2004). A randomized trial of electronic versus paper pain diaries in children: Impact on compliance, accuracy, and acceptability. *Pain, 107*(3), 213–219.

Papp, L. A., Goetz, R., Cole, R., Klein, D. F., Jordan, F., Liebowitz, M. R., et al. (1989). Hypersensitivity to carbon dioxide in panic disorder. *American Journal of Psychiatry, 146*, 779–781.

Pardey, J., Moulden, M., & Redman, C. W. (2002). A computer system for the numerical analysis of nonstress tests. *Am J Obstetric Gynecol, 186*(5), 1095–1103.

Picard, R. W., Vyzas, E., & Healey, J. (2001). Toward machine emotional intelligence: Analysis of affective physiological state. *IEEE Transactions on Pattern Analysis and Machine Intelligence, 23*(10), 1175–1191.

Pine, D. S., Coplan, J. D., Papp, L. A., Klein, R. G., Martinez, J. M., Kovalenko, P., et al. (1998). Ventilatory physiology of children and adolescents with anxiety disorders. *Archives of General Psychiatry, 55*, 123–129.

Pine, D. S., Klein, R. G., Roberson-Nay, R., Mannuzza, S., Moulton, J. L., 3rd, Woldehawariat, G., et al. (2005). Response to 5% carbon dioxide in children and adolescents: Relationship to panic disorder in parents and anxiety disorders in subjects. *Arch Gen Psychiatry, 62*(1), 73–80.

Plutchik, R. (1980). A general psychoevolutionary theory of emotion. In R. Plutchik & H. Kellerman (Eds.), *Emotion: Theory, research, and experience: Vol. 1. Theories of emotion* (pp. 3–33). New York: Academic Press.

Porges, S. W., & Byrne, E. A. (1992). Research methods for measurement of heart rate and respiration. *Biol Psychol, 34*(2–3), 93–130.

Porges, S. W., Doussard-Roosevelt, J. A., Portales, A. L., & Greenspan, S. I. (1996). Infant regulation of the vagal "brake" predicts child behavior problems: A psychobiological model of social behavior. *Dev Psychobiol, 29*(8), 697–712.

Porges, S. W., Doussard-Roosevelt, J. A., Portales, A. L., & Suess, P. E. (1994). Cardiac vagal tone: Stability and relation to difficultness in infants and 3-year-olds. *Dev Psychobiol, 27*(5), 289–300.

Putnam, L. E., Johnson, R., Jr., & Roth, W. T. (1992). Guidelines for reducing the risk of disease transmission in the psychophysiology laboratory. SPR Ad Hoc Committee on the Prevention of Disease Transmission. *Psychophysiology, 29*(2), 127–141.

Ridderinkhof, K. R., & van der Stelt, O. (2000). Attention and selection in the growing child: Views derived from developmental psychophysiology. *Biol Psychol, 54*(1–3), 55–106.

Rosenbaum, J. F., Biederman, J., Bolduc-Murphy, E. A., Faraone, S. V., Chaloff, J., Hirshfeld, D. R., et al. (1993). Behavioral inhibition in childhood: A risk factor for anxiety disorders. *Harv Rev Psychiatry, 1*(1), 2–16.

Roth, W. T. (1998). Applying psychophysiology in the clinic. *Psychophysiology, 35*, S9.

Roth, W. T., Wilhelm, F. H., & Trabert, W. (1998). Autonomic instability during relaxation in panic disorder. *Psychiatry Research, 80*(2), 155–164.

Salomon, K., Matthews, K. A., & Allen, M. T. (2000). Patterns of sympathetic and parasympathetic reactivity in a sample of children and adolescents. *Psychophysiology, 37*(6), 842–849.

Schmidt, N. A. (1998). Salivary cortisol testing in children. *Issues Compr Pediatr Nurs, 20*(3), 183–190.

Schneider, C. (1987). Cost effectiveness of biofeedback and behavioral medicine treatments: A review of the literature. *Biofeedback Self-Regulation, 12*(2), 71–92.

Schneider, S., Wilhelm, F. H., & Martin, I. J. (2005). *Scales for Iconic Self-Assessment of Anxiety in Children (ISAAC)*. Basel, Switzerland: University of Basel, Institute for Psychology.

Schwartz, M. S. (2003). Nocturnal or sleep enuresis: The urine alarm as a biofeedback treatment. In M. S. Schwartz & F. Andrasik (Eds.), *Biofeedback: A practitioner's guide* (3rd ed.). New York: Guilford Press.

Schwartz, M. S., & Andrasik, F. (Eds.). (2003). *Biofeedback: A practitioner's guide* (3rd ed.). New York: Guilford Press.

Spangler, G., & Grossmann, K. E. (1993). Biobehavioral organization in securely and insecurely attached infants. *Child Dev, 64*(5), 1439–1450.

Stern, R. M., Ray, W. J., & Quigley, K. S. (2000). *Psychophysiological Recording* (2nd ed.). Oxford, UK: Oxford University Press.

Task Force of the European Society of Cardiology and the North American Society of Pacing and Electrophysiology. (1996). Heart rate variability: Standards of measurement, physiological interpretation and clinical use. *Circulation, 93*(5), 1043–1065.

Teicher, M. (1995). Actigraphy and motion analysis: New tools for psychiatry. *Harv Rev Psychiatry, 3*(1), 18–35.

Wilhelm, F. H., Gerlach, A. L., & Roth, W. T. (2001). Slow recovery from voluntary hyperventilation in panic disorder. *Psychosomatic Medicine, 63*, 638–649.

Wilhelm, F. H., Gevirtz, R., & Roth, W. T. (2001). Respiratory dysregulation in anxiety, functional cardiac, and pain disorders: Assessment, phenomenology, and treatment. *Behavior Modification*, 513–545.

Wilhelm, F. H., & Grossman, P. (in press). Continuous electronic data capture of cardiopulmonary physiology, motor behavior, and subjective experience: Towards ecological momentary assessment of emotion. *Interacting with Computers*.

Wilhelm, F. H., Grossman, P., & Coyle, M. A. (2004). Improving estimation of cardiac vagal tone during spontaneous breathing using a paced breathing calibration. *Biomedical Sciences Instrumentation, 40,* 317–324.

Wilhelm, F. H., Grossman, P., & Roth, W. T. (2005). Assessment of heart rate variability during alterations in stress: Complex demodulation vs. spectral analysis. *Biomedical Sciences Instrumentation, 41,* 346–351.

Wilhelm, F. H., & Roth, W. T. (1996). Ambulatory assessment of clinical anxiety. In J. Fahrenberg & M. Myrtek (Eds.), *Ambulatory assessment: Computer-assisted psychological and psychophysiological methods in monitoring and field studies* (pp. 317–345). Gottingen, Germany: Hogrefe & Huber.

Wilhelm, F. H., & Roth, W. T. (1998a). Taking the laboratory to the skies: Ambulatory assessment of self-report, autonomic, and respiratory responses in flying phobia. *Psychophysiology, 35*(5), 596–606.

Wilhelm, F. H., & Roth, W. T. (1998b). Using minute ventilation for ambulatory estimation of additional heart rate. *Biological Psychology, 49*(1–2), 137–150.

Wilhelm, F. H., & Roth, W. T. (2001). The somatic symptom paradox in DSM-IV anxiety disorders: Suggestions for a clinical focus in psychophysiology. *Biological Psychology, 57*(1–3), 105–140.

Wilhelm, F. H., Roth, W. T., & Sackner, M. A. (2003). The LifeShirt: An advanced system for ambulatory measurement of respiratory and cardiac function. *Behavior Modification, 27*(5), 671–691.

Wilhelm, F. H., Trabert, W., & Roth, W. T. (2001a). Characteristics of sighing in panic disorder. *Biological Psychiatry, 49*(7), 606–614.

Wilhelm, F. H., Trabert, W., & Roth, W. T. (2001b). Physiological instability in panic disorder and generalized anxiety disorder. *Biological Psychiatry, 49*(7), 596–605.

10

Peer Sociometric Assessment

Elias Mpofu
JoLynn Carney
Department of Counselor Education
Counseling Psychology and Rehabilitation Services
The Pennsylvania State University

Michael C. Lambert
Department of Human Development and Family Services
University of Missouri
Columbia, Missouri

INTRODUCTION

How children are perceived by peers and children's relationships within social networks have been a preoccupation of educators, clinicians, and researchers for decades (Bukowski & Cillessen, 1998; Cillessen & Bukowski, 2000; De Jung & Kuntz, 1962; Eilbert & Glaser, 1959). The preoccupation with the study of the nature and quality of the relationships that children have with peers is premised on the belief that their social standing (or social status) with peers is an important indicator of social development or adjustment (Ladd, 1999; Newcomb & Bagwell, 1996; Hartup & Stevens, 1997; Newcomb, Bukowski, & Bagwell, 1999). For instance, children with higher peer social acceptance may have superior social skills or leadership qualities (Mpofu, 1997; Mpofu & Watkins, 1997). They are also more likely to engage in mutually beneficial social interactions with peers, which could boost their school achievement (Ladd, Buhs, & Troop, 1999). Children with lower social acceptance (or less liked) are at greater risk for school failure and dropout than those with higher social acceptance (Berndt, Hawkins,

& Jiao, 1999). Children with emotional behavioral disorders are likely to be less accepted by peers, although emotional behavioral disorders could result from or be accentuated in children with lower peer social acceptance (Deptula & Cohen, 2004; Miller-Johnson, Coie, Maumary-Gremaud, Lockman, & Terry, 1999; Ray, Cohen, Secrist, & Duncan, 1997). Moreover, children with poor social acceptance are at an elevated risk for delinquency or significant mood disorder in adulthood (Bagwell, Newcomb, & Bukowski, 1998; Deptula & Cohen, 2004; Nelson & Dishion, 2004).

The preoccupation with children's peer relationships is attested to by the sheer volume of published scholarship on the topic. More than 1000 works and studies have been published on peer relations in children since the year 1900, with as many as 250 citations since the year 2000 alone. Interest in the study of peer relations in children and their measurement is on the increase.

Assessment is the cornerstone of effective relationship interventions with children. For instance, an increasing number of social enhancement programs for children include assessment of peer relations as outcome measures (e.g., Asher, Parker, & Walker, 1996; Conduct Problems Research Group, 1999; Mpofu, 2003; Murphy & Schneider, 1994). Data on children's peer relations may also be useful to corroborate clinical diagnosis for emotional-behavioral or adjustment disorders (Cillessen & Bukowski, 2000; Zakriski et al., 1999) or referral for specialized sociobehavioral services (Merrill, 2001). In school settings, measures of children's social relations are an important index of the extent to which schools meet social justice expectations, such as equitable quality of school life for all students, regardless of sociocultural background (Ladd, Buhs, Troop, 2003; Mpofu, 1997; Mpofu, Thomas, & Chan, 2004). Peer sociometric assessment provides a unique perspective into student social relationships beyond that possible with self-report.

The word *sociometry* derives from the Latin terms *socius*, which means "social," and *metrum*, which translates to "measure" (Hoffman, 2001). By definition, sociometry is the measurement of the social standing of individuals within a group (Wu, Hart, Draper, & Oslen, 2001). It is used to study intergroup relationships, mostly involving children in school settings (Ray, Cohen, & Secrist, 1995; Zakriski et al., 1999). In those settings, social relations (e.g., acceptance, preference, popularity, visibility) among intact social cohorts of children (i.e., classmates) are assessed through the use of nomination or rating scale sociometric procedures. Informants are peers and sometimes teachers. The purposes for which sociometric data are collected determine the specific questions that are asked and the level of analysis and interpretations to follow. For example, questions about peer acceptance tend to be of a more general nature, whereas those on social preference may specify a context of performance or activity. Regardless of the specific questions under consideration, peer sociometric assessments are measures of social performance and interpersonal perception. In this chapter we discuss three aspects of peer sociometric assessment: procedures, psychometrics, and prospects.

PROCEDURES IN PEER SOCIOMETRIC ASSESSMENT

Several peer sociometric assessment procedures are identifiable: nomination, rating scale, and ranking. These approaches are used to assess various aspects of peer relationships, including friendship, acceptance, preferences, and acquaintance (Cillessen & Bukowski, 2000; Mpofu, 1997, 1999). Participants may be asked to express their peer relationship statuses in general (e.g., "Name three people in your class you would like to be.") or specific to settings (e.g., "Whom would you like to play with at break time?"). The data from sociometric measures are presented to express the relative social position of each child in the cohort using standardized scores or classification systems based on such scores. Peer sociometric data can also be presented to show social networks within a group and via sociograms. There are more sociometric measures of how individuals are perceived by peers (outsider perspectives) than of how they perceive their social status with peers (insider perspectives). In the following sections, we provide a brief overview of nomination, rating, and ranking sociometric procedures. We also present approaches used by the first author to assess self-perceived social status with nomination and rating scale procedures. In addition, we describe the use of sociograms and sociomatrices.

PEER NOMINATION PROCEDURES

Peer nomination is a popular sociometric procedure (Merrill, 2003). Peer nominations are commonly used to determine children's popularity or social status within a cohort. In school settings, the basic peer nomination procedure is to ask classmates to name peers whom they like ("like most" nominations) and do not like ("like least" nominations) or whom they prefer for specified activities (e.g., project work, play). Children may also respond to prompts, such as name three classmates (a) "whom you admire most; (b) whom others look up to; (c) whom you would like to be like; (d) who get angry most of the time; (e) whom you would least like to be like; (f) who do not try hard enough and get poor grades." Some studies use even more negative prompts, such as (a) "Whom would you least like to play with?" and (b) "Whom would you not want to be friends with?" (Chan & Mpofu, 2001, p. 47). The use of negative nominations may be a concern to parents, administrators, and possibly the children, in that the children may inadvertently learn negative attitudes toward others. Nonetheless, there is no evidence of any adverse impact from the use of negative nominations with children.

Children can also be asked to nominate up to three sets of three children they prefer for particular activities, excluding previous nominees. For instance, Mpofu (2003) asked adolescents to nominate up to three sets of classmates with whom they would like to interact, without repeating names. The assumption is that students would be relatively unconstrained in their choices (which would optimize selection for each student) while at the same time not forced to make superficial choices (which would reduce measurement error from false endorsements). Each of the adolescents nominated at least five peers with the relatively unconstrained nomination procedure. Limited-choice nomination procedures have the advantage of ease of administration, particularly with younger children. Older children or adolescents are better able to do flexible or unlimited nominations.

The "guess who" technique is an adaptation of the standard peer nomination procedure as previously described. With the "guess who" technique, children are provided with descriptive sentences and asked to write down the names of classmates (three or fewer) who they think would best fit the description. Prompts include statements such as "Guess who no one knows well, or guess who does the best job, or guess who is often angry at others" (Merrill, 1998, p. 265). The picture sociometric technique is also an adaptation of the standard peer nomination technique and is for use with preschool through second-grade students (Landau & Milich, 1990). Each student is shown an arbitrary array of classmates' pictures and asked to respond to a series of prompts by selecting a photograph of a peer. The prompts are statements very similar to those used in peer nomination studies, such as "Who would you like to play with most?"

A variety of scoring rubrics and interpretive frameworks is used with peer nomination data (Asher & Dodge, 1986; Coie, Dodge, & Coppotelli, 1982; Elksunin & Elksunin, 1997; Mpofu, 1999; Newcomb, Bukowski, William, & Patee, 1995; Worthen, Borg, & White, 1993). For example, socially accepted children are those with a high number of positive nominations, socially rejected children have a high number of negative nominations, socially neglected children have received very few or no nominations, and socially preferred children have more positive than negative nominations (Elksunin & Elksunin, 1997; Newcomb & Bukowski, 1983). The total number of nominations that a child receives is a measure of his or her social impact or visibility (Terry, 2000). With the "guess who" technique, scoring can be as simple as adding up frequencies for each descriptor or more sophisticated by obtaining frequencies on categories created from items of similar content (e.g., category of all items assessing peer popularity) (Merrill, 2003).

Several approaches are used to scale data from peer nomination for quantitative analysis and description. Those by Coie et al. (1982), Newcomb and Bukowski (1983), and Asher and Dodge (1986) are among the better known or studied. A commonly used procedure in scaling nomination data is to compute the proportion of students who are "most liked" and "least liked" by each child by summing nominations across students and dividing by the number of raters. Scores are often standardized within classroom and may be followed by the application of a peer status classification system. The classification systems of Coie et al. and Newcomb and Dodge (1982) yield five types of peer social statuses: popular, rejected, neglected, controversial, average. *Popular* children are highly liked and rarely disliked; *rejected* children are highly disliked and are rejected; *neglected* children are rarely liked and not actively disliked; *controversial* children are both highly disliked and highly liked; and *average* children are rated at the mean or neither liked nor disliked. The Coie et al. and Newcomb and Bukowski classification systems use different statistical algorithms to determine cutoff points for peer social status categories. The Coie et al. system uses deviation scores from the mean and on a *z*-scale, taking into account individual children's social preference and social impact statuses. The Newcomb and Bukowski method uses a probabilistic model to determine the cutoff scores for the various peer statuses. Using only positive nomination data, Worthen, Borg, and White (1993) classify and interpret results into categories of *stars* (frequently nominated peers), *isolates* (never-nominated peers), and *neglectees* (occasionally nominated peers).

The data for the peer sociometric classifications proposed by Coie et al. (1982) are interpreted within the context of the particular cohort (e.g., classmates). The lower social status (e.g., isolate, neglected, rejected) does not necessarily translate to a different population of children (e.g., children attending a school; nonschool children). For example, socially rejected children in a classroom setting may have as many friends as nonrejected students in community settings (Deptula & Cohen, 2004; Ray et al., 1997). Children with lower acceptance in individual classrooms made more out of class choices for friends as compared to those with higher social acceptance (Mpofu, 1997; Mpofu & Watkins, 1998). Socially rejected children perceived their social status to be higher than from peer ratings (Mpofu, 2003; Ray & Cohen, 1995) or were satisfied with the quality of their friendships (Brendgen, Littlet, & Krappmann, 2002; Poulin & Boivin, 1999). Children who are relatively new to a cohort may receive fewer nominations simply for being less well known to peers rather than for their likeability (Newcomb, Bukowski, & Pattee, 1993). In large cohorts, and particularly with limited nomination, children who are liked by peers may not be nominated to the extent commensurate with their actual social acceptance or standing. Many of the children who are apparently liked by peers would be categorized as average or neglected. Thus, the children's peer-rated social statuses within a cohort provide only a partial picture of their actual peer social standing or their social capital with peers.

PEER RATING PROCEDURE

Peer rating procedures or roster rating methods are also used to assess peer social status. The major difference with peer nomination procedures is that with peer rating all students rate all fellow students. Typically, peers are asked to circle a number from 1 to 5 (e.g., 1 = "not at all" to 5 = "very much") that is listed next to each child's name and in response to a socially oriented prompt. Younger children are often asked to circle a number from 1 to 3 or a face ranging from frowning to smiling and that are also anchored on a numeric scale. For example, classmates are asked to rate their peers on such items as degree to which they would like to play with that child and degree to which they would like to work with that child (Bierman, 2004). Other statement prompts are: "I consider him/her to be one of my best friends" and "He/she is a person with whom I can share my secrets" (Mpofu, 1997, 1999).

Peer ratings can be collected from children using an item *x* person matrix. There are several ways of presenting an item *x* person matrix. In general, names of the children and items are presented on a grid. An approach that the first author has used is presented in Table 10.1. The approach, an adaptation of that by Hall and Gaerddert (1960), presents a number of prosocial items on which children must rate peers. The instructions to the children include the scoring key for the items (1 = lowest; 5 = highest) and the code for each of the items, in Roman numerals (I–VII). The item codes are presented at the top and children's names to the left side of a spreadsheet. The children draw a line through own names to avoid displacement of ratings from unintended self-rating. They are asked to work down the item columns rather than across items so as to consider all peers on one sociometric criterion at a time. The requirement to rate all peers one item at a time is also intended to minimize rating errors by focusing the children on a single peer criterion.

Several scoring and interpretation options apply to peer rating data (Chan & Mpofu, 2001). The most frequently used scoring method is 1 = "least liked" and 5 = "most liked." For instance, the data from peer ratings are standardized, and a mean peer rating score is computed for each child. The child's mean rating serves as an index of social preference within the group. Alternatively, results are interpreted as those students receiving above the median *frequency* of 5 scale ratings being popular and those who receive above the median *frequency* of 1 scale rating being rejected. However, as noted previously, children may receive lower ratings because they are not well known to the cohort and not necessarily because they are liked or rejected (Bukowski, Sippola, Hoza, & Newcomb, 2000; Chan & Mpofu, 2001). Children who receive high scores are liked by their peers. Children may give a positive rating to others they did not rate highly either out of sympathy or indifference (Maassen, van der Linden, Goosens, & Bokhorst, 2000).

Chan and Mpofu (2001) proposed a method for combining the advantages of peer rating and peer nomination techniques by adding an additional rating to the 1–5 scale of "I don't know this student well" (DK category), which could help identify students who are either ignored or neglected by peers (p. 50). These authors suggest that this adaptation provides information on all classmates (a peer rating advantage) while at the same time identifying children who may be neglected because they are less known to the group. "Incorporating the DK category also allows scores to be interpreted for students who receive above the median frequency of DKs as neglected and those students who receive scores of 1 and 5 above the median in frequency as controversial" (p. 51).

Peer ratings have a number of distinct advantages over other sociometric techniques. First, they provide social acceptance data on all children in a cohort, since all children rate every child (Merrill, 2003; Mpofu, 1997). As a result, they yield more data on the peer relationships of each child as compared to peer nomina-

TABLE 10.1 Example Peer Rating Procedure

Instructions to Students

Rate every member of your class on each of the seven statements printed below. Look at these statements as often as you wish. Work as quickly as possible; your first idea as to the proper rating for any one person is likely the best one.

Rate every person. If you feel you do not know a boy or girl well enough to give the proper rating, make a guess anyway, then draw a circle around the rating.

Draw a line through your own name. Don't rate yourself by your name but on the special space on another page.

Rate every boy and girl by giving him or her a number for each of the seven items. The numbers you will use will be from 1 to 5. The numbers you will give will mean the following:

5 (the highest rating)
4 (above average)
3 (average)
2 (below average)
1 (the lowest possible rating)

Description

He/she fits the following description:

I. Very cheerful and has a sense of humor; always tries to help someone who may have trouble.
II. He/she greets other people when he/she sees them.
III. He/she is a person with whom I would talk over my personal affairs or secrets.
IV. I consider him or her to be one of my best friends.
V. He/she is a person who I would like to have as president of our class or other group in which I am active.
VI. I am more like him/her.
VII. He/she is more like me.

Names	Male/Female (M/F)	Date of Birth	Statements						
			I	II	III	IV	V	VI	VII

tion. Second, peer-rating procedures provide both positive and negative information without using negative prompts. This could make the method more acceptable to caregivers and the children (Asher & Dodge, 1986). A drawback of peer ratings is that they may lack the sensitivity to measure a broader range of social statuses. For instance, there may be a loss of measurement sensitivity from the fact that children rate those they particularly like or dislike more reliably than many peers with whom they are not actively involved (Haselager, Hartup, van Lieshout, & Riksen-Walraven, 1998; Hundley & Cohen, 1999). Combining nomination and rating procedures produces more powerful differentiations between children's social statuses in cohorts than either method alone (Merrill; Mpofu, 1999, 2003). For example, rating scale data can be scored to be functionally equivalent to nomination data by ascribing rejection status to children with a high frequency of "least liked" ratings and popular status to those with a high frequency of "most liked" ratings (Bukowski et al., 2000).

SOCIOMETRIC RANKING PROCEDURE

Sociometric ranking procedures provide information on each child as perceived by the informants in the social environment, who could be caregivers or peers. There are three general methods for collecting sociometric rankings: full ranking, partial ranking, and paired comparisons (Cillessen & Bukowski, 2000; Merrill). With the *full ranking* procedure, an informant (e.g., a teacher) could rank-order all students in the classroom on specific sociometric criteria such as popularity or positive interactions with peers. On the one hand, the method has the advantage of providing sociometric data on all children in a classroom. On the other hand, informant fatigue may compromise the quality of rankings, particularly with large cohorts. Informants may also be forced to differentiate between participants they may consider equivalent on the criterion in question. Moreover, the quality of the data is enhanced with the use of multiple informants familiar with or participants of the cohort (e.g., peers). Rankings from multiple informants compensate for biases associated with those by a single informant.

The full ranking procedure could be used to determine children's standing in specific social domains and relative to the whole group. The *partial ranking* method requires informants to determine which children in a cohort match a given set of social-behavioral criteria and then to rank-order those students in terms of severity or strength of fit with established criteria (Merrell, 2003). Thus, partial ranking is restricted to only those judged to specific criteria. Multiple informants (e.g., peers) add value to the data from partial ranking because combining their perspectives enhances the chances of including children who may meet the target criteria. Partial ranking contributes to sensitivity of measurement by combining nomination with rankings. It also does not force informants to rank participants on criteria that may not apply.

The *paired comparisons* method involves having informants rank each person against every other person in the cohort on specified social criteria. The method produces an exhaustive ranking of all participants. Scores from the rankings or paired comparisons are expressed as a standard scale for normative interpretations. The full, partial, and paired comparison methods are rarely used in sociometric research, mostly because they are labor intensive and more susceptible to response tendencies than alternative methods. Subsequent discussion of peer sociometric methods will consider peer nomination and rating only.

INSIDER AND OUTSIDER PEER SOCIOMETRIC PROCEDURES

A majority of current peer sociometric assessment procedures measure outsider views of peer social status rather than how the individual perceives his or her own social status within a group setting (or insider views) (Cillessen & Bukowski, 2000; Mpofu, 1997). A major limitation from ignoring the individual's view of his or her own social status is that an entire insider perspective is missed, and, with it, information important to individualizing social interventions. Mpofu (1999, 2003, 2004) distinguished between actual and perceived peer social status. *Actual* peer social status is the individual's social status from sociometric assessment by peers (an outsider view). *Perceived* social status is the individual's own perception of how he or she is viewed by peers (insider view). Perceived peer social status is important for social participation, in that it mediates the online processing of social stimuli by individuals and customizes their response to the stimuli (see also Crick & Dodge, 1996). In other words, actual social status as interpreted by the social actor from the lens of his or her own perception as a social agent accounts, in part, for the sociobehavioral consequences that individuals experience.

Mpofu (1999, 2003) used both peer nomination and peer rating sociometric procedures to measure actual and perceived social status in adolescents. He further differentiated between same-gender and opposite-gender social status, in view of the fact that children's perception of peers is significantly influenced by gender. For example, children give higher sociometric ratings to those of their own gender (Graham & Cohen, 1997; Mpofu, 1997). To account for gender differences in peer sociometric assessment, Mpofu proposed a sociometric assessment procedure comprising a 2 social status (actual, perceived) × 2 gender (same, opposite) matrix, resulting in four peer social statuses: actual same-gender social status, actual opposite-gender social status, perceived same-gender social status, perceived opposite-gender social status. This matrix also represents four levels of insider and outsider perspectives from the two for each of the social statuses by gender. For example, one insider perspective is from the individual's subjective social world (i.e., perceived social status) and another from membership of a gender category (i.e., same-gender social status).

To measure actual social status with peer nomination, Mpofu (2003) had adolescents make unlimited nominations of peers on any of 12 statements of social behavior (7 positive; 5 negative). Following Mpofu's procedure, the person's actual social status is the mean difference between the positive and negative nomination by peers adjusted by adding a nonzero positive constant. The constant is added to adjust negative values to positive. Scores can be standardized to a preferred metric for normative interpretation or other analyses. These social status scores are then split into same and opposite gender. For perceived social acceptance, Mpofu asked the adolescents to nominate themselves to 12 statements of social behavior as they would be perceived by boys in their class and then by girls in their class. (With multiple samples, the perceived social status measure is administered with counterbalancing for gender.) The individual's perceived social acceptance score is the difference between the positive and negative self-nominations adjusted by a positive constant. Same- and opposite-gender social status are derived as previously described.

A peer rating procedure used by Mpofu (1997, 1999, 2004) to assess actual social status was described previously (see Table 10.1). To measure perceived social acceptance, Mpofu asked adolescents to rate themselves on the same five to seven prosocial items as (1) "the boys in their class would" and (2) "as the girls in their class would." The standardized mean self-social perception within gender is the measure of perceived same- and opposite-gender social statuses. The combined mean from self-rated social perception for boys and girls is the overall measure of perceived social status. Reliability information on the measures by Mpofu and their validity for supporting social enhancement interventions with children are presented in a later section.

SOCIOGRAMS AND SOCIOMATRICES

A *sociogram* is a graphic presentation of the pattern of relationships within a social cohort. These patterns can be discerned from sociometric data from both peer nomination and peer rating. Various types of relationships can be charted on a sociogram: reciprocal, cluster, cleavage, simple, and complex (see Figure 10.1). *Reciprocal* (or mutual) relationships are those in which two children mutually choose each other on a criterion (e.g., best friend) or rate each other similarly on a sociometric rating scale. Unreciprocated relationships are those in which a choice or quality of rating by a participant rater is not returned by the receiver. These may suggest an aspired, emerging, or terminating mutual relationship (Hundley & Cohen, 1999). A cluster is a tightly knit pattern of mutual or reciprocated choices involving a small group of people who make or receive fewer choices outside the group. A cleavage comprises one or more networks within a cohort that do not make any choices outside the specific grouping. Social cleavages can be explained by many factors, including affinity by age, race, culture, gender, socioeconomic class, behavioral style, and ability (Graham & Cohen, 1997; Mpofu, 1997). For example, children with aggression may choose for peers others with aggression and exclude from their network any nonaggressive children. This peer preference may show as a cleavage in a sociogram.

Sociograms can also be described as comprising stars, chains, pairs, power, isolates, bridging ties, and cut points. A *star* is a formation of arrow lines point-

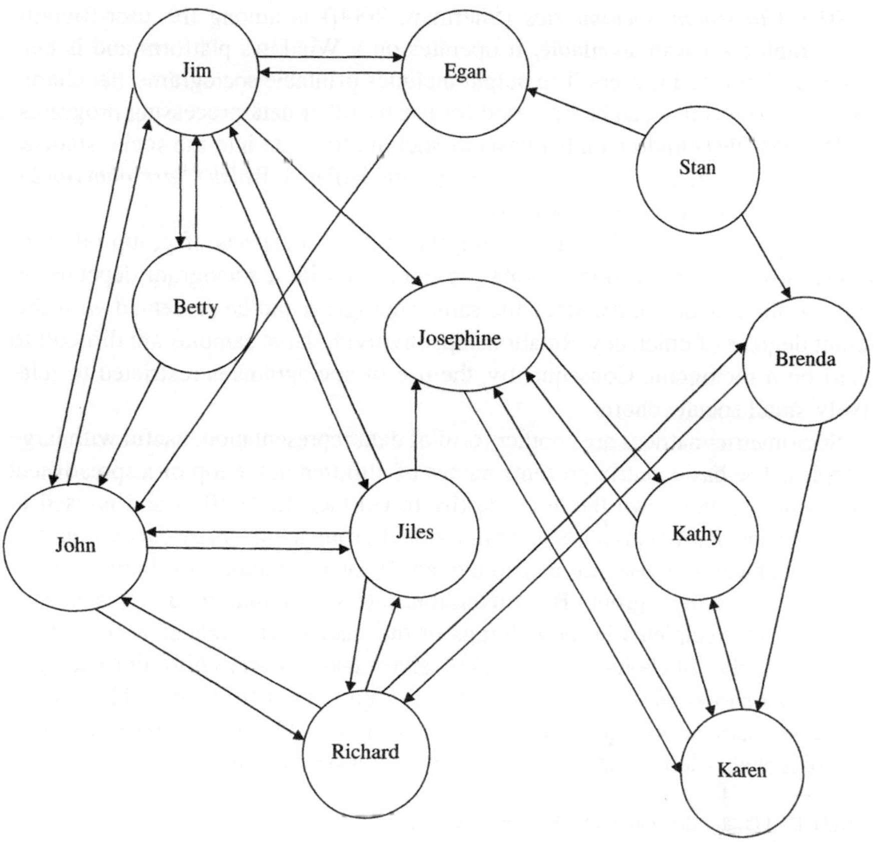

FIGURE 10.1 Sociogram illustrating a cleavage (Josephine, Karen, and Kathy), reciprocal/mutual relationship (e.g., Brenda and Richard), cluster (e.g., John, Jiles, Richard), and isolate (e.g., Stan).

ing either toward or away from a focal point representing a person (e.g., person receiving many choices or giving many choices). A *chain* is a sequence of one-direction arrows linking several persons (e.g., string of unreciprocated choices). A *pair* is a reciprocated choice. *Power* is the cluster of arrows depicting an individual chosen by highly popular individuals within a cohort. An *isolate* is represented by a focal with no choices received. A *bridging tie* is a link person for two or more otherwise-separate clusters. A *cut point* is the focal person who, if removed from a socionetwork, results in a lack of contact between several groupings. *Simple* networks are those comprising largely unreciprocated relationships and/or a few clusters (or mix of stars, chains, pairs, and power). *Complex* networks combine a number of relationships, such as reciprocated and unreciprocated relationships involving clusters and cleavages.

Several software programs for constructing sociograms are available; they require a small fraction of the effort it takes to draw a sociogram manually.

Walsh's Classroom Sociometrics (Sherman, 2000) is among the user-friendly sociographic software available. It operates on a Windows platform and is currently available to PC users. The output includes printable sociograms, bar charts, and scatter plots that can be imported for use by other data-processing programs. It also classifies children on the basis of sociometric data into the social statuses of popular, rejected, controversial, average, and isolated. *Walsh Classroom Sociometrics* includes a *help* file for users.

Sociograms are helpful for showing the structural aspects of group relationships. However, the quality of data presentation with a sociogram depends, in part, on the artistic ability, since the same sociogram can be presented with different degrees of efficiency. Relationships involving large samples are difficult to chart on a sociogram. Consequently, the use of sociograms is restricted to relatively small social cohorts.

Sociometric matrices are another form of data representation, useful with large samples. The basic matrix presents names of children at the top of a spreadsheet (by columns) and down the left side (by rows) (see Table 10.2) and is used to represent social relations among the individual group members. *Adjacency matrix* is the technical term used to refer to the tabulation of relationships between individuals comprising a group. By convention, raters (or initiators) are presented in the rows and recipients in the columns of the matrix. This makes it possible to plot the number of choices each child receives against every child. For example, Table 10.2 shows an 8 (column) × 8 (rows) adjacency matrix for 8 children and their endorsements for peers on a social criterion (e.g., "I am more like him/her."). The diagonal is left blank since the rater cannot be a receiver at the same time.

TABLE 10.2 Illustration of a Sociomatrix[1]

	Auxilia	Judy	Hanuza	Megan	Tom	Blanco	Rose	Scholastica
Auxilia		0	–	+	–	+	0	0
Judy	+		–	+	0	+	0	0
Hanuza	–	0		0	–	0	0	+
Megan	0	+	0		0	+	+	+
Tom	0	0	+	0		+	–	0
Blanco	0	+	+	+	+		–	+
Rose	+	0	–	–	–	–		–
Scholastica	0	0	+	+	+	+	–	
Totals								
Total +	2	2	3	4	2	5	1	3
Total 0	4	5	1	2	2	1	3	3
Total –	1	0	3	1	3	1	3	1
Total received	7	7	7	7	7	7	7	7
Mutuals								
+	0	2	1	2	1	4	0	3
0	1	3	1	2	2	0	1	2
–	1	0	1	0	1	1	2	1

[1]Social criterion: "I am more like him/her."

A plus sign (+) shows agreement, a zero (0) moderate agreement, and a negative sign (–) disagreement. The sociomatrix can also be used with limited or unlimited nomination procedures, with choices scored "1" and nonchoices "0."

Social network analysis with an adjacency matrix involves computing the out-degree and in-degree values for each individual. In-degree values are derived from summing up the column values per person (or how the person was rated by other group members). For example, the endorsement totals each member of a social is calculated down the columns and is an in-degree measure. These in-degree totals can be used to classify the group members into social statuses following conventional peer social status procedures, such as by Coie et al. (1982), Newcomb, Bukowski, and Pattee (1993). Out-degree measures are the row totals for each person (or how the individual rated other group members). The analysis of mutuals is based on out-degree measures.

Network analysis for mutuals is important for identifying individuals who are accepted, rejected, or neglected by a group. For example, Blanco and Scholastica (from Table 10.2) have above the median positive endorsements and could be informal leaders in the group. Judy and Megan are generally accepted by the group, in that they have no negative endorsements. Rose, with no positive endorsement and two negatives, is rejected by the group, while Auxilia, who has no positive endorsement and a single negative endorsement, may be neglected. Hanuza and Auxilia, Rose and Blanco, and Scholastica and Rose appear to be in conflict. A social enhancement intervention with this group would use as outcome criteria a positive shift in the group social statuses of Auxilia and Rose as well as in the dyadic relationships between Rose and Blanco and between Scholastica and Rose. With a fully inclusive adjacency matrix or one comprising reciprocated endorsements only, the out-degree and in-degree values are equal for each person. This means that every person in the social cohort has an error-free perception of his or her mutuality, a relatively rare event.

Density is a commonly used measure of adjacency. The density of lines in a social network is also an index of its complexity. *Density* is defined as the number of lines in a sociogram relative to the total lines if all points are connected (Scott, in press) or the proportion of actual ties to possible ties (Cook, 2001). It is a measure of the proportion of reciprocated relationships in a sociogram. There are several ways to calculate density. Using a probabilistic approach, the total number of bidirectional (or nondirectional) lines possible for a finite array of points is given by ${}_nC_2 = n!/(n-2)!2!$, where n = number of points and $C = n - 2$. For a sociogram with 10 points and connecting two points at time, the formula translates to $10!/[(10 - 2)!2!] = 3{,}628{,}800/(40{,}320 \times 2) = 45$. If the sociogram comprised 35 people, the density would be .77. The latter result means that about three-quarters of the social network are ties. Density values range from 0 to 1. With complete or inclusive sociograms, every point is connected directly to every other point, so the density is 1. Most sociograms would combine bidirectional and unidirectional lines, and the algorithms of the density use of the formula would be adapted to account for that complexity. As a general rule, the higher the density, the more complex the social network. With large samples, the utility of density as a measure of complexity of social network is reduced. Studies that report density as an index of social network complexity are more prevalent in the sociological rather than the psychological literature. Branden, Kenis, Raab, Schneider, and Wagner (1999) and Wasserman and Faust (1994) offer a cogent overview for the reader who wants to learn more about network data representation.

PSYCHOMETRIC CHARACTERISTICS OF PEER ASSESSMENT PROCEDURES

Reliability indices expected for peer sociometric assessments include measures of stability, such as test–retest correlations and interrater agreement for a composite social cohort or social status classification within a cohort. Internal consistency reliabilities for peer rating scales are infrequently reported. This may be because a majority of peer sociometric ratings use only a single item or too few items to comprise a coherent scale. As discussed later, the reliability of peer sociometric assessments is likely to be higher if the social criterion is specific to context, event, ability, or group (e.g., "Name three people you would like to play poker with.") than with less specific criterion (e.g., "Name three people you like."). Most of the published studies do not provide enough information about the reliability of the peer sociometric assessment nomination procedures used. The following sections review the evidence for the reliability of peer sociometric assessments, and the validity of interpretations or decisions based on them.

RELIABILITY OF PEER SOCIOMETRIC MEASURES

Reliability studies that use stability indices are based on the assumption that peer sociometric assessments measure enduring characteristics of children as participants of social cohorts. From the perspective of stability of measures as an aspect of reliability, a lack of stability would suggest measurement error. However, and as discussed later, a lack of stability in peer sociometric measures over time could suggest a reliable change in children's social statuses from maturation and/or experience. Thus, the reliability of peer sociometric assessments should be understood within the context of other information on the children's social participation.

Children's peer sociometric assessments are relatively stable across occasions. For example, short-term test–retest correlations in the margin of .23 to .61 have been observed between peer sociometric assessments over a period spanning 1 to 12 months (Cillessen, Bukowski, & Haselager, 2000). Short-term stability indices for rating scale data (.44 to .51) tend to be higher than for nomination data (.28 to .30) (Maassen et al., 2000). These reliabilities are less than the minimum of .90 required for individual counseling. Comparisons between procedures indicate that peer rating measures tend to (a) yield higher reliability coefficients and (b) provide distributions that are less skewed than from peer nomination measures (Merrill, 2003). However, there is evidence that average rating scores received on these measures do not distinguish well between rejected and neglected peers, since both receive ratings at the low end of the distribution (Bierman, 2004).

The long-term stability of peer sociometric measures is typically lower than their short-term stability (.11 to .29, median = .19) and relatively higher within peer social statuses, notably among popular and rejected children (.29 to .74) (Cillessen et al., 2000). Investigations into temporal stability indicate that the stability of peer status may result from several factors: stability of (a) underlying child characteristics (e.g., behavioral, social, emotional), and (b) social experiences of children. For example, children may maintain a view of themselves as social agents that projects a consistent social perception to peers. Moreover, children's social self-perceptions, such as the belief that others will like them, appear to positively impact interactions with new acquaintances (Phillipsen, Deptula, & Cohen, 1999). Impressions previously developed by the group about peers remain stable and influence group expectations more than actual behaviors of peers (e.g., peers' negative expectations and stereotypes of a rejected child are related to that child's rejected status from one school year to the next) (Bierman, 2004). Children may also be socialized to a consistent peer social status. For example, rejected children may maintain a stable peer status through the socialization to aggression by similar others (Houtzager & Baaerveldt, 1999; Warman & Cohen, 2000). Popular children may become better able to attract friends over time due to the enhancement of social skills through practice (Bierman; Cillessen et al.). Peer sociometric statuses are also relatively stable within gender, more so among younger children (Graham & Cohen, 1997; Mpofu et al., 2004).

Conversely, the factors that lower the stability of peer sociometric measures include a change in the underlying characteristics and/or contingencies of social behavior. For example, children may, as a result of differences in interpersonal perception from development, maturation, and/or experience exhibit more within-group variability in social performance, which could lower the stability of their social status. Changes in the contingencies of social behavior such as a child's friendship network may influence the stability of peer sociometric measures. For example, nonaggressive children who have aggressive peers for friends gravitate toward the social status of their aggressive peers (Deptula & Cohen, 2002). Children who participate in a social circle may be perceived as similar in social status from that association (Haselager et al., 1998). Goffman (1963) referred to *courtesy social status* to describe the social phenomenon in which people were perceived to share similar characteristics with their associates.

The reliability of peer sociometric assessment varies little by sample size. For instance, peer sociometric data are usually collected from at least 70% to 80% of a cohort. However, peer sociometric data from as few as 10 students correlated about .61 with data from 100 children, whereas those from 25 children correlated about .80 with data from a total sample of 100 (Zakriski et al., 1999). Thus, peer sociometric data of comparable reliability with that from whole class administrations may be possible from a subsample of classmates.

Mpofu (1999, 2003) reported interrater reliability indices ranging from .79 to .98 from peer nomination data and involving a variety of sociometric criteria. Reliability was higher with nominations on restricted rather than general criteria. For example, Mpofu (1999) used a restricted sociometric criterion with a peer nomination procedure. He asked adolescents attending schools with full integration for special education needs students to nominate three people in their class who were "in need of help." This resulted in an observed interrater agreement index of .98 from peers nominating classmates with disabilities as needing help. The sociometric criterion "in need of help" may have been interpreted by the students as referring to the special population of students with disabilities. With more general sociometric criteria (e.g., "nominate classmates who are helpful"), Mpofu observed an interrater reliability of around .79.

In a previous section, reference was made to the studies by Mpofu (1997, 1999, 2004) in which adolescents used a peer rating procedure (see Table 10.1) to assess the actual social status of classmates based on five to seven prosocial items. Internal consistency reliabilities ranging from .89 to .90 were observed for the actual social status measure. The observed internal consistency reliabilities for perceived social status based on the same prosocial items ranged from .40 to .77. This evidence suggests that peer sociometric ratings are more reliable than self-sociometric ratings. Moreover, reliability is enhanced with ratings on several social criteria.

VALIDITY ISSUES WITH PEER SOCIOMETRIC MEASURES

The available evidence for the valid use of peer assessment procedures has come from studies that examined the stability of peer sociometric assessment, their concurrent validity, predictive validity, and responsiveness to change following appropriate intervention. The stability of peer sociometric assessments can be interpreted as evidence of their validity for measuring interpersonal perception as an underlying or latent construct (Terry, 2000). Very few studies have investigated the stability of social statuses within cohorts, despite their importance for understanding types of peer relationships (Cillessen et al., 2000). However, there is a growing body of evidence for the usefulness of peer sociometric assessments as outcome measures.

STABILITY AS EVIDENCE OF VALIDITY

The evidence for the stability of peer sociometric measures as an index of reliability was considered in a previous section. If peer sociometric assessment measures an underlying construct (e.g., interpersonal perception), then behaviors that predict membership to a status category should also predict stable category membership with children. For example, Cillessen et al. (2000) concluded on the basis of extensive study that "children receiving the most extreme scores for behavior" were "the most likely to remain in the status group with which the behavior is associated" (p. 87). As discussed in a previous section, social status associated with extreme scores on peer sociometric assessments (e.g., most liked/least liked) and related peer social status (i.e., rejected, popular) are quite stable, especially through grade school (Bierman, 2004). The evidence appears to support the notion that peer sociometric assessments are measures of a latent construct in children, such as interpersonal perception (Terry, 2000).

The evidence for the predictive validity of peer sociometric assessments is from studies on correlational and causal effects of peer social status on relationship outcomes over time (e.g., Boulton, Trueman, Chan, Whitehand, & Amatya, 1999; Phillipsen et al., 1999; Ray et al., 1997). For example, Boulton et al. studied the protective function of friendship to experiencing peer victimization by examining the association between peer reports of victimization and self-reported friendship among early adolescents. These researchers defined victimization to include being hit or kicked, being called names, and/or being left out. Data were collected at two points during the school year. Findings from the first data-collection point indicated that those early adolescents who had a reciprocated best friend among their classmates received significantly fewer peer nominations for victimization than did the peers without a reciprocated best friend. Those who did not have a best friend at either data-collection time showed the highest increase in victimization over the course of the study, while those who did have a best friend at both data-collection times showed the highest decreases in victimization. Their analysis also indicated that a decrease in conflict and betrayal reported to characterize the participants' best friendship was associated with decreases in victimization. An earlier study by Ray et al. (1997) also found that children with mutual friends were perceived by peers to experience less victimization over the school year. Studies that predicted school adjustment and mood disorders from peer sociometric data were reviewed previously.

Evidence for the responsiveness of peer sociometric measures is from intervention studies that used peer sociometric measures as outcomes. For example, Mpofu (2003; Mpofu & Thomas, 2004) found evidence for the utility of peer nomination as a social enhancement intervention outcome measure. The interventions were designed to reduce disability stigma in adolescents, and they involved randomly assigning classrooms with adolescents with physical disabilities to one or more of the following interventions: peer interaction, role salience, academic support, and control. *Peer interaction* involved active participation in structured school curricula activities with other adolescents. *Role salience* referred to the enactment of a socially desired classroom and/or school position of responsibility (e.g., class president, soccer captain). *Academic support* was extra tuition in school subjects that presented difficulties. Data on actual (i.e., peer) social acceptance and perceived (i.e., self-) social acceptance were collected from 8342 adolescents with disabilities (n = 218) and without disabilities (n = 8124) attending 194 classrooms. Peer nomination and self-nomination measures of social acceptance were taken at baseline and at 12-week intervals over a period of 6 months. Repeated-measures analysis of the actual and perceived social acceptance measures showed significant reductions in disability stigma in both the adolescents with and without disabilities, particularly with interventions involving peer interaction. Evidence for the responsiveness of the peer nomination measures was from the fact that peer interaction, which is directly related to social status through effective use of social skills, was singularly the most effective intervention. Interventions involving role salience were effective in raising their perceived social status. The positive changes in disability stigma in both adolescents with and without disabilities over the intervention period provided evidence for the efficacy of peer nominations as outcome measures.

CONCURRENT VALIDITY

Current research suggests a considerable lack of concurrent validity among peer, teacher, and parent sociometric measures of peer status (Chan & Mpofu, 2001; Newcomb & Bagwell, 1995; Younger, Schneider, Wadson, Guirguis, & Bergeronen, 2000; Wu et al., 2001). For instance, whereas the reliability of teacher sociometric ratings are generally in the range of .50 to .70, the correlation between peer and teacher sociometric assessments is typically between .17 and .70, with a median of about .45 (Wu et al.; Mpofu, 1999; Zakriski et al., 1999). Peer picture sociometric techniques appear to produce more effective discrimination of peer social status than ratings provided by teachers (Merrill, 1998). The difference in reliability between peer and teacher sociometric ratings is explained, in part, by the fact that teachers and child peers may have different perspectives on the behavior of individual children from differences in the amount and context of observation. For example, teachers may not observe low-frequency behaviors that may be salient to peer social status.

Correlated or parallel forms of peer and teacher sociometric ratings are rarely reported in the literature, which limits the evidence available to evaluate the comparability of teacher and peer sociometric evaluations. Mpofu (1997) observed a correlation of .17 between teacher and student ratings of classmates using a rating scale with similar items. Teachers can be regarded as providing more objective observations of an individual child's behavior from their accumulated experience with child behavior in school settings (Merrill, 2003). Teacher sociometric assessment data are the next best alternative for the assessment of peer acceptance and rejection when peer sociometric data are not available (Bierman, 2004). The more comprehensive sociometric assessments utilize both peer and teacher sociometric measures.

A few studies have examined the concurrent validity of peer sociometric assessments with social adjustment measures. For example, Mpofu (1999) studied the concurrent validity of peer ratings data from 142 adolescents and teacher ratings of the same students on the Social Skills Questionnaire (SSQ) and the Academic Competence Questionnaire (ACQ) (Gresham & Elliot, 1990). He observed a mean correlation of .23 between actual same-gender peer social acceptance and social skills, as measured on the SSQ, and a mean correlation of .10 between perceived opposite-gender peer social acceptance and social skills, as measured on the same scale. The mean correlations between the actual same-gender peer social acceptance and academic competence as measured on the ACQ was .36; that for perceived peer social acceptance and the ACQ was at .13. Actual peer social acceptance explained about 5% of the variance in social skills as rated by teachers, and perceived peer social acceptance accounted for 1% of the variance in social skills from teacher ratings. The variance in academic competence explained by the peer social acceptance measures was between 2% and 13%. The very low concurrent validity between the peer sociometric measures and teacher ratings of social skills and academic competence is explained, in part, by the different perspectives from which students and teachers view social relationships in classrooms (Mpofu et al., 2004).

PROSPECTS OF PEER SOCIOMETRIC ASSESSMENT

Peer sociometric assessment has served and continues to serve the need to understand the quality of children's relationships quite admirably. The evidence for their reliability and appropriateness for providing social-group-level data for a variety of purposes, including initial behavioral screening for more intensive investigation, classification, and responsiveness, is encouraging. The utility of peer sociometric assessments could be enhanced in several ways: use within a multimethod, context-sensitive framework, sensitivity to cultural diversity, greater use of social network representational methodologies, and application of modern test theory. Each of these prospects is discussed next.

A MULTIMETHOD, CONTEXT-SENSITIVE ASSESSMENT FRAMEWORK IS ADVOCATED

Numerous and different needs are served through the assessment of child social behavior. Sociometric techniques can be used as one prong of a multi-layered approach in assessing the complex construct of children's social status and peer relationships (Bierman, 2004; Merrill, 2001, 2003), together with behavioral observations, role-plays, checklists, and other informant surveys. For example, Zakrisky and Coie (1996) demonstrated the use of video to collect data on peer relations. Merrill (2001) has proposed that first-line choices for social skills assessment are naturalistic behavioral observation and behavior rating scales, which directly assess social skills. Second-line assessment choices would be sociometric techniques and interviewing. These second-line choices act as supplemental assessment procedures providing rich data on children's social functioning. A combination of nomination and rating-scale peer sociometric measures appears to hold great promise from the strengths of each of these time-tested sociometric methods. The convergence of peer social status data from complementary sociometric assessments results in more reliable assessment and more valid decisions. In a later section, we propose the development of a new generation of peer sociometric assessments from the application of modern test theory.

A criticism of peer sociometric assessments is that they measure acceptance or reputation rather than the social skills for which the observed social statuses are the products (Merrell, 2001). Another shortcoming of peer sociometric assessments is that they have lower reliability to predict social performance in real-world settings when compared to observational or behavioral data (Cavell, Mehan, & Fiala, 2003; Merrell, 1999). Use of behaviorally and contextually anchored peer sociometric measures may enhance the quality of outcomes with these measures. Behaviorally and contextually anchored peer sociometric measures ask children to nominate or rate peers on social criteria that are directly related to social performance (social skills) in specific contexts (e.g., sharing resources for homework). Peer sociometric measures that are behaviorally and contextually anchored are likely to support a seamless transition between the results of assessment and the interventions from the assessment. Counselors and other caregivers who use the results from behaviorally and contextually anchored peer sociometric measures can directly teach to the skills and context of performance, which would enhance the social learning and transfer in children. In a previous section, we reviewed the evidence to the effect that the reliability of peer sociometric assessments was higher with restricted, context-specific social criteria than with unrestricted or general criteria.

PEER SOCIOMETRIC ASSESSMENTS SHOULD BE CULTURALLY SENSITIVE

Although research literature on peer sociometric assessment has been done in different countries, little by way of cross-cultural research exists. Furthermore, most existing research in international settings focus mainly on general issues of peer nomination, without much reference to the cultural issues associated with such work. When such comparisons are made, this research focuses mainly on interpreting the findings from such studies within the context of the United States. For example, there is interest in how well the peer sociometric assessments designed in the United States can function elsewhere (e.g., Cohen, Zhou, Hsueh, & Hancock, 2004; Hsueh, Zhou, Cohen, Hundley, & Deptula, 2004; Ezpeleta, Poliano, Domenech, & Domenech, 1990). Nonetheless, studies have been carried out involving comparisons of peer social status among blacks and whites and sometimes with consideration of gender and socioeconomic status (e.g., Kupersmidt, Greisler, DeRosier, Patterson, & Davis, 1995; Phillipsen et al., 2000).

The study by Kupersmidt et al. (1995) is particularly noteworthy for its use of a complex factorial design and peer nominations in examining the effects of race, SES, and neighborhood characteristics and children's adjustment. Kupersmidt et al. observed that low-income African American children living in single-parent homes were more aggressive than most other children, regardless of household composition. Middle-income white children, on the other hand, were least aggressive, according to their peers. Intriguingly, Kupersmidt et al. also found that this result was moderated by the neighborhood in which the child lived, where African American children in single-parent households in low-SES neighborhoods were most aggressive. The converse was true for low-income black children living in middle-class neighborhoods, where aggressiveness levels were comparable to those of all other children studied. Equally significant was the finding that white lower-SES children from single-parent families living in middle-class neighborhoods were significantly likely to be rejected by their peers. Thus, SES seemed to mediate peer social status, beyond that explained by race alone.

Comparative studies on peer social status could be enhanced by controlling for the effects on peer sociometric assessments of group differences in interpersonal perception thresholds. Black and white children in the United States seem to have different thresholds in judgment regarding peer nominations. For example, African American children tend to overestimate favorable nominations, whereas white children underestimate such nominations (Ray et al., 1995; Zakrisky & Coie, 1996). The peer social status of black children attending racially integrated schools may be influenced by their perceived friendliness, whereas that for white children may be influenced by their perceived leadership potential (Mpofu et al., 2004; Phillipsen et al., 1999). Thus, black and white children may be held to different social standards by peers or in ways that may bias their peer social status. We infer that there may be less within-race differences in peer sociometric assessments from shared interpersonal perception thresholds. Peer sociometric measures should be studied for their equitability in assessing peer social status with culturally diverse participants.

Children are more likely to give favorable ratings to same-sex peers than to opposite-sex peers (Cohen, Budesheim et al., 1997; Duncan & Cohen, 1995; Graham & Cohen, 1997; Kovacs, Parker, & Hoffman, 1996; Mpofu, 1997, 2003). That is, the prevalence of cross-sex relationships among many children is relatively rare. However, cross-sex friendships are moderated by race, in that African American children are more likely to have cross-sex friends than are their white peers (Kovacs et al., 1996). Use of limited nomination procedures may also bias children's peer evaluations, in that children are more likely to make choices from among others who are similar in race and/or gender (Schofield & Whitely, 1983). Use of unlimited nominations and rating scales may help reduce the confounds on peer social status associated with limited nominations. Nonetheless, there is a need to develop evidence-based protocols for the use of peer sociometric assessment with children with diverse gender, race, and other social attributes.

SOCIAL-NETWORK-REPRESENTATION APPROACHES ENHANCE THE QUALITY OF PEER SOCIOMETRIC ASSESSMENT

There are two levels for analyzing peer sociometric data: group and individual (Terry, 2000). Group-level approaches include social network analysis using sociomatrices (Wasserman & Faust, 1994). They reference observations to the structural aspects of the group. Individual-level approaches focus almost exclusively on the individual's relationship to the group. A majority of peer sociometric assessments from a psychological tradition are oriented to the individual level. The examination of multiple levels of complexity in children's peer relationships is encouraged (Duncan & Cohen, 1995; Mpofu, Thomas, & Chan, 2004; Phillipsen et al., 1999; Rubin, Bukowiski, & Parker, 1998). We are of the view that comprehensive peer sociometric assessment should combine both group- and individual-level analysis. In particular, practices in peer sociometric assessment in the psychological tradition could incorporate more structural-level analysis than hitherto.

Specifically, we advocate the wider use by practitioners of affiliation matrices to understand and predict the cohesion of social groups from those shared behaviors, experiences, and events that bridge the social worlds of the participants. An *affiliation matrix* describes relations between individuals or groups and social units (Cook, 2001; Wasserman & Faust, 1994). It enables the discernment of experiences or events common to some members of a social cohort. The identified shared experiences may be resources or benchmarks for planning social interventions in several ways. For example, a person-by-experience matrix would enable the identification of individuals whose qualities of group participation may be influenced by a common experience that may be relevant to social intervention planning. Table 10.3 presents a person-by-experience matrix for seven children and four experiences. On the basis of the data from a person-by-experience matrix, a person-by-person adjacency matrix can be imputed showing the prevalence of shared experiences among the group members (see Table 10.4). For example, Table 10.4 shows that Kelvin and Janis have above-the-median shared experiences, and this may explain, in part, any affinity between them or any behavioral similarity. The individuals sharing an experience may be in various peer statuses with each other and with members of the larger group (e.g., mutual, unreciprocated) and help bridge a targeted intervention for others for which their particular experience is a resource. Affiliation matrices can be similarly applied to person-by-behavior peer sociometric data involving social skills, for example (see Table 10.1). Person-by-person data can then be imputed for constructing social optimal-enhancement intervention for groups involving the identified

TABLE 10.3 Illustration of a Person-by-Experience Affiliation Matrix

	Divorce	Single Parent	Low SES	Summer Camp	HeadStart
Roger	1	0	0	1	0
Janis	1	1	0	1	0
Tracy	0	0	1	0	0
Nina	0	1	0	1	0
Sach	0	0	1	0	1
Kelvin	0	1	1	1	1
Rose	0	0	0	0	0

TABLE 10.4 Imputed Person-by-Person Adjacency Matrix for Experience

	Roger	Janis	Tracy	Nina	Sach	Kelvin	Rose
Roger	2	1	0	1	0	1	0
Janis	1	3	0	1	0	1	0
Tracy	0	0	1	0	1	0	0
Nina	1	1	0	2	0	2	0
Sach	0	0	1	0	2	1	0
Kelvin	1	1	1	2	2	4	0
Rose	0	0	0	0	0	0	0

The diagonal shows the total number of experiences per person.

persons with bridging experiences. Furthermore, studies that use affiliation data can enhance understanding of children's peer social statuses by examining possible mediator effects on children's peer status from their affiliation statuses (see Phillipsen et al., 1999, for example).

THERE IS NEED TO DEVELOP OBJECTIVE MEASURES OF PEER SOCIAL STATUS

A majority of existing peer sociometric measures have been developed using a rational approach to item construction, where experts unilaterally derive test items that they administer to and norm on individual classrooms. With these measures, experts may have derived the items based on specific theories of social behavior in children or simply on the need to cover important social outcomes as adjudged by peer review. The extant measures of peer social status also share considerable redundancy of items, in part from borrowing of "good" items by authors from exiting measures. Item redundancy between and within peer sociometric measures may also be explained by the need by researchers to maximize the likelihood that important social behaviors or dispositions are adequately sampled. These are clearly defensible methods to develop measures and are very useful for classifying children by their peer statuses. Nonetheless, the measures developed from these methods tend to be sample dependent and with ordinal-scale rather than interval-scale properties. They lack comparability, even within samples, because they do not share a common equal-interval metric or take into account cultural differences among the respondents.

We believe, however, that for the purposes of developing peer sociometric measures that are objective and responsive to change from maturation or experience, the use of a probabilistic model is stronger and more valid. Objective measures of peer social status should enable separation of an individual's peer social status from the particular test items used to measure that person's social status. This means that a child's peer social status can be reliably established from peer responses to any set of questions that are equivalent in measuring peer social status. In other words, the child's peer social status should be reliably established even though the peer informants took different test items on different occasions and/or skipped some questions. Furthermore, peer informant responses to an item should provide direct evidence on an individual's peer social status independent of the sample on which the test was normed.

The independence of interpretation of items from the specific instruments used has been referred to as the *transparency* of measures (Smith & Taylor, 2004). According to Smith and Taylor, transparent measures are constructed to be like those for physical properties, such as temperature, volume, and length, in objectivity, in that they "do not require the knowledge of the measuring instrument for interpretation" (p. 230). These strengths of objective measures enable reliable interpretation of scores at the item level to infer a relational status of interest (e.g., peer status).

Based on item response theory (IRT) (e.g., the Rasch models; van der Linden & Hambleton, 1997; Wright & Mok, 2000), peer sociometric measures could be developed that are both objective and predictive of future peer social status (prospective peer social status) in the absence of intervention. IRT is a method for determining the worth of a test item (or group of items) from the information that the item or group of items contributes toward estimating a person's ability on an underlying construct (or latent trait) (Andrich, 1988; Gierl, Henderson, Jodoin, & Klinger, 2001; Rasch, 1980). That latent trait estimation is possible because with IRT, test item characteristics (e.g., item difficulty, item discrimination) and person ability are placed on a common scale (or metric) using log-odd units, or logits, so that item statistics are established while taking into account person ability estimation.

Objective measures of prospective peer social status are especially relevant to social enhancement interventions, in that they enable a probabilistic estimation of a child's peer sociometric status. With a probabilistically derived measure, it is possible to reliably infer many other peer social statuses for an individual because the social criterion is positioned on a continuum of social status criteria that are possible (some below it, some above it), given a particular peer evaluation on a social criterion. For example, children perceived by peers to be withdrawn run objective risks for isolation, neglect, even rejection. If we knew from the results of an objective peer sociometric measure a particular child's peer social status on a social criterion of social withdrawal, we could reliably infer how that person would be rated by peers on likeability, friendliness, etc. This is possible because objective measures place all these social citeria on a continuum (high–low), with each social criterion maintaining its location on the hierarchy of social status–related behaviors, regardless of respondents.

Unlike objective measures (as previously described), current peer sociometric measures index an individual's past performance in peer relationships (because they are deterministic rather than probabilistic). Consequently, they do not make it possible to reliably predict individual peer social status for behaviors that were not observed or surveyed on the basis of a sample of observations of behaviors that are equivalent in mapping the peer social status. For example, a measure of perceived friendliness among children constructed using traditional approaches says more about the current likeability of a child than it does about the child's potential peer social status independent of intervention. This is because the measure does not locate peer-rated friendliness within a continuum of social criteria with known probabilities for peer social status. Thus, inferences about the meaning of observed social acceptance are constrained to the occasion, sample, and items.

Several models of test development based on IRT have been proposed (Andrich, 1996; Bond & Fox, 2001). The Rasch model is clearly the most known and studied among the IRT models. With the Rasch model, the probability that a person of certain ability will endorse an item as keyed is given by the difference between the trait level and the item difficulty logits. This is given by the formula

$$P_{ni}(X_{ni} = 1/B_n, D_i) = \frac{e^{(B_n - D_i)}}{1 + e^{(B_n - D_i)}}$$

where $P_{ni}(X_{ni} = 1/B_n, D_i)$ is the probability of that person n on item i will score correctly ($x = 1$) and with person ability B_n and item difficulty D_i. This probability is equal to the log transformation $e(2.7183)$ raised to the difference between a person's ability and an item's difficulty ($B_n - D_i$), divided by 1 plus the log transformed and raised difference. The observed item response is determined by the latent trait and the difficulty of the item. Item difficulty values are commonly expressed on the z-score metric.

We are not aware of any peer sociometric measures that were developed from cocalibration of peer social status data and that used the approach we suggest. Briefly stated, we propose an approach to calibrate peer sociometric measures using behaviorally anchored items selected from existing peer relations measures and with (1) evidence of good psychometric properties and/or (2) wide use in peer sociometric assessments. Peer social status data could be collected using such measures with unlimited nomination or rating scale. If using peer ratings data with polytomously scored items, the peer ratings can be calibrated using any available Rasch software (e.g., WINSTEPS; Linacre & Wright, 2000). With peer nomination data, item difficulty would be the endorsability of a particular social criterion item by peers for an individual. It would be a measure of how easy it was for a group of respondents to endorse a social criterion for a given individual. Data from out-degree measures of an adjacency matrix could be used to calibrate item difficulty values. A person peer relation's abilities will be estimated from peer-perceived social performance on the set of items that measure the latent construct of peer social status. The data for the peer relation ability calibration would be from the in-degree measures of an adjacency matrix. The difference between the in-degree and out-degree measures for each person per item converted to log-odd units should yield an objective measure of peer social status as previously defined. The feasibility of calibrating peer nomination data using in-degree and out-degree measures of an adjacency matrix remains to be demonstrated.

The work by Terry (2000) exemplifies an alternative latent-trait approach to peer sociometric assessment. Terry proposed a latent-trait model of interpersonal perception (LaTRIPP) that has great promise for the objective scaling of peer nomination sociometric measures. The model is based on the premise that peer sociometric assessments involve making social judgments on the latent trait of interpersonal perception. Based on that assumption, Terry hypothesized that peer sociometric assessment is a function of three parameters: the interpersonal perception ability of the person nominated (voter) = θ_i, the social sensitivity of respondent (voter) j to the social criterion $\theta = \beta_j$, the social threshold of respondent j to the social criterion = θ. Algebraically, the model translates to the following formula:

$$\pi_{ij} = \{1 + \exp[-1.7\alpha_j(\theta_i - \beta_j)]\}^{-1} \tag{1}$$

If social sensitivity is assumed to be constant or invariant across respondents (i.e., $\alpha = j$), the equation simplified to the Rasch model as described earlier. Terry demonstrated that the model was a good fit for the peer nomination data from 102 eight-grade students responding to a likeability item. The model by Terry appears to be an instance of the multifacets IRT model proposed by Linacre and Wright (1996), in which measure parameters are estimated from data from multiple judges (who may vary in reliability of ratings), participants (with varying levels of the attribute of interest), settings, and/or occasions. Future research should attempt to explore the feasibility of using the multifacets model by Linacre and Wright to calibrate peer sociometric data. The multifacets model and the IRT program have been used successfully to calibrate measures of health outcomes in hospital settings and more recently to calibrate the performance of judges at the 2004 Olympics (Linacre, 2004).

SUMMARY

Peer sociometric assessments have been described as "one of the most valid and useful sources of data regarding children's social adjustment as they are perceived by their peers" (Cavell, Meehan, & Fiala, 2003, p. 444). This is a significant endorsement of their worth as an approach to understanding peer social status in children. While sociometric assessment techniques are usually not norm referenced or commercially published, they do have a long history of use and provide a rich source of data that have commendable degrees of reliability and validity for the purposes for which they are used: determining peer social status for screening, classification, and social-enhancement intervention. Sociometric assessment translates quite readily to the school environment where they are commonly used; however, these techniques cannot be applied to the classroom setting without administrative and parental/guardian consent, which can be difficult to gain.

A variety of sociometric techniques provides unique information about peer relationships and has differing degrees of strengths and limitations. Researchers interested in using sociometric techniques will need to carefully consider the advantages and disadvantages of each when choosing a primary method for their study based on the type of data they are interested in collecting. For example, the data from peer sociometric assessment tend to emphasize traitlike qualities of children's peer relationships (e.g., friendliness) rather than specific social skills. Behaviorally anchored items may be a better choice for supporting social-enhancement interventions. However, trait-based measures will remain important for a variety of purposes, including screening of those at risk for social liability within the cohort.

The data from peer sociometric measures are sample dependent and on an ordinal scale. Consequently, they are difficult to interpret in terms of the individual child's objective peer status and regardless of the sample or scale of measurement. Applications of modern test theory such as IRT to peer sociometric assessment are possible. Several possibilities for constructing objective measures of peer social status are outlined in this chapter.

We have suggested that future trends in sociometric assessment techniques should incorporate a multimethod, context-sensitive assessment framework. This multipronged approach will be most productive when it is culturally sensitive, makes greater use of social-network-representational methodologies, and applies modern test theory. We believe that by advancing a multimethod framework of study, researchers can best serve counselors and caregivers, who in turn can be more effective in their interventions by utilizing information gained from this approach.

REFERENCES AND RESOURCES

Andrich, D. (1988). *Rasch models for measurement.* Newbury Park, CA: Sage Publications.

Andrich, D. (1996). Measurement criteria for choosing among models for graded responses. In A. Von Eye & C. C. Clogg (Eds.), *Analysis of categorical variables in developmental research (pp. 3–35).* Orlando, FL: Academic Press.

Asher, S. R., & Dodge, K. A. (1986). Identifying children who are rejected by their peers. *Developmental Psychology, 22,* 444–449.

Asher, S. R., & Dodge, K. A. (1996). Identifying children who are rejected by their peers. *Developmental Psychology, 22,* 444–449.

Asher, S. R., Parker, J. G., & Walker, D. L. (1996). Distinguishing friendship from acceptance: Implications for intervention and assessment. In W. M. Bukowski & A. Newcomb (Eds.), *The company they keep: Friendship in childhood and adolescence* (pp. 366–405). New York: Cambridge University Press.

Bagwell, C. L., Newcomb, A. F., & Bukowski, W. M. (1998). Preadolescent friendship and peer rejection as predictors of adult adjustment. *Child Development, 69,* 140–153.

Bierman, K. L. (2004). *Peer rejection: Developmental processes and intervention strategies.* New York: Guilford Press.

Bond, T. G., & Fox, C. M. (2001). *Applying the Rasch model: Fundamental measurement in the human sciences.* Mahwah, NJ: Erlbaum.

Boulton, M. J., Trueman, M., Chau, C., Whitehand, C., & Amatya, K. (1999). Concurrent and longitudinal links between friendship and peer victimization: Implications for befriending interventions. *Journal of Adolescence, 22,* 461–466.

Branden, U., Kenis, P., Raab, J., Schneider, V., & Wagner, D. (1999). Explorations into the visualization of policy networks. *Journal of Theoretical Politics, 11*(1), 75–106.

Bredgen, M., Little, T. D., & Krappman, L. (2000). Rejected children and their friends: A shared evaluation of friendship quality? *Merrill-Palmer Quarterly, 46,* 45–70.

Buhs, E. S., & Ladd, G. W. (2001). Peer rejection as an antecedent of young children's school adjustment: An examination of mediating processes. *Developmental Psychology, 37,* 550–560.

Bukowski, W. M., & Cillessen, A. H. (Eds.). (1998). *Sociometry then and now: Building on six decades of measuring children's experience with the peer group.* San Francisco: Jossey-Bass.

Bukowski, W. M., Sippola, L., Hoza, A. F., & Newcomb, A. F. (2000). Pages from a sociometric notebook: An analysis of nomination and rating scale measures of acceptance, rejection, and social preference. In A. H. N. Cillessen & W. M. Bukowski (Eds.), *Recent advances in the measurement of acceptance and rejection in the peer system* (pp. 11–26). San Franciso: Jossey-Bass.

Cavell, T. A., Meehan, B. T., & Fiala, S. E. (2003). Assessing social competence in children and adolescents. In C. R. Reynolds & R. W. Kamphaus (Eds.), *Handbook of psychological and educational assessment of children: Personality, behavior, and context* (2nd ed., pp. 433–454). New York: Guilford Press.

Chan, S., & Mpofu, E. (2001). Children's peer status in school settings: Current and prospective assessment procedures. *School Psychology International, 22,* 43–52.

Cillessen, H. N., & Bukowski, W. M. (2000). Conceptualizing and measuring peer acceptance and rejection. In A. H. N. Cillessen & W. M. Bukowski (Eds.), *Recent advances in the measurement of acceptance and rejection in the peer system* (pp. 3–10). San Franciso: Jossey-Bass.

Cillesen, A. H. N., & Bukowski, W. M. (2000). *Introduction: Conceptualizing and measuring peer acceptance and rejection.* In A. H. N. Cillessen & W. M. Bukowski (Eds.), Recent advances in the measurement of acceptance and rejection in the peer system (New Directions for Child Development No. 88, pp. 3–10). San Francisco: Jossey-Bass.

Cillessen, A. H. N., Bukowski, W. M., & Haselarger, G. J. T. (2000). Stability of sociometric categories. In A. H. N. Cillessen & W. M. Bukowski (Eds.), *Recent advances in the measurement of acceptance and rejection in the peer system* (pp. 75–93). San Franciso: Jossey-Bass.

Coie, J. D., Dodge, K. A., & Coppotelli, H. (1982). Dimensions and types of social status. A cross-age perspective. *Developmental Psychology, 18,* 557–570.

Cohen, R., Budesheim, T. L., MacDonald, C. D., & Eymard, L. A. (1997). Weighing the evidence: Likeability and trait attributions of a peer as a function of behavioral characteristics, body weight, and sex. *Child Study Journal, 27,* 69–93.

Cohen, R., Zhou, Z. K., Hsueh, Y., & Hancock, M. (2004, August). *Distinguishing among respect, liking, and friendships as measures of peer social competence.* Paper presented at the 28th International Congress of Psychology, Beijing, China.

Conduct Problems Research Group. (1999). Initial impact of the Fast Track prevention trial for conduct problems: 1. The high-risk sample. *Journal of Consulting and Clinical Psychology, 67,* 631–647.

Cook, J. (2001). Social networks: A primer. Retrieved November 24, 2004, from http://www.soc.duke.edu/~jcook/networks.html

Crick, N. R., & Dodge, K. A. (1996). Social information-processing mechanism on reactive and proactive aggression. *Child Development, 67,* 710–722.

De Jung, J. E., & Kuntz, A. H. (1962). Peer status indices from nomination and rating procedures in regular homogeneous ability grouped sixth graders. *Psychological Reports, 11,* 693–702.

Deptula, D. P., & Cohen, R. (2004). Aggressive, rejected and delinquent adolescents: A comparison of their friendships. *Aggression and Violent Behavior, 9,* 75–104.

Deptula, D. P., & Cohen, R. (2002). Aggressive, rejected, and delinquent children and adolescents: A comparison of their friendships. *Aggression and Violent Behavior, 9,* 75–104.

Duncan, M. K., & Cohen, R. (1995). Liking within peer group as a function of children's sociometric status and sex. *Child Study Journal, 25,* 265–288.

Eilbert, L. R., & Glaser, R. (1959). Differences between well and poorly adjusted groups in an isolated environment. *Journal of Applied Psychology, 4,* 271–274.

Elksnin, L. K., & Elksnin, N. (1997). Issues in the assessment of children's social skills. *Diagnostique, 22,* 75–86.

Espelage, D. L., Holt, M. K., & Henkel, R. R. (2003). Examination of peer group contextual effects on aggressive behavior during early adolescence. *Child Development, 74,* 205–220.

Ezpeleta, L., Poliano, A., Domenech, E., & Domenech, J. M. (1990). Peer Nomination Inventory of Depression in a Spanish sample. *Journal of Abnormal Child Psychology, 18,* 373–391.

Gierl, M. L., Henderson, D., Jodoin, M., & Klinger, D. (2001). Minimizing the influence of item parameter estimation errors in test development: A comparison of three selection procedures. *Journal of Experimental Education, 69,* 261–279.

Goffman, E. (1963). *Stigma: Notes on the management of spoiled identity.* Englewood Cliffs, NJ: Prentice Hall.

Graham, J. A., & Cohen, R. (1997). Race and sex as factors in children's sociometric ratings and friendship choices. *Social Development, 6,* 355–372.

Hall. W. F., & Gaerddert, W. (1960). Social skills and their relationship to scholastic achievement. *Journal of Genetic Psychology, 97,* 269–273.

Hartup, W. W., & Stevens, N. (1997). Friendships and adaptation in the life course. *Psychological Bulletin, 121,* 355–370.

Haselager, G. J. T., Hartup, W. W., van Lieshout, C. F. M., & Riksen-Walraven, J. M. A. (1998). Similarities between friends and nonfriends in middle childhood. *Child Development, 69,* 1198–1208.

Hoffman, C. (2001). Introduction to sociometry. Retrieved November 22, 2004, from http://www.hooppandtree.org/sociometry.htm.

Houtzager, B., & Baerveldt, C. (1999). Just like normal: A social network study of the relation between petty crime and the intimacy of adolescent friendships. *Social Behavior and Personality, 27,* 177–192.

Hsueh, Y., Zhou, Z. K., Cohen, R., Hundley, R. J., & Deptula, D. P. (2004, August). *Knowing and showing respect by Chinese and U.S. children: Relating children's understanding of respect to friendships.* Paper presented at the 28th International Congress of Psychology, Beijing, China.

Hundley, R. J., & Cohen, R. (1999). Children's relationship with classmates: A comprehensive analysis of friendship nominations and liking. *Child Study Journal, 29,* 233–247.

Kovacs, D. M., Parker, J. G., & Hoffman, L. W. (1996). Behavioral affective, and social correlates of involvement in cross-sex friendship in elementary school. *Child Development, 67,* 2269–2286.

Kupersmidt, J. B., Greisler, P. C., DeRosier, M. E., Patterson, C. J., & Davis, P. W. (1995). Childhood aggression and peer relationships in the context of family and neighborhood factors. *Child Development, 66,* 360–375.

Ladd, G. (1999). Peer relationships and social competence during early and middle childhood. *Annual Review of Psychology, 50,* 333–359.

Ladd, G. W., Buhs, E. S., & Troop, W. (2003). Children's interpersonal skills and relationships in school settings: Adaptive significance and implications for school-based prevention and intervention programs. In P. K. Smith & C. H. Hart (Eds.), *Blackwell handbook of childhood social development* (pp. 394–415). Oxford, UK: Blackwell.

Landau, S., & Milich, R. (1990). Assessment of children's social status and peer relations. In A. M. LaCreca (Ed.), *Through the eyes of the child* (pp. 259–291). Boston: Allyn & Bacon.

Linacre, J. M. (2004, October). *Winsteps and Facets: Basic and advanced workshops.* Raleigh, NC.

Linacre, J. M., & Wright, B. D. (1996). *Facets: Many-facet Rasch analysis.* Chicago: MESA Press.

Linacre, J. M., & Wright, J. D. (2000). WINSTEPS: Multiple-choice, rating scale, and partial credit Rasch analysis [Computer software]. Chicago: MESA Press.

Maassen, G. H., van der Linden, F. A., Goossens, J., & Bokhorst, J. (2000). A ratings-based approach to two-dimensional sociometric status determination. In A. H. N. Cillessen & W. M. Bukowski (Eds.), *Recent advances in the measurement of acceptance and rejection in the peer system* (pp. 55–74). San Franciso: Jossey-Bass.

Merrill, K. W. (1998). Assessing social skills and peer relations. In H. B. Vance (Ed.), *Psychological assessment of children: Best practices for school and clinical setting* (pp. 246–276). New York: Wiley.

Merrill, K. W. (1999). Behavioral, social, and emotional assessment of children and adolescents, Mahwah, NJ: Lawrence Erlbaum Associates.

Merrill, K. W. (2001). Assessment of children's social skills: Recent developments, best practices, and new directions. *Exceptionality, 9,* 3–18.

Merrill, K. W. (2003). *Behavioral, social, and emotional assessment of children and adolescents* (2nd ed.). Mahwah, NJ: Erlbaum.

Miller-Johnson, S., Coie, J. D., Maumary-Gremaud, A., Lockman, J., & Terry, R. (1999). Relationship between childhood rejection and aggression and adolescent delinquency severity and type among African American youth. *Journal of Emotional and Behavioral Disorders, 7,* 137–146.

Mpofu, E. (1997). Children's social competence and academic achievement in Zimbabwean multicultural school settings. *Journal of Genetic Psychology, 158,* 5–24.

Mpofu, E. (1999). *Social acceptance of early adolescents with physical disabilities.* Ann Arbor, MI: UMI Dissertation Services.

Mpofu, E. (2003). Enhancing social acceptance of early adolescents with physical disabilities: Effects of role salience, peer interaction, and academic support interventions. *International Journal of Disability, Development and Education, 50,* 435–454.

Mpofu, E. (2004, July). *Contextual and developmental factors in the experience of stigma by adolescents.* American Psychological Association 2004 Convention, Honolulu, Hawaii.

Mpofu, E., & Thomas, K. R. (2004, July). *Randomized, school-based disability stigma reduction intervention with adolescents.* American Psychological Association 2004 Convention, Honolulu, Hawaii.

Mpofu, E., Thomas, K., & Chan, F. (2004). Social competence in multicultural schools: Effects of ethnic and gender differences. *International Journal of Psychology,* 169–178.

Mpofu, E., & Watkins, D. (1997). Self-concept and social acceptance in African multiracial schools: A test of the insulation, subjective culture and bicultural competence hypotheses. *Cross-Cultural Research, 31,* 331–355.

Murphy, K., & Schneider, B. (1994). Coaching socially rejected early adolescents regarding behaviors used by peers to infer liking: A dyad-specific intervention. *Journal of Early Adolescence, 14,* 83–95.

Nelson, S. E., & Dishion, T. J. (2004). From boys to men: Predicting adult adaptation from middle childhood sociometric status. *Development and Psychopathology, 16,* 441–459.

Newcomb, A. F., & Bagwell, C. L. (1995). Children's friendship relations: A meta-analytic review. *Psychological Bulletin, 117,* 306–347.

Newcomb, A. F., & Bagwell, C. L. (1996). The developmental significance of children's friendship relations. In W. M. Bukowski, A. F. Newcomb, & W. W. Hartup (Eds.), *The company they keep: Friendship in childhood and adolescence* (pp. 289–231). Cambridge, UK: Cambridge University Press.

Newcomb, A. F., & Bukowski, W. M. (1983). Social impact and social preference as determinants of children's peer group status. *Developmental Psychology, 19,* 856–867.

Newcomb, A. F., Bukowski, W. M., & Pattee, L. (1993). Children's peer relations: A meta-analytic review of popular, rejected, neglected, controversial, and average sociometric status. *Psychological Bulletin, 113,* 99–128.

Newcomb, A. E., Bukowski, W. W., & Bagwell, C. L. (1999). Knowing the sounds: Friendship as a developmental context. In W. A. Collins, & B. Laursen (Eds.), *Relationships as developmental contexts: The Minnesota symposia on child psychology, Vol. 30* (pp. 63–84). Mahwah, NJ: Erbaum.

Newcomb, A. F., Bukowski, W. M., & Pattee, L. (1993). Children's peer relations: A meta-analytic review of popular, rejected, neglected, controversial, and average sociometric status. *Psychological Bulletin, 113,* 99–129.

Phillipsen, L. C., Deptula, D. P., & Cohen, R. (1999). Relating characteristics of children and their friends to relational and overt aggression. *Child Study Journal, 29,* 269–289.

Poulin, F., & Boivin, M. (1999). Proactive and reactive aggression and boys' friendship quality inmainstean classrooms. *Journal of Emotional and Behavioral Disorders, 7,* 168–177.

Poulin, F., & Boivin, M. (2000). The role of proactive and reactive aggression in the formation and development of boy's friendships. *Developmental Psychology, 36,* 233–240.

Rasch, G. (1980). *Probabilistic models for some intelligence and attainment tests.* Chicago: University of Chicago Press.

Ray, G. E., & Cohen, R. (1997). Children's evaluation of provocation between peers. *Aggressive Behavior, 23,* 417–431.

Ray, G. E., Cohen, R., & Secrist, M. E. (1995). Best-friend networks of children across settings. *Child Study Journal, 25,* 169–187.

Ray, G. E., Cohen, R., Secrist, M. E., & Duncan, M. K. (1997). Relating aggressive and victimization behaviors to children's sociometric status and friendships. *Journal of Social and Personal Relationships, 14,* 95–108.

Rubin, K. H., Bukowski, W. M., & Parker, J. G. (1998). Peer interactions, relationships, and groups. *Social, emotional, and personality development* (5th ed.), pp. 619–700, New York: Wiley.

Schofield, J. W., & Whitely, B. E. (1983). Peer nomination vs. rating scale measurement of children's peer preferences. *Social Psychology Quarterly, 46,* 241–251.

Schwartz, D., McFadyen-Ketchum, S., Dodge, K. A., & Pettit, G. S. (1999). Early behavior problems as a predictor of later peer group victimization: Moderators and mediators in the pathways of social risk. *Journal of Abnormal Child Psychology, 27,* 191–201.

Scott, J. (in press). *Social network analysis: A handbook.* Retrieved November 24, 2004, from http://www.analytictech.com.

Sherman, L. (2000). *Classroom sociometrics.* Retrieved November 22, 2004, from http://www.classroomsociometrics.com.

Smith, R. M., & Taylor, P. A. (2004). Equating rehabilitation outcome scales: Developing common metrices. *Journal of Applied Measurement, 5,* 229–242.

Terry, R. (2000). Recent advances in measurement theory and the use of sociometric techniques. In A. H. N. Cillessen & W. M. Bukowski (Eds.), *Recent advances in the measurement of acceptance and rejection in the peer system* (pp. 27–53). San Francisco: Jossey-Bass.

van der Linden, W., & Hambleton, R. K. (1997). *Handbook of modern item response theory.* New York: Springer.

Warman, D. M., & Cohen, R. (2000). Stability of aggressive behaviors and children's peer relationships. *Aggressive Behavior, 26,* 277–290.

Wasserman, S., & Faust, K. (1994). *Social network analysis: Methods and applications.* New York: Cambridge University Press.

Worthen, B. R., Borg, W. R., & White, K. R. (1993). Measurement and evaluation in the schools: A practical guide. White Plains, NY: Longman.

Wright, B. D., & Mok, M. (2000). Rasch models overview. *Journal of Applied Measurement, 1,* 83–106.

Wu, X., Hart, C. H., Draper, T. W., & Olsen, J. A. (2001). Peer and teacher sociometrics for preschool children: Cross-informant concordance, temporal stability, and reliability. *Merrill-Palmer Quarterly, 47,* 416–443.

Younger, A. J., Schneider, B. H., Wadson, R., Guirguis, M., & Bergeron, N. (2000). A behavior-based peer nomination measure of social withdrawal in children. *Social Development, 9,* 544–564.

Zakriski, A. L., & Coie, J. D. (1996). A comparison of aggressive-rejected and nonaggressive-rejected children's interpretation of self-directed and other-directed regression. *Child Development, 67,* 1048–1070.

Zakriski, A. L., Seifer, R., Sheldrick, R. C., Prinstein, M. J., Dickstein, S., & Sameroff, A. J. (1999). Child-focused versus school-focused sociometrics: A challenge for the applied researcher. *Journal of Applied Developmental Psychology, 20,* 481–499.

PART II

EVALUATION OF SPECIFIC DISORDERS AND PROBLEMS

11

ANXIETY AND FEAR

JANET WOODRUFF-BORDEN
OVSANNA T. LEYFER
Department of Psychological and Brain Sciences
University of Louisville
Louisville, Kentucky

INTRODUCTION

Anxiety and fear are ubiquitous aspects of childhood. Indeed, anxiety is conceptualized as adaptive (Barlow, 2001) and as a feature of normal development, with children progressing through developmentally appropriate stages of normal anxiety (Beidel & Stanley, 1993). Yet, despite its developmental significance and course, for a significant proportion of children anxiety is not a transient epiphenomenon of childhood and indeed is of clinical import. Epidemiological studies indicate that anxiety disorders are among the most common disorders of childhood and adolescence (Fergusson, Horwood, & Lynskey, 1993; Verhulst, van der Ende, Ferdinand, & Kasius, 1997). The prevalence of anxiety in children raises the question of whether childhood anxiety persists in its same form into adulthood. For example, Kendall et al. (1992) suggest that children who display anxiety symptoms will mature into adults suffering from an anxiety disorder. Work to date would argue that although anxiety tends to persist, its form also tends to change over time (e.g., Beidel, Flink, & Turner, 1996; Cantwell & Baker, 1987; Last, Perrin, Hersen, & Kazdin, 1996). These issues underscore the need for accurate and developmentally informed assessment, conceptualization, and treatment planning. Additionally, reliable and valid diagnostic tools are critical for further studies of epidemiology of anxiety disorders and their comorbidity as well as genetic and other familial factors of the disorders. This chapter focuses on current methods of assessment of anxiety in children and demonstrates their clinical application in a case study.

DSM-IV ANXIETY DISORDERS OF CHILDHOOD

The DSM-IV-TR (APA, 2000) specifies the following types of anxiety disorders in children: Separation Anxiety, Specific Phobia, Social Anxiety Disorder, Generalized Anxiety Disorder, Panic Disorder, Obsessive-Compulsive Disorder, Post-Traumatic Stress Disorder (PTSD), and Acute Stress Disorder. This represents a significant shift from earlier versions of the DSM, with Separation Anxiety the only disorder still considered a disorder first diagnosed in childhood. The diagnostic changes underscore the current view of childhood anxiety as "essentially downward extensions" of the adult anxiety disorders (Schniering, Hudson, & Rapee, 2000, p. 454).

Separation Anxiety is a rather common disorder found in approximately 4% of children (APA, 2000). It is characterized by excessive worry about separation from caregivers and/or from home. One of the main characteristics of the disorder is that the fear is not age appropriate; hence, the knowledge of the child's developmental level is very important in its diagnosis. Specific Phobia is associated with apparent strong or unreasonable fear of a specific object or situation, which leads to avoidance of the object or situation and/or distress when exposed to it (APA). It is important to note that the fear is in excess of what would be expected given the child's developmental level. The DSM criteria do not require the child to recognize that the fear is excessive (APA). The prevalence rates of Specific Phobia in children and adolescents range from 7.5% to 10%, with slightly higher prevalence in girls than boys (Lichtenstein & Annas, 2000). One of the main challenges in diagnosing specific phobias is differentiating phobias from fears that are developmentally appropriate, with the degree to which the fear is maladaptive an important factor in making the differentiation (Robinson, 2003).

Social Anxiety Disorder (SAD) is associated with a strong and unreasonable fear of social and performance situations, which subsequently leads to avoidance of the situation and/or distress when exposed to the situation (APA, 2000). The DSM requirement to recognize that the fear is excessive is suspended for children, but the fear must extend beyond interactions with adults and can only be diagnosed in children who have a capacity to form age-appropriate relations. SAD is rare in children younger than 10, and there are no gender differences in its prevalence (Albano, Chorpita, & Barlow, 1996). The prevalence of Social Phobia in children and adolescents is estimated to be approximately 1% (summarized in Beidel & Morris, 1995). Generalized Anxiety Disorder (GAD) is characterized by excessive, uncontrollable worry or anxiety across a number of situations and events (APA). The anxiety is accompanied by symptoms of restlessness, difficulty concentrating, sleep disturbance, muscle tension, fatigue, and/or irritability. For child diagnosis it is sufficient for the child to experience only one of the symptoms (APA). Studies using DSM-III or DSM-III-R criteria have found the rate of GAD in children to range from 2% to 4% (Achenbach, Connors, Quay, Verhulst, & Howell, 1989; Anderson, Williams, McGee, & Silva, 1987; Bowen, Offord, & Boyle, 1990). It is more prevalent in older children, with a mean onset between 10 and 13 years of age (Last, Strauss, & Francis, 1987; Strauss, Lease, Last, & Francis, 1988). GAD is more prevalent in female children (e.g., Bowen et al., 1990). Panic disorder is characterized by unexpected panic attacks, followed by at least one month of worrying about the occurrence of more attacks in the future and the consequences of the panic. Panic Disorder may include agoraphobia, which is the fear of being in certain situations or places from which it would be difficult to escape if one experiences a panic attack (APA, 2000). Few studies have focused on epidemiology of panic disorders in children. A study by Whitaker et al. (1990) found a prevalence of 0.6% in adolescents.

Obsessive-Compulsive Disorder (OCD) is characterized by having either obsessions or compulsions or both. Obsessions are defined as intrusive persistent thoughts or impulses that may not make sense; compulsions are defined as repetitive driven behaviors an individual performs in response to the obsession. Children do not have to recognize that the obsessions or compulsions are unreasonable or excessive (APA, 2000). The prevalence of OCD has been reported to be 0.4% in adolescents (Flament et al., 1988). Younger children are more likely to have compulsions rather than obsessions (Rettew, Swedo, Leonard, Lenane, & Rapoport, 1992). When diagnosing OCD in children, it is important to be aware of repetitive behaviors or rituals that are developmentally appropriate or are more characteristic of the stereotyped behaviors found in children with pervasive developmental disorders, for these have a different content than rituals characteristic of anxiety. The developmentally appropriate behaviors will generally disappear by the age of 10 (Swedo, Rapoport, Leonard, Lenane, & Cheslow, 1989). One can make the distinction based on how distressed the child gets when prevented from performing the behavior (Albano et al., 1996) as well as on close examination of the function of the behavior (e.g., specifically as a means of reducing anxiety).

PTSD usually is diagnosed after an individual is exposed to a traumatic or life-threatening event and as a result experiences helplessness, intense fear, or on inability to control the event. The traumatic event is then re-experienced consistently in the form of flashbacks, dreams, and/or intrusive memories specific to the traumatic event (APA, 2000). Children often may re-experience the event through bad dreams, which may even go beyond the scope of the event and take on a more general form. They may also relive the event through play (Robinson, 2003). No epidemiological studies have examined rates of PTSD in children and adolescents (Amaya-Jackson & March, 1995), but prevalence reports in adults have varied from 1% to 8% (APA; Helzer, Robins, & McEvoy, 1987; Kessler, Sonnega, Bromet, Hughes, & Nelson, 1995).

ASSESSMENT STRATEGIES

Currently, several methods exist for assessing anxiety in children: diagnostic interviews, both self-report and informant-based rating scales and checklists, as well as behavioral, cognitive, and psychophysiological measures.

DIAGNOSTIC INTERVIEWS

Structured and semistructured interviews are designed to make specific diagnoses according to current diagnostic classification systems, such as DSM-IV or ICD-10. This type of diagnostic interview groups symptoms and behaviors into diagnostically meaningful clusters, and the onset and duration of the symptoms are taken into account. Several interviews have been designed to target anxiety and other disorders in children, the most used ones including the Anxiety Disorders Interview Schedule for DSM-IV: Child and Parent Versions (ADIS-C/P; Silverman & Albano, 1996), the Diagnostic Interview Schedule for Children (DISC-IV; Shaffer, Fisher, Lucas, Dulcan, & Schwab-Stone, 2000), the Diagnostic Interview Schedule for Children and Adolescents (DICA; Reich, 2000), and the Schedule for Affective Disorders and Schizophrenia for School-Age Children (K-SADS; Ambrosini, 2000).

Anxiety Disorders Interview Schedule for DSM-IV

The ADIS-C/P is a semistructured interview developed to diagnose DSM-IV anxiety and related disorders in children and adolescents from ages 6 to 17 years. The ADIS-C/P provides current diagnoses based on both parent report and child report as well as a composite diagnosis based on both reports. Silverman, Saavedra, and Pina (2001) examined the reliability of the ADIS, finding good to excellent reliability for Separation Anxiety Disorder, Social Anxiety Disorder, Specific Phobia, and Generalized Anxiety Disorder. The ADIS has been shown to have good to excellent interrater reliability for these disorders for both the Child and Parent Interview as well as for the composite diagnoses of these disorders (Silverman et al.). Wood, Piacentini, Verbman, McCracken, and Barrios (2002) evaluated the concurrent validity of the ADIS with the Multidimensional Anxiety Scale for Children (MASC; March, Parker, Sullivan, Stallings, & Conners, 1997) and found support for its concurrent validity. A study of the DSM-III-R version of the ADIS-C/P indicated moderate to excellent interrater agreement for all the anxiety disorders; in contrast, the parent–child agreement was poor for the majority of the diagnoses (kappas ranging from .11 to .44; Rapee, Barrett, Dadds, & Evans, 1994).

Diagnostic Interview Schedule for Children and Adolescents

The DICA is a semistructured diagnostic interview comprised of questions appropriate to *DSM-III-R*, *DSM-IV*, and most of *ICD-10* diagnostic criteria (Reich, 2000). In contrast to the ADIS-C/P, which focuses on current diagnoses, the DICA assesses lifetime diagnoses. Currently two separate versions of the interview exist: one for younger children (6–12) and another for older children (13–17). The interview solicits information from both the parent and the child (Silverman, 1994).

Reich (2000) reported kappas of .55–.65 for overanxious, separation anxiety, and simple phobia in a mixed community and clinical group of young children and kappas of .72 and .75 for overanxious and separation anxiety (past) for 13- to 18-year-olds. Earlier, Welner, Reich, Herjanic, Jung, and Amado (1987) studied reliability, validity, and parent–child agreement for the child version of DICA in a group of psychiatric inpatients, finding high test–retest reliability. The parent–child agreement ranged from good to moderate for the majority of the diagnoses. Validity was examined by comparing the interview with diagnoses in the physician's discharge chart, finding that physicians agreed with the DICA diagnosis in 81.5% of the cases. In contrast, Ezpeleta, de la Osa, Domenech, Navarro, Losilla, and Judez (1997) reported low to moderate agreement between clinician and DICA diagnosis.

Diagnostic Interview Schedule for Children

The DISC is a structured diagnostic interview designed for use by lay interviewers in epidemiological studies. The current version of the DISC is based on the *DSM-IV* and *ICD-10*. Currently there are two versions of the DISC: DISC-P, for parents of children ages 6–17 years, and DISC-Y, which is administered to children and adolescents ages 9–17. The present version assesses the diagnoses within the past 4 weeks and within the past 12 months. It also has a "whole-life" module, the administration of which is optional. The psychometric properties of the DISC-IV have been investigated in a clinical sample (Shaffer et al., 2000). The test–retest reliability of the parent version for anxiety disorders is moderate for Social Anxiety Disorder, Separation Anxiety, and Generalized Anxiety (kappas = .54 to .65). Kappa for specific phobia was .96. Results were similar for the child version, Specific Phobia yielding the highest kappa (.68) and Social Phobia the lowest (.25). For combined diagnosis, Specific Phobia yielded a kappa of .86, while the kappas for the rest of the anxiety disorders ranged from low to moderate. The test–retest reliability of the previous version of the DISC with a community sample yielded similar results (kappa = .49; Schwab-Stone et al., 1996). Agreement between the DISC and clinician ratings (concurrent validity) was poor for Separation Anxiety and Social Anxiety in the parent version but was moderate for the composite category of anxiety disorders and Overanxious Anxious Disorder separately. On the child version, the agreement was poor (.31–.49) for anxiety disorders as a category and for Overanxious Anxiety Disorder and Social Phobia separately, but it was moderate for Separation Anxiety. The agreement was moderate on the combined diagnoses from the two versions, the best being the one for Overanxious Anxious Disorder.

Schedule for Affective Disorders and Schizophrenia for School-Age Children

There are two versions of the K-SADS: Present State (KSADS-P), which assesses diagnoses within the past 12 months, and Epidemiological (K-SADS-E), which assesses the most severe past episode as well as the current state at the time of the interview (Ambrosini, 2000). With the DSM revisions, the KSADS-P has undergone several revisions, the latest one done by Ambrosini and Dixon in 1996 (Ambrosini) and matching DSM-III-R and DSM-IV criteria. Also, after the introduction of the DSM-IV, the Present and Lifetime version of the K-SADS (K-SADS-P/L) was introduced, which was based on the DSM-III-R and DSM-IV criteria (Kaufman et al., 1997).

All versions are semistructured and administered by a trained clinician and solicit information from both the parent and the child. They are intended for children and adolescents ages 6–18. Interrater reliability for the most recent version of the K-SADS-P has been perfect for Generalized Anxiety Disorder and Separation Anxiety. On previous versions of K-SADS-P/L and E it has ranged from .24 to .80 (reviewed in Ambrosini, 2000). Data support the reliability and validity of the K-SADS, yet the sample sizes have been small; hence the instrument's psychometric properties need further evaluation (Ambrosini).

SELF-REPORT MEASURES

Several self-report instruments are available to assess fear and anxiety in children and adolescents. Self-reports have several advantages over diagnostic interviews: They are quick and easy to administer, and yet they permit the collection of information about a wide range of symptoms related to anxiety; they usually have high levels of test–retest reliability; and they are able to assess change over time, which is useful in measuring treatment progress. However, the self-report measures are not based on diagnostic criteria and hence are unable to differentiate between various diagnostic clusters. In addition, self-reports depend heavily on one's ability to read and understand questions (Stallings & March, 1995) and are potentially influenced by response bias (Anastasi & Urbina, 1977). The most widely used instruments include the Multidimensional Anxiety Scale for Children (MASC; March, Parker, Sullivan, et al., 1997), the Revised Children's Manifest Anxiety Scale (RCMAS, Reynolds & Richmond, 1978), the State–Trait Anxiety Inventory for Children (STAIC; Spielberger, Edwards & Lushene, 1973), and the Fear Survey Schedule for Children–Revised (FSSC-R; Ollendick, 1983).

Multidimensional Anxiety Scale for Children

The MASC (March et al., 1997) is a four-point Likert-type scale consisting of 39 items assessing four aspects of anxiety in children and adolescents ages 8–19: physical, cognitive, subjective, and behavioral. When the items were factor analyzed (March et al., 1997), the following four factors emerged: physical anxiety, harm avoidance, social anxiety, and separation anxiety. The first three factors are further divided into two subfactors each: tense and somatic for the physical anxiety factor, humiliation fears and performance fears for the social anxiety factor, and perfectionism and anxious coping for the harm avoidance factor. The internal reliability of the MASC is acceptable (alpha = 0.6–0.85) for the factor and subfactor scores and excellent (0.9) for the total score (March et al., 1997). Test–retest reliability has also ranged from adequate to good (March & Sullivan, 1999). Convergent and divergent validity studies of the MASC relative to other measures of anxiety, depression, and disruptive behaviors have demonstrated that the MASC is a valid measure of child anxiety symptoms (March et al., 1997). Finally, March and Sullivan (1999) demonstrate that the MASC is able to differentiate between anxious and nonanxious children and children with other psychiatric disorders.

Revised Children's Manifest Anxiety Scale

The RCMAS is a 37-item checklist designed to assess anxiety in children and adolescents ages 6–19. It consists of yes/no response items describing feelings and actions indicative of various aspects of anxiety. The scale can be further divided into three empirically derived subscales (physiological anxiety, worry/oversensitivity, and social concerns/concentration) and a lie scale. The internal consistency coefficient (alpha) has been found to be .60–.70 or lower for the physiological anxiety and the social concerns/concentration subscale, .70–.80 for the worry/oversensitivity scale, and in the .80 range for the total anxiety score (summarized in Gerard & Reynolds, 1999). Test–retest reliability has been found to be moderate (.68) for the total score (Reynolds, 1981). Validity studies of the RCMAS have compared the scores on the instrument with those on the STAIC, finding high correlation with the trait subscale, but very low correlation with the state subscale, suggesting that it is a measure of manifest anxiety (Reynolds, 1980, 1982, 1985).

State–Trait Anxiety Inventory for Children

The STAIC consists of two separate 20-item scales. The state scale targets present-state anxiety, and the trait scale targets anxiety that is stable across situations. The instrument has been standardized on a sample of children ages 8–12 (Spielberger, Edwards, & Lushene, 1973). Consistent with the state-trait distinction, test–retest reliability of the trait scale is better (.65 for males and .71 for females) than that for the state scale (.31 for males and .47 for females; Spielberger et al.). Finch, Montgomery, and Deardorff (1974) found that the STAIC has low test–retest reliability but high internal consistency. The correlations have been found to be low or moderate between the state and the trait scales and the Children's Manifest Anxiety Scale (.27 and .54, respectively; Finch & Nelson, 1974), suggesting perhaps that state and trait anxiety cannot be validly distinguished in children with emotional problems. Whereas Strauss et al. (1988) have reported that children with Overanxious Disorder received higher scores on both the state and trait scales than children without any disorder, others (Hoehn-Saric, Maisami, & Wiegand, 1987) found that the STAIC did not discriminate between children with anxiety diagnoses and those with other psychiatric disorders in a sample of psychiatric inpatients.

Fear Survey Schedule for Children—Revised

This instrument is a revision of the Fear Survey Schedule for Children (Scherer & Nakamura, 1968) and is designed to determine specific types of fears in school-aged children. It consists of 80 fear items that are rated on a three-point scale. A factor analysis of the FSSC-R has yielded five factors: fear of failure and criticism, fear of the unknown, fear of injury and small animals, fear of danger and death, and medical fears (Ollendick, 1995). The instrument has been found to be useful in distinguishing separation anxiety–related fears and other school situation–related fears in children who had school-related fears (Ollendick & Mayer, 1984). It also differentiates between various types of specific phobias (Weems, Silverman, Saavedra, Pina, & Lumpkin, 1999).

BEHAVIORAL OBSERVATION

Behavioral assessment of anxiety in children and adolescents incorporates direct observation, behavioral avoidance tests (BATs; Schniering et al., 2000), and, more recently, observation of familial interaction. Each approach to behavioral assessment allows for an ideographic understanding of a child's anxiety. Behavioral observations are useful objective additions to the assessment of anxiety because they are void of some of the limitations of interviews and self-reports, such as desire to project a more favorable image of self. They enable researchers and clinicians to track how anxiety is manifested across different situations. They are also flexible and allow identification and tracking of treatment targets. However, the relative lack of information regarding subjective experiences of anxiety and the lack of standardization somewhat limit their utility.

In BATs, rather than observing the child's behavior in a particular setting, the child's behaviors are recorded when he or she is exposed to the feared stimulus (Robinson, 2003). With some types of anxiety disorders, such as GAD, it is difficult to create the anxiety-provoking situations, and, therefore, BATs are not very practical in many cases (Schniering et al., 2000).

Self-monitoring is another method of behavioral assessment. Here the child records his or her anxiety responses, their severity, events immediately before and after the anxiety-provoking event, as well as thoughts associated with it (Robinson, 2003). However, Kearney and Wadiak (1999) suggest that self-monitoring will be strongly affected by the child's verbal and cognitive level and his or her motivation to follow the procedure.

A recent development is the behavioral observation of familial interactions of anxious children and their parents (Barrett, Rapee, Dadds, & Ryan, 1996). The role of the family in childhood anxiety has emerged as critical for several reasons. Children of anxious parents are up to seven times more likely than children of control parents to develop an anxiety disorder (Turner, Beidel, & Costello, 1987). Thus, the probability is high that an anxious child has an anxious parent whose report of the child is likely influenced by anxiety. Further, parental behavior has an impact on the child; in particular, parental control and lack of warmth have been highlighted as important constructs in the interactions of anxious parents and their children (Moore, Whaley, & Sigman, 2004; Rapee, 1997; Whaley, Pinto, & Sigman, 1999; Woodruff-Borden, Morrow, Bourland, & Cambron, 2002). In addition, Dadds, Barrett, Rapee, and Ryan (1996) demonstrated the impact of parents on anxious children selecting more avoidant strategies to cope with problem situations. Several coding systems have been published (e.g., Dadds, Rapee, & Barrett, 1994; Whaley et al., 1999; Woodruff-Borden et al., 2002) that allow for various dimensions of the parent–child interaction to be coded. The Family Anxiety Coding Schedule (Dadds et al., 1994) has been shown to be sensitive to changes when treating anxious children with a family-based adjunct to treatment.

There are no data supporting that behavioral observations are more efficacious in assessment than interviews or self-report. There also are no data to suggest that behavioral observations can distinguish among the anxiety disorders or between children with other psychiatric diagnoses. However, their ideographic application makes them an especially important aspect of an individualized assessment and treatment plan; when feasible, they can be used as an adjunct to interview and self-report data.

COGNITIVE ASSESSMENT

A large body of research supports the presence of biased information processing in anxious adults (see Matthews & MacLeod, 1994; Williams, Watts, MacLeod, & Matthews, 1997). Recent attention has been devoted to information processing of anxious children, with experimental results suggesting that anxious children tend to interpret ambiguous situations as more negative or threatening than do nonanxious controls (Barrett et al., 1996; Bell-Dolan, 1995; Chorpita, Brown, Albano, & Barlow, 1996). Assessment of these cognitive components of anxiety in children is in the most preliminary stages, and few measures specifically for children have been developed. Ambrose and Rholes (1993) modified an adult cognitive measure (Cognitions Checklist; Beck, Brown, Steer, Eidelson, & Riskind, 1987). Children's anxiety was associated with threat-related cognitions, although higher levels of threat were more associated with depression. Laurent and Stark (1993) created the Thought Checklist for Children based on the Cognitions Checklist. Similar to the findings of Ambrose and Rholes, threat-related cognitions differentiated anxious and nonanxious children but not anxious and depressed children. Although promising, questions remain regarding the psychometric properties of these measures, including the important issue of construct validity. That is, do measures based on "scaled-down" adult anxiety measures assess the same construct in adult and child samples. To address this, Ronan, Kendall, and Rowe (1994) developed the Negative Affect Self-Statement Questionnaire. Children's self-statements were used to create the measure of thoughts that "pop" into a child's head. According to the authors, one advantage of the measure is that it uses child language to define negative affect. Ronan (1996) suggests that the measure is also useful clinically to help children express cognitions early in treatment, when they may be unable or reticent to identify cognitions. Although preliminary, initial psychometrics appear promising. Test–retest reliabilities are good to excellent (Ronan et al., 1994), factors meaningfully differentiate anxiety and depression (Lerner et al., 1999), and the measure appears sensitive to treatment outcome (Kendall, 1994; Kendall et al., 1997). Further development and validation of cognitive measures for anxious children will continue to build on these important initial findings.

PHYSIOLOGICAL ASSESSMENT

The physiological responses of anxious children make physiological assessment seem particularly pertinent. In particular, assessment of common features of anxiety, such as heart rate, heart rate variability, blood pressure, muscle tension, and respiration, would seem informative (Kearney & Wadiak, 1999). Beyond utility in assessing one of the response channels of anxiety, physiological assessments obviate the issues associated with self- and other report. Children diagnosed with an anxiety disorder demonstrate elevated adrenergic responses (Rogeness, Cepeda, Macedo, Fischer, & Harris, 1990), increased physiological reactivity (Beidel, 1991), and elevated baseline zygomatic muscle tension (Turner, Beidel, & Epstein, 1991). Despite these promising findings, standardized methodological approaches, norms, and psychometric properties of physiological assessments have yet to be established in the child anxiety literature.

RESEARCH BASIS

Self-report and structured interviews are the most frequently used assessment strategies for child anxiety. Despite their obvious conceptual relevance, physiological and cognitive assessments are not routinely incorporated, and additional psychometric development would aid their more routine application. As noted earlier, behavioral observations contribute an important adjunct to assessment and treatment, though they share similar limited psychometric study and validation.

Some researchers have noted an insufficiency of studies on the validity of the DSM-IV categories for child anxiety disorders (Silverman, 1992; Werry, 1994). Additionally, very high comorbidity rates of anxiety disorders in children have been reported (as high as 50% in clinical samples; Anderson, 1994), suggesting that the subcategories of anxiety disorders are not valid. However, Spence (1997) found that a six-factor model where anxiety symptoms clustered along factors related to panic-agoraphobia, Social Anxiety, Separation Anxiety, Generalized Anxiety, Obsessive-Compulsive Disorder, and fear of physical injury best explained the data, supporting the DSM-IV model. In preschoolers, a five-factor structure was later found, including all the aforementioned factors except for panic-agoraphobia (Spence, Rapee, McDonald, & Ingram, 2001). The covariation of these factors was explained by a higher-order-factor model, on which the types of anxiety loaded on a factor of general anxiety.

Despite support for the general diagnostic categories, childhood anxiety is generally viewed on a continuum, with developmentally appropriate and transient experiences of anxiety being quantitatively different from diagnostically significant anxiety states. Critical for assessment is the ability of instruments to distinguish anxious from nonanxious children, among the anxiety disorders, and between the anxiety disorders and other psychiatric disorders.

The structured interviews already detailed generally have moderate to high interrater reliability (e.g., Rapee et al., 1994). Child report on structured interviews tends to be somewhat stable over time, with moderate test–retest reliability on diagnoses and less stability for symptoms (Boyle et al., 1993; Silverman & Eisen, 1992). It is not clear whether this is an artifact of a child's reporting on a complex phenomenon or whether these are actual changes in the experience of symptoms. Younger children (6–11 years) demonstrate poorer reliability, and boys tend to be less reliable than girls (Silverman & Eisen). Noteworthy, agreement between parent report and child report tends to be poor to moderate, regardless of interview used (Boyle et al.; Rapee et al.; Weissman et al., 1987). In general, children tend to report fewer symptoms than their parents report. This may be a reflection of a lack of understanding by children, or it may reflect a true difference between sources about the experience of anxiety by the child and the observation by the parent.

Self-report measures of child anxiety tend to have good to excellent test–retest reliability, as reviewed earlier, with correlations ranging from .44 to .98 (Beidel, Turner, & Morris, 1995; Finch et al., 1974; Ollendick, 1983; Reynolds & Richmond, 1985). As with interviews, agreement between children and parents on self-report measures tends to be fairly poor (Engel, Rodrique, & Geffken, 1994). Again, it is not clear if this is artifactual or an accurate reflection of different sources of information (Kazdin, French, & Unis, 1983). The impact of parental anxiety on report of the child also needs to be examined.

Validity of interviews and self-report is less well established than reliability. Concurrent validity, as reviewed earlier, has been established between interviews and clinician ratings. Interviews are also able to reasonably diffentiate anxious from nonanxious children, among the anxiety disorders, and between anxious and other diagnoses (e.g., Fisher et al., 1993; Sylvester, Hyde, & Reichler, 1987). Convergent validity has been established for the self-report measures, as detailed earlier. However, self-report measures have shown poor discriminant validity and are not particularly effective in differentiating among the anxiety disorders and between anxiety and other disorders (Hodges, 1990; Perrin & Last, 1992), suggesting that the anxiety disorders are likely more diffuse in childhood. An important aspect of validity not yet addressed is construct validity, an issue that crosses the current diagnostic system, interviews, and self-report. Specifically, examination is needed for the use of "scaled-down" adult disorders and whether these are accurate representations of anxiety experienced by children. That is, do the constructs define anxiety consistently from childhood to adulthood?

CLINICAL UTILITY

Several factors impact the clinical utility of child anxiety assessment strategies. As already noted, child report of anxiety is affected by age, gender, and level of cognitive development. Children's report of broad constructs seems relatively reliable, while report of more discrete information is less so. In addition, a child's cultural background is an important consideration in the assessment process. Anxiety and fear are clearly cross-cultural experiences, although their expression differs (Ollendick, King, & Frary, 1989). To adequately assess anxiety in children, the clinician needs an understanding of how anxiety and fear, as well as expected development, are defined in a child's culture (Canino, Bird, & Canino, 1997).

Familial factors of anxious children also impact clinical utility. Anxious children tend to have anxious parents, whose report may be impacted significantly by their own anxiety. Use of multiple informants is critical, and it allows a more complete assessment of the child. However, use of multiple sources often introduces tremendous variance. Children tend to report fewer symptoms than their parents, and clinical decisions must be made regarding the composite of the different reports, with particular attention to factors influencing parent report and the child's access to internal experiences and language to explain these.

DEVELOPMENTAL CONSIDERATIONS

DEVELOPMENTAL PROGRESSION OF FEARS AND ANXIETY

While fears and anxieties are quite common in children and adolescents, the task for the clinician becomes differentiation between fears and anxieties that are pathological from those that are developmentally appropriate. As the child grows older, the content of fears and anxieties changes (reviewed in Gullone, 2000). An infant is fearful of loud noises; as he or she gets older, this fear changes into fear of unfamiliar faces. At around preschool age, children are fearful of being alone and of darkness. Research has also suggested that the intensity of fears decreases with age (e.g., Gullone & King, 1997). The content of anxieties changes as well, from physical concrete threats to more abstract ones (Vasey, 1993), as the child gets older and develops the capacity for abstract thinking. Therefore, assessment of childhood anxiety disorders requires an understanding of the developmentally appropriate anxieties and fears in the course of development.

STABILITY OF ANXIETY

Given the expected developmental changes in anxiety over time, an important consideration is how stable anxiety disorders are in children. Do they remain the same over time, remit, or change to another type of anxiety? Retrospective work suggests anxious adults recall being anxious children (Pollack et al., 1996), implying continuity of anxiety over time. However, evidence for stability of specific childhood anxiety disorders appears less robust. Beidel, Flink, and Turner (1996) followed anxious children for 6 months and found that while most remained anxious, their specific diagnoses changed. Longitudinal studies are needed to address factors linked to changes in anxiety over time and whether these are a function of development or the lack of validity for separate child diagnostic categories.

APPLICATION OF ADULT CONSTRUCTS OF ANXIETY

The DSM-IV defines childhood anxiety disorders consistent with the definition of adult anxiety, with the exception of separation anxiety. As such, anxiety in children is defined by the adult construct. Given their inherent link to diagnostic systems, the same is true for structured interviews. It is also true for a number of self-report measures, which are child versions of the adult measures (e.g., STAIC, RCMAS). Children's understanding of anxiety may coincide with their developing ability to introspect, which appears to progress throughout childhood and to become well developed in adolescence (Harter, 1990). Thus, a child's age and developmental level will affect the construct validity of assessment measures, and an important clinical consideration is the child's understanding of the questions and constructs being assessed as well as his or her ability to introspect and access internal experiences.

ASSESSMENT, CONCEPTUALIZATION, AND TREATMENT PLANNING

Clinicians have a variety of assessment strategies from which to select an appropriate battery for a given child. Use of structured interviews, self-report, and other report (generally parents and teachers) is most common, with some anxieties and fears lending themselves readily to behavioral observation and BATs. Older children are also able to self-monitor, providing important observational data. The critical role of family factors was discussed earlier, and extant literature would argue for the importance of including an assessment of this important parameter for child anxiety. Considerations inherent in the use of multiple informants are highlighted with child anxiety, because the differences in parent report and child report are predictable.

Consideration of how the child experiences anxiety is necessary for a functional analysis, and examination of behavioral, physiological, cognitive, and affective parameters is critical. Children with the same anxiety disorder will experience and express their anxiety in individualized ways. For example, some children tend to avoid (behavioral), whereas others endure situations with physiological sensations such as stomach aches. Events and experiences antecedent and consequent to anxiety, such as familial factors, developmental considerations, and conditioning, are also identified through the assessment, yielding a functional analysis and conceptualization of the child's anxiety that leads to a treatment plan. As part of the treatment plan, planned ongoing data collection and assessment allows examination of the efficacy of treatment over time. The following case illustrates the assessment of childhood anxiety and highlights several factors critical for conceptualization and treatment planning, including discrepant parent–child reports, differences in self-report and diagnostic information, and parental factors in assessment and treatment.

CASE STUDY

IDENTIFICATION

John is a 10-year-old Caucasian boy. He lives with his parents, who are married and college educated. He has two siblings; he is the middle child. John's younger sibling has significant developmental delays and requires considerable attention from the mother.

PRESENTING COMPLAINTS

John presented to an anxiety specialty clinic with "test anxiety" and worries linked to perfectionism. At the time of the intake, John's mother reported that he worried when unable to understand the teacher in class. She also noted that the test anxiety interfered with John's taking a mathematics placement test. He became so distressed when confronted with the test that teachers eventually administered it in a surreptitious manner through gym class. Per John's initial report, he worried about a significant number of health-related issues, including contracting a disease, particularly tetanus, his health, his mother's health, and the clogging of his arteries. He also reported numerous fears, including fear of spiders, asteroids, tornadoes, poisonous minerals, and sharks.

John and his mother were administered the ADIS-C and ADIS-P (Silverman & Albano, 1996). In addition, John completed the MASC, STAIC-State, and STAIC-Trait. On the ADIS-P, John's mother reported that he has significant fear and avoidance of storms and tornadoes, getting shots, having blood tests, seeing blood, as well as of contracting an illness or disease. These fears caused John a great deal of distress and impairment. His mother also reported that John frequently worried about children bullying him in school and about his health, which he had difficulty stopping. She stated that he exhibited a range of physiological symptoms associated with anxiety, for example, restlessness and difficulty sleeping, and that these symptoms were moderately impairing. While John did not meet the diagnostic criteria for Oppositional Defiant Disorder, his mother stated that he frequently refused to comply and that he screamed at her in response to her requests. Per his mother's report, John also met the diagnostic criteria for Attention Deficit Hyperactivity Disorder, predominantly inattentive type.

On the ADIS-C, John endorsed very severe fear and avoidance of dogs and bees as well as of getting shots, but not of blood tests or seeing blood. He also reported a past fear of elevators. Similar to his mother's report, he endorsed a severe fear of catching an illness or disease. Overall, it appeared that reports from both John and his mother suggested a diagnosis of Specific Phobia. However, the types that they reported were different, with the exception of the Other type, which includes phobia of catching an illness or disease. John also reported worrying about performance-related issues, particularly related to sports. He did not endorse any physiological symptoms of anxiety, except for prior difficulty sleeping when he was 8 years old. Similar to his mother's report, John endorsed sufficient symptoms to meet criteria for ADHD, predominantly inattentive type, and he reported interference caused by these symptoms.

Results of the ADIS-P and ADIS-C in this case are characteristic of the low-moderate agreement between parent report and child report. While agreeing on global issues, clear differences emerged between John and his mother, specifically around the presence of physiological symptoms, the nature of fears, and the presence of oppositional behaviors. During his first session, John was also asked to fill out the MASC. The MASC scores were not elevated for any of the subscales, and his inconsistency score was below the cutoff, suggesting that his responses were fairly consistent. Lack of MASC elevations was contrary to both John's and his mother's ADIS reports. The STAIC-State was used to monitor John's progress in therapy. The score rose significantly from a baseline of 49 (while on medication) to a peak of 65 and then started decreasing, eventually reaching a plateau (a return to baseline levels of 49, but without medication). Based on the information collected, John received diagnoses of GAD, ADHD-predominately inattentive type, and a number of specific phobias.

HISTORY

No significant medical history was reported. While John had no known family history of anxiety, his mother described him as being anxious in different situations since early childhood. He had avoided some of these situations and had endured others with a great deal of distress. John's parents had noticed behaviors related to difficulty paying attention since he was approximately 5 years old. Two years prior to presenting for the current treatment, John's teacher complained that he was distracted during class and was not following directions. He was evaluated and subsequently diagnosed with ADHD, Combined type. He was prescribed Aderoll by his pediatrician, which was very effective per his teacher's report. One year prior to presenting for the current treatment, John's pediatrician prescribed Zoloft to address his anxiety. Per mother report, it was minimally effective, and she stopped administering it to John as the current treatment began.

DEVELOPMENTAL ISSUES

Upon presentation, John was fearful or anxious of a number of situations and events. It appears that while specific situations or areas of worrying have changed over time, John has remained anxious and fearful throughout his life. As already noted, when diagnosing a child with an anxiety disorder, one must differentiate between worries and fears that are developmentally appropriate and those that are not. For example, as an infant, John was fearful of loud noises, per his medical reports. Currently, he reports no fear of them. Also, he and his mother report his fear of shots being worse when he was younger than currently. In the OCD section of the ADIS-C, John endorsed a period of one year when he was 8 when he was concerned that something bad would happen if he touched things or opened doors with his left hand. This was "annoying," per his report, and "did not make any sense." However, it diminished over time. Currently he reports no compulsive behaviors, consistent with the findings by Swedo et al. (1989). Thus, John appeared to be an anxious and fearful child whose anxiety caused significant interference. The nature of the fears at times was developmentally appropriate but always excessive. Further, the types of fears changed rapidly, with a common factor of worrying or catastrophizing that something bad was going to happen.

PEER AND SCHOOL ISSUES

Overall, both John and his mother reported him as having excellent relationships with peers. He has several close friends with whom he spends time on a regular basis. However, in school John was frequently teased by his peers. This did not appear to be related to his fears and anxieties, but rather to his desire to correct other children's mistakes and a "know-it-all attitude," as reported by his mother. Outside school, John did not have conflicts with his peers, although during interactions with a friend who has a form of Pervasive Developmental Disorder, he had at times been impatient and volatile. This issue has not appeared to affect his relationship with that particular friend.

At the beginning of treatment John experienced many difficulties in school that went beyond his problems with attention and concentration. He was unable to take tests, and they had to be modified for him in order for John not to know these were tests. He reported one occasion when he threw his water bottle against the wall in school, because he was unable to complete a task in class. Also, he worried about not understanding his teacher and falling behind the class and subsequently of not being able to catch up.

BEHAVIORAL ASSESSMENT RESULTS

Developing an understanding of how John's perception of threat of danger contributed to his feelings of anxiety and to behaviors associated with it was a critical aspect of conceptualizing and treatment planning. Because John had excellent verbal abilities, self-monitoring appeared to be an appropriate method of behavioral assessment for him. He was asked to keep a daily worry log with the help of his mother, carefully outlining the incidents of worrying, situations or thoughts precipitating them, and the consequences of the worry, enabling the clinician to perform a functional behavioral analysis.

During therapy sessions, *in vivo* and imaginal exposures were conducted targeting some of John's fears. He was also taught muscular and breathing relaxation techniques. He was taught to measure his heart rate prior to and immediately after the exposure as well as after completing the relaxation and breathing exercise.

It became apparent that while John's worries emerged in a variety of different settings (school, home, playing with a friend, and others), they had one underlying theme: his physical health and safety. The obvious precipitants of these worries were encountering any health-related information. Further, every time John would worry, his parents would spend a great deal of time reassuring him. While John recognized that some of his worries were not reasonable, he reportedly would get so overwhelmed by them when they emerged that he was unable to reason. Subsequently he was taught through exposures to revert to relaxation and deep breathing when confronted with a worry-provoking situation and then to attempt to resolve it.

ETHICAL AND LEGAL ISSUES AND COMPLICATIONS

John and his mother attended the first several sessions together. His mother strongly believed that she needed to follow the flow of the sessions in order to remind John to practice the skills learned during the therapy and also to learn some of the cognitive-behavioral therapy concepts. John and his mother had one common goal for the therapy, agreeing that John worried a great deal about performance and health-related issues and that he needed to learn to cope with these worries. However, she also wanted John to work on his "defiant" behavior at home in response to her requests. John disagreed with his mother's reports of his defiance, maintaining that these were only isolated episodes that were short-lived. This created some conflict between the two of them during sessions, and after several sessions it was decided that, in part, these conflicts were likely linked to familial issues involving the relative lack of attention that John received in the household, given the demands on his mother to care for a developmentally disabled child, and also to maternal levels of negative affect. Thus, the therapist worked to balance the mother's right to know what happened during the therapy sessions with modeling of appropriate parental responses to John's symptoms and behaviors.

John presented with significant anxiety, fears, and attentional problems, in addition to behaviors, reported as oppositional by his mother, that seemed functional in garnering her attention in a household otherwise, of necessity, largely focused on another sibling. His presentation reflected a number of important issues in the assessment of child anxiety: differences in child report and parent report of problems and symptoms, lack of agreement between various types of assessment methods, parental factors in the assessment and treatment of children, family issues, and significant comorbidity of anxiety states in children, all of which require considerable attention in effectively assessing and treating child anxiety.

SUMMARY

Anxiety is a common experience of childhood, and for a subset of children it becomes interfering and clinically significant. Indeed, epidemiological studies indicate that anxiety disorders are among the most common disorders of childhood and adolescence, underscoring the need for accurate and developmentally informed assessment, conceptualization, and treatment planning. This chapter examined assessment strategies, including their research basis, clinical utility, and illustrative use in a case study. Considerations in assessing anxiety in children were highlighted; in particular, familial factors and developmental and cultural issues need to be considered. A critical issue for further examination is the construct validity of "anxiety" as it is currently defined. Assessment approaches and diagnostic nomenclature view anxiety in children as a younger version of adult anxiety. However, although the experience of anxiety tends to persist, its form often changes over time in children. Whether the separate diagnostic categories adequately define childhood anxiety awaits further examination of the longitudinal experience of childhood anxiety, which will further inform approaches to assessment as more is known about the construct of anxiety and its expression in childhood.

REFERENCES AND RESOURCES

Achenbach, T. M., Conners, C. K., Quay, H. C., Verhulst, F. C., & Howell, C. T. (1989). Replication of empirically derived syndromes as a basis for taxonomy of child/adolescent psychopathology. *Journal of Abnormal Child Psychology, 17,* 299–323.

Albano, A. M., Chorpita, B. F., & Barlow, D. L. (1996). Childhood anxiety disorders. In E. J. Mash & R. A. Barkley (Eds.), *Child psychopathology* (pp. 196–241). New York: Guilford Press.

Amaya-Jackson, L., & March, J. S. (1995). Posttraumatic Stress Disorder. In J. S. March (Ed.), *Anxiety disorders in children and adolescents* (pp. 276–301). New York: Guilford Press.

Ambrose, B., & Rholes, W. S. (1993). Automatic cognitions and symptoms of depression and anxiety in children and adolescents. An examination of the control specificity hypothesis. *Cognitive Therapy and Research, 17,* 289–309.

Ambrosini, P. J. (2000). Historical development and present status of the schedule for affective disorders and schizophrenia for school-age children (K-SADS). *Journal of the American Academy of Child and Adolescent Psychiatry, 39,* 49–58.

American Psychiatric Association. (2000). *Diagnostic and statistical manual of mental disorders, 4th edition, text revision* (DSM-IV-TR). Washington, DC: Author.

Anastasi, A., & Urbina, S. (1977). *Psychological testing* (7th ed.) Upper Saddle River, NJ: Prentice Hall.

Anderson, J. C. (1994). Epidemiological issues. In T. H. Ollendick, N. J. King, & W. Yule (Eds.), *International handbook of phobic and anxiety disorders in children and adolescents* (pp. 43–66). New York: Plenum Press.

Anderson, J. C., Williams, S., McGee, R., & Silva, P. A. (1987). DSM-III disorders in preadolescent children. Prevalence in a large sample from the general population. *Archives of General Psychiatry, 44,* 69–76.

Barlow, D. L. (2001). *Anxiety and its disorders* (2nd ed.). New York: Guilford.

Barrett, P. M., Rapee, R. M., Dadds, M. R., & Ryan, S. (1996). Family enhancement of cognitive styles in anxious and aggressive children: The FEAR effect. *Journal of Abnormal Child Psychology, 24,* 187–203.

Beck, A. T., Brown, G., Steer, R. A., Eidelson, T. J., & Riskind, J. H. (1987). Differentiating anxiety and depression: A test of the cognitive content-specificity hypothesis. *Journal of Abnormal Psychology, 96,* 179–183.

Beidel, D. C. (1991). Social phobia and overanxious disorder in school-aged children. *Journal of Child and Adolescent Psychiatry, 97,* 80–82.

Beidel, D. C., Flink, C. M., & Turner, S. M. (1996). Stability of anxious symptomatology in children. *Journal of Abnormal Child Psychology, 24,* 257–269.

Beidel, D. C., & Morris, T. L. (1995). Social phobia. In J. S. March (Ed.), *Anxiety disorders in children and adolescents* (pp. 181–212). New York: Guilford Press.

Beidel, D. C., & Stanley, M. A. (1993). Developmental issues in the measurement of anxiety. In C. G. Last (Ed.), *Anxiety across the lifespan: A developmental perspective* (pp. 167–203). New York: Springer.

Beidel, D. C., Turner, S. M., & Morris, T. L. (1995). A new inventory to assess childhood social anxiety and phobia: The Social Phobia and Anxiety Inventory for Children. *Psychological Assessment, 7,* 73–79.

Bell-Dolan, D. J. (1995). Social cue interpretation of anxious children. *Journal of Clinical Child Psychology, 24,* 1–10.

Boyle, M. H., Offord, D. R., Racine, Y., Sanford, M., Szatmari, P., Fleming, J. E., et al. (1993). Evaluation of the Diagnostic Interview for Children and Adolescents for use in general population samples. *Journal of Abnormal Child Psychology, 21,* 663–681.

Bowen, R. C., Offord, D. R., & Boyle, M. H. (1990). The prevalence of overanxious disorder and separation anxiety disorder: Results from the Ontario Child Health Study. *Journal of the American Academy of Child and Adolescent Psychiatry, 29,* 753–758.

Canino, G., Bird, H. R., & Canino, I. A. (1997). Methodological challenges in evaluating cross-cultural research of child psychopathology. In C. T. Nixon & D. A. Northruo (Eds.), *Evaluating mental health services* (pp. 259–276). London: Sage Publications.

Cantwell, D. P., & Baker, L. (1987). The prevalence of anxiety in children with communication disorders. *Journal of Anxiety Disorders, 1,* 239–248.

Chorpita, B. F., Brown, T. A., Albano, A. M., & Barlow, D. H. (1996). *The influence of parenting style on psychological vulnerability for the development of anxiety disorders.* New York: Association for Advancement of Behavior Therapy.

Dadds, M. R., Barrett, P. M., Rapee, R. M., & Ryan, S. (1996). Family process and child anxiety and aggression: An observational analysis. *Journal of Abnormal Child Psychology, 24,* 715–734.

Dadds, M. R., Rapee, R. M., & Barrett, P. M. (1994). Behavioral observation. In T. H. Ollendick, N. J. King, & W. Yule (Eds.), *International handbook of phobic and anxiety disorders in children and adolescents* (pp. 349–364). New York: Plenum Press.

Engel, N. A., Rodrigue, J. R., & Geffken, G. R. (1994). Parent–child agreement on ratings of anxiety in children. *Psychological Reports, 75,* 1251–1260.

Ezpeleta, L., de la Osa, N., Domenech, J. M., Navarro, J. B., Losilla, J. M., & Judez, J. (1997). Diagnostic agreement between clinicians and the Diagnostic Interview for Children and Adolescents—

DICA-R—in an outpatient sample. *Journal of Child Psychology and Psychiatry and Allied Disciplines, 38,* 431–440.

Fergusson, D. M., Horwood, Z. L. J., & Lynskey, M. T. (1993). Prevalence and comorbidity of DSM-III-R diagnoses of a birth cohort of 15-year-olds. *Journal of the American Academy of Child and Adolescent Psychiatry, 32,* 1127–1134.

Finch, A. J., Jr., Montogomery, L. E., & Deanrdorff, P. A. (1974). Reliability of state-trait anxiety with emotionally disturbed children. *Journal of Abnormal Child Psychology, 2,* 67–69.

Finch, A. J., Jr., & Nelson, W. M., 3rd. (1974). Locus of control and anxiety in emotionally disturbed children. *Psychological Reports, 35,* 469–470.

Fisher, P. W., Shaffer, D., Piacentini, J., Lapkin, J., Kafantaris, L. H., & Herzog, D. B. (1993). Sensitivity of the Diagnostic Interview Schedule for Children, 2nd edition (DISC-2.1) for specific diagnoses of children and adolescents. *Journal of the American Academy of Child and Adolescent Psychiatry, 32,* 666–673.

Flament, M. F., Whitaker, A., Rapoport, J. L., Davies, M., Berg, C. Z., Kalikow, K., et al. (1988). Obsessive compulsive disorder in adolescence: An epidemiological study. *Journal of the American Academy of Child and Adolescent Psychiatry, 27,* 764–771.

Gerard, A. B., & Reynolds, C. R. (1999). Characteristics and applications of the Revised Children's Manifest Anxiety Scale (RCMAS). In M. E. Maruish (Ed.), *The use of psychological testing for treatment planning and outcomes assessment* (pp. 323–340). Mahwah, NJ: Erlbaum.

Gullone, E. (2000). The development of normal fear: A century of research. *Clinical Psychology Review, 20,* 429–451.

Gullone, E., & King, N. J. (1997). Three year follow-up of normal fear in children and adolescents aged 7 to 18 years. *British Journal of Developmental Psychology, 15,* 97–111.

Harter, S. (1990). Issues in the self-concept of children and adolescents. In A. M. LaGreca (Ed.), *Through the eyes of the child: Obtaining self-reports from children and adolescents* (pp. 292–325). Boston: Allyn & Bacon.

Helzer, J. E., Robins, L. N., & McEvoy, L. (1987). Post-traumatic stress disorder in the general population. Findings of the epidemiologic catchment area survey. *New England Journal of Medicine, 317,* 1630–1634.

Hodges, K. (1990). Depression and anxiety in children: A comparison of self-report questionnaires to clinical interview. *Psychological Assessment, 2,* 376–381.

Hoehn-Saric, E., Maisami, M., & Wiegand, D. (1987). Measurement of anxiety in children and adolescents using semistructured interviews. *Journal of the American Academy of Child and Adolescent Psychiatry, 26,* 541–545.

Kaufman, J., Birmaher, B., Brent, D., Rao, U., Flynn, C., Moreci, P., et al. (1997). Schedule for Affective Disorders and Schizophrenia for School-Age Children-Present and Lifetime Version (K-SADS-PL): Initial reliability and validity data. *Journal of the American Academy of Child and Adolescent Psychiatry, 36,* 980–988.

Kazdin, A. E., French, N. H., & Unis, A. S. (1983). Child, mother, and father evaluations of depression in psychiatric inpatient children. *Journal of Abnormal Child Psychology, 11,* 167–180.

Kearney, C. A., & Wadiak, C. (1999). Anxiety disorders. In S. D. Netherton, D. Holmes, & C. E. Walker (Eds.), *Clinical handbook of anxiety disorders in children and adolescents* (pp. 251–281). Northvale, NJ: Jason Aronson.

Kendall, P. C. (1994). Treating anxiety disorders in children: Results of a randomized clinical trial. *Journal of Consulting and Clinical Psychology, 62,* 100–110.

Kendall, P. C., Chansky, T. E., Kane, M. T., Kortlander, E., Ronan, K., Sessa, F. M., & Siqueland, L. (1992). *Anxiety disorders in youth.* Boston: Allyn & Bacon.

Kendall, P. C., Flannery-Schroeder, E., Panichelli-Mindel, S. M., Southam-Gerow, M., Henin, A., & Warman, M. (1997). Therapy for youths with anxiety disorders: A second randomized clinical trial. *Journal of Consulting and Clinical Psychology, 65,* 366–380.

Kessler, R. C., Sonnega, A., Bromet, E., Hughes, M., & Nelson, C. B. (1995). Posttraumatic stress disorder in the National Comorbidity Survey. *Archives of General Psychiatry, 52,* 1048–1060.

Last, C. G., Perrin, S., Hersen, M., & Kazdin, A. E. (1996). A prospective study of childhood anxiety disorders. *Journal of the American Academy of Child and Adolescent Psychiatry, 35,* 1502–1510.

Last, C. G., Strauss, C. C., & Francis, G. (1987). Comorbidity among childhood anxiety disorders. *Journal of Nervous and Mental Disease, 175,* 726–730.

Laurent, J., & Stark, K. D. (1993). Testing the cognitive content-specificity hypothesis with anxious and depressed youngsters. *Journal of Abnormal Psychology, 102,* 226–237.

Lerner, J., Safren, S. A., Henin, A., Warman, M., Heimberg, R. G., & Kendall, P. C. (1999). Differentiating anxious and depressive self-statements in youth: Factor structure of the Negative Affect Self-Statement Questionnaire among youth referred to an anxiety disorders clinic. *Journal of Clinical Child Psychology, 28,* 82–93.

Lichtenstein, P., & Annas, P. (2000). Heritability and prevalence of specific fears and phobias in childhood. *Journal of Child Psychology and Psychiatry and Allied Disciplines, 41,* 927–937.

March, J. S., Parker, J. D., Sullivan, K., Stallings, P., & Conners, C. K. (1997). The Multidimensional Anxiety Scale for Children (MASC): Factor structure, reliability, and validity. *Journal of the American Academy of Child and Adolescent Psychiatry, 36,* 554–565.

March, J. S., & Sullivan, K. (1999). Test–retest reliability of the Multidimensional Anxiety Scale for Children. *Journal of Anxiety Disorders, 13,* 349–358.

Matthews, A., & MacLeod, C. (1994). Cognitive approaches to emotion and emotional disorders. *Annual Review of Psychology, 45,* 25–50.

Moore, P. S., Whaley, S. E., & Sigman, M. (2004). Interactions between mothers and children: Impacts of maternal and child anxiety. *Abnormal Psychology, 113,* 471–476.

Ollendick, T. H. (1983). Reliability and validity of the Revised Fear Survey Schedule for Children (FSSC-R). *Behaviour Research and Therapy, 21,* 685–692.

Ollendick, T. H. (1995). Assessment of anxiety and phobic disorders in children. In K. D. Craig & K. S. Dobson (Eds.), *Anxiety and depression in adults and children* (pp. 99–124). Thousand Oaks, CA: Sage Publications.

Ollendick, T. O., King, N. J., & Frary, R. B. (1989). Fears in children and adolescents: Reliability and generalizability across gender, age, and nationality. *Behavior Research and Therapy, 27,* 19–26.

Ollendick, T. H., & Mayer, T. H. (1984). School phobia. In S. M. Turner (Ed.), *Behavioral treatment of anxiety disorders* (pp. 367–411). New York: Plenum Press.

Perrin, S., & Last, C. G. (1992). Do childhood anxiety measures measure anxiety? *Journal of Abnormal Child Psychology, 20,* 567–578.

Pollack, M. H., Otto, M. W., Sabatino, S., Majcher, D., Worthington, J. J., McArdle, E. T., et al. (1996). Relationship of childhood anxiety to adult panic disorder: Correlates and influence on course. *American Journal of Psychiatry, 153,* 376–381.

Rapee, R. M. (1997). Potential role of childrearing practices in the development of anxiety and depression. *Clinical Psychology Review, 17,* 47–67.

Rapee, R. M., Barrett, P. M., Dadds, M. R., & Evans, L. (1994). Reliability of the DSM-III-R childhood anxiety disorders using structured interviews: Interrater and parent–child agreement. *Journal of the American Academy of Child and Adolescent Psychiatry, 33,* 984–992.

Reich, W. (2000). Diagnostic interview for children and adolescents (DICA). *Journal of the American Academy of Child and Adolescent Psychiatry, 39,* 59–66.

Rettew, D. C., Swedo, S. E., Leonard, H. L., Lenane, M. C., & Rapoport, J. L. (1992). Obsessions and compulsions across time in 79 children and adolescents with obsessive-compulsive disorder. *Journal of the American Academy of Child and Adolescent Psychiatry, 31,* 1050–1056.

Reynolds, C. R. (1980). Concurrent validity of "What I think and feel": The Revised Children's Manifest Anxiety Scale. *Journal of Consulting and Clinical Psychology, 48,* 774–775.

Reynolds, C. R. (1981). Long-term stability of scores on the Revised Children's Manifest Anxiety Scale. *Perceptual Motor Skills, 53,* 702.

Reynolds, C. R. (1982). Convergent and divergent validity of the Revised Children's Manifest Anxiety Scale. *Educational and Psychological Measurement, 42,* 1205–1212.

Reynolds, C. R. (1985). Multitrait validation of the Revised Children's Manifest Anxiety Scale for children of high intelligence. *Psychological Reports, 56,* 402.

Reynolds, C. R., & Richmond, B. O. (1978). "What I think and feel": A revised measure of children's manifest anxiety. *Journal of Abnormal Child Psychology, 6,* 271–280.

Reynolds, C. R., & Richmond, B. O. (1985). *Revised Children's Manifest Anxiety Scale: Manual.* Los Angeles, CA: Western Psychological Services.

Robinson, K. (2003). Assessment of childhood anxiety. In C. R. Reynolds & R. W. Kamphaus (Eds.), *Handbook of psychological and educational assessment* (pp. 508–525). New York: Guilford Press.

Rogeness, G. A., Cepeda, C., Macedo, C. A., Fischer, C., & Harris, W. R. (1990). Differences in heart rate and blood pressure in children with conduct disorder, major depression, and separation anxiety. *Psychiatry Research, 33,* 199–206.

Ronan, K. R. (1996). Building a reasonable bridge in childhood anxiety assessment: A practitioner's resource guide. *Cognitive and Behavioral Practice, 3,* 63–90.

Ronan, K. R., Kendall, P. C., & Rowe, M. (1994). Negative affectivity in children: Development and validation of a self-statement questionnaire. *Cognitive Therapy and Research, 18,* 509–528.

Scherer, M. W., & Nakamura, C. Y. (1968). A fear Survey Schedule for Children (FSS-FC): A factor analytic comparison with manifest anxiety (CMAS). *Behavior Research and Therapy, 6,* 173–182.

Schniering, C. A., Hudson, J. L., & Rapee, R. M. (2000). Issues in the diagnosis and assessment of anxiety disorders in children and adolescents. *Clinical Psychology Review, 20,* 453–478.

Schwab-Stone, M. E., Shaffer, D., Dulcan, M. K., Jensen, P. S., Fisher, P., Bird, H. R., et al. (1996). Criterion validity of the NIMH Diagnostic Interview Schedule for Children Version 2.3 (DISC-2.3). *Journal of the American Academy of Child and Adolescent Psychiatry, 35,* 878–888.

Shaffer, D., Fisher, P., Lucas, C. P., Dulcan, M. K., & Schwab-Stone, M. E. (2000). NIMH Diagnostic Interview Schedule for Children Version IV (NIMH DISC-IV): Description, differences from previous versions, and reliability of some common diagnoses. *Journal of the American Academy of Child and Adolescent Psychiatry, 39,* 28–38.

Silverman, W. K. (1992). Taxonomy of anxiety disorders in children. In G. D. Burrows, R. Noyes, & S. M. Roth (Eds.), *Handbook of anxiety* (Vol. 5). Amsterdam: Elsevier.

Silverman, W. K. (1994). Structured diagnostic interviews. In T. H. Ollendick, N. J. King, & W. Yule (Eds.), *International handbook of phobic and anxiety disorders in children and adolescents (pp. 293–315).* New York: Plenum.

Silverman, W. K., & Albano, A. M. (1996). *The Anxiety Disorders Interview Schedule for DSM-IV—Child and Parent Versions.* San Antonio, TX: Psychological Corporation.

Silverman, W. K., & Eisen, A. R. (1992). Age differences in the reliability of parent and child reports of child anxious symptomatology using a structured interview. *Journal of the American Academy of Child and Adolescent Psychiatry, 31,* 117–124.

Silverman, W. K., Saavedra, L. M., & Pina, A. A. (2001). Test–retest reliability of anxiety symptoms and diagnoses with the Anxiety Disorders Interview Schedule for DSM-IV: Child and parent versions. *Journal of the American Academy of Child and Adolescent Psychiatry, 40,* 937–944.

Spence, S. H. (1997). Structure of anxiety symptoms among children: A confirmatory factor-analytic study. *Journal of Abnormal Psychology, 106,* 280–297.

Spence, S. H., Rapee, R., McDonald, C., & Ingram, M. (2001). The structure of anxiety symptoms among preschoolers. *Behavior Research and Therapy, 39,* 1293–1316.

Spielberger, C. D., Edwards, C. D., & Lushene, R. E. (1973). *State-Trait Anxiety Inventory for Children.* Palo Alto, CA: Consulting Psychologists Press.

Stallings, P., & March, J. S. (1995). Assessment. In J. S. March (Ed.), *Anxiety Disorders in Children and Adolescents (pp. 125–147).* New York: Guilford.

Strauss, C. C., Lease, C. A., Last, C. G., & Francis, G. (1988). Overanxious disorder: An examination of developmental differences. *Journal of Abnormal Child Psychology, 16,* 433–443.

Swedo, S. E., Rapoport, J. L., Leonard, H., Lenane, M., & Cheslow, D. (1989). Obsessive-compulsive disorder in children and adolescents. Clinical phenomenology of 70 consecutive cases. *Archives of General Psychiatry, 46,* 335–341.

Sylvester, C. E., Hyde, T. S., & Reichler, R. J. (1987). The Diagnostic Interview for Children and Personality Inventory for Children in studies of children at risk for anxiety disorders or depression. *Journal of the Academy of Child and Adolescent Psychiatry, 26,* 668–675.

Turner, S. M., Beidel, D. C., & Costello, A. (1987). Psychopathology in the offspring of anxiety disorders patients. *Journal of Consulting and Clinical Psychology, 55,* 229–235.

Turner, S. M., Beidel, D. C., & Epstein, L. H. (1991). Vulnerability and risk for anxiety disorders. *Journal of Anxiety Disorders, 5,* 151–166.

Vasey, M. W. (1993). Development and cognition in childhood anxiety: The example of worry. In T. H. Ollendick & R. J. Prinz (Eds.), *Advances in clinical child psychology (vol 15, pp. 1–39).* New York: Plenum.

Verhulst, F. C., van der Ende, J., Ferdinand, R. F., & Kasius, M. C. (1997). The prevalence of DSM-III-R diagnoses in a sample of Dutch adolescents. *Archives of General Psychiatry, 54,* 329–336.

Weems, C. F., Silverman, W. K., Saavedra, L. M., Pina, A. A., & Lumpkin, P. W. (1999). The discrimination of children's phobias using the Revised Fear Survey Schedule for children. *Journal of Child Psychology and Psychiatry and Allied Disciplines, 40,* 941–952.

Weissman, M. M., Wickramaratne, P., Warner, V., John, K., Prusoff, B. A., Merikangas, K. R., et al. (1987). Assessing psychiatric disorders in children. Discrepancies between mothers' and children's reports. *Archives of General Psychiatry, 44,* 747–753.

Welner, Z., Reich, W., Herjanic, B., Jung, K. G., & Amado, H. (1987). Reliability, validity, and parent–child agreement studies of the Diagnostic Interview for Children and Adolescents (DICA). *Journal of the American Academy of Child and Adolescent Psychiatry, 26,* 649–653.

Werry, J. S. (1994). Diagnostic and classification issues. In T. H. Ollendick, N. J. King, & W. Yule (Eds.), *International handbook of phobic and anxiety disorders in children and adolescents* (pp. 21–42). New York: Plenum Press.

Whaley, S. E., Pinto, A., & Sigman, M. (1999). Characterizing interactions between anxious mothers and their children. *Journal of Consulting and Clinical Psychology, 67,* 826–836.

Whitaker, A., Johnson, J., Shaffer, D., Rapoport, J. L., Kalikow, K., Walsh, B. T., et al. (1990). Uncommon troubles in young people: Prevalence estimates of selected psychiatric disorders in a nonreferred adolescent population. *Archives of General Psychiatry, 47,* 487–496.

Williams, J. M. G., Watts, F. N., MacLeod, C., & Matthews, A. (1997). *Cognitive psychology and emotional disorders* (2nd ed.). New York: Wiley.

Wood, J. J., Piacentini, J. C., Bergman, R. L., McCracken, J., & Barrios, V. (2002). Concurrent validity of the anxiety disorders section of the Anxiety Disorders Interview Schedule for DSM-IV: Child and parent versions. *Journal of Clinical Child and Adolescent Psychology, 31,* 335–342.

Woodruff-Borden, J., Morrow, C., Bourland, S., & Cambron, S. (2002). The behavior of anxious parents: Examining mechanisms of the transmission of anxiety from parent to child. *Journal of Clinical Child and Adolescent Psychology, 31,* 364–374.

12

DEPRESSION

WILLIAM M. REYNOLDS

Department of Psychology
Humboldt State University
Arcata, California

INTRODUCTION

Assessment is critical for research and clinical work with depressed children and adolescents. Reliable and valid assessment procedures allow for determining the presence or absence of depression and depressive symptoms in children and adolescents. In this manner, assessment, whether by self-report, clinical interview, or other methodology, provides a method for the clinical evaluation of individuals as well as for research designed to enhance our understanding of depression in young people. To help children and youth who are depressed and in a state of significant psychological distress, we must first identify these youngsters. This is an important goal of professionals dedicated to the psychological well-being of children and adolescents. In this manner, the tools we use to identify depressed youngsters must be psychometrically sound and linguistically appropriate; otherwise we risk missing those children and adolescents who may be in need of psychological assistance.

This chapter describes measures for the assessment of depression in young persons. Assessment of depression in children and adolescents encompasses multimodal procedures for making decisions about persons. Likewise, it should be recognized that assessment as a process does not occur in isolation. Assessment of depression in children and adolescents, as with other clinical domains and populations, is a complex interaction of the individual being evaluated, the assessment methods, the clinician or evaluators, the setting events, as well as prior experiences and the reasons for the assessment.

Assessment provides us with a means to evaluate the effectiveness of interventions designed to ameliorate depression in young people. This is an important application, whether for the evaluation of an individual who is treated or a major investigation of psychotherapy and pharmacotherapeutic interventions, such as the Treatment for Adolescents with Depression Study (TADS Team, 2004). The effectiveness of treatments for psychological disorders such as depression can best be determined by the utilization of valid and reliable assessment procedures (Reynolds & Stark, 1983). This suggests that outcome measures of depression used in treatment research must demonstrate high levels of reliability and validity.

There are a number of characteristics unique to depression that impact the use and format of depression assessment procedures. Depression is an internalizing disorder (Reynolds, 1992; Reynolds & Johnston, 1994) that encompasses many symptoms that are not easily observable. Cognitive symptoms of guilt, self-deprecation, suicidal ideation, hopelessness, and feelings of worthlessness are among the symptoms of depression that are hard to notice unless a formal evaluation is conducted. Similarly, some somatic symptoms, such as insomnia and appetite loss, and other problems are sometimes difficult to observe and may go undetected by parents and significant others. The clinical distress or severity level associated with many of these symptoms is subjective to the individual. Suicidal ideation is an example of a covert symptom whose presence and severity can only be ascertained from the youngster. Because of the internalizing nature of depression, caution must be used when gathering assessment data from significant others.

Another aspect of depression in children and adolescents that supports the need for assessment is the generally limited self-awareness of their psychological condition, along with the lack of self-referral for mental health problems by children and adolescents. The outcome of this is that many youngsters feel their life is quite miserable but are unaware that they may have a mental health problem or that they should let someone know of their condition so that treatment can be provided. We cannot expect children to know the symptoms of depression and, if these symptoms occur, to tell an adult.

ASSESSMENT STRATEGIES

Depression in children, and to a lesser extent in adolescents, is generally best evaluated from a multidimensional perspective, with different measures using diverse sources of information (e.g., parent, child) as well as different methods (e.g., self-report questionnaires versus clinical interview) (Reynolds, 1992). As discussed by Kazdin (1994), difficulties are inherent in the combination and interpretation of the outcome of depression measures using multiple informants. However, use of multiple informants, particularly with children, provides a much richer picture of the nature of depressive symptoms.

A number of assessment modalities have been used to evaluate depression in children and adolescents. The two primary modes of assessment are clinical interviews and paper-and-pencil self-report measures. Table 12.1 lists those measures

TABLE 12.1 Modes of Assessment Described in This Chapter

Diagnostic Clinical Interviews	Severity Clinical Interviews	Self-Report Questionnaires
Diagnostic Interview for Children and Adolescents (DICA; Reich, 2000)	Child Depression Rating Scale—Revised (CDRS-R; Poznanski & Mokros, 1996)	Children's Depression Inventory (CDI; Kovacs, 1992)
Diagnostic Interview Schedule for Children—Revised (DISC-R; Shaffer, Fisher, Lucas, Dulcan, & Schwab-Stone, 2000)	Hamilton Depression Rating Scale (HDRS; Hamilton, 1967)	Reynolds Child Depression Scale (RCDS; Reynolds, 1989)
Schedule for Affective and Schizophrenic Disorders (SADS; Endicott & Spitzer, 1978)		Reynolds Adolescent Depression Scale—2nd ed. (RADS-2; Reynolds, 2002)
Schedule for Affective and Schizophrenic Disorders for School Age Children (K-SADS-PL; Kaufman et al., 1997)		Beck Depression Inventory—II (BDI-II; Beck, Steer, & Brown, 1996)

that are described in this chapter. There are also procedures that utilize parent and teacher checklists and peer reports, although these methods are limited in their ability to assess internalizing disorders in children and adolescents. Clinical interview measures can be further differentiated between diagnostic interviews that include the evaluation of depression along with other disorders and severity interviews that are specific to the assessment of depression.

DIFFERENTIATION BETWEEN THE ASSESSMENT OF DEPRESSION SYMPTOM SEVERITY AND DIAGNOSIS

The assessment of depression as a clinical state in children and adolescents as well as adults is generally accomplished by one of two measurement perspectives: (a) the assessment of the severity of a range or depth of depressive symptoms to evaluate the "clinical level" of depression experienced by the individual; and (b) the formal diagnosis of depression manifested by the person according to a specified set of rules or classification criteria. These two measurement perspectives typically use different assessment procedures and provide different information on the nature of depression in persons. Although these approaches are not mutually exclusive, they are different in their focus and outcome. Both of these approaches provide valid and useful information and are, to some extent, complementary. Both have applications dictated by the type and level of information required to make a specific decision about depression in a child or adolescent. In research applications it is not uncommon to find both diagnostic and severity measures used for the study of depression in young people (e.g., TADS Team, 2004).

Assessment of the depth or severity of depressive symptoms is typically conducted using self-report measures and rater checklists and provides useful information as to the clinical distress level of depressive symptomatology experienced by the youngster. Clinical severity measures include paper-and-pencil depression scales as well as semistructured clinical interviews, such as the Children's Depression Rating Scale—Revised (Poznanski & Mokros, 1996). In the severity assessment approach, a cutoff score is used to delineate a clinically relevant level of depressive symptomatology. A score at or above this level may result in the child's being considered depressed. It is important to recognize that this cutoff-score method is not the equivalent of providing a diagnosis of a depressive disorder according to recognized classification systems. The formal diagnosis of depression requires more extensive evaluation procedures, incorporating structured diagnostic interviews or other in-depth diagnostic methodologies. For the most part, the use of self-report, clinical interviews, and other measures that focus on assessment of severity is limited to the perspective of depression as a unipolar mood disturbance that represents an internalizing domain of psychological distress.

CLINICAL INTERVIEWS

The clinical interview, particularly if it is structured or semistructured, is generally considered to be the most sensitive and selective assessment methodology for the measurement of depression (Hamilton, 1982; Puig-Antich & Gittelman, 1982). The interview format allows for the clinical evaluation and probing of youngsters' symptoms, including the severity of symptoms, frequency, and duration of occurrence and the determination of whether symptom endorsement is a function of depression or factors extraneous to the disorder. For example, a child or adolescent who indicates significant difficulty sleeping or delay in falling asleep may be manifesting a symptom of depression, or it may be due to an extraneous factor, such as being kept up at night because of the crying or feeding schedule of a newborn sibling. After conducting hundreds of interviews with children and adolescents, the author has found many youngsters who appeared somewhat symptomatic but for whom, upon further inquiry as to the cause of the symptom, it was determined that it was for reasons other than depression.

The clinical interview also allows for insight into whether delusions or psychosis may be present. Although rare, the latter do occur and may confound the interpretation of symptom endorsement as specific to depression. By using a trained clinician to determine the presence and severity of the symptom, rather than leaving it to the distressed child or adolescent, the clinical relevance of symptoms and their constellation can be determined. It is evident that the clinical interview has the potential for an accurate and valid assessment of depression. Because the clinical interview is individualized to each child, this assessment format allows for the accommodation of developmental and cognitive restrictions in children (Kovacs, 1986).

The clinical interview is typically a more sensitive and specific procedure than other methods, such as paper-and-pencil measures, for the assessment of depression. However, there are costs to this increased utility. One is the requirement of time. Interviews are individual assessments that require between 30 and 90 minutes, depending on the interview measure and the severity of depression (and potential comorbid disorders) experienced by the child or adolescent. In cases involving severe psychomotor retardation, an interview may be painstakingly long. Clinical interviews also require trained examiners capable of providing reliable and valid assessments. Nevertheless, clinical interviews provide for a thorough evaluation of depression in children and adolescents.

DIAGNOSTIC INTERVIEWS

For determination of depression according to formal classification criteria that includes inclusion and exclusion components, the standard practice has been the use of structured clinical interviews. Structured clinical interviews are designed to evaluate all symptoms, their duration, and potential exclusion criteria as specified by a formal set of diagnostic criteria. In this manner, the Schedule for Affective Disorders and Schizophrenia—Children's Version, referred to as the Kiddie SADS or K-SADS (Puig-Antich & Chambers, 1978), was originally designed to provide diagnostic information on disorders in children according to Research Diagnostic Criteria (RDC; Spitzer, Endicott, & Robins, 1978). Revisions of the K-SADS, as well as revisions of other interviews, such as the Diagnostic Interview for Children and Adolescents (Herjanic & Reich, 1982) and the Diagnostic Interview Schedule for Children (Costello, Edelbrock, & Costello, 1985), have focused on assessment of symptoms as specified by the *Diagnostic and Statistical Manual of Mental Disorders* (DSM; American Psychiatric Association, 1994) criteria for psychiatric disorders. All of these diagnostic interviews are briefly described next.

Schedule for Affective Disorders and Schizophrenia

The Schedule for Affective Disorders and Schizophrenia (SADS; Endicott & Spitzer, 1978) was developed to assess Research Diagnostic Criteria (RDC) disorder classifications (Spitzer et al., 1978) and has been a much used research interview for deriving formal diagnoses of psychopathology in clinical and research studies with adults and to some extent with adolescents. There are several forms of the SADS, distinguished by whether the resulting diagnosis is of current psychopathology, change, or lifetime occurrence. As noted, the SADS has been used with adolescents, for whom symptoms of depression bear greater similarity to those of adults than do those of younger children. Unlike the child version of the SADS discussed next, parental report is typically not utilized in the evaluation of depression in adolescents as it is with younger children. The SADS and the child version of this interview presented here are highly structured clinical interviews that require extensive training and clinical practice prior to their use with young persons. It should be noted that the most recent child version was developed to assess both children and adolescents.

Schedule of Affective Disorders and Schizophrenia for School-Age Children

The Schedule for Affective Disorders and Schizophrenia for School-Age Children (Puig-Antich & Chambers, 1978; Puig-Antich & Ryan, 1986), or K-SADS, is a downward extension of the Schedule for Affective Disorders and Schizophrenia (SADS) developed by Endicott and Spitzer (1978) for the clinical evaluation of Research Diagnostic Criteria disorders. As noted earlier, the K-SADS is a diagnostic interview schedule that requires extensive training on the part of interviewers. As with the SADS, a number of versions are available, differing primarily on the time of episode. For example, the Present Episode version (K-SADS-PE) is designed to assess current psychiatric problems in children (Chambers et al., 1985), while the K-SADS-E (Epidemiological version) was developed to evaluate past and current psychiatric problems (Orvaschel, Puig-Antich, Chambers, Tabrizi, & Johnson, 1982).

The most recent revision of the K-SADS is by Kaufman and colleagues (1997) and incorporates present and lifetime versions of 32 DSM-IV Axis I psychiatric disorders. It is designed for obtaining information from children and adolescents ages 7–18 years and from their parents as informants.

Diagnostic Interview Schedule for Children

The Diagnostic Interview Schedule for Children (DISC; Costello, Edelbrock, Kalas, Kessler, & Klaric, 1982) was developed under the auspices of the National Institute of Mental Health and was patterned after the adult Diagnostic Interview Schedule and included parallel child and parent interview forms. Initial research with the DISC (e.g., Costello & Edelbrock, 1985) suggested the need for improvement. Subsequently, NIMH pursued revisions, which were undertaken by Shaffer and colleagues, with several versions developed, beginning with the Diagnostic Interview Schedule for Children—Revised Version (DISC-R; Shaffer et al., 1993). Shaffer, Fisher, Lucas, Dulcan, and Schwab-Stone (2000) developed the DISC-IV, the latest version of the DISC. The current version includes computer software to assist in the administration and scoring of the interview. There is also a computer administered version. The DISC-IV evaluates 36 DSM-IV disorders in children and adolescents, with versions available for both child and adolescent report (ages 9–17 years) and parent (caretaker) report (for ages 6–17 years). The DISC-IV has also been modified for use with preschool children as young as 3 years of age (Luby, Mrakotsky, Heffelfinger, Brown, & Spitznagel, 2004).

Diagnostic Interview for Children and Adolescents

Similar to the DISC, the Diagnostic Interview for Children and Adolescents (DICA; Herjanic & Reich, 1982) has evolved over the past two decades, with the most current version designed to assess DSM-IV disorders in children and adolescents (Reich, 2000). The author suggests that the DICA is best used as a semistructured clinical interview that may be administered by well-trained lay interviewers. There is also a computer-administered version of the DICA, although the authors (Rourke & Reich, 2004) note that the clinician-administered version is preferable, given the ability of the clinician to answer questions and present the interview in a manner tailored to the needs of the child. There are separate interview versions for children ages 6–12 years and adolescents 13–17 years and a version for parents that includes ages 6–17 years.

CLINICAL SEVERITY INTERVIEWS

Several semistructured interviews have as their focus the assessment of the severity of depressive symptoms. Similar to paper-and-pencil measures of depression, these clinical interviews utilize cutoff scores for the identification of a clinical level of depression in children and adolescents. However, as in the case of paper-and-pencil self-report measures, cutoff scores on these severity interviews are not intended for use as a diagnostic indicator but rather as a level of symptom severity that is clinically relevant, particularly as a screener for depressive disorders. In this regard, these measures have demonstrated reasonable levels of sensitivity and specificity in the identification of youngsters who are likely to have a diagnosis of major depression.

For the most part, these interviews have been used as child or adolescent informant measures. When additional assessment information is obtained from parents, the interviewer should be cognizant that positive parental responses to questions dealing with covert, internalizing symptoms should be supported whenever possible with behavioral or other empirical evidence for their report. Parental report of no symptom presence may be a function of their ignorance or difficulty in observing the symptom.

Children's Depression Rating Scale—Revised

The Children's Depression Rating Scale—Revised (CDRS-R; Poznanski et al., 1984), originally developed in 1979 (Poznanski, Cook, & Carroll, 1979), is a semistructured clinical interview measure of the severity of symptoms of depression designed for use with children ages 6–12 years. The CDRS-R consists of 17 items, each representing a depressive symptom and rated on a scale of 1 (normal) to 7 (severe). On the CDRS-R, 14 of the items are presented in a direct interview question format, and three items (depressed affect, tempo of language, and hypoactivity) are scored based on the interviewer's observations of the child during the interview. The CDRS-R typically requires 20–30 minutes to administer. A manual for the CDRS-R has been published by Poznanski and Mokros (1996). Several cutoff scores have been used with the CDRS-R. Poznanski,

Freeman, and Mokros (1985) recommended a score of 40 and above on the CDRS-R as a clinical cutoff for depression in children; the TADS team used a cutoff of 45 and above as inclusion criteria along with a diagnosis of Major Depressive Disorder.

Hamilton Depression Rating Scale

The Hamilton Depression Rating Scale (HDRS; Hamilton, 1960, 1967) is a clinical interview measure of the severity of depressive symptoms and one of the most frequently used outcome measures in psychiatric studies of depression in adults. There are several versions of the HDRS, the most popular being the 17-item form. Items are evaluated by the clinician as to their severity, with higher scores indicative of greater depressive pathology. Two items that assess psychomotor retardation and psychomotor agitation are observational and are rated by the interviewer based on the adolescent's behavior during the interview. Items on the HDRS are scored from 0 to 4 or 0 to 2, depending on the symptom assessed, with higher scores indicating greater symptom pathology. Researchers have utilized a number of cutoff scores to delineate a clinical level of depressive symptomatology, with such scores typically ranging from 15 to 20. There are a number of caveats to the use of the HDRS. In particular, a number of contemporary symptoms of depression are not evident on the HDRS (e.g., low self-esteem, self-deprecation). Likewise, items dealing with loss of insight, hypochondriasis, and several anxiety items are tangentially related to depression. Nevertheless, as a severity measure of depression, the HDRS, with minor adjustments for age differences, works quite well with adolescents.

SELF-REPORT MEASURES

A number of self-report measures has been developed for the assessment of depression in children and adolescents. Several measures designed for use with adults have also been used with adolescents. Use of self-report questionnaires for assessment of depressive symptomatology in children and adolescents has seen a rapid growth in research and clinical applications. From a few reports in the early 1980s to the routine use of self-report depression measures in a wide range of child and adolescent mental health disciplines (Archer & Newsom, 2000), self-report measures provide a simple and direct method for the evaluation of the clinical severity of depressive symptoms in young people. The measures described next are among the most frequently used self-report scales for the assessment of depressive symptomatology in children and adolescents. In addition to these measures, a number of other scales have been developed; they are listed at the end of this section.

Children's Depression Inventory

The Children's Depression Inventory (CDI; Kovacs, 1979, 1992) was originally developed by Kovacs and Beck (1977) as a downward revision of the Beck

Depression Inventory (BDI; Beck, Ward, Mendelson, Mock, & Erbaugh, 1961). The CDI, one of the most frequently used research measures of depression in children, consists of 27 items, each evaluating a symptom of depression or related affect. Items are presented as three statements of varying symptom severity. The child responds by selecting the statement that best describes the youngster's feelings and behavior over the past two weeks. The CDI manual (Kovacs, 1992) presents normative data based on a sample of 1266 children and young adolescents in grades 2 through 8 from an unspecified number of schools in Florida. Data appear to be a subsample of youngsters from a previously published study by Finch, Saylor, and Edwards (1985). Norms are not provided for high school students.

Reynolds Child Depression Scale

The Reynolds Child Depression Scale (RCDS; Reynolds, 1989) is a 30-item self-report measure designed for use with children ages 8–13 years. On the RCDS, 29 items are rated as to the frequency of their occurrence during the past two weeks using a four-point response format of "almost never" to "all the time." Items are worded to evaluate current symptom status (e.g., item 8: "I feel like crying, item 14: I feel like hurting myself"). Seven items are reverse keyed (e.g., item 25: "I feel like having fun"), with a negative response indicative of depressive symptom status. Item 30 consists of five "smiley-type" faces, ranging from sad to happy, that the child completes by placing an X over the face that indicates how he or she feels and represents an evaluation of dysphoric mood. The manual for the RCDS provides normative information on over 1600 children representing heterogeneous ethnic and socioeconomic backgrounds, along with procedures for administration, scoring and interpretation, and data on reliability and validity.

Reynolds Adolescent Depression Scale

The Reynolds Adolescent Depression Scale (RADS; Reynolds, 1986a, 1987) was developed to evaluate the severity of depressive symptoms in adolescents ages 12–18 years and subsequently renormed (RADS-2; Reynolds, 2002), with the age range expanded to include youngsters ages 11–20. The RADS consists of 30 items and uses a four-point ("almost never" to "most of the time") response format. Items on the RADS were written to reflect symptomatology specified by the DSM for Major Depression and Dysthymic Disorder, as well as additional symptoms delineated by the RDC. Items on the RADS-2 require a third-grade reading level.

The RADS-2 presents a number of significant developments over the RADS. These developments include a new standardization sample of 3300 adolescents, stratified to mirror year 2000 U.S. Census data for gender and ethnic background and the inclusion of younger adolescents in grade six. Also new is the provision of standard scores (*T* scores with a mean of 50 and a standard deviation of 10) in addition to percentile ranks. The RADS-2 also includes four factorially derived subscales that provide scores on scales of Dysphoric Mood, Anhedonia/Negative Affect, Negative Self-Evaluation, and Somatic Complaints. Item placement on the RADS-2 subscales was based on the results of a factor analysis that resulted in a nearly equal number of items (7 or 8) on each of the four subscales. Finally, the RADS protocol was improved, with a new self-scoring carbonless answer sheet that provides for easy scoring as well as for plotting a profile of RADS-2 subscale scores. The RADS-2 Manual provides extensive documentation of the psychometric characteristics of the RADS-2 depression total and subscale scores. The manual also provides information on the interpretation of the RADS-2 total and subscale scores as well as several case illustrations.

Beck Depression Inventory—II

The Beck Depression Inventory (BDI; Beck et al., 1961) was developed for adults and comprises 21 items, each consisting of four statements (scored from 0 to 3) of varying degrees of symptom severity. Beck and colleagues (Beck, Steer, & Brown, 1996) revised the BDI to include symptoms consistent with DSM-IV diagnostic criteria for depressive disorders. Changes were made to 15 of the 21 BDI items. In addition, the time frame for rating symptoms was changed from one week to two weeks, consistent with symptom duration criteria specified by the DSM for Major Depression. Several investigators have used the BDI with adolescents, although the reading requirements and format of the scale may be challenging for some youngsters. Krefetz, Steer, Gulab, and Beck (2002) reported on the convergent validity of the BDI-II with the Reynolds Adolescent Depression Scale in a sample of 100 psychiatric inpatients. They reported a high correlation between the two measures, with both scales effective in differentiating inpatients who were and were not diagnosed with a major depressive disorder. Osman, Kopper, Barrios, Gutierrez, and Bagge (2004) have also provided evidence for the reliability and validity of the BDI-II with psychiatric inpatient samples of adolescents.

OTHER SELF-REPORT MEASURES

Center for Epidemiological Studies—Depression Scale

The Center for Epidemiological Studies—Depression Scale (CES-D; Radloff, 1977) consists of 20 items, was designed for use with adults, and has been used by a number of investigators with adolescents (e.g., Doerfler, Felner, Rowlison, Evans, & Raley, 1988; Garrison, Jackson, Marsteller, McKeown, & Addy, 1990; Hops, Lewinsohn, Andrews, & Roberts, 1990; Radloff, 1991).

Adolescent Psychopathology Scales—Major Depression and Dysthymia Scales

The Adolescent Psychopathology Scales (APS; Reynolds, 1998) is a multidimensional self-report measure of psychopathology designed for use with adolescents ages 13–19. The APS consists of 20 clinical disorder scales, 5 personality scales, and 11 content scales as well as several validity indicators. The development of the APS was based on a clinical sample of over 500 adolescents from 31 inpatient and outpatient treatment settings in 21 states and a nonclinical sample of over 2800 adolescents drawn from 11 public junior and senior high schools in eight states. The APS includes scales of Major Depression and Dysthymic Disorder. The Major Depression scale consists of 29 items reflecting DSM-IV symptoms, with items rated on the basis of their occurrence over the past two weeks. The Dysthymic Disorder scale consists of 16 items rated as to their occurrence over the past six months. Reynolds (1993b) reported an internal consistency reliability of .95 for both the normal and clinical samples for the Major Depression scale. The Dysthymia Disorder scale demonstrated internal consistency reliability coefficients of .89 and .88 for the clinical and school samples, respectively. Validity evidence in the form of content validity, contrasted groups validity (normal adolescents versus those with a diagnosis of major depression), and criterion-related validity as demonstrated by correlations with other self-report (MMPI, RADS) and clinical interview (SADS, HDRS) measures of depression are presented in the APS manual and support the validity of the Major Depression and Dysthymia scales of the APS with adolescents.

Other Scales

In addition to the measures just described, a number of other self-report measures of depression have been reported in the research and clinical literature. These include the Children's Depression Adjective Check Lists (Eddy & Lubin, 1988); the Depression Self-Rating Scale by Birleson (1981); the Multiscore Depression Inventory, originally designed for use with adults (Berndt, Petzel, & Berndt, 1980); the Children's Depression Scale by Lang and Tisher (1978); the Childhood Depression Assessment Tool (Brady, Nelms, Albright, & Murphy, 1984), a 26-item yes–no-format questionnaire; the Rating Scale of Dysphoria (Lefkowitz, Tesiny, & Solodow, 1989), a 12-item self-rating adaptation of the Peer Nomination Inventory of Depression (Lefkowitz & Tesiny, 1980); the 66-item Depressive Experiences Questionnaire for Adolescents (Blatt, Schaffer, Bers, & Quinlan, 1992); the six-item Depressive Affect self-report scale by Rosenberg (1965); the depression subscale of the Youth Self-Report (Achenbach & Edelbrock, 1987); and the revised self-report version of the depression scale from the Child Behavior Checklist (Achenbach & Edelbrock, 1983) developed by Clarke, Lewinsohn, Hops, and Seeley (1992).

RESEARCH BASIS

All of the measures just described have demonstrated acceptable levels of reliability and validity. All of the self-report measures (e.g., the CDI, RCDS, RADS, BDI) have dozens, and in some cases, such as with the CDI and RADS, hundreds, of publications reporting on the reliability and validity of these measures with clinical and nonclinical samples of children and adolescents in the United States as well as other countries. Similarly, the diagnostic clinical interviews have undergone continued development and refinement for over two decades, with researchers attending to changes in diagnostic criteria as well as procedures to enhance reliability and validity.

CLINICAL UTILITY

The clinical utility of the measures of depression described earlier in this chapter vary as a function of their purpose and potential applications. For example, the paper-and-pencil self-report measures are ideal for both individual as well as large group screening of children and adolescents in school settings. Reynolds (1986b) described a multigate procedure for the screening of depression in children and adolescents. The relatively high levels of specificity and sensitivity of cutoff scores on the RADS-2 and the ability to screen an entire school in less than 15 minutes and identify those youngsters who may have a depressive disorder and are in need of further evaluation point to the high levels of clinical utility these measures provide psychologists and other mental health professionals. Likewise, the use of structured and semistructured clinical interviews provides a reliable template for professionals to obtain diagnostic information as to the presence of depressive disorders in children and adolescents.

DEVELOPMENTAL CONSIDERATIONS

There are a number of developmental considerations in the assessment of depression, particularly when evaluating young children. Linguistic competence, including reading and comprehension ability, is an important consideration when using self-report measures. These task demands suggest that most children ages 9 years and above who do not have learning problems can respond to self-report measures that include language at a third-grade reading level. To avoid confounding with reading, it is recommended that measures be read to children in grades three and four. Likewise, it is important to consider metacognitive demands of the measure, including interviews and self-report assessments. Thus, task demands such as the ability to recognize one's emotional and behavioral characteristics as they apply to a specified time frame and to evaluate the frequency, severity, or nature of these characteristics may limit the reports of younger-aged children. The ability of the youngsters to self-monitor their behavior and emotions as well as self-evaluate these facets is a requirement of most measures.

Additional developmental aspects specific to the assessment of depression in children are of primary concern to the assessment of young children rather than adolescents and address both the reliability and validity of measures of depression in youngsters. Many of these issues are generic to the direct assessment of children and have been described in more detail elsewhere (Reynolds, 1992). Because of the task demands of these assessment measures, the utilization of reports by others (in particular, parents) is important. However, when there are differences in symptom report between a child and parent, it is up to the clinician to evaluate all available assessment data and integrate this information to determine the child's current symptom status.

As a function of the limitations just noted, there are few self-report measures that can be used with children below the age of 8 years, although some research suggests that self-report measures of depression can be used with children as young as those in the first grade (Ialongo, Edelsohn, Werthamer-Larsson, Crockett, & Kellam, 1993). For children ages 6 and above, clinical interviews, such as the CDRS-R, may be used, although some children's metacognitive ability for emotions may limit their response. Thus, for young children, parent reports using clinical interviews are a primary source of information. Parent reports are also of value for school-age children, assuming reliable and valid reporting on the part of the parent.

ASSESSMENT, CONCEPTUALIZATION, AND TREATMENT PLANNING

Assessment is critical for the determination of appropriate treatment and for monitoring treatment progress. Multiple studies have demonstrated the efficacy of treatments for depression in children and adolescents (e.g., Kahn, Kehle, Jenson, & Clark, 1990; Lewinsohn, Clarke, Hops, & Andrews, 1990; Mufson et al., 1994; Reynolds & Coats, 1986; Stark, Reynolds, & Kaslow, 1987; Stark, 1990; TADS Team, 2004). In all studies, multiple measures of depression were utilized for the selection of depressed children and adolescents as well as to show the outcome of treatments.

In clinical practice, it is useful to examine the nature of significant symptom endorsement of severity measures and the presence of subtypes of depression when using diagnostic interviews. For example, when somatic symptoms are endorsed or a diagnosis of melancholic subtype is given, treatment of depression is likely to be most effective if antidepressant medications are included in therapy. Similarly, significant levels of depressive symptomatology in a youngster who reports more cognitive and emotional symptoms of depression with limited somatic involvement should suggest an initial trial of psychotherapy (e.g., cognitive-behavioral, interpersonal).

CASE STUDY

IDENTIFICATION

The case reported here is taken from an actual evaluation, with changes made to the student description, demographic information, and other modifications to ensure anonymity and provide sufficient information to illustrate the assessment of depression in children and adolescents. The case described is of Jenny, a Caucasian female who at the time of the initial school assessment was 14 years old and in the eighth grade at a small middle school in a suburban community.

PRESENTING COMPLAINT

Jenny, as described next, has a history of behavior and emotional problems. The present complaint stems from a noticeable decline in her behavior at school as well as the observation of dysphoric mood by her homeroom teacher and concerns expressed by her mother. Of particular note was a recent episode of peer aggression in which Jenny started a fight with a younger girl. Jenny was suspended from school; upon her return, her mother reported to the school that she was worried that Jenny might hurt herself and that she was out of control at home.

HISTORY

Jenny's mother had been married and divorced three times, her second husband being Jenny's natural father. Jenny has no contact with her natural father, who is reported by her mother to be an alcoholic. Following her last divorce, which occurred when Jenny was 10 years old, Jenny's mother reported becoming involved in heavy drug and alcohol use, for several years. When Jenny was 12 years old, her mother caught her using marijuana. This in part prompted her mother to seek drug rehabilitation counseling. Her mother reports she occasionally will have one or two drinks, but states she no longer uses drugs. She is not certain whether Jenny uses drugs but would not rule it out. Jenny has one younger sister, offspring of her mother's third marriage. Jenny's mother, currently unmarried, is a maintenance worker in a wood-products company.

Jenny did not attend preschool and has a history of relatively poor academic performance in school. She was evaluated for a learning disability in third grade, but did not meet school standards for this educational classification. Nevertheless, Jenny has been considered a slow learner in school, with teachers frequently noting that she does not pay attention and shows minimal commitment to learning.

Jenny had a relatively unremarkable social history until she entered sixth grade at the local middle school. Until that time, Jenny got along well with peers and had a group of friends who, her mother reported, had a positive influence on Jenny. Shortly after Jenny started sixth grade, her mother noticed that Jenny changed her group of friends to a more "tough" crowd, started swearing and throwing things at home, and frequently lost her temper.

When Jenny was 13, her mother noticed cuts on Jenny's arm and also on her leg; Jenny denied knowing how they were caused. Shortly thereafter Jenny came home with a tattoo of a cross on the index finger of her left hand. When her mother confronted her, Jenny indicated that she had other tattoos and ran from the house. When she returned two days later, her mother felt that Jenny was at risk to herself and had her hospitalized in a psychiatric inpatient unit of a local hospital. Jenny stayed 30 days and was discharged with diagnoses of Substance Abuse, Conduct Disorder, and possible Major Depression. Suicidal ideation and school and behavioral/emotional problems were also noted. Hospital staff consultation with school psychological personnel was also provided. It was decided not to pursue formal school classification procedures for emotional disturbance at that time but to revisit the possibility in four months. During this time Jenny would meet on a weekly basis with a counselor in school. After four months, it was decided that Jenny was improving in her behavior at school and at home and that she would maintain her current class placement and her meetings with the school counselor.

The following year Jenny's behavior in school rapidly deteriorated. Her teachers noted that she was sullen and at times belligerent toward other students as well as teachers. She was sent to the school office for bullying (physical aggression against a sixth-grade girl) as well as for truancy. This resulted in a three-day suspension. This also created a major source of conflict between her mother and Jenny. When Jenny returned to school she was evaluated by the school psychologist, who on the basis of her evaluation recommended that Jenny be further evaluated by the county community mental health agency. Results of these assessments are described later.

DEVELOPMENTAL ISSUES

Jenny's natural mother and father were married two years following Jenny's birth. Pregnancy and birth were normal, although her mother reports moderate use of alcohol during her pregnancy. Jenny's developmental milestones (e.g., sitting up, speech, toilet training, walking) were within a normal range, although a bit below average in relationship to age norms. Jenny's social relationships with other children were good until several years ago, as already noted. When Jenny was hospitalized in the inpatient psychiatric unit at age 13, a psychiatric social worker reported that Jenny may have been sexually abused by her mother's third husband when Jenny was 9 years old.

PEER AND SCHOOL ISSUES

Jenny has few friends, except for a group of girls considered to be discipline problems by the school. Her teachers report that, for the most part, Jenny is unpopular with most of the other students in her classes. Jenny has been sent to the school office on numerous occasions. In addition to the most recent behavioral problems described earlier, she has a history of truancy, smoking on the school grounds, swearing, and talking back to teachers.

ASSESSMENT RESULTS

The school psychologist conducted an informal clinical interview and administered several self-report measures to Jenny. She also collected assessment information from several of Jenny's teachers and her mother as well as direct observations of Jenny's behavior on the playground at recess and at lunch. The school psychologist had previously established a positive relationship with Jenny and believed that the assessment results were valid. The interview with Jenny suggested that, in addition to her externalizing problem behaviors, Jenny reported feelings of depression and reported that she has been thinking of suicide. Based on her initial interview with Jenny, the school psychologist administered the Reynolds Adolescent Depression Scale—2nd Edition, the Suicidal Ideation Questionnaire (SIQ; Reynolds, 1988), and several other measures.

On the RADS-2, Jenny obtained a raw score of 89, which is above the RADS-2 clinical cutoff raw score of 76. In comparison to the standardization sample of 3300 adolescents, Jenny obtained a standard score of 70*T* on the RADS-2 Depression Total, which is at the 97th percentile. This score is in the severe clinical symptom range and well above the recommended cutoff score of 61*T*. Jenny answered all of the items on the RADS-2. Clinically significant elevations were found on all four of the RADS-2 subscales.

Similar levels of standard score elevation were found on the Anhedonia/Negative Affect, Somatic Complaints, and Negative Self-Evaluation subscales, with a somewhat lower score on the Dysphoric Mood subscale. Jenny obtained a raw score of 22 on the Dysphoric Mood subscale, which equates to a *T* score of 59 and a percentile rank of 82nd, with item endorsement indicative of feelings of sadness, crying and general distress, along with a pervasive sense of loneliness. On the Anhedonia/Negative Affect subscale Jenny obtained a *T* score of 65 and a percentile rank of 92nd. On this subscale she reported a lack of interest in engaging in fun activities, interacting with others, and engaging in other pleasant activities. On the Negative Self-Evaluation subscale, Jenny had a score of 72*T*, which was at the 98th percentile. This was a significant domain of problems for Jenny, with reports of low self-worth, self-denigration, and helplessness. Jenny endorsed RADS-2 item 14, which evaluates feeling of hurting oneself at a clinically severe level. Her response to this item, which is also one of the RADS-2 critical items, suggests the need for further, more direct evaluation of possible suicidal ideation and suicide attempt planning. On the Somatic Concerns subscale, Jenny received a *T* score of 65, which is at the 95th percentile in relation to the national standardization sample. Jenny endorsed feeling tired and other somatic concerns.

Jenny's *T* score of 70 on the Depression Total scale suggests a clinically significant level of depression, which may be considered severe in her level of symptom endorsement. Overall, Jenny reported a severe level of depression on the RADS-2. Scores on the RADS-2 in this range are generally found in adolescents who manifest a depressive disorder. By symptom domain, Jenny's highest score was on the RADS-2 subscale indicative of low self-worth and self-denigration. This is consistent with Jenny's statements to the school psychologist that she feels worthless and that no one cares about her, especially her mother. These statements also related to her feelings of helplessness and that she wishes she were dead.

On the 30-item form of the SIQ, Jenny received a total score of 71, which is significantly above the cutoff score of 41 and at the 95th percentile in relation to the SIQ standardization sample. This score is indicative of a clinically significant level of suicidal ideation. Jenny indicated that a majority of the SIQ items occurred a couple of times a month. She did not endorse any of the SIQ items as occurring on a daily or weekly basis in the past month, with the exception of item 5 (dealing with morbid ideation), which she reported as occurring about once a week.

A follow-up interview by the school psychologist focusing on Jenny's suicidality suggested that, although Jenny had thoughts of harming herself, she did not have a plan nor did she have current thoughts that she would kill herself. Based on Jenny's scores on the RADS-2, SIQ, and the interview as well as her conduct problems and history of psychiatric care, Jenny was referred to the county mental health office for further evaluation and treatment. A subsequent psychiatric interview resulted in a diagnosis of Conduct Disorder with Major Depression probable.

ETHICAL AND LEGAL ISSUES OR COMPLICATIONS

One of the primary ethical and legal issues related to the assessment of depression is ensuring that sufficient information on current level of suicidality is obtained, given the association between depression and suicidal behavior. Suicidal behavior should also be monitored once treatment is initiated, especially when treatment includes the use of antidepressant medications. The use of reliable and valid assessment measures of suicidality, such as the SIQ, which was also used in the TADS study, provides for formal documentation of a youngster's current reported level of risk.

SUMMARY

Assessment of depression in children and adolescents is a complex and often multifaceted procedure. This chapter has presented information on measures of depression designed for or used with children and adolescents. A requirement for determining if a child or adolescent is depressed is the availability of objective and valid assessment instruments as well as appropriate procedures for the integration of these measures. Identification of depressed children and adolescents is a primary concern for psychologists, psychiatrists, counselors, social workers, and school and mental health service providers. It is important that professionals who utilize depression measures be trained in the application and interpretation of these measures as well as knowledgeable as to the limitations inherent in each measure.

REFERENCES AND RESOURCES

Achenbach, T. M., & Edelbrock, C. (1983). *Manual for the Child Behavior Checklist and Revised Child Behavior Profile*. Burlington, VT: University of Vermont Department of Psychiatry.

Achenbach, T. M., & Edelbrock, C. (1987). *Manual for the Youth Self-Report and Profile*. Burlington, VT: University of Vermont Department of Psychiatry.

American Psychiatric Association. (1994). *Diagnostic and statistical manual of mental disorders—4th Edition*. Washington, DC: Author.

Archer, R. P., & Newsom, C. R. (2000). Psychological test usage with adolescent clients: Survey update. *Assessment, 7,* 227–235.

Beck, A. T., Steer, R. A., & Brown, G. K. (1996). *Manual for the Beck Depression Inventory—II*. San Antonio, TX: Psychological Corporation.

Beck, A. T., Ward, C., Mendelson, M., Mock, J., & Erbaugh, J. (1961). An inventory for measuring depression. *Archives of General Psychiatry, 4,* 561–571.

Berndt, D. J., Petzel, T., & Berndt, S. M. (1980). Development and initial evaluation of a multiscore depression inventory. *Journal of Personality Assessment, 44,* 396–404.

Birleson, P. (1981). The validity of depressive disorder in childhood and the development of a self-rating scale: A research report. *Journal of Child Psychology and Psychiatry, 22,* 73–88.

Blatt, S. J., Schaffer, C. E., Bers, S. A., & Quinlan, D. M. (1992). Psychometric properties of the Depressive Experiences Questionnaire for Adolescents. *Journal of Personality Assessment, 59,* 82–98.

Chambers, W. J., Puig-Antich, J., Hirsch, M., Paez, P., Ambrosini, P. J., Tabrizi, M. A., & Davies, M. (1985). The assessment of affective disorders in children and adolescents by semistructured interview: Test–retest reliability. *Archives of General Psychiatry, 42,* 696–702.

Clarke, G. N., Lewinsohn, P. M., Hops, H., & Seeley, J. R. (1992). A self- and parent-report measure of adolescent depression: The Child Behavior Checklist Depression Scale (CBCL-D). *Behavioral Assessment, 14,* 443–463.

Costello, E. J., & Edelbrock, C. S. (1985). Detection of psychiatric disorders in pediatric primary care: A preliminary report. *Journal of the American Academy of Child Psychiatry, 24,* 771–774.

Costello, E. J., Edelbrock, C. S., & Costello, A. J. (1985). Validity of the NIMH Diagnostic Interview Schedule for Children: A comparison between psychiatric and pediatric referrals. *Journal of Abnormal Child Psychology, 13,* 579–595.

Costello, E. J., Edelbrock, C. S., Duncan, M. K., Kalas, R., & Klaric, S. H. (1984). *Report on the NIMH Diagnostic Interview Schedule for Children (DISC)*. Washington, DC: National Institute of Mental Health.

Doerfler, L. A., Felner, R. D., Rowlison, R. T., Evans, E., & Raley, P. A. (1988). Depression in children and adolescents: A comparative analysis of the utility and construct validity of two assessment measures. *Journal of Consulting and Clinical Psychology, 56,* 769–772.

Eddy, B. A., & Lubin, B. (1988). The Children's Depression Adjective Check Lists (C-DACL) with emotionally disturbed adolescent boys. *Journal of Abnormal Psychology, 16,* 83–88.

Endicott, J., & Spitzer, R. L. (1978). A diagnostic interview: The schedule for affective disorders and schizophrenia. *Archives of General Psychiatry, 35,* 837–844.

Finch, A. J., Saylor, C. F., & Edwards, G. L. (1985). Children's Depression Inventory: Sex and grade norms for normal children. *Journal of Consulting and Clinical Psychology, 53,* 424–425.

Garrison, C. Z., Jackson, K. L., Marsteller, F., McKeown, R., & Addy, C. (1990). A longitudinal study of depressive symptomatology in young adolescents. *Journal of the American Academy of Child and Adolescent Psychiatry, 29,* 581–585.

Hamilton, M. (1960). A rating scale for depression. *Journal of Neurology, Neurosurgery, and Psychiatry, 23,* 56–62.

Hamilton, M. (1967). Development of a rating scale for primary depressive illness. *British Journal of Social and Clinical Psychology, 6,* 278–296.

Hamilton, M. (1982). Symptoms and assessment of depression. In E. S. Paykel (Ed.), *Handbook of affective disorders* (pp. 3–11). New York: Guilford Press.

Herjanic, B., & Reich, W. (1982). Development of a structured psychiatric interview for children: Agreement between child and parent on individual symptoms. *Journal of Abnormal Child Psychology, 10,* 307–324.

Hops, H., Lewinsohn, P. M., Andrews, J. A., & Roberts, R. E. (1990). Psychosocial correlates of depressive symptomatology among high school students. *Journal of Clinical Child Psychology, 19,* 211–220.

Ialongo, N., Edelsohn, G., Werthamer-Larsson, L., Crockett, L., & Kellam, S. (1993). Are self-reported depressive symptoms in first-grade children developmentally transient phenomena? A further look. *Development and Psychopathology, 5,* 433–457.

Kahn, J. S., Kehle, T. J., Jenson, W. R., & Clark, E. (1990). Comparison of cognitive-behavioral, relaxation, and self-modeling interventions for depression among middle-school students. *School Psychology Review, 19,* 196–211.

Kaufman, J., Birmaher, B., Brent, D. A., Rao, U., Flynn, C., & Moreci, P. (1997). Schedule for Affective Disorders and Schizophrenia for School-Age Children—Present and Lifetime Version (K-SADS-PL). *Journal of the American Academy of Child and Adolescent Psychiatry, 36,* 980–988.

Kazdin, A. E. (1994). Informant variability in the assessment of childhood depression. In W. M. Reynolds and H. F. Johnston (Eds.), *Handbook of depression in children and adolescents* (pp. 249–271). New York: Plenum Press.

Kovacs, M. (1979). *Children's Depression Inventory.* University of Pittsburgh School of Medicine.

Kovacs, M. (1986). A developmental perspective on methods and measures in the assessment of depressive disorders: The clinical interview. In M. Rutter, C. E. Izard, & P. B. Read (Eds.), *Depression in young people: Developmental and clinical perspectives* (pp. 435–465). New York: Guilford Press.

Kovacs, M. (1992). *Children's Depression Inventory manual.* North Tonawanda, NY: Multi-Health Systems.

Kovacs, M., & Beck, A. T. (1977). An empirical-clinical approach toward a definition of childhood depression. In J. G. Schulterbrandt & A. Raskin (Eds.), *Depression in childhood: Diagnosis, treatment and conceptual models* (pp. 1–25). New York: Raven Press.

Krefetz, D. G., Steer, R. A., Gulab, N, A., & Beck, A. T. (2002). Convergent validity of the Beck Depression Inventory—II with the Reynolds Adolescent Depression Scale in psychiatric inpatients. *Journal of Personality Assessment, 78,* 451–460.

Lang, M., & Tisher, M. (1978). *Children's Depression Scale.* Victoria, Australia: Australian Council for Educational Research.

Lefkowitz, M. M., & Tesiny, E. P. (1980). Assessment of childhood depression. *Journal of Consulting and Clinical Psychology, 48,* 43–50.

Lefkowitz, M. M., Tesiny, E. P., & Solodow, W. (1989). A rating scale for assessing dysphoria in youth. *Journal of Abnormal Child Psychology, 17,* 337–347.

Lewinsohn, P. M., Clarke, G. N., Hops, H., & Andrews, J. (1990). Cognitive-behavioral treatment for depressed adolescents. *Behavior Therapy, 21,* 385–401.

Luby, J. L., Mrakotsky, C., Heffelfinger, A., Brown, K., & Spitznagel, E. (2004). Characteristics of depressed preschoolers with and without Anhedonia: Evidence for a melancholic depressive subtype in young children. *American Journal of Psychiatry, 161,* 2004.

Mufson, L., Moreau, D., Weissman, M. M., Wickramaratne, P., Martin, J., & Samoilov, A. (1994). The modification of interpersonal psychotherapy with depressed adolescents (IPT-A): Phase I and Phase II studies. *Journal of the American Academy of Child and Adolescent Psychiatry, 33,* 695–705.

Orvaschel, H., Puig-Antich, J., Chambers, W., Tabrizi, M. A., & Johnson, R. (1982). Retrospective assessment of prepubertal major depression with the Kiddie-SADS-E. *Journal of the American Academy of Child Psychiatry, 21,* 392–397.

Osman, A., Kopper, B. A., Barrios, F., Gutierrez, P. M., & Bagge, C. L. (2004). Reliability and validity of the Beck Depression Inventory—II with adolescent psychiatric inpatients. *Psychological Assessment, 16,* 120–132.

Poznanski, E. O., Cook, S. C., & Carroll, B. J. (1979). A depression rating scale for children. *Pediatrics, 64,* 442–450.

Poznanski, E. O., Freeman, L. N., & Mokros, H. B. (1985). Children's Depression Rating Scale—Revised. *Psychopharmacology Bulletin, 21,* 979–989.

Poznanski, E. O., & Mokros, H. (1996). *Children's Depression Rating Scale—Revised (CDRS-R).* Los Angeles: Western Psychological Services.

Poznanski, E. O., Grossman, J. A., Buchsbaum, Y., Banegas, M., Freeman, L., & Gibbons, R. (1984). Preliminary studies of the reliability and validity of the Children's Depression Rating Scale. *Journal of the American Academy of Child Psychiatry, 23,* 191–197.

Puig-Antich, J., & Chambers, W. (1978). *The Schedule for Affective Disorders and Schizophrenia for School-age Children (Kiddie-SADS).* New York: New York State Psychiatric Institute.

Puig-Antich, J., & Gittelman, R. (1982). Depression in childhood and adolescence. In E. S. Paykel (Ed.), *Handbook of affective disorders* (pp. 379–392). New York: Guilford Press.

Radloff, L. S. (1977). The CES-D Scale: A self-report scale for research in the general population. *Applied Psychological Measurement, 1,* 385–401.

Radloff, L. S. (1991). The use of the Center for Epidemiologic Studies Depression Scale in adolescents and young adults. *Journal of Youth and Adolescence, 20,* 149–166.

Reich, W. (2000). Diagnostic Interview for Children and Adolescents (DICA). *Journal of the American Academy of Child and Adolescent Psychiatry, 39,* 59–66.

Reich, W., Herjanic, B., Welner, Z., & Gandhy, P. R. (1982). Development of a structured psychiatric interview for children: Agreement in diagnosis comparing child and parent interviews. *Journal of Abnormal Child Psychology, 10,* 325–336.

Reynolds, W. M. (1986a). *Reynolds Adolescent Depression Scale.* Odessa, FL: Psychological Assessment Resources.

Reynolds, W. M. (1986b). A model for the screening and identification of depressed children and adolescents in school settings. *Professional School Psychology, 1,* 117–129.

Reynolds, W. M. (1987). *Reynolds Adolescent Depression Scale: Professional manual.* Odessa, FL: Psychological Assessment Resources.

Reynolds, W. M. (1988). *Suicidal Ideation Questionnaire: Professional manual.* Odessa, FL: Psychological Assessment Resources.

Reynolds, W. M. (1989). *Reynolds Child Depression Scale: Professional manual.* Odessa, FL: Psychological Assessment Resources.

Reynolds, W. M. (1992). Depression in children and adolescents. In W. M. Reynolds (Ed.), *Internalizing disorders in children and adolescents* (pp. 149–254). New York: John Wiley & Sons.

Reynolds, W. M. (1998). *Adolescent Psychopathology Scale.* Odessa, FL: Psychological Assessment Resources.

Reynolds, W. M. (2002). *Reynolds Adolescent Depression Scale—2nd Edition.* Odessa, FL: Psychological Assessment Resources.

Reynolds, W. M., & Coats, K. I. (1986). A comparison of cognitive-behavioral therapy and relaxation training for the treatment of depression in adolescents. *Journal of Consulting and Clinical Psychology, 54,* 653–660.

Reynolds, W. M., & Johnston, H. F. (1994). The nature and study of depression in children and adolescents. In W. M. Reynolds & H. F. Johnston (Eds.), *Handbook of depression in children and adolescents* (pp. 3–17). New York: Plenum Press.

Reynolds, W. M., & Stark, K. D. (1983). Cognitive behavior modification: The clinical application of cognitive strategies. In M. Pressley & J. R. Levin (Eds.), *Cognitive strategy research: Psychological foundations* (pp. 221–266). New York: Springer-Verlag.

Robbins, D. R., Alessi, N. E., Colfer, M. V., & Yanchyshyn, G. W. (1985). Use of the Hamilton Rating Scale for Depression and the Carroll Self-Rating Scale in adolescents. *Psychiatry Research, 14,* 123–129.

Rosenberg, M. (1965). *Society and the adolescent self-image*. Princeton, NJ: Princeton University Press.

Rourke, K. M., & Reich, W. (2004). The Diagnostic Interview for Children and Adolescents (DICA). In M. J. Hilsenroth & D. L. Segal (Vol. Eds.), M. Hersen (Ed. in Chief), *Comprehensive handbook of psychological assessment, Vol 2: Personality assessment* (pp. 271–280). Hoboken, NJ: John Wiley & Sons.

Shaffer, D., Fisher, P., Lucas, C., Dulcan, M., & Schwab-Stone, M. (2000). The Diagnostic Interview Schedule for Children, Version IV (DISC-IV): Description, differences from previous versions, and reliability of some common diagnoses. *Journal of the American Academy of Child and Adolescent Psychiatry, 39,* 28–38.

Shaffer, D., Schwab-Stone, M., Fisher, P., Cohen, P., Piacentini, J., Davies, M., Conners, C. K., & Reiger, D. (1993). The Diagnostic Interview Schedule for Children—Revised Version (DISC-R): I. Preparation, field testing, interrater reliability, and acceptability. *Journal of the American Academy of Child and Adolescent Psychiatry, 32,* 643–650.

Spitzer, R. L., Endicott, J., & Robins, E. (1978). Research diagnostic criteria: Rationale and reliability. *Archives of General Psychiatry, 35,* 773–782.

Stark, K. D. (1990). *Childhood depression: School-based intervention*. New York: Guilford Press.

Stark, K. D., Reynolds, W. M., & Kaslow, N. J. (1987). A comparison of the relative efficacy of self-control therapy and behavioral problem-solving therapy for depression in children. *Journal of Abnormal Child Psychology, 15,* 91–113.

Treatment for Adolescents with Depression Study (TADS) Team (2004). Fluoxetine, cognitive-behavioral therapy, and their combination for adolescents with depression: Treatment for adolescents with depression study (TADS) randomized controlled trial. *Journal of the American Medical Association, 292,* 807–820.

13

SOCIAL SKILLS DEFICITS

MEGAN M. McCLELLAND

Department of Human Development and Family Sciences
Oregon State University
Corvallis, Oregon

CORI SCALZO

Cognitive Assessment Services, Inc. (CAS)
Bronxville, New York

INTRODUCTION

A large body of research has highlighted the importance of children's early social skills for adjustment and school success (e.g., DeRosier, Kupersmidt, & Patterson, 1994; Dishion, 1990; Ladd, 1990). Children in elementary school who have poor social skills often have a number of problems, including peer rejection, behavior problems, and low levels of academic achievement (Alexander, Entwisle, & Dauber, 1993; Cooper & Farran, 1988; McClelland, Morrison, & Holmes, 2000). In addition, teachers report that children come into school with differing levels of social skills and that these skills are critical for social competence (Foulks & Morrow, 1989). For example, in one study some teachers reported that at least 50% of children entering kindergarten did not have the basic social competencies needed to do well in school, such as cooperating, following directions, and working independently (Rimm-Kaufman, Pianta, & Cox, 2000). Moreover, a recent recommendation from the Committee on Integrating the Science of Early Childhood Development called for promoting aspects of young children's social competence, such as self-direction, persistence, cooperation, and motivation (Shonkoff & Phillips, 2000).

One of the main issues regarding children's social behavior has been how to adequately define social skills. Some research has moved from general conceptualizations of social skills to defining specific aspects of social skills important for different child outcomes. For example, a differentiation can be made between *interpersonal social skills*, which are important for social competence, and *learning-related social skills*, which are important for academic success in school (Cooper & Farran, 1988; McClelland et al., 2000; McClelland & Morrison, 2003).

When looking at broader *interpersonal social skills*, two conceptualizations are useful. First, researchers and clinicians have focused much attention on children's *sociometric status*, or *peer acceptance*. This conceptualization examines children's acceptance or rejection by their peers. The peer acceptance literature has been a major focus of social development theory, and research has found that peer rejection is a major indicator of later antisocial problems in children (e.g., Coie & Dodge, 1998; Dodge et al., 2003). For example, a recent study found that children's poor social skills and peer rejection in early elementary school predicted later antisocial behavior when children were 10–12 years old, but only for children who were initially more aggressive. These rejected children were also more likely to develop hostile attributional biases when interpreting social situations, which contributed to further behavior problems (Dodge et al.).

The second definition of interpersonal social skills can be viewed from a *social validity* conceptualization (Gresham, 2001). This definition focuses on the behaviors that are important for children's positive acceptance in a variety of contexts, such as with teachers, peers, and parents. The social validity of social skills incorporates McFall's (1982) differentiation of *competence* and *skill*. According to McFall, *social competence* can be defined as an evaluation of a person's performance on a social task, and *social skill* is the actual ability to perform a social task competently. This is important in assessing children's social skills because a child may not have the skills required to successfully negotiate a social situation, and intervention can help improve these skills. In addition, a child could be judged as having social skills deficits as compared to a group of his or her peers, which can provide insight into the broader factors influencing that child's peer acceptance. Together, the social validity conceptualization includes children's ability to perform competently in social situations as well as how others perceive those skills.

In addition to social skills that assess children's interpersonal competence, there are social skills related to children's academic and classroom success. Research has indicated that children's *learning-related social skills*, including self-regulation, responsibility, independence, and cooperation, are particularly important for early school performance and adaptation (Blair, 2002; Cooper & Farran, 1988; McClelland et al., 2000; McClelland & Morrison, 2003). In recent research, children rated as having poor learning-related social skills at the beginning of kindergarten performed worse on academic indices between kindergarten and sixth grade as compared to their peers. The children with poor learning-related social skills also shared a number of problematic characteristics, including having significantly lower IQs, more behavior difficulties, poorer family learning environments, and more medical problems, such as hearing and language problems (McClelland et al., 2000; McClelland, Morrison & Acock, 2005).

These studies call attention to the importance of children's early learning-related social skills and interpersonal social skills for long-term social and academic adjustment. Researchers, clinicians, and other professionals working with children and families need to reliably and accurately assess, conceptualize, and treat children who have social skills deficits. The present chapter discusses children's social skills assessment from a comprehensive research and clinical framework. First, we describe the primary assessment strategies available for children with social skills deficits as well as the research basis for those strategies. We then discuss the clinical utility of the assessment strategies and the developmental considerations that are important when assessing children's social skills. Next, we outline the assessment, conceptualization, and treatment planning in measuring children's social skills. Finally, we provide a case study to illustrate the assessment of a child with social skills deficits, other important issues to consider, and treatment recommendations.

RESEARCH BASIS AND DESCRIPTION OF ASSESSMENT STRATEGIES

Researchers and clinicians have used a number of methods to assess children's social skills. In recent years, the literature on the different types of assessment strategies has grown, and considerable progress has been made in the reliability and validity of these methods. However, the types of assessment strategies vary in their usefulness for assessing children's social skills. According to Merrell (2001), there are three lines of social skills assessment: Naturalistic observations and behavior rating scales are recommended as first choices for assessment; interviewing methods and sociometric techniques are suggested as second choices; and projective techniques and self-report may be useful but are not recommended as primary means of assessing social skills.

In general, research on social skills assessment recommends multiple forms of assessment, starting with a screening tool, such as behavioral rating scale, and following with more in-depth observational techniques and interviews (Gresham, 2001; Merrell, 2001). In this section, we provide brief descriptions of the first two lines of recommended assessment strategies and the research basis for those methods. Those interested in more detailed coverage of social skills assessment strategies are referred to reviews such as Merrell (1999).

NATURALISTIC OBSERVATION

Naturalistic observation of children's behavior is one of the best methods for assessing children's social skills deficits. Observing children's behavior in context provides a rich source of information about specific behaviors as well as information about other ecological factors included in the child's social environment. Often the best setting to assess children's social skills is the school environment, where children have opportunities to interact with peers, especially during recess, free play, or lunch. Some of the key components important for behavioral observations include having a clear definition of the behavior being assessed, using observers who are trained and objective, and using an adequate behavioral coding system that minimizes interpretation from observers (Gresham, 2001; Merrell, 2001).

In order to adequately observe children's behavior, researchers and practitioners must decide how a behavior will be recorded and coded. Often observations are conducted according to the *frequency* of the behavior (i.e., how often a child shows a particular behavior during an observation period, *duration* (i.e., how long a behavior lasts), and *interval recording* (i.e., whether specific behaviors are seen during a time interval). Gresham (2001) asserts that "the most important aspect of what makes a behavior 'socially skilled' is its quality and not its frequency or temporal dimensions" (p. 337). In order to judge the quality of a behavior, observers can be trained to rate behaviors using videotaped examples of a targeted behavior. Although not many observational instruments are available to assess children's social skills, the Peer Social Behavior Code and the Bronson Social and Task Skill Profile are two recommended examples.

Peer Social Behavior Code (PSBC)

The PSBC is one example of an observational tool for assessing children's interpersonal social skills. It was developed by Walker and Severson (1992; Walker et al., 1994) as part of the *Systematic Screening for Behavior Disorders* (SSBD), which is a screening system for children's behavior disorders in elementary school (grades 1–6). The PSBC includes six categories of assessing social behavior: social engagement, social involvement, participation, parallel play, alone, and no codable response. Observations are conducted in a series of 10-second intervals during unstructured, free play time, and behaviors are coded as positive or negative in the categories of social engagement, social involvement, and participation. The research basis for the PSBC is comprehensive and the psychometric properties are strong. In one study, the average interrater reliability in percent agreement for the PSBC was 95% for observations in classrooms and 88% for observations in the playground. Results also indicated that the PSBS and the SSBD system correctly and efficiently identified children who needed special services (Walker et al., 1994).

Bronson Social and Task Skill Profile (BSTSP)

The BSTSP is an example of an observational tool assessing children's learning-related social skills and interpersonal social skills (Bronson, 1996). The measure records children's social and mastery behaviors, including their ability to use self-regulatory skills to plan, organize, and complete tasks and to cooperate successfully with peers in the classroom. The BSTSP uses structured categories of Use of Time, Social Behavior, and Mastery Behaviors to record children's behavior in a modified interval sampling method during unstructured free play time. The tool can be used with children in preschool through grade 2.

The research basis for the BSTSP indicates that the reliability and validity information is strong, and the measure has been used in a number of studies (Bronson, 1994; Bronson, Tivnan, & Seppanen, 1995). Interobserver reliability in terms of the percent agreement among raters ranges from 84% to 100% in the Use of Time, Social Behavior, and Mastery Behaviors categories, and the manual recommends that new observers be trained to 90% interobserver agreement in each category. There is also a teacher rating version of the BSTSP available called the Child Behavior Rating Scale (Bronson et al., 1995).

Research on children's social skills supports naturalistic observations as a primary means of assessing social skills deficits, but there are disadvantages that limit their usefulness. First, naturalistic observations can be very time intensive, which can be a practical drawback. In addition to the actual observation time, careful planning is required to identify what behaviors to target, to decide on the specific observation and coding system to use, and to train observers. This time commitment is important because prior planning can do much to strengthen the validity of naturalistic observations. A second potential disadvantage is deciding on the number of observations required to get data that are representative of a child's behavior in a specific setting. Often, multiple observations are required to adequately sample the behavior, and Gresham (2001) suggests that two to three observations be conducted in a setting of concern. Given these limitations, although naturalistic observations are a strong method for social skills assessment, many researchers suggest that they be used after administering an initial screening tool, such as a behavior rating scale. Behavior rating scales have emerged as one of the best strategies for assessing children's social competence; they are discussed next.

BEHAVIOR RATING SCALES

Behavior rating scales have improved markedly in their psychometric properties in recent years and provide an efficient method for assessing social skills deficits. Behavior rating scales have many advantages. They are less time intensive than naturalistic observations and are an effective way to collect data across a number of situations over time. In addition, rating scales provide data that can be more reliable than information gathered through interviewing and projective techniques. Parent and teacher rating scales provide information on children's behavior from people who are familiar with a particular child. Finally, parent and teacher rating scales are good methods for assessing children who are too young or who are unable to report on their own behavior. This can be important because research has found that self-reports may not be a reliable strategy for assessing social skills deficits, especially for young children (Merrell, 2001). A wide variety of social skills behavior rating scales are available today for researchers and practitioners. We present a few measures that have strong psychometric properties and have been shown to be useful in assessing children's interpersonal social skills and learning-related social skills: the Social Skills Rating System; the School Social Behavior Scales; the Walker–McConnell Scales of Social Competence and School Adjustment; and the Cooper–Farran Behavioral Rating Scale.

Social Skills Rating System (SRRS)

The SSRS is a comprehensive rating system for assessing social skills, problem behaviors, and academic competence, with different scales for parents and teachers to complete as well as a self-report version for older students (Gresham & Elliott, 1990). There are Preschool (ages 3–5), Elementary (grades K–6), and Secondary (grades 7–12) versions of the system. In general, the SSRS measures the interpersonal and learning-related skill domains of Cooperation, Assertion, and Self-Control (for parent and teacher versions), Responsibility (parent version only) and Empathy (student version only) in a Total Social Skills domain. The Problem Behaviors domain assesses Externalizing, Internalizing, and Hyperactivity behaviors (teacher and parent versions). There is also an Academic Competence version for teachers to complete at the Elementary and Secondary levels according to a five-point scale. For the Social Skills and Problem Behaviors domains of the scale, items are rated on frequency and importance (each according to a three-point scale).

In terms of the research basis for this measure, the SSRS has adequate-to-strong psychometric properties. Internal reliabilities for items in the Total Social Skills domain range from .83 (student versions) to .94 (teacher versions for Preschool and Elementary). Internal reliabilities for the Problem Behaviors domain range from .73 (parent Preschool version) to .88 (teacher version for Elementary; Gresham & Elliott, 1990). Although the reliability and validity information for the SSRS is a strength of the measure, a weakness is the restricted range of the Social Skills and Problem Behaviors domains. Items for these domains are rated on a three-point scale, which can limit the variability in the responses from raters. In addition, the standardization sample is underrepresentative of children from less educated and minority families (Gresham & Elliott). However, a strength of the SSRS is that it assesses aspects of children's interpersonal social skills and learning-related social skills.

School Social Behavior Scales (SSBS)

The SSBS was developed by Merrell (1993) specifically for use in school settings to measure children's interpersonal skills and learning-related social skills between kindergarten and grade 12. The SSBS is a 65-item teacher rating scale with two scales: the Social Competence scale (32 items), including Interpersonal Skills, Self-Management Skills, and Academic Skills; and the Antisocial Behavior scale (33 items), including Hostile-Irritable behaviors, Antisocial-Aggressive behaviors, and Disruptive-Demanding behaviors. Items on the SSBS are rated on a five-point scale according to frequency (1 = never to 5 = frequently). The research basis for the SSBS indicates adequate-to-strong psychometric qualities. Internal reliabilities for items on the SSBS range from .91 to .98, and three-week test–retest reliabilities range from .76 to .83 for items in the Social Competence scale and .60 to .73 for items in the Antisocial Behavior scale (Merrell, 1993, 2001). Strengths for the SSBS include the five-point scale that allows for a greater range of scores and assessing both interpersonal skills and learning-related social skills. The rating scale is limited by having only a teacher version and by being focused solely on social behavior. Thus, the SSBS does not adequately screen for other problems, such as Attention-Deficit Hyperactivity Disorder or internalizing disorders.

Walker–McConnell Scales of Social Competence and School Adjustment (SSCSA)

The SSCSA is another behavior rating scale designed for teachers and school professionals to measure aspects of children's interpersonal and learning-related social skills (Walker & McConnell, 1995a, 1995b). The scales can be used with children in elementary school (grades K–6) and with adolescents (grades 7–12) and has a teacher version available. The elementary version of the scale assesses Teacher-Preferred Social Behavior, Peer-Preferred Social Behavior, and School Adjustment. The adolescent version includes the same scales as well as Empathy, Self-Control, and Peer Relations scales. Items are rated on a five-point scale to indicate the frequency of the behaviors, ranging from 1 (never occurs) to 5 (frequently occurs). The research basis for the SSCSA is well documented, with excellent psychometric properties. The internal reliabilities for total scores in the SSCSA range from .92 to .98, and three-week test–retest reliabilities range from .88 to .92. Limitations with the SSCSA include having only a teacher version of the scales and not assessing problem behavior.

Cooper–Farran Behavioral Rating Scale (CFBRS)

The CFBRS is a teacher-rated scale consisting of 37 items rated on seven-point Likert scales assessing interpersonal and learning-related social skills for children in early elementary school (Cooper & Farran, 1991). The measure has separate scales for interpersonal social skills and work-related skills (including self-regulation, independence, and responsibility) and has adequate reliability and validity. Cooper and Farran found that intrarater reliability in the CFBRS ranged from .49 to .80 and that interrater reliability ranged from .31 to .68. Interrater reliabilities for the subscales are .78 for interpersonal skills and .79 for work-related skills. A strength of the CFBRS as compared to other scales such as the Social Skills Rating Scale (SSRS) is the use of a seven-point scale, which can capture more variability in scores. In addition, the CFBRS differentiates between children's interpersonal social skills and their learning-related social skills, which is useful in assessing specific social skills deficits. However, some weaknesses with the measure are that it has been used primarily with children in kindergarten through second grade and that it only has a teacher-rated version.

In general, behavior rating scales present an efficient, reliable, and economical way to assess children's social skills deficits. However, to get a comprehensive picture of a child's social skills strengths and weaknesses, it is important to use behavior rating scales in conjunction with other forms of assessment, such as naturalistic observations, interviewing, and role-play. We discuss the assessment strategies and the research bases for interviewing and role-play techniques next.

INTERVIEWING

Interviewing techniques have long been a popular form of assessing children's social competence. According to Merrell (2001), interviewing "is perhaps the oldest and most widely used social-emotional assessment method" (p. 5). After the primary means of assessing social skills with observations and behavior rating scales, interviewing methods represent a critical second line of assessment. Interviews are a flexible assessment strategy that can be either structured or free-flowing and unstructured. Interviewing is a useful tool to obtain information about the context and ecological environment in which a child lives, including details of the child's family, parents, peers, and school. This is a particularly important component of assessment because recent theoretical conceptualizations indicate that children's development occurs within a dynamic, multilevel, and interactive framework. These theories argue that children's social competence is influenced by a complex set of interacting factors, including the child's individual characteristics such as temperament, family factors such as parenting and the home environment, and schooling factors such as teacher–child relationships and peers (Gottlieb, Wahlsten, & Lickliter, 1998; McClelland, Kessenich, & Morrison, 2003). Thus, interviews can provide important contextual information and specific data about difficult situations on which intervention and treatment can be based.

Although interviews are a vital strategy for social skills assessment in children, little empirical research has examined their effectiveness. A major limitation of interviewing is the possibility that social desirability will influence the responses from a child (Meier & Hope, 1998). Young children in particular can be suggestible and may answer questions in ways they think the interviewer wants them to answer (Ceci & Bruck, 1998). In addition, research has found that children with social skills deficits often have problems with social information processing, where they misinterpret social cues and see situations as more hostile than they are in reality (Dodge et al., 2003). Thus, the information children give in an interview may be biased. Overall, interviews are an important aspect of assessing children's social skills, but research underscores the need for multiple forms of assessment strategies.

ROLE-PLAY TECHNIQUES

Role-play techniques are closely linked to interviewing and can take place in the context of the interview. Often role-plays take the form of a scenario presented to a child, who then gives responses, or a situation involving a confederate or a clinician, who engages the child in a staged interaction. A benefit of role-play assessments is that they can be used within an interview situation to obtain information about social skills and deficits when direct observation is not possible. In addition, role-plays can be used to elicit behavior that occurs infrequently in children (Meier & Hope, 1998; Torgrud & Holborn, 1992). Role-play strategies are also an important part of intervention techniques and allow children an opportunity to practice appropriate behaviors in different situations.

The research basis for role-play techniques is limited, and the literature highlights a number of limitations. First, research indicates that, in general, role-plays have poor reliability and validity (Torgrud & Holborn, 1992; Van Hasselt, Hersen, & Bellack, 1981). The degree to which role-plays are reliable and valid depend on how much the behavior in the role-play situation reflects real behavior. Often what children say they will do may not be what they actually do in a real-world situation. Children may respond in ways they think they should respond but not make actual changes in behavior or in the way they interpret social situations. As discussed earlier, children's social competence is influenced by a number of factors that may be context specific; thus, the role-play may not match a real situation. Together, role-play techniques and interviewing strategies are components of the assessment process but reflect secondary methods for adequately measuring children's social skills.

SOCIOMETRIC TECHNIQUES

Sociometric techniques have been used predominantly in the research arena to study children's peer relations and social competence. Examples of sociometric techniques include peer ratings, peer rankings, and peer nomination, which involve children rating how much they like each child in their class, identifying peers they especially like or dislike, and nominating peers who are aggressive or start fights. The research basis for this assessment technique is extensive and indicates that sociometric procedures are strong predictors of current and future social acceptance (e.g., Coie & Dodge, 1998; Dodge et al., 2003). However, the main reasons these techniques have remained mostly in the research domain are due to practical constraints. Sociometric procedures often involve all the children in a classroom, which requires the consent of school administrators and every parent in a classroom. In addition, school administrators and parents may be reluctant to give consent because of fears that social rejection will be reinforced by the sociometric procedures (Merrell, 2001). These issues make sociometric procedures an impractical means of assessing social skills in children for clinicians. Thus, although sociometric assessment strategies are psychometrically very strong, they are considered a secondary form of assessment. In general, the assorted assessment strategies for children's social skills vary in their recommendation, based on their research support and psychometric properties.

CLINICAL UTILITY

To be clinically useful, assessment instruments must be reliable and valid. Beyond that, other factors, including specificity, cost effectiveness, and efficiency, must be considered. In this section, the clinical utility of the assessment tools just discussed will be reviewed.

NATURALISTIC OBSERVATION

As previously stated, naturalistic observation is the gold standard of social skills assessment (Elliott, Sheridan, & Gresham, 1989). A primary reason for this is its clinical utility. While it is time consuming and, therefore, not particularly cost effective or efficient, naturalistic observation provides the most detailed, specific, and ecologically valid information about target behaviors. Naturalistic observation allows the clinician to gain direct information about target behaviors as well as their antecedents and sustaining consequences. In this way, the clinician is able to assess the "function" of the problem behaviors (Gresham, 2001; Sheridan & Elliott, 1991). The clinician can also obtain information about other cues or related factors (such as anxiety and a poor temperament fit between a teacher and child) that parents or teachers might not otherwise provide in the context of interviews or rating scales. Direct observation of the problem behaviors limits the number of assumptions that need to be made about the causes and effects of the behaviors (Gresham, 1988). However, in the case of more covert behaviors, some inferences and assumptions remain (Gresham & Lambros, 1998).

Naturalistic observation is also useful for the clinician in terms of understanding the skills and interests of the child's peers (e.g., movies, playground games, sports). In addition, each peer group differs in terms of sophistication and/or cohesiveness. Information about these issues can be useful for case conceptualization as well as treatment planning. The transfer of skills will be most successful when there is a specific match between the social skills training and the application setting. Because naturalistic observation is time consuming, it is typically used as part of the initial assessment and may not be practical for ongoing evaluation of treatment progress. For these interim evaluations, behavior rating scales are more efficient (Gresham, 2001).

BEHAVIOR RATING SCALES

As previously mentioned, behavior rating scales can have good reliability and validity and are cost effective and efficient. An additional strength is the availability of normative data, which allow for meaningful comparisons with typical same-aged peers. This can be very useful for parents or other adults who may not have exposure to the range of same-aged peers and may have a poor concept of typical behaviors for a certain-age child. For these reasons, they can be used frequently and may be the best tools for assessing progress throughout treatment. It has also been suggested that when administration of the full measure or rating scale is too cumbersome, critical items or subscales can be administered to evaluate progress at frequent intervals (Gresham, 2001). Behavior rating scales are particularly useful to the clinician when multiple raters are involved and the clinician can glean information about which behaviors are present and most problematic in the various settings. The raters may not agree because behaviors vary across settings, but this information is useful for the clinician when specific behaviors are targeted for treatment.

Despite these strengths, behavioral rating scales are not highly useful for providing information about antecedents and consequences of behaviors, which are central to developing an effective treatment plan (Gresham, 2001). In other words, the behavior ratings scales simply indicate which behaviors are occurring and their severity or frequency. The scales do not give information about what triggers or occurs before the behavior(s) or what responses are provided to the child following the behavior(s).

INTERVIEWING

Like behavior rating scales, interviews can cover a broad range of behaviors across settings. For example, a parent typically sees more problem behaviors than can be assessed during observation, and they are more likely to see the children in a variety of contexts. In this way, the interview provides unique information that can be used to conceptualize the case and to plan for treatment. Compared to naturalistic observation, the interview may also be a more realistic and efficient tool for assessing progress following or during intervention.

The Functional Assessment Interview (FAI) is often used by clinicians to understand which behaviors are most socially relevant to the child. The FAI is a semistructured interview used for clarifying and prioritizing the primary social skills problems as well as for generating an initial analysis of the antecedents, consequences, and environmental specifics related to the problem behaviors. For example, a child's peers might be highly interested in a certain video game. Teaching the child the language of the video game and how to play might provide him or her with a tool to successfully engage his or her peers in conversation or play. In some social settings, physical skills are most salient and necessary for joining in group play, whereas conversational skills might be more important in other settings. This information is important for treatment planning, so the most socially relevant behaviors can be prioritized in treatment. However, despite these clinical strengths, interviewing techniques are not widely researched and often lack reliability and validity (Kratochwill, Sheridan, Carlson, & Lasecki, 1999).

ROLE-PLAY TECHNIQUES

Theoretically, role-play techniques are useful for clinicians, and they can provide an opportunity for direct observation of social skills when naturalistic observation is not feasible. Role-plays can be used to elicit low-frequency behaviors that might otherwise be difficult to observe. The use of in-office role-plays also skirts issues of confidentiality related to assessment in applied settings (Meier & Hope, 1998). However, the clinical utility of the role-play technique is limited by relatively poor reliability and validity (Merrell, 2001). In addition, the information obtained during role-play assessments may be too specific and not highly generalizable (Matson & Ollendick, 1988).

SOCIOMETRIC TECHNIQUES

As previously discussed, the reliability and validity of sociometric techniques are strong. For clinical purposes, the pragmatic constraints significantly limit the clinical utility of this assessment tool. It is unrealistic that clinicians working with individuals or small groups would have the time or resources to conduct this type of assessment. Another limitation is that ratings by peers tend to be fairly static and are not typically reflective of subtle changes made during social skills training (Meier & Hope, 1998). On the other hand, there is evidence that sociometric ratings, more than other techniques, provide powerful information about a child's acceptance or position in a social group (Sheridan & Elliott, 1991).

DEVELOPMENTAL CONSIDERATIONS

In addition to considering the research basis and clinical utility of social skills assessment strategies, using measures that are appropriate for the targeted child or population is critical. Some of the developmental considerations for social skills assessment tools include the child's age and developmental stage and sociocultural sensitivity.

First, it is important to use assessment strategies that are appropriate for a child's age and developmental stage. For example, young children may have difficulty communicating, so an in-depth interview may not be the best method unless it is supplemented by other strategies, such as naturalistic observation and behavior rating scales, or by interviewing parents or teachers. In addition, using an age-appropriate measure eliminates problems with ceiling and floor effects, particularly with behavior rating scales. Ceiling effects occur when a measure assesses skills that most children are scored as successfully having. In contrast, floor effects occur when a measure assesses skills that most children in the age group or developmental stage have not yet attained, so scores are clustered at the bottom of a scale (Miller, 1998). Fortunately, most behavior ratings scales, such as the SSRS, SSBS, and SSCSA, have age-appropriate versions.

Second, the sociocultural sensitivity of measures is important when deciding among social skills assessment methods. Some behavior rating scales are written at a high literacy level, which may make it difficult for less educated parents to understand and complete. This issue is also relevant for children who complete self-report measures, where their reading level can interfere with their understanding of the questions. In addition, cultural differences in norms and values can influence the rating of children's behavior by observers, teachers, and parents. For example, research by Rimm-Kaufman and colleagues (2000) found that nonminority teachers rated minority children as having more social and academic difficulties in the transition to kindergarten than nonminority children. These issues emphasize the need to choose social skills instruments that have been validated on diverse populations and for researchers and clinicians to be aware of cultural differences in the observation and evaluation of children's behavior.

ASSESSMENT, CONCEPTUALIZATION, AND TREATMENT PLANNING

Assessment, conceptualization, and treatment planning are three distinct phases for identification and remediation of social skill deficits. *Assessment* is the process of identification whether a problem exists as well as the specific nature of the problem. Case *conceptualization* is the process by which the clinician organizes and makes sense of the data collected during the assessment phase. During the conceptualization phase, target behaviors are selected and the antecedents and consequences of the behaviors clearly identified. During the *treatment planning* phase, the target behaviors, order of behaviors, and most appropriate treatment are determined. In addition, the therapists and other professionals who will be involved are selected and a plan is delineated for integrating the treatment into other aspects of the child's life. Both the case conceptualization and the treatment planning should be considered flexible and dynamic processes that change in response to the needs of the child and new information gained during the treatment.

Assessment lays the groundwork for conceptualization of the case and subsequently for treatment planning (Merrell, 2001). The more detailed and accurate the information from the assessment, the more tailored and specific the treatment plan can be. Assessment should proceed from the global to the specific, with hypothesis testing at each step (Elliott, Sheridan, & Gresham, 1989). A useful three-step paradigm for linking assessment to conceptualization and treatment planning was proposed by Gresham (2001). First, it is useful to get a broad overview of the different behaviors present using a social skills rating form. Once it is clear that social skills are a problem area and a general sense of the social skills deficits have been obtained, the Functional Assessment Interview (FAI) is recommended as the next assessment step. The FAI is particularly useful for generating the specific information to develop an effective plan for the naturalistic observation, which is the third recommended step. Naturalistic observation provides the detailed information most useful for case conceptualization and treatment planning (Gresham, 2001). In addition, understanding the function of the problem behaviors in a particular setting (through the observation and assessment of the antecedents and consequences) provides some of the most useful information for creating an effective treatment plan.

One method to determine which program of intervention best targets the main problems identified is the Keystone Behavior Strategy, which links specific assessment to intervention planning (Nelson & Hayes, 1986). During the case conceptualization phase, it is important to receive input from the parents, teachers, and those implementing the treatment in order to prioritize the target behaviors and the settings in which the treatment will be applied. Assessment is also used at the close of treatment to assess clinical progress as well as to ensure treatment integrity (Elliott & Busse, 1991; Kratochwill et al., 1999). Assessment should be conducted in applied settings to determine the generalization of the interventions. For example, children often will make adequate progress in a therapeutic setting but have difficulty generalizing the skills to applied settings (Berler, Gross, & Drabman, 1982).

An important component of assessment and treatment planning is the dissemination of relevant data to parents, teachers, and other professionals working with the child. Just as obtaining data from multiple sources is necessary for a valid and complete assessment, the sharing of those findings and the integration of treatment across settings is also critical. This integration provides additional support for the child and those working with the child. Finally, the social skills assessment should be part of a larger assessment, including cognitive, academic, and medical assessment. Communication between professionals conducting each aspect of the assessment is critical for accurate diagnosis as well as for successful treatment and monitoring of the problems.

CASE STUDY

IDENTIFICATION

Joe S. is a 13-and-a-half year-old Caucasian male who was referred for a complete neuropsychological evaluation, conducted over the course of four days. The evaluation was intended to address a variety of cognitive and social-emotional issues. Most relevant to Joe's social skills, and included in this case description, are his test results in the areas of general intellectual functioning and language skills. Social skills assessment was a special focus of the evaluation. Joe had been evaluated by a neurologist and developmental pediatrician, and neurological problems, other than those related to attention and depression, were ruled out.

Presenting Complaints

Joe presented with a history of academic problems, particularly in the areas of verbal and written expression and reading comprehension, and social skills deficits. Joe's learning problems are compounded by a low frustration tolerance and performance anxiety. He also has a history of Attention Deficit/Hyperactivity Disorder, for which he takes Concerta, and Depression, for which he takes Zoloft. Socially, Joe has become isolated and somewhat withdrawn.

History and Developmental Issues

Joe reportedly met all developmental milestones within normal limits but was described as an irritable and very active baby. From infancy to 6 years of age, he suffered severe ear infections. Joe sees a psychiatrist, who has treated him with Concerta for ADHD and Zoloft for Depression, both of which have reportedly been effective.

Peer and Social Issues

Joe is an only child, who reportedly has a strong relationship with both parents. Emotionally, Joe has been somewhat fragile. He has a history of Depression and suicidal ideation, and he has received individual psychotherapy to address these issues. Joe has made a few friends at school, and he occasionally has friends over to his house. He participated in a social skills group in kindergarten, per the teacher's recommendation, which was reportedly helpful. Nevertheless, Joe has never had a large circle of friends, and he struggles to initiate new friendships. Joe's mother, Mrs. S., reported some difficulties with peer interactions, specifically related to problems reading social cues and weak pragmatic language. Joe enjoys music, and his father is teaching him to play the guitar. In sum, Joe is a sensitive and caring young man who has had significant, long-standing learning problems that interfere with his adaptation to a mainstream academic setting and compromise his social functioning.

BEHAVIORAL ASSESSMENT RESULTS

Neuropsychological testing measures included but were not limited to the Wechsler Intelligence Scales for Children—Fourth Edition (WISC-IV); Comprehensive Assessment of Spoken Language (CASL); Behavior Assessment System for Children (BASC)—Parent Form; Clinical Interview—Student and parent; Social Skills Rating System—Student (SSRS-S), Parent (SSRS-P), and Teacher (SSRS-T); Functional Assessment Interview—Parent; Functional Assessment Observation: Classroom and Lunchroom.

Results of the cognitive testing are provided first, for they provide a global framework for the understanding of the cognitive and language-based underpinnings of Joe's social skill deficits.

General Intellectual Functioning

The Wechsler Intelligence Scale for Children—Fourth Edition (WISC-IV; Wechsler, 2003) was administered as a general index of Joe's intellectual functioning. He performed in the *Very Superior* range (98th percentile) for nonverbal, visual-perceptual abilities, and in the *Average* range (50th percentile) for verbal abilities. This significant discrepancy indicates that Joe's nonverbal reasoning abilities are much better developed than his verbal reasoning abilities, and he meets criteria for a mild Verbal Learning Disability.

Language Ability

In addition to the WISC-IV, subtests of the CASL, which assesses several components of language, including expressive and nonliteral language (Carrow-Woolfolk, 1999), indicated that Joe performed at the average level on all subtests, including generating synonyms, idiomatic language, grammaticality judgment, nonliteral language, and getting meaning from context. Results suggested that Joe could benefit from the teaching of social scripts to enhance his interactions with his peers, but he will need a social skills group to practice the correct implementation of these scripts. It will be insufficient to teach him what to say if he is unable to practice these tools during peer interactions. Joe performed the weakest on the pragmatic judgment subtest. Joe's difficulty on this task was consistent with parent, teacher, and examiner observation of his social skills and ability to use language in context. In general, Joe's knowledge of and use of language on this measure was better than in more applied contexts. Since language is a relative weakness for him, his ability to demonstrate what he does know declines when combined with other task demands.

These and other cognitive, neuropsychological test instruments provided the foundation for more detailed assessment of Joe's social skill deficits. Before proceeding with further social skill measures, there was a need to clarify the extent to which Joe continued to suffer from symptoms of depression and possibly anxiety. If left unaddressed, these symptoms can significantly impact social skills and interfere with the remediation of social skills deficits.

Adaptive Functioning

Joe's social skills and his social/emotional functioning were assessed more broadly. Parent report and the child clinical interview were used to assess Joe's emotional and adaptive functioning. In general, Joe presented as an anxious young man who displayed a significant amount of performance anxiety as well as frustration. Joe reported a generally positive relationship with both parents. Joe expressed concern about not having many friends and did not feel that he had the skills or ability to make new friends. Joe did not have insight into the nature of his social difficulties and could not articulate typical aspects of a friendship. For example, he was unable to articulate "what a friend is" or "how to make a friend." In addition, Joe was unable to describe common interests he might share with other people his age, without prompting.

Parent questionnaire responses on the BASC (Reynolds & Kamphaus, 1992), which is a general behavior assessment scale, indicated several areas of *At-Risk* and *Clinically Significant* emotional or behavior concerns. Joe's mother's responses placed Joe in the *Clinically Significant* range for Withdrawal and Anxiety and in the *At-Risk* range for Depression, Attention, and Atypicality.

Social Skills Clinical Interview

With other cognitive and emotional issues clarified, the clinical interview with Joe's mother, Mrs. S., was focused on social skills and preceded the use of behavior rating forms and a more detailed functional assessment interview. Mrs. S. reported that Joe had a few childhood friends, who were often neighborhood or family friends rather than school friends. However, in some grades, he had one or two children in the class with whom he was able to eat lunch and to whom he talked at recess. Once he is one on one with a peer, he is able to make some conversation, and at times he enjoys himself.

When asked about which aspects of social situations are most difficult for Joe, Mrs. S. indicated that he has particular difficulty with the language or conversational aspects of social interactions, including initiating conversation, selecting conversation topics that are appealing to the others his age, articulating his thoughts, and letting the other children speak in turn. Mrs. S. indicated that Joe also could be disruptive in a small group or classroom settings (e.g., humming, tapping), which further alienates him. However, she reported that medication has helped diminish these disruptive behaviors. The maternal report indicated that Joe has never enjoyed group activities. He is also not athletic, so sports are not enjoyable for him. Joe's anxiety and resistance to change further increases his discomfort with joining new groups or entering new social situations. He typically chooses activities that minimize interpersonal conflict, such as playing the guitar, watching television, and playing video games. Mrs. S. stated that she hopes that Joe can learn to speak appropriately with peers, become more comfortable in group settings, and establish friendships that include visiting friends' houses.

Social Skills Behavior Ratings

Once it was determined that both Joe and Mrs. S. considered Joe to have significant social deficits, the Social Skills Rating System (SSRS) was given, based on its strong psychometric properties, the availability of multiple rater forms, and normative data for peers his age (Gresham & Elliott, 1990). Mrs. S. completed the SSRS-P, and Joe obtained a Total Social Skills score below the 1st percentile, indicating significant deficits in learning-related social skills, including difficulties with cooperation, assertion, responsibility, and self-control.

Joe's teacher, Ms. K., completed the SSRS-T, and her ratings were consistent with those by Joe's mother. Joe's Total Social Skills were at the 4th percentile, and his Total Problem Behaviors were at the 92nd percentile (for problem behaviors, the higher percentages indicate more problem behaviors). Ms. K.'s ratings also indicated difficulties with learning-related social skills in cooperation, assertion, and self-control. Joe's externalizing problems included arguing and low frustration tolerance; his internalizing problems included loneliness, anxiety, sadness, and low self-esteem. More specific data were gathered through the Functional Assessment Interview.

Functional Assessment Interview

The more general clinical interviews and the social skills rating scales were used to clarify the most problematic and developmentally relevant skill deficits. The semistructured functional assessment interview (FAI) was useful for further clarifying these deficits and for determining the conditions under which these problems were most likely to occur. Additional information about the nature, antecedents, and consequences of these social skill problems was used to inform the functional assessment observations. Joe's mother, Mrs. S., identified the following social skills deficits as most problematic and as the most important targets for intervention: (1) does not initiate social conversation, (2) avoids group activities, (3) is argumentative in conversations with peers and adults, (4) perseverates on conversation topics, and (5) asks excessive questions.

The FAI indicated that Joe is a slow information processor, and much of the language presented socially comes too quickly for him to process. He has acquisition skill deficits and needs to become more skilled at reading nonverbal social cues and at processing language. His failure to initiate conversation was viewed as related to poor expressive language skills, which is considered to be both an acquisition weakness and a performance weakness. It is an acquisition weakness in that his expressive language skills, particularly nonliteral language skills, need to be improved. However, he has adequate language skills to initiate basic conversation and sustain a brief conversation at an age-appropriate level. Joe has learned to avoid group activities and conversations with others, which seems to reduce anxiety. He perseverates during conversation, argues, and asks questions, which seem to be attempts to deal with unstructured situations, to increase clarity and purpose of tasks/situations, and to reduce anxiety. The latter three behaviors have increased social isolation and rejection from his peers, and even adults working with Joe find these behaviors irritating.

Functional Assessment Observations

Direct observation of social skill problems in naturalistic settings is one of the most useful tools for treatment planning (Gresham, 2001). This method of assessment was used to directly inform the clinician(s) who will work with Joe regarding the specific nature, antecedents, and sustaining consequences of the behavior. Similar to the behavior rating scales, which provide normative data, the functional assessment was also conducted using a "typical" comparison peer, to help determine the extent of Joe's difficulties relative to other peers in his actual social setting. Functional assessment observations were conducted at school on two separate days. One assessment was conducted during a lunch period, and the other was conducted during a class period. Two sets of behaviors were observed, which encompassed the five target behaviors described in the FAI: (1) social engagement (i.e., initiation of social conversation, voluntary participation in social groups, and acceptance of social overtures from peers); (2) controlling behaviors (i.e., perseveration on a topic or ignoring prompts to change topic, asking excessive questions, and arguing with peers/adults).

During the first observation period (lunch), Joe transitioned to the cafeteria on his own, without initiating conversation, and sat alone. Another peer sat close to him, but neither boy acknowledged the other. On the walk back to class, another boy said "Hello" to Joe and he responded with "Hi," but did not continue the conversation. In contrast, the peer comparison was engaged in conversation during transition to the cafeteria and sat with a group of three other boys. They shared conversation throughout the lunch period. The peer comparison left the lunchroom before his group of friends and transitioned to the next class on his own. During the walks to and from class, Joe did not initiate conversation or join a group of peers. A classmate walked next to Joe for several paces, but Joe did not respond. Joe's peer comparison walked to and from class with the same peer. On the way to class, they were finishing their conversation from lunch; and after class, they walked next to each other without talking. During the classroom observation period, the students were instructed to get into their pre-formed groups to continue work on a group project. During the group project, Joe was called on to describe his progress. He was quite perseverative in his description of what he had learned, and ignored two attempts at redirection from the group members. Joe was argumentative when he was asked more directly to stop his contribution. In contrast, the peer comparison shared his contribution in the group and participated appropriately.

The 50-minute school periods were broken down into 10-minute intervals. A point was given for both sets of behaviors for each 10-minute interval in which they occurred. The total percent time voluntarily engaged in social interactions and total percent time engaged in controlling behaviors was calculated for both Joe and his "typical" classmate. Across the 12 10-minute intervals, Joe was voluntarily socially engaged 8% of the time, while his peer was voluntarily socially engaged 50% of the time. Across the 12 intervals, Joe exhibited controlling behaviors 25% of the time compared to 8% for the peer's behavior.

ETHICAL AND LEGAL COMPLICATIONS

Legal issues were not directly related to this case. The primary ethical consideration in this case was confidentiality. For this reason, behavior observations were done in a highly discrete manner. Consent from the parent and assent from the child were obtained prior to the assessment. When consent for observation was obtained for the typical peer, Joe's identifying information was not disclosed.

Further, the identifying information for this case was changed so as not to breech the confidentiality of the client involved.

CONCEPTUALIZATION AND TREATMENT RECOMMENDATIONS

Joe is a 13-and-a-half-year-old male with long-standing academic, emotional, and social concerns. He was referred for a comprehensive neuropsychological and social skills evaluation to assist with educational and social treatment planning. Specific assessment of Joe's social skills pointed to two primary areas of social skill deficits: (1) social engagement (i.e., initiation of social conversation, voluntary participation in social groups, and acceptance of social overtures from peers); (2) controlling behaviors (i.e., perseveration on a topic or ignoring prompts to change topic, asking excessive questions, and arguing with peers/adults). Joe is significantly more likely than his peers to avoid social situations and to reject social overtures. He also struggles once engaged in social interactions, especially with expressive language demands, which makes him frustrated and anxious. Further, he engages in controlling behaviors (e.g., arguing, persisting with a topic despite cues for redirection, and asking many questions), presumably to reduce the ambiguity of the situation and to reduce anxiety. Joe also lacks more effective and socially acceptable means of structuring social situations. He needs help in relaxing during social situations, and he can be taught more effective means of structuring and decreasing the ambiguity of social situations. The better he becomes at reading social cues and understanding social language, the less overwhelming and anxiety producing social situations will be. Based on these findings, the following social skills recommendations were made.

1. Joe should obtain speech-language therapy to improve his ability to understand both nonverbal and verbal communication. Speech-language therapy should be integrated with social skills training. Scripts for initiating social conversations or for receiving social overtures can be practiced.
2. Social skills training should take place in a group setting. Those working with Joe can help facilitate newly learned material in naturalistic settings because generalization of skills is often problematic (Berler et al., 1982).
3. At school, Joe should be placed in groups with peers who will be tolerant of his behaviors and who will encourage him to interact socially. Joe's teachers should monitor Joe's group participation carefully and facilitate social interactions and socially acceptable behavior.
4. Those working with Joe on social skills will need to be aware of *Clinically Significant* levels of Anxiety and persistent symptoms of Depression. These symptoms typically manifest themselves in perfectionism, performance anxiety, low frustration tolerance, sadness, and emotional lability.
5. Joe's psychiatrist and psychologists should assess his current medication and therapeutic interventions and work in conjunction with those administering

social skills training and speech-language therapy. Strategies for increasing frustration tolerance and self-esteem should be generated and implemented.

6. Joe should be encouraged to continue his interest in guitar and to seek out other activities that interest him. Participation in activities outside of school, particularly group activities, will facilitate peer relationships and increase his self-esteem.

SUMMARY

Recent advances in assessment have produced a vast array of tools for researchers and practitioners to choose from when treating children with social skills deficits. However, it is critical that there be a connection between the research literature and clinical application. This chapter sought to assist researchers and clinicians in how to reliably and accurately assess, conceptualize, and treat children with social skills deficits. We outlined recommendations for social skills assessments and described the research basis and clinical utility of each method. In particular, naturalistic observations and behavioral rating scales were identified as primary assessment choices, and interviewing and sociometric strategies were suggested as important secondary choices. We also discussed key developmental considerations and the assessment, conceptualization, and treatment planning involved with treating children with social skills deficits. Finally, we provided a case study to illustrate the assessing of a child with social skills problems. By presenting a comprehensive framework of social skills assessment, we hope to bridge the gap between research and clinical practice to successfully treat children with behavioral difficulties.

REFERENCES AND RESOURCES

Alexander, K. L., Entwisle, D. R., & Dauber, S. L. (1993). First-grade classroom behavior: Its short- and long-term consequences for school performance. *Child Development, 64,* 801–814.

Berler, E. S., Gross, A. M., & Drabman, R. S. (1982). Social skills training with children: Proceed with caution. *Journal of Applied Behavior Analysis, 15,* 41–53.

Blair, C. (2002). School readiness: Integrating cognition and emotion in a neurobiological conceptualization of children's functioning at school entry. *American Psychologist, 57,* 111–127.

Bronson, M. B. (1994). The usefulness of an observational measure of young children's social and mastery behaviors in early childhood classrooms. *Early Childhood Research Quarterly, 9,* 19–43.

Bronson, M. B. (1996). *Manual for the Bronson Social and Task Skill Profile (teacher version).* Chestnut Hill, MA: Boston College.

Bronson, M. B., Tivnan, T., & Seppanen, P. S. (1995). Relations between teacher and classroom activity variables and the classroom behaviors of prekindergarten children in Chapter 1 funded programs. *Journal of Applied Developmental Psychology, 16,* 253–282.

Carrow-Woolfolk, E. (1999). *Comprehensive assessment of spoken language.* Circle Pines, MN: American Guidance Service.

Ceci, S. J., & Bruck, M. (1998). Children's testimony: Applied and basic issues. In W. Damon (Series Ed.), I. Sigel, K. Renninger (Vol. Eds.), *Handbook of child psychology: Vol. 4. Child psychology in practice* (5th ed., pp. 713–774). New York: John Wiley & Sons.

Coie, J. D., & Dodge, K. A. (1998). Aggression and antisocial behavior. In W. Damon (Series Ed.) & N. Eisenberg (Vol. Ed.), *Handbook of child psychology: Vol. 3. Social, emotional, and personality development* (5th ed., pp. 779–862). New York: John Wiley & Sons.

Cooper, D. H., & Farran, D. C. (1988). Behavioral risk factors in kindergarten. *Early Childhood Research Quarterly, 3,* 1–19.

Cooper, D. H., & Farran, D. C. (1991). *The Cooper–Farran Behavioral Rating Scales.* Brandon, VT: Clinical Psychology Publishing Co.

DeRosier, M. E., Kupersmidt, J. B., & Patterson, C. J. (1994). Children's academic and behavioral adjustment as a function of the chronicity and proximity of peer rejection. *Child Development, 65,* 1799–1813.

Dishion, T. J. (1990). The family ecology of boys' peer relations in middle childhood. *Child Development, 61,* 874–892.

Dodge, K. A., Lansford, J. E., Burks, V. S., Bates, J. E., Petit, G. S., Fontaine, R., & Price, J. M. (2003). Peer rejection and social information-processing factors in the development of aggressive behavior problems in children. *Child Development, 74,* 374–393.

Elliott, S. N., & Busse, R. T. (1991). Social skills assessment and intervention with children and adolescents: Guidelines for assessment and training procedures. *School Psychology International, 12,* 63–83.

Elliott, S. N., Sheridan, S. M., & Gresham, F. M. (1989). Assessing and treating social skills deficits: A case study for the scientist-practitioner. *Journal of School Psychology, 27,* 197–222.

Foulks, B., & Morrow, R. D. (1989). Academic survival skills for the young child at risk for school failure. *Journal of Educational Research, 82,* 158–165.

Gottlieb, G., Wahlsten, D., & Lickliter, R. (1998). The significance of biology for human development: A developmental psychobiological systems view. In W. Damon (Series Ed.) & R. M. Lerner (Vol. Ed.), *Handbook of child psychology: Vol. 1. Theoretical models of human development* (5th ed., pp. 233–273). New York: John Wiley & Sons.

Gresham, F. M. (1988). Social skills: Conceptual and applied aspects of assessment, training, and social validation. In J. C. Witt, S. N. Elliott, & F. M. Gresham (Eds.), *Handbook of behavior therapy in education.* New York: Plenum Press.

Gresham, F. M. (2001). Assessment of social skills in children and adolescents. In J. J. Andrews, D. H. Saklofske, & H. L. Janzen (Eds.), *Handbook of psychoeducational assessment: Ability, achievement, and behavior in children* (pp. 325–355). San Diego, CA: Academic Press.

Gresham, F. M., & Elliott, S. N. (1990). *Social Skills Rating System.* Circle Pines, MN: American Guidance Service.

Gresham, F. M., & Lambros, K. M. (1998). Behavioral and functional assessment. In T. Watson & F. Gresham (Eds.), *Handbook of child behavior therapy* (pp. 3–22). New York: Plenum Press.

Kratochwill, T. R., Sheridan, S. M., Carlson, J., & Lasecki, K. (1999). Advances in behavioral assessment. In C. R. Reynolds & T. B. Gutkin (Eds.), *The handbook of school psychology* (3rd ed., pp. 350–382). New York: John Wiley & Sons.

Ladd, G. W. (1990). Having friends, keeping friends, making friends, and being liked by peers in the classroom: Predictors of children's early school adjustment? *Child Development, 61,* 1081–1100.

Matson, J. L., & Ollendick, T. H. (1988). *Enhancing children's social skills: Assessment and training.* New York: Pergamon Press.

McClelland, M. M., Kessenich, M., & Morrison, F. J. (2003). Pathways to early literacy: The complex interplay of child, family, and sociocultural factors. In R. V. Kail & H. W. Reese (Eds.), *Advances in child development and behavior: Vol. 31* (pp. 411–447). New York: Academic Press.

McClelland, M. M., & Morrison, F. J. (2003). The emergence of learning-related social skills in preschool children. *Early Childhood Research Quarterly, 18,* 206–224.

McClelland, M. M., Morrison, F. J., & Acock, A. C. (2005). *The impact of kindergarten learning-related social skills on academic trajectories at the end of elementary school.* Manuscript submitted for publication.

McClelland, M. M., Morrison, F. J., & Holmes, D. H. (2000). Children at-risk for early academic problems: The role of learning-related social skills. *Early Childhood Research Quarterly, 15,* 307–329.

McFall, R. M. (1982). A review and reformulation of the concept of social skills. *Behavioral Assessment, 4,* 1–33.

Meier, V. J., & Hope, D. A. (1998). Assessment of social skills. In A. S. Bellack & M. Hersen (Eds.), *Behavioral assessment: A practical handbook* (4th ed., pp. 232–255). Boston: Allyn & Bacon.

Merrell, K. W. (1993). *School social behavior scales.* Austin, TX: Pro-Ed.

Merrell, K. W. (1999). *Behavioral, social, and emotional assessment of children and adolescents.* Mahwah, NJ: Erlbaum.

Merrell, K. W. (2001). Assessment of children's social skills: Recent developments, best practices, and new directions. *Exceptionality, 9,* 3–18.

Miller, S. A. (1998). *Developmental research methods.* Upper Saddle River, NY: Prentice-Hall.

Nelson, R. O., & Hayes, S. C. (Eds.). (1986). *Conceptual foundations of behavioral assessment.* New York: Guilford Press.

Raver, C. C. (2002). Emotions matter: Making the case for the role of young children's emotional development for early school readiness. *Social Policy Report, 16,* 3–18.

Reynolds, C. R., & Kamphaus, R. W. (1992). *Behavioral Assessment System for Children.* Circle Pines, MN: American Guidance Service.

Rimm-Kaufman, S. E., Pianta, R. C., & Cox, M. J. (2000). Teachers' judgments of problems in the transition to kindergarten. *Early Childhood Research Quarterly, 15,* 147–166.

Sheridan, S. M., & Elliott, S. N. (1991). Behavioral consultation as a process for linking the assessment and treatment of social skills. *Journal of Educational and Psychological Consultation, 2,* 151–173.

Shonkoff, J. P., & Phillips, D. A. (Eds.). (2000). *From neurons to neighborhoods: The science of early childhood development.* Washington, DC: National Academy Press.

Torgrud, L. J., & Holborn, S. W. (1992). Developing externally valid role-play for assessment of social skills: A behavior analytic perspective. *Behavioral Assessment, 14,* 245–277.

Van Hasselt, V. B., Hersen, M., & Bellack, A. S. (1981). The validity of role play tests for assessing social skills in children. *Behavior Therapy, 12,* 202–216.

Walker, H. M., & McConnell, S. R. (1995a). *Walker–McConnell Scale of Social Competence and School Adjustment: Elementary version.* San Diego, CA: Singular.

Walker, H. M., & McConnell, S. R. (1995b). *Walker–McConnell Scale of Social Competence and School Adjustment: Adolescent version.* San Diego, CA: Singular.

Walker, H. M., & Severson, H. H. (1992). *Systematic screening for behavior disorders.* Longmont, CO: Sopris West.

Walker, H. M., Severson, H. H., Nicholson, F., Kehle, T., et al. (1994). Replication of the Systematic Screening for Behavior Disorders (SSBD) procedure for the identification of at-risk children. *Journal of Emotional and Behavioral Disorders, 2,* 66–77.

Wechsler, D. (2003). *Wechsler Intelligence Scale for Children* (4th ed.). San Antonio, TX: Psychological Corporation.

14

Alcohol and Drug Abuse

Brad C. Donohue
Jennifer Karmely
Marilyn J. Strada

Department of Psychology
University of Nevada, Las Vegas, Nevada

INTRODUCTION

According to a recent survey by the United States Department of Health and Human Services (Johnston, O'Malley, Bachman, & Schulenberg, 2004), the use of alcohol and illicit drugs among adolescents in America appears to be on the decline. The prevalence of substance use in the adolescent population, however, remains relatively high, as compared with most mental health–related disorders. For instance, according the United States Centers for Disease Control (CDC, 2003), 45% of the adolescent population reported having used alcohol during the past 30 days, and 75% reported alcohol use at least once during their lifetime. Twenty-two percent of youth reported marijuana use during the past 30 days, and 40% reported having used marijuana. Lifetime use of the comparatively less prevalent "hard drugs" (i.e., illicit drugs other than marijuana) also continues to be relatively high (about 5% to 9%), with past 30-day use of most hard drugs being around 2% to 5%. Aarons, Brown, Hough, Garland, and Wood (2001) found similar consumption rates, with about a quarter of their youth sample evidencing criteria for either substance abuse or substance dependence.

According to the *Diagnostic and Statistical Manual of Mental Disorders* (DSM-IV-TR; APA, 2000), alcohol and drug abuse are each diagnosed when at least one of the following occur: (a) substance use interferes with responsibilities at home or work, (b) use of substance in hazardous situations, (c) use results in legal problems, and (d) continuing to use substance despite recurring problems related to use. Substance dependence is more severe than substance abuse and includes hallmark biological symptoms of tolerance and withdrawal. Tolerance occurs when the adolescent requires increasing amounts of the respective substance to experience intoxication. Some substances lead to extremely quick development of tolerance (e.g., cocaine may lead to tolerance after only one dosage), which assists in biologically protecting youth from potential fatalities resulting from overdose. Conversely, withdrawal occurs when uncomfortable, and potentially dangerous, physiological symptoms occur consequent to the abrupt decrease or cessation of intake of the respective substance. Each substance or class of substances (e.g., amphetamines, benzodiazapines, barbiturates) will elicit particular withdrawal symptoms. For instance, withdrawal symptoms for alcohol, a central nervous system depressant, often include anxiety, tremors, increased blood pressure, and potential strokes. Other DSM-IV-TR symptoms of dependence include (a) unintended increase in amount and frequency of use, (b) unsuccessful attempts to reduce or eliminate use, (c) spending a significant amount of time obtaining, using, and recovering from the substance, (d) significant decrease in accustomed activities, and (e) continued use despite negative mental and physical health symptoms that are influenced by the substance. Thus, adolescent substance abuse is a widespread and significant problem necessitating empirically validated assessment and treatment methods.

The assessment of substance abuse and dependence is complicated. For instance, these disorders consistently present with severe behavioral problems (e.g., academic problems, disengagement from school, family and former peers, loss of interest or functioning in extracurricular activities, relationship problems with family and authority figures) and psychiatric disorders (Conduct Disorder, Oppositional Defiant Disorder, Major Depression and Dysthymia, Attention-Deficit Hyperactivity Disorder; Garland et al., 2001; Kennedy, 1993). Moreover, these youth (and sometimes their family) are very often not motivated to engage in the assessment process and are notoriously poor informants.

This chapter describes various behavioral assessment procedures and strategies that are appropriate for use in substance-abusing and -dependent youth, including their research support and clinical utility. A behavioral conceptualization of substance abuse will occur within the context of assessment, including a systematic method of utilizing assessment results in the process of treatment planning. As will be emphasized, the assessment of adolescent substance abuse and substance dependence is a comprehensive process that includes psychological evaluation of various comorbid disorders and related problems. From the point of initial contact with the family, assessment is ongoing and may occur in a variety of settings, including outpatient and inpatient medical facilities, homes, psychiatric hospitals, psychological practices, detention centers, and correctional facilities.

DESCRIPTION OF ASSESSMENT STRATEGIES

GENERAL OVERVIEW OF ASSESSMENT PROCESS AND STRUCTURE

Initial Telephone Contact with Youth and Parent

Although substance-abusing and -dependent youth are often referred to treatment programs by school or court representatives, the first contact with the family typically occurs in a telephone call with the legal guardian. During this initial interaction the appropriateness of the referral is determined with the parent, and a session is potentially scheduled to occur with the referred youth and relevant family members. Attendance at the initial scheduled session in this population is often less than 50% (Gariti et al., 1995), delaying assessment and leading to poor outcomes (Matas, Staley, & Griffin, 1992). Interestingly, however, assessing both the parent and youth two or three days prior to the initial scheduled session for 10–15 minutes about the nature and success of the program, briefly assessing their perspectives on the presenting problem, providing empathy, reviewing benefits of program participation, problem solving potential obstacles to attending the session, and reviewing specific directions to the facility have been found to increase initial session attendance 29%, relative to a less involved control group (Donohue et al., 1998). The aforementioned study also demonstrated similar attendance improvement rates in subsequent sessions utilizing similar procedures.

Intake Session

The initial meeting with the youth and family is traditionally referred to as an intake session. The primary objectives in this session are to enlist family support and to gather a broad base of information to assist in identifying specific areas to assess in subsequent sessions. Clinical areas that are initially assessed include identifying the reasons for seeking treatment, past psychiatric and medical history and treatment (including medications), behavior problems and skills, family and peer support, developmental milestones, drug use/abuse history, and current mental status. In general, this session usually lasts up to 90 minutes, whereas remaining assessment sessions typically last about an hour. Although it is ideal to have the therapist who will eventually treat the family conduct the intake session, it may be more cost effective to have a trained paraprofessional with good enlistment skills implement this session. The assessment process may be expedited through the concurrent administration of standardized measures that can be completed either in the waiting room while a family member is being seen individually or during the wait prior to the session. The intake should ideally begin with a behavioral observation of the youth and family in the waiting area, including their manner of communication, posture, dress, hygiene, and seating arrangements. In general, we recommend you spend the initial part of this session assessing the reasons for referral with the entire family so that interactions can be observed while these issues are discussed and subsequently assess the youth and family separately to provide opportunities for family members to express themselves without potential interruption, arguments, or audience control. In doing so, the family should be asked to decide who should be seen individually first, and session time should be distributed equally for each family member. It is important to recognize that substance-abusing adolescents are almost always influenced to participate in the assessment process by their parents, academic administrators, or legal authorities. Therefore, these youth are likely to have preconceived ideas about how the information they provide may be used to enforce severe sanctions from others (e.g., academic suspension or expulsion, legal probation, discontinuance from employment, restriction of privileges at home). As such, they may be unmotivated to provide information about their use of substances and other problem behaviors. In these situations, more time should be spent with the youth establishing rapport by soliciting, and subsequently descriptively praising, their perspectives on the presenting problem, pro-social interests, activities with friends, strengths, and past achievements.

Although the specific protocol and organization of intake procedures differ among agencies, some procedures are essential. Indeed, a description of the assessment process should be fully delineated to the family, including the consequences of their providing consent to be assessed, the purpose of the assessment process, and how the obtained information will be used to conceptualize presenting concerns and to develop the treatment plan. Consent to conduct the assessment, including credentials of the treatment provider, hours of clinician availability and emergency contact information, duration of sessions, and procedures for canceling sessions, must be obtained from the legal guardian prior to conducting any assessment procedures. Although typically not legally required, study assent should be attempted to enlist youth in the assessment process, and, whenever possible, an attempt should be made to mutually determine what assessment information will be shared (e.g., parents may be provided urine test results), and what specific information will be confidential, as well as the specific exclusions to confidentiality that are mandated by law (e.g., danger to self or others, court orders).

The intake session should ideally conclude with an assessment of each participating family member's satisfaction with the assessment process so that potential concerns may be addressed. A business appointment card with agency contact information and time of the next mutually determined appointment should be provided to both the youth and the legal guardian. A routine 5-minute follow-up telephone call should be provided to both the parent and the youth within 24 hours of the session, to reinforce their participation, express positive qualities about their family, and answer any questions that may have been derived during the ride home. As already mentioned, these procedures have effectively been utilized to increase subsequent session attendance (Donohue et al., 1998).

First Behavioral Assessment Session

Depending on the nature, setting, and purpose of assessment, the first assessment session following intake is almost always performed by the therapist who will be later conducting treatment with the substance-abusing youth and family. These sessions usually include administration of various behavioral assessment methods (e.g., behavioral observation, role-plays, standardized inventories) and a clinical interview with the youth, and relevant family members, emphasizing areas that are pertinent to substance use as well as a comprehensive assessment of important domains that were briefly assessed during the intake session. Motivational interviewing techniques may be helpful in establishing rapport during the interview and in increasing the youth's motivation to provide relevant information (W. R. Miller & Rollnick, 2002). While the youth elaborates on presenting issues, the assessor expresses genuine empathy when distress is indicated and acknowledges obstacles that are mentioned in establishing abstinence from substances (i.e., "rolling with the resistance"). Questionnaires should be administered to augment clinical interviews during this session.

Second Behavioral Assessment Session

After data from the clinical interview and other measures are incorporated, the next assessment session should involve a detailed query of specific factors acting to maintain substance use (i.e., functional analysis). This procedure entails determining both the antecedent stimuli that trigger drug use and other problem behavior as well as consequences that act to reinforce these behaviors. The results of this assessment are directly relevant to treatment, as the assessor begins to formulate specific stimuli that will need to be replaced with competing repertoires and stimuli that are incompatible with drug use (Azrin, Donohue, Besalel, Kogan, & Acierno, 1994).

Third Behavioral Assessment Session

The third session generally marks the conclusion of formal assessment, dissemination of assessment results, and development of the treatment plan. Primary concerns are addressed, and assessment results are conveyed comprehensibly to the family. Because the parent and the youth often have very different treatment goals, it is sometimes prudent to report assessment findings to the youth and family separately. It is important to encourage questions and attempt to solicit potential concerns regarding the assessment results and to formalize treatment goals that are acceptable to the entire family.

Ongoing Behavioral Assessment Sessions

Behavioral assessment is ongoing and should be integrated within and between treatment sessions to monitor and guide treatment planning and to evaluate the effectiveness of treatment. For instance, youth can monitor stimuli (e.g., persons, places, activities) that put them at increased risk to use substances as well as those stimuli that put them at decreased risk. Later, associations with these stimuli can be reviewed to identify competing stimuli and to learn skills that may be utilized to decrease risk associated with drug and alcohol use. Thus, ongoing assessment may influence changes in treatment protocol or the level of care (i.e., can be intensified or reduced). Measures that were initially administered (e.g., questionnaires, urinalysis) are often readministered immediately prior to the start of some sessions, for results of these measures are often directly related to treatment goals, the appropriateness of treatment termination, and booster sessions.

GENERAL ASSESSMENT STRATEGIES

Assessment tools should be selected to yield unique information, unless data need to be confirmed or supported. These methods should also complement the reasons for referral. When there is uncertainty about the informant's accuracy and openness, which is often the case in adolescent substance abusers, "lie scales" should be employed that measure the youth's likelihood of denying pathology. These scales usually include content that reflects undesired behaviors that have been found to exist in most people (e.g., "I have stolen at least once in my lifetime," "I have told a lie more than once"). Therefore, denial of a significant number of these items is associated with attempts to present oneself in a favorable light, and greater likelihood of denying pathology (i.e., drug use). The negative interaction of substance-abusing adolescents with their community, coupled with the surreptitious nature underlying this disorder, necessitates a comprehensive assessment utilizing multiple assessment methods and informants (e.g., parents, teachers, probation officers, ministers, siblings, friends, coaches, physicians). Assessment methods most often include semistructured and structured interviews, standardized questionnaires, role-plays, behavioral observation, examination of professional records (e.g., school, court, medical, psychological), self-monitoring, and biological assessments to detect the presence of substances (e.g., urinalysis testing). It is also important to conduct assessment procedures across multiple settings, times, and situations. A complete medical exam is essential to identify potential effects of substance misuse and to assist in ruling out medical conditions that may mask, exacerbate, or mimic symptoms of drug or alcohol use, particularly if the youth reports symptoms that appear to be consistent with withdrawal or tolerance. Medical referrals to a physician or psychiatrist should also be made when the assessment indicates medication may be an appropriate component of the treatment plan (e.g., Ritalin for ADHD), and these referrals should be documented.

Establishing Rapport

Nonspecific factors related to the relationship between practitioners and their clients are essential to the therapeutic process (Chatoor & Krupnick, 2001) and may be particularly important among families that have been affected by substance abuse. Specific methods have been identified to facilitate rapport, including the incorporation of questions and statements that express interest in activities, hobbies, and relative strengths of the youth that may be rarely discussed at home. It may be helpful to distribute small token awards (e.g., candy bars, donuts, soda, costume jewelry) for attending sessions and actively participating in the assessment process. Complimenting youth consequent to their evidencing desired pro-social behaviors during therapy is a practical method of achieving rapport and revealing that their strengths are being considered along with their presenting problems. It is also important to remain neutral and nonjudgmental, for substance-abusing youth are often negatively judged by authority figures. Similarly, their parents may have a history of being blamed for contributing to the problems of these youth, leading to excessive defensiveness in responding to certain questions. Therefore, questions and statements should be phrased so that negative connotations for substance use and related problem behaviors are difficult to insinuate. For instance, instead of asking a youth to disclose the reasons drugs are used (e.g., "Why do you do drugs?"), the youth should be asked to disclose reinforcers that are derived consequent to drug use (e.g., "What are some positive things drug use is able to provide you?"). It is also prudent to refrain from expressing hypotheses or interpretations of the youth's behavior until the formal assessment is complete.

Assessment of Suicide

Substance-abusing and -dependent youth are at heightened risk to commit suicide, particularly when these youth are actively using central nervous system depressants (e.g., alcohol, barbiturates, opiates) or experiencing withdrawal symptoms consequent to the cessation of intake of central nervous system stimulants (e.g., cocaine, amphetamines; Maskey, Crown, & Oyebode, 2004; Rowan, 2001; Tapert, Colby, & Barnett, 2003). Therefore, an empirically validated plan for assessing suicidal ideation should be employed when evaluating these youth. Along these lines, it is first important to assess demographic indicators of suicide (i.e., being a male, 15–24 years old, Caucasian, low socioeconomic status, few social supports) and to utilize semistructured interviews to determine the presence of additional risk factors, such as a history of suicide attempts, a well-developed plan to commit suicide, intent, a means to commit suicide (e.g., pills, guns, knives; which are usually easy for substance-abusing youth to access), a lack of future orientation, social isolation, negative life events or significant stressors, chronic illness that is painful, a recent loss of a significant other, and use of alcohol or drugs. Other signs include persistently flat affect, negative self-appraisal, and problems with cognitive processing (i.e., disorganized, irrational, or psychotic thought patterns). Along these lines, it is important to recognize that many of these symptoms are sometimes elicited during intoxication. A counterintuitive risk factor for suicide is a rapid shift from severe depression to calm, elevated mood. Although many of these indicators are common in substance-abusing and -dependent youth in general, it should be clear that as the number and severity of these factors intensify, the risk of suicide is known to increase. If an adolescent is conservatively judged to be at risk to commit suicide, standardized inventories with normative data (e.g., Suicide Probability Scale; Cull & Gill, 1990) should be administered to provide a quantifiable assessment of risk and to assist in guiding the extent of protection that is warranted to ensure the adolescent's safety.

Assessment of Child Maltreatment

Child maltreatment is frequently indicated in substance-abusing and -dependent youth. Indeed, the majority of adolescent substance abusers have been abused or neglected by their parents (see Dennis & Stevens, 2003, for review), and the majority of perpetrators of child maltreatment have been identified to abuse substances (see Donohue, 2004). Therefore, child maltreatment is a salient issue in the assessment of adolescent substance abuse and is likely to be revealed in these families, if thoroughly assessed. However, like other professionals mandated to report child maltreatment to state authorities (CAPTA; U.S. Department of Health and Human Services, 2003), many substance abuse counselors avoid such assessment, for various reasons that are beyond the scope of this chapter (see Alvarez, Donohue, Kenny, Cavanagh, & Romero, 2004, for review). Regardless, mental health providers should be aware of the specific definitions of child abuse and neglect, including reporting policies and procedures, because they will inevitably assess child maltreatment, whether intended or not. To assist in this process, Donohue, Carpin, and Alvarez (2002) developed, and favorably evaluated utilizing a controlled design, a standardized method of diplomatically reporting child maltreatment to state authorities when indicated. This standardized process involves solicitation of concerns regarding the consequences of reporting child maltreatment with a nonperpetrating caregiver, informing the caregiver why the report must occur, involving the caregiver in the reporting process, determining the optimum method of informing the perpetrator that the report was performed, and an assessment of the safety of all family members living in the perpetrator's home, including the implementation of safety precautions.

BEHAVIORAL ASSESSMENT OF SUBSTANCE ABUSE AND DEPENDENCE

The primary purpose of the behavioral assessment of adolescent substance abuse and dependence is to identify and understand behaviors and thoughts that maintain substance use. Functional analysis is a critical component of behavioral assessment and has received greater empirical validation than its less directive counterparts (Haynes, 1998; Newcomer & Lewis, 2004). Consistent with the tenets of functional analysis, the "ABC" model is often utilized to assist in providing a framework in which to understand why substance use occurs (i.e., its "function"). In this model the "A" represents antecedent stimuli that precede the target behavior ("B," i.e., substance use), whereas the "C" represents consequences that occur after the target behavior is performed. In this way, behavior can be conceptualized to occur as a result of its interactions with environmental antecedents and consequences, which act to maintain the frequency of its occurrence. Thus substance use is maintained by antecedent stimuli that precede (e.g., drug-using friends, smell of marijuana) and follow (e.g., reduction of anxiety, pleasurable physiological sensations) its occurrence. Behavioral assessment is systems oriented and quite involved, because many stimuli interact across various environmental settings (e.g., school, home), times (e.g., early morning, late afternoon), and conditions (e.g., tired, rested) to influence the frequency of behavior. In therapy contexts, a comprehensive functional analysis consists of four stages: problem identification, problem analysis, intervention, and progress assessment. *Problem identification* entails gathering all available information regarding the presenting problems through a variety of clinical activities, including the examination of patient records, obtaining background information, interviewing, standardized self-report measures, self-report monitoring, behavioral observation, and role-playing. *Problem analysis*, the consolidation of all information obtained in the problem identification phase, is employed to prioritize problems and establish an outline of the behavioral chain of events leading to substance use and other targeted problems. Examination of the behavioral chain is often used to identify which *interventions* will likely disrupt the problem behavior (i.e., substance use). The final phase entails readministering relevant *assessment* measures throughout therapy to establish treatment efficacy and make necessary alterations in the treatment plan (the measures of which are considered behavioral progress indicators in this phase). The functional analysis is reviewed more fully later in this chapter to demonstrate how behavioral assessment may be utilized to conceptualize substance abuse and to develop a standardized treatment plan.

RESEARCH BASIS

Behavioral assessment is heavily grounded in research, in terms of both its reliance on reliable and valid measures as well as its objectivity in determining case success. Indeed, two key components of research are (a) peer replication of assessment procedures and (b) the dissemination of quantified results obtained through standardized assessment procedures. Although behavioral therapy has historically relied on objective behavioral measures, it is becoming increasingly evident that various standardized self-report measures of substance use patterns as well as relevant measures of thoughts and satisfaction have been found to closely correspond with objective biological indicators of substance use. The former measures are easily administered to assist in determining treatment efficacy, necessary effect sizes, and optimal course of treatment. However, relative to the objective behavioral measures, assessment results derived from self-report must be interpreted with particular caution, for adolescent substance abusers and their families are often exposed to environmental factors that may influence them to distort their reports.

As indicated in extensive reviews of the assessment literature involving adolescent substance abusers (e.g., Winters, Latimer, & Stinchfield, 2001), dozens of psychometrically supported assessment measures for adolescent substance abuse now exist. Some of these standardized measures are listed in Table 14.1, along with their supporting information and application.

Structured and Semistructured Interviews

Structured interviews have excellent psychometric support and are particularly effective in establishing substance abuse diagnoses in research settings or in clinics in which reliable diagnostic information is critical (e.g., forensic or court settings). A structured interview comprises a prearranged set of questions to be administered in a prearranged and specific order. An example of a commonly utilized structured interview is the Structured Clinical Interview for DSM-IV (SCID-IV; Spitzer, Williams, & Gibbon, 1990). The SCID-IV includes a diagnostic assessment of prevalent disorders, including substance abuse (i.e., section E) and has been utilized in controlled trials funded by the National Institutes of Health to reliably diagnose youths as substance-abusing and -dependent youths (e.g., Azrin, Donohue, & Teichner, 2001). During implementation of structured interviews, clinicians are instructed to read questions verbatim and to record answers according to the standard response formats (e.g., Likert scales). In "semistructured" interview formats, the interviewer is permitted to choose which questions will be utilized among a prearranged set of questions. The interviewer is free to query additional questions or to modify the method of inquiry to some extent. Thus, these interviews have less psychometric support than their structured counterparts, but they offer greater flexibility.

Measures of Substance Use

The mechanisms for quantifying the frequency and duration of substance use include both standardized self-report procedures and biological substance–detection methods. Perhaps the most psychometrically validated measure of substance use frequency is the Timeline Followback procedure (TLFB; Sobell & Sobell, 1996). In this procedure, the substance abuser is presented with a calendar that goes back in time up to 4–6 months. The calendar initially includes significant experiences that are relatively common (e.g., holidays). The substance abuser is then instructed to add memorable activities and events that have personal significance (e.g., birthdays, parties, sporting events) to the calendar in the appropriate dates. The recorded events and activities serve to anchor memories of substance use occurring in the assessed time period. The youth is subsequently queried to record the days in which particular substances were used in the calendar, including the specific amounts. Thus, this method offers great clinical utility, because it permits an assessment of substance use patterns in association with significant activities and events during the assessed months. Reliability and validity of the TLFB are excellent (Donohue et al., 2004; see Sobell & Sobell,

1996). Although adolescent TLFB reports of the frequency of marijuana and "hard drugs" have evidenced significant correlations with objective urinalysis tests in controlled clinical trials involving adolescent substance abusers (e.g., Azrin, Donohue, et al., 1994; Azrin, McMahon, et al., 1994), this procedure is particularly influenced by self-report biases. Indeed, youth may have a tendency to deny "hard drug" use, relative to marijuana or alcohol use, because these youth are typically not criticized for their use of the latter substances, as compared with hard drugs. Therefore, a useful strategy to increase the likelihood of detection of drug use in adolescents, particularly hard drug use, is to administer the TLFB to parents regarding their recollections of adolescent substance use (Donohue et al., 2004).

Illicit drugs and alcohol are metabolized in the kidneys. Therefore, the by-products or metabolites of these substances can be detected through analysis of the breath, urine, blood, and hair follicles consequent to use (Baselt, 2002). These analyses can be broad screens of multiple substances or single assay tests of specific substances. The window of detection varies according to the metabolic rate of the specific substance. For instance, marijuana, which is fat soluble, can usually be detected in urinalysis testing up to 2 or 3 weeks in most adolescents of average activity level and weight, whereas alcohol, a water-soluble substance, is usually impossible to detect after a day. Most hard drugs (e.g., cocaine, LSD, MDMA, benzodiazapines) are also difficult to detect a few days after use. Other problems related to detection of substances via biological testing procedures, include the youth's utilization of techniques to avoid detection (i.e., using the abused substance outside the known window of detection if testing is relatively infrequent and routine, putting cleansing agents into the urine sample if administration is unmonitored, ingesting water excessively prior to testing, ingesting agents that are known to invalidate detection procedures, of which some are undetectable, substituting urine if administration is unmonitored). Relative to the use of illicit drugs, urine-testing procedures remain the most cost-effective option in biological detection procedures, particularly when analyzed by the service provider (i.e., "stick test"). However, breathalyzer tests (i.e., breathing into a tube to determine the presence or absence of use) are the most cost-effective test of alcohol, and these tests are widely employed by law enforcement officers to assist in determining alcohol intoxication. The breathalyzer is also less invasive than other biological testing procedures, particularly blood tests. The window of detection for hair follicle tests of illicit drug use may be up to three or four months, although these tests have difficulty reliably determining when the drug use occurred and are relatively expensive. It is important to utilize biological tests frequently if resources permit (or to test randomly) and to maintain strict monitoring of the youth during collection procedures. When the youth reports difficulties urinating, it may be helpful to encourage the youth to drink water and eat salted foods throughout the session and, while the youth attempts to urinate, to run water from the faucet, flush toilets, and wet the youth's hand.

TABLE 14.1 Measures of Adolescent Substance Abuse

Instrument	Assessment Domain/Purpose	Description	Administration	Psychometric Properties
Assessment of Alcohol Use				
Adolescent Alcohol Involvement Scale (AAIS) Mayer & Filstead, 1979	Indicates alcohol use frequency and degree of problem severity related to psychological functioning, social relations, and family living	Screening instrument 14 items Score range: 0–79 Score categories: nonuser/normal user, misuser, abuser/dependent Normed on youth ages 13–19 Copyright status unknown	Self-report, paper-and-pencil Individual or group admin. Admin. time: 5 min Scoring time: 10 min	Scores related to substance use diagnosis and youth's use according to parents and clinical assessments Internal consistency (IC) range: .55–.76
Adolescent Drinking Index (ADI) Harrell & Wirtz, 1999	Measures severity of drinking problem, as evidenced by psychological, physical, social symptoms and loss of control	Screening instrument 24 items Subscales: self-medicating drinking, rebellious drinking Normed on youth ages 12–17 Copyright-protected scale	Self-report, paper-and-pencil Individual or group admin. Admin. time: 5 min	IC: greater than .90; 2-week test–retest: .78 Moderate correlation with alcohol consumption level
Adolescent Obsessive-Compulsive Drinking Scale (A-OCDS) Deas, Roberts, Randall, & Anton, 2001	Identifies degree of craving and problem alcohol drinking, assesses presence of alcohol-related thoughts, distress about and resistance to obsessive thoughts, compulsive alcohol drinking	14 items For use with youth 14–20 years old Subscales: Irresistibility, Interference Copyright-protected scale	Self-report, paper-and-pencil Admin. time: 5 min	IC: .81 Differentiates between experimental and problem alcohol drinkers
Alcohol Expectancy Questionnaire—Adolescent Version (AEQ-A) Brown, Christiansen, Goldman, & Inn, 1980	Provides insight into adolescents' perceived reinforcements from alcohol use and possible factors that help maintain alcohol consumption	90 items Expectancies measured: global positive effects (i.e., social behavior change, improvement of cognitive/motor abilities, sexual enhancement, increase arousal, relaxation/tension reduction) and	Self-report, paper-and-pencil or computer version Admin. time: 20–30 min	IC for all scales: range .37–.81 Drinking consumption negatively related to negative expectancies and positively related to positive expectancies

		negative expectancy of cognitive and behavioral functioning Normed on youth 12–19 years old Free use of this copyright-protected scale is allowed by test developers		
Rutgers Alcohol Problem Index (RAPI) White & Labouvie, 1989	Assesses impact of alcohol use on family life, social relations, psychological functioning, delinquency, physical problems, and neuropsychological functioning	Screening instrument 23 items Score range: 0–69 Normed on youth ages 14–18 (clinical sample mean scores range: 21–25; nonclinical sample scores range: 5–8) Public-domain scale	Self-report, paper-and-pencil Admin. time: 10 min Scoring time: 3 min	IC: .92 Relation between heavy alcohol users and diagnosis of substance use disorders: r = .75–.95 3-year stability coefficient: .40
Assessment of Drug Use				
Adolescent Drug Abuse Diagnosis (ADAD) Friedman & Utada, 1989	Assesses youth's experiences, attitudes, feelings, behaviors related to drug and alcohol use	Structured interview 150 items Modeled after ASI adult version Domains: medical, school, employment, social, family, psychological, legal, alcohol, and drug use Shorter form with 83 items available Public-domain scale	Self-report Score category: no problem, slight, moderate, considerable, extreme problem	Interrater reliability: range .85–.97 Test–retest reliability: .71
Adolescent Drug Involvement Scale (ADIS) Moberg & Hahn, 1991	Measures drug use problem severity in same manner as AAIS	Screening instrument 13 items Score range: 0–98 Public-domain scale	Self-report, paper-and-pencil Individual or group admin. Admin. time: 5 min Scoring time: 2 min	IC: .85 Good validity (r = .72 with self-reported levels of drug use, r = .79 with youth's perceived drug use severity

(continues)

TABLE 14.1 *(continued)*

Instrument	Assessment Domain/Purpose	Description	Administration	Psychometric Properties
Circumstances, Motivation, Readiness, and Suitability Scales (CMRS) De Leon, Melnick, Kressel, & Jainchill, 1994	Predicts perceived degree of circumstantial pressures to enter and leave treatment, motivation to change, and readiness for treatment	25 items Scales: external votivation, internal motivation, readiness for treatment, perceived appropriateness of the treatment modality Copyright-protected scale	Self-report Admin. time: 5–10 min	IC: range .77–.80 Predict short-term retention
Drug Use Screening Inventory–Revised (DUSI-R) Tarter, 1990	Measures involvement and severity of drug-related problems, current status; identifies prevention areas; can be used as treatment-outcome measure	Screening instrument 159 items Score range: 0–100% for severity of the disorder Subscales: Substance Abuse, Psychiatric Disorder, Behavior Problems, School Problems, Health Status, Work Adjustment, Peer Relations, Social Competency, Family Adjustment, Leisure/Recreation, Lie (validity scale) Normed on youth ages 10–16 Copyright-protected scale	Self-report, paper-and-pencil Individual interview or self-administered computer version. Admin. time: 20 min Scoring time: 10 min or 0 for computer version	Drug users score higher than nondrug users (Kirisci, Mezich, & Tarter, 1995)
Personal Experience Screening Questionnaire (PESQ) Winters, 1992	Determines need for further assessment and provides overview of drug use history and psychosocial problems	Screening instrument 40 items Subscales: Problem Severity, Drug Use History, Select Psychosocial Problems, Response Distortion Tendencies (validity scale) Normed on normal, juvenile offenders, and drug-abusing youth ages 12–18 Copyright-protected scale	Self-report, paper-and-pencil Admin. time: 10 min Scoring time: 10 min	Accuracy rate of predicting need to assess further: 87%

Assessment of Substance Use				
Adolescent Diagnostic Interview (ADI) Winters & Henley, 1993	Assesses for symptoms of psychoactive substance use, obtains sociodemographic information, substance use history, psychosocial functioning and stressors, school and interpersonal functioning, and cognitive functioning	Structured interview format 213 questions Appropriate for ages 12–18 Copyright-protected scale	Self-report Admin. time: 50 min	Interrater agreement: kappa = .66–.96 Test–retest reliability: kappa = .53–.79 Concurrent and criterion validity
Client Substance Index (CSI) Moore, 1983	Assesses for symptoms of substance dependence based on Jellinek's model	Screening instrument 113 items Score categories: no problem, misuse and abuse of substances, chemical dependency Copyright status unknown	Self-report, paper-and-pencil Short form, CSI-S normed on juvenile offenders, with 15 items available (Thomas, 1990)	Discriminates between clinical and nonclinical samples
Customary Drinking and Drug Use Record (CDDR) Brown et al., 1998	Measures current and lifetime alcohol and other drug use consumption, diagnostic criteria for substance dependence symptoms and severity of problems related to alcohol and drug use.	Structured interview format Domains: Level of involvement, withdrawal, characteristics, psychological/behavioral dependence symptoms, and negative consequences Public-domain scale	Self-report Admin. time: 15–30 min	Convergence with Time-Line Follow Back, $r = .68–.74$ IC: .72–.94 Test–retest: .70–.92

(*continues*)

TABLE 14.1 *(continued)*

Instrument	Assessment Domain/Purpose	Description	Administration	Psychometric Properties
Life Satisfaction Scale for Problem Youth (LSSPY) Donohue et al., 2003	Assesses degree of satisfaction with various aspects of life	12 items Assessment domains: friendships, family, school, employment/work, fun activities, appearance, sex life/dating, use of drugs, use of alcohol, money/material possessions, transportation, control over one's life Score range: 0–100%	Self-report Paper-and-pencil form Admin. time: <1 min Scoring time: <1 min	IC: Cronbach's alpha: .74 Significantly correlated with relevant measures; predictor of overall life satisfaction
National Institute of Mental Health Diagnostic Interview Schedule for Children (NIMH DISC-IV) Shaffer, Fisher, Lucas, Dulcan, & Schwab-Stone, 2000	Obtains information from both parent and child to assess for the presence of symptoms related to 30 psychiatric disorders (including substance use disorders), experienced over the past 4 weeks to 12 months	Structured interview Approximately 3000 questions for entire interview Versions: Parent version (DISC-P) for children 6–17 years old; child/adolescent version (DISC-Y) for ages 9–17 Information can be interpreted combined or separately Spanish version available	Self-report and collateral report Computer version available Admin. time: 70 min with nonclinical interviewees, 90–120 min with known substance abusers Interview administration training needed	Psychometric properties of DISC-IV substance use scale have not been examined, but information available for prior versions of the instrument
Parent Satisfaction with Youth Scale (PSYS) Donohue, DeCato, Azrin, & Teichner, 2001	Assesses parents' degree of satisfaction with their youth	11 items Behavioral domains: communication, friends and activities, curfew, household rules, school work, response to rewards, response to discipline, chores, alcohol use, drug use, illegal behavior, overall happiness with youth Score range: 0–100% happiness	Self-report Paper-and-pencil form Admin. time: 5 min Scoring time: 3 min	IC: Cronbach's alpha: .84 Interitem correlation: .35 Item-total correlation: median .59, mean item-total correlation: .54 Significantly correlated with relevant measures

Personal Experience Inventory (PEI) Winters & Henly, 1989	Provides comprehensive, standardized assessment of problems related to substance use	276 items Subscales: Substance use problem severity, substance use onset/frequency, personal and environmental risk and protective factors, school problems, family problems, psychiatric disorders, validity of responses Normed on youth ages 12–18 Spanish version available Copyright-protected scale	Self-report, paper-and-pencil Admin. time: 45–60 min Manual or computerized scoring	IC: .70–.97 Relation between PEI and other related scales (i.e., AAIS, Alcohol Dependence Scale) range from .35 to .87
Problem Oriented Screening Instrument for Teenagers (POSIT) Rahdert, 1991	Identifies need for further assessment of problem areas and treatment needs related to substance abuse, mental and physical health, and social relations	Screening instrument 139 items, of which 17 are specific to substance abuse Substance Abuse Scale Score Range: 0–17 Short version of 64 items available Spanish version available Public-domain scale	Self-report, paper-and-pencil Admin. time: 20–30 min Scoring time: 2–5 min if scored manually, 2 sec if scored in computer	Internal reliability: .94, differentiates between substance users and nonusers
Role-Play Test Donohue, Van Hasselt, Hersen, & Perrin, 1999	Assess substance refusal skills	Role-play format Four scenarios about drug and alcohol use. Responses are rated on 7-point scale (range: extremely unskilled to extremely skilled). Domains assessed: denies first offer to use substance, avoids going to place where substance is present, states why cannot/will not use substance, makes derogatory statement about substance use/involvement, suggests	Admin. time: 10 min	Performance ratings for molecular behaviors in the role-play scenarios are significantly correlated with overall ratings of performance

(*continues*)

TABLE 14.1 *(continued)*

Instrument	Assessment Domain/Purpose	Description	Administration	Psychometric Properties
		alternative activity, denies second offer to use substance, does not make plan to engage in substance use/activity later, concerned/neutral affect, speech fluency		
Structured Clinical Interview for the DSM Adapted for Adolescents (SCID) Martin, Kaczynski, Maisto, Bukstein, & Moss, 1995	Interview instrument to identify the presence or absence of substance use symptoms to make diagnosis	Structured interview Six self-contained modules, including substance use disorders, mood episodes, psychotic symptoms, psychotic disorders, mood disorders, anxiety, and adjustment disorder Computerized version available Available in Spanish, French, German, Danish, Italian, Hebrew, Zulu, Turkish, Portuguese, and Greek	Self-report Admin. time: 30–90 min with nonclinical interviewees, 60–120 min with clinical patients Can administer specific modules for areas of concern or relevant screening questions	Interrater reliability for alcohol DSM-IV symptoms: kappa range .84–1.0; for other substance use disorders: kappa range .82–1.0; for other substances in a 7- to 10-day test–retest interval: kappa .76
Substance Abuse Subtle Screening Inventory—Adolescent Form (SASSI-A) G. A. Miller, 1985	Identifies individuals who may have a substance use disorder	Screening instrument 81 items Score categories: chemical dependent, nonchemical dependent Subscales: face-valid alcohol, face-valid other drug, obvious attributes, subtle attributes, defensiveness Spanish version available Copyright-protected scale	Self-report, paper-and-pencil, computer version, optical scanning form, or audiotape version Individual or group admin. Admin. time: 15 min Scoring time: 5 min if scored manually	Scores related to MMPI scales Cutoff score related to diagnosis of substance use disorder Accuracy to identify substance abusers: 90%

Teen Addiction Severity Index (T-ASI) Kaminer, Bukstein, & Tarter, 1991	Indicates need for treatment and problem severity based on assessment of chemical use, school status, employment-support status, family relationships, legal status, peer-social relationships, and psychiatric status	Structured interview format 70 items Used in 13- to 18-year-olds Public-domain scale	Self-report Admin. time: 30–45 min Scoring time: 5 min if manual scoring, 1 min if computer scoring	Interrater agreement: .78
Timeline Followback (TLFB) Sobell & Sobell, 1996	Provides estimates of daily alcohol drinking and/or drug use	Semistructured interview 12-month calendar, with memory aids to help adolescent recall past alcohol and/or drug use Appropriate for ages 14 years and older Spanish, French, Swedish, Polish versions available Free use of this copyright-protected scale is allowed by test developers	Self-report, paper-and-pencil or computer version Admin. time: 10–30 min	Strong correlations with biological measures and collateral reports in adult samples and parent reports in adolescent samples for both alcohol and drug use up to 6 mo Good test–retest reliability
Youth Happiness with Parent Scale (YHPS) DeCato, Donohue, Azrin, & Teichner, 2001	Assesses adolescents' degree of satisfaction with their parents	11 items Behavioral domains: communication, friends and activities, curfew, household rules, school work, rewards, discipline, chores, alcohol use, drug use, illegal behavior, overall happiness with parent score range: 0–100% happiness	Self-report Paper-and-pencil form Admin. time: 5 min Scoring time: 3 min	IC: Cronbach's alpha: .78 Interitem correlation: .35 Interitem correlation:mean: .26 Median item-total correlation: .46; mean item-total correlation: .45

Standardized Inventories

Standardized behavioral rating scales and problem-behavior checklists include inventories of behaviors or traits (e.g., substance use, vandalism), which assess particular clinical domains (e.g., substance abuse, conduct disorders). These measures are usually administered in questionnaire "paper-and-pencil" formats, although computerized administration versions are sometimes available. Response options are usually Likert-type scales (e.g., 1 = extremely agree, 5 = extremely disagree) or dichotomous forced-choice options (e.g., yes or no, true or false). Administration procedures are standard, and scores are often compared to samples in the population at large that evidence similar demographics (e.g., age, gender). Thus, these self-report scales permit standard administration and objective interpretation of responses. There are numerous scales available for the assessment of substance abuse that have established acceptable reliability and validity (see Table 14.1).

Self-Monitoring

Self-monitoring is a hallmark behavioral assessment procedure that may be utilized to assess thoughts and behaviors on an ongoing basis. For instance, a drug-abusing adolescent might be asked to indicate the duration of time spent (a) with persons who abuse drugs, (b) in places drug use is known to occur, (c) or engaging in activities that involve drug use (see Azrin, McMahon, et al., 1994). Instructions can focus on self-monitoring during specific times (e.g., between 5 p.m. and 1 a.m. on weekend evenings) or during specific situations (e.g., at parties). The behaviors being monitored should be observable and objective (e.g., swearing or yelling instead of "being disrespectful"). Thoughts are a vital part of the behavioral chain of behaviors leading to substance use and should be recorded verbatim (e.g., "I can't wait to get paid and go . . ."). Associated stimuli or events may be monitored to assist the youth in gaining insight regarding the factors that act to maintain substance use. In addition to monitoring behaviors and thoughts qualitatively, the occurrence, frequency, and duration of specific or quantified details, as well as subjective ratings of mood and demonstrated skills, have all been used effectively to understand substance abuse–related problems and progress in therapy.

Although not as important prior to treatment, the behaviors, thoughts, and feelings being monitored should ideally be goals for therapy. Indeed, self-monitoring strategies have been found to produce genuine improvements in the things being monitored by consistently focusing attention on desired behavior, thus providing greater opportunities to understand behavior and receive positive feedback and recognition from others. Of course, improvements in self-monitored behaviors may be influenced by social desirability or memory deficits. Along these lines, accuracy may be compromised if praise or material rewards are contingent on the report of pro-social responses. Although this may not be ideal during the initial stages of assessment, treatment clinicians may be willing to sacrifice accuracy in self-monitoring reports to permit greater opportunities for reinforcement, as consistent with shaping.

Behavioral Observation

As indicated, the aforementioned self-report assessment methods have all demonstrated psychometric support in adolescent substance abusers. However, self-report methods are biased due to concerns regarding social desirability and distortions in memory, as indicated. Therefore, behavioral observation of adolescent substance abusers as well as of their family is an essential component in the assessment process. Behavioral observation methods range in complexity. Some observations casually target nonspecified behaviors during informal situations, such as the waiting room prior to the formal assessment session, whereas other observations are highly structured and directed at molecular behaviors that may be clearly defined (e.g., eye contact). Of course, *in vivo* formal behavioral observation of illicit substance use is not possible (unless it is candid), although it is sometimes possible to observe behavioral patterns that occur before or after substance use. Indeed, in their extensive review of the literature, Donohue, Van Hasselt, Hersen, and Perrin (1999) identified numerous studies that have convincingly demonstrated how skill deficits contribute to the progression of adolescent substance abuse. It is customary to conduct informal observation initially and to move on to formal observation of specified behaviors. For instance, observing a youth shaking hands softly while looking to the floor during an initial greeting may lead to formal observation of the youth in a social gathering at a recreational center with unknown peers. In conducting formal behavioral observation procedures, there may be initial reactivity to the assessor's presence that is not typical of the event. Although response reactivity to the observer generally goes away with continued presence, the desensitization process is facilitated if the observer attempts to be inconspicuous, for instance, utilizing videotape technology, shifting vision to multiple areas, or avoiding notations immediately after the behavior occurs. In substance-abusing adolescents, common observation scenarios include formal lectures, lunch, gym class, or recess at school or participation in activities at home or work. When observation is cost prohibited, the assessor can teach reliable significant others to conduct observations (e.g., teachers), although this is not ideal because self-reporting biases may occur. Another method of increasing the efficiency of behavioral observation procedures is to reliably identify when and where targeted behaviors are most likely to occur and to schedule observation only during these times. However, varying observations (time, setting) may provide valuable information that might otherwise be overlooked. The common methods of recording observational data include dichotomous ratings (e.g., presence or absence, appropriate or inappropriate), Likert-type ratings (e.g., 7 = extremely skilled, 1 = extremely unskilled), frequency recording (e.g., tally marks every time a specified behavior occurs), qualitative statements (e.g., yells at nurse after being told to put out cigarette), and interval recording (e.g., frequency during a specified time).

Role-Playing

Although behavioral observations offer increased confidence in the generalizability of observed behaviors to the assessment process, it is not possible to use these strategies in substance use situations or in situations that involve other illicit behaviors (e.g., responding to encouragement from friends to rob a pharmacy to obtain materials that will be used to create methamphetamine). Therefore, role-plays complement the assessment process, for they may be utilized to examine interpersonal skills in scenarios that attempt to simulate real-world scenarios, which may be otherwise unavailable. For instance, if a drug-dependent youth reported difficulties assertively refusing offers to use marijuana at parties, the party scenario could be enacted during the session, with the therapist portraying a friend assertively offering drugs to the youth. During the role-play, the therapist is able to observe behaviors, mannerisms, and statements from the youth that may be modified to increase the likelihood of future drug refusal. In general, role-play assessment of substance abuse–related behavior involves (a) querying the youth to describe the circumstances that were relevant to recent use of substances, (b) determining a key person in the scenario who influenced the youth to engage in drug-associated behavior, (c) simulating the scenario while enacting the role of the key person as the youth repeats his or her conduct, (d) querying the youth about feelings and thoughts that may have occurred during the role-play encounter.

CLINICAL UTILITY

Clinical utility involves the extent to which assessment procedures are able to assist in ameliorating clinical problems and disorders. As reported by Haynes and Lench (2003), clinical utility concerns the respective measures' validity, cost effectiveness, applicability, practicality, transportability across assessors and settings, and acceptability to assessors and respondents. Therefore, behavioral assessment procedures generally offer excellent clinical utility in families who are affected by adolescent substance abuse and dependence, because these methods are directly applicable to the remediation of problem behaviors and thoughts, rely upon standardized procedures that are replicable, and may be utilized during every stage of treatment across a wide variety of settings. However, the particular aspects of clinical utility vary between and among the different behavioral assessment methods, thus requiring closer examination. For instance, various standardized behavioral observation methods, the hallmark of behavioral assessment, have reliably been found to evidence outstanding validity. Assessors also consistently report these measures as both acceptable and easy to implement. Similarly, excepting initial anxiety or discomfort, most persons readily permit to being observed, appreciate the benefits gained from observational procedures, and report that these procedures do not interfere with their ongoing monitored activities. However, unless the observations are informal or conducted within the treatment facility, behavioral observation will incur costs associated with travel to *in vivo* locations. Therefore, expected gains associated with increased generalizability of assessment findings must be considered in light of costs that are likely to occur when choosing assessment strategies. Behavioral observation procedures are generally transportable across assessors when response formats are relatively simple (e.g., frequency counts of specified behavior) but not when these methods require extensive training in specific coding strategies (e.g., qualitative responses). Also related to transportability, observations are limited to behaviors that may be observed in their natural occurrence. Therefore, situations that involve substance use or related behaviors for which youth are highly motivated to conceal will not be appropriate for behavioral observation, unless application is candid (e.g., hidden videotape monitoring). Of course, videotaping an adolescent substance abuser without consent may decrease the acceptability of this approach.

Role-play tests vary in their degree of validity evidenced, and performance in role-plays may sometimes fail to generalize to *in vivo* situations due to factors associated with anxiety, motivation, fatigue, etc. For instance, a youth may demonstrate satisfactory skills in refusing a contrived offer to smoke marijuana but continue to accept offers in his natural environment. Role-play tests are generally effective in the identification of skill deficits that are relevant to substance-abusing youth across a wide array of behavioral domains that involve social interaction. Similar to behavioral monitoring procedures, role-play tests are relatively easy to learn, although their response formats vary considerably, with some being more involved (and requiring more costs associated with training) than others. A relative strength of role-play testing is that behavioral skills may be observed in situations that approximate real-life encounters for which it is difficult or impractical to utilize other assessment methods (i.e., applicability). Self-report measures (including structured and semistructured interviews), particularly when brief, offer outstanding cost effectiveness and acceptability by assessors and respondents and are easily administered in (transportable to) almost any setting. However, specific to the assessment of drug use behavior, self-report measures are notoriously biased and have demonstrated small-to-modest correlations with biological measures of substance use. Nevertheless, the advantages of utilizing self-report measures with adolescent substance abusers, in conjunction with biological measures and lie scales, strongly enhance the utility of these measures.

DEVELOPMENTAL CONSIDERATIONS

Recognizing that the onset of substance abuse and dependence usually occurs during adolescence but is influenced by earlier events, Tarter, Sambrano, and Dunn (2002) explicated a developmental trajectory in the progression of substance use disorders based on epidemiological risk factors. Although substance use rarely occurs prior to 10 years, in their model underlying factors can be identified as early as infancy and early childhood. For instance, infants who are genetically predisposed to have "difficult" temperaments have been found to experience later emotional instability, as evidenced through fussiness and irregular biorhythms later in development (Lerner & Vicary, 1984). Tarter et al. note genetic predispositions interact with the environment in a bidirectional manner to influence substance abuse and dependence. For instance, infants are highly dependent on parents during earlier stages of their development. Thus, parental factors (e.g., parental substance abuse and pathology, poor parenting skills) are very likely to influence poor adjustment in the early development of their children. Indeed, parent-relevant risk factors have been found to be associated with poor attachment between parents and their infants, which often later contribute to problems establishing strong parent–child relationships that buffer against substance-abusive behavior, as indicated later.

Middle and late childhood is marked by an increase in time spent away from the immediate home environment, most often at school or outside play with peers. Children of caregivers who evidence the aforementioned parenting risk factors are more likely to miss opportunities to develop skills and other repertoires, resulting in poor behavioral and academic performance (Maziade, 1989). Failing to meet performance expectations of positive role models (parents, teachers, well-adjusted peers), these youth are also more likely to withdraw from well-monitored pro-social activities with these individuals (e.g., school work) and to pursue friendships with peers who are especially inclined to have lower standards of conduct outside the home and school environments (Ary, Duncan, Duncan, & Hops, 1999). With the passage of time, problems of conduct (e.g., disengagement from school, coercive arguments with parents) are exacerbated in a process called *epigenesis*. Access to drugs usually occurs during adolescence and is initiated with peers outside the home. Therefore, if youth spend less time engaged in adult-monitored activities with positive role models, they are at particular risk of developing substance abuse.

Other risk factors of substance use include self-regulation, which is directly related to a shift from Piaget's concrete operations to his formal operations stage of cognitive development. Formal operations involve higher-level thought processes, such as abstract thought, logic, and a self-evaluation of thought patterns. These changes are initiated at the onset of adolescence, with a second surge occurring during late adolescence (Dacey & Kenney, 1997). Formal operations are related to brain maturation occurring in the dorsal portion of the frontal lobe, resulting in a decrease in gray matter density and dendrite connections (i.e., synaptic pruning) and axon mediation (Giedd et al., 1999). These developments are necessary for self-regulation of behaviors and emotions through increases in reasoning, attention, and forethought. Familial history of substance abuse has been found to correlate with lower levels of executive functioning in several self-regulatory tasks (i.e., response suppression, response regulation, and delayed gratification) (Nigg et al., 2004), all of which have been indicated in adolescent substance abusers.

As might be inferred, there is a strong link between substance abuse and both poor academic performance (Diego, Field, & Sanders, 2003) and poor motivation to do well in school (Hawkins & Catalano, 1992). According to Tarter et al. (2002) this pattern is also associated with low self-esteem, low future expectations, conformity with peer deviance, and negative parental appraisal, all of which increase the likelihood of substance abuse. The family continues to be the primary source of support for most youth during adolescence. Parenting marked by passivity or minimal levels of involvement is, therefore, associated with a variety of problems, which are commonly concurrent with substance abuse, including delinquency (Gorman-Smith, Tolan, Loeber, & Henry, 1998) and poor academic performance (Bogenschnieder, 1997). Negative outcomes are associated with specific negative parenting behaviors, such as low maternal participation, erratic rules and contingencies, authoritarian or permissive styles of parenting, insufficient monitoring of the youth, and vague expectancies with regard to age-appropriate behaviors (Kendel & Andrews, 1987; Shedler & Block, 1990). Poor communication and conflict between the parent and youth during childhood precedes the onset of these behaviors in adolescence (Hawkins & Catalano, 1992), particularly when parental alcohol dependence or abuse is present (Nathan, Skinstad, & Dolan, 2001).

ASSESSMENT, CONCEPTUALIZATION, AND TREATMENT PLANNING

A review of professional records should be conducted prior to meeting the substance-abusing youth and family to assist in the identification and conceptualization of problems. Medical charts, psychiatric reports, and school records can provide a variety of information relevant to effective treatment planning, including developmental history (e.g., achievement of developmental milestones), medical history (e.g., seizures, head injury, illness/disease), current and past onset, duration, dose, and response to prescribed medications, psychiatric history (e.g., hospitalizations, response to psychological interventions, substance use), family history (e.g., relationships with all relevant significant others), educational history (e.g., highest level achieved, grades in school, standardized tests, educational placement), and social history (e.g., family constellation and quality of relationships, social supports). However, the primary method of understanding the development and maintenance of substance abusive behavior is the behavioral interview, which is usually the first time family members have an opportunity to fully express their concerns regarding the myriad problem behaviors typically found in their homes. Therefore, prior to conducting the interview, it is important to establish an agenda with the family, including the purpose of the interview and the estimated duration of time for each topic area. The latter strategy involves each family member in the initial planning stages of assessment and assists in informing them about their expectations for assessment, thus preventing unnecessary "venting" of problem behaviors that may be assessed utilizing other assessment tools. The initial stages of the interview should be focused on identifying and broadly understanding problems, whereas latter stages involve a detailed functional analysis (i.e., ABCs) of substance use and related problem behaviors. Along these lines, the youth's substance use is conceptualized to serve an immediate purpose or function in reducing distress (e.g., anxiety, social introversion) and increasing a desired state (e.g., relaxation, disinhibition), which outweighs the delayed negative consequences of use. The immediate pleasurable consequences are particularly powerful when antecedent skills that could normally assist in obtaining desired states (e.g., coping skills, social and academic repertoires, non-drug-abusing social networks) are absent or lacking. Therefore, in addition to identifying problem behaviors, it is important to assess domains that may include antecedent and consequent stimuli that can be later incorporated in the treatment plan to prevent substance use, including activities and hobbies, perceived strengths, friends and social support systems, and academic functioning. Specific areas worthy of exploration with the parent include methods of discipline, the youth's response to discipline, relative strengths and weakness of the parent–youth relationship, activities with the youth, medical conditions, parental job satisfaction, social supports, health care, financial status, stressors, social skills, coping abilities, and relevant cultural factors (e.g., fluency with English, attitude toward seeking and accepting mental health services).

The functional analysis should be focused on clearly defining problem behaviors that were identified in formal assessment (e.g., interviews, behavioral observation, role-plays, standardized inventories). Relevant to substance abuse, this process includes noting when the substance use occurs and when it is absent, antecedent thoughts and behaviors (i.e., what occurs prior to use), associated events and feelings (i.e., what happens during use), and consequent thoughts and behaviors (i.e., what occurs after use). This should also include the youth's and the parents' thoughts regarding the maintenance of substance use and their expectancies regarding resolution of the problem. The youth and parents should also be asked to list the methods of addressing substance abuse that have already been attempted as well as resources and motivation of each individual in resolving the problem situation.

Functional analyses always include a "problem analysis," in which data are initially examined so that hypotheses may be formulated about the function of problem behavior (i.e., substance-abusive behavior). Problem behaviors that were identified during the interviews are grouped into related actions, whenever appropriate. For example, use of cocaine and alcohol as well as driving while intoxicated would appropriately be listed together as "substance abuse behaviors," whereas swearing and kicking staff members might be clustered together as "aggressive behaviors." These lists provide a solid organizational structure in which to understand contributing factors of substance abuse and to assist in determining which empirically validated interventions are most economically appropriate for implementation. Similar steps may be performed to interpret and organize data from other assessment measures (e.g., role-playing, behavioral observation, standardized inventories). For instance, problem behaviors represented within elevated subscales from standardized measures can be grouped together. Thus, information from interviews and other assessments can be integrated.

Once problem behaviors are organized into their respective problem domains, problem behaviors that appear to be most important (e.g., use of cocaine) may be selected for problem analysis. Specifically, the antecedent and consequent stimuli, supported by obtained information from the family, may be written to the left and right of the selected problem behavior. For instance, if the problem behavior consisted of Mary's using marijuana at a party, antecedent stimuli would be listed to the left of yelling (e.g., nervous around boys) and the consequences (e.g., feels comfortable with boys) would be listed to the right of yelling. The initial hypothesis regarding the development and maintenance of problem behaviors can then be confirmed or disconfirmed. For example, Mary uses marijuana at a party (target behavior) because she feels uncomfortable talking with boys (antecedent) and marijuana results in her feeling comfortable with boys (consequence). It is clear that social skills training focused on initiating conversation with boys may help Mary eliminate substance use at parties. However, additional assessment needs may also be identified in reviewing this process with the youth and the parents. That is, there may be problem behaviors that need greater specification or antecedent and consequent stimuli that were not recognized or fully assessed. In any event, the problem analysis should result in well-established hypotheses and behavioral chains for each problem domain, thus assisting in a well-formulated treatment plan.

Upon successful integration of the assessment information, a postassessment interview with the youth and the parents is scheduled to review assessment results. Utilization of an agenda assists in maintaining structure and in reviewing necessary information within the allotted time. The clinician should query what the youth and parents were most interested in knowing at the outset of the session. In presenting assessment results, the assessor should be careful to initiate discussion by reporting positive qualities, including the importance of building on the reported strengths. The dissemination of information should start with an overall impression of the youth and should include specific scores and percentiles only if queried by a family member. Indeed, it is usually sufficient to state that the youth is functioning like most children her age, rather than mention that she is functioning at the 45th percentile. It is also important to assess the youth and parents' understanding and acceptance of diagnostic impressions and assessment findings. The assessor should conceptualize the ABCs of substance use, make specific recommendations, and obtain feedback from the family regarding their motivation to pursue recommendations for treatment, including benefits and potential obstacles. Finally, a prognosis should be provided, including interventions that have evidenced success in the substance abuse treatment outcome literature (e.g., Behavioral Therapies, Multisystemic Therapy, Community Reinforcement Approach) as well as variables that have been associated with successful prognosis (e.g., attendance, successful completion of therapy assignments).

Many clinics require that a tentative treatment plan be completed after the first or second contact with the client. This treatment plan is usually one or more vague goals to address in treatment, and youth are typically encouraged to emphasize substance abuse to some extent (e.g., to be clean from drugs). More specific and formal treatment plans are usually completed within the first month. This plan should include objective behavioral indicators of successful completion and dates targeted for goal completion. The behavioral indicators should be within the youth's control, and the goals should be realistic. As treatment progresses, the effects of intervention are assessed through ongoing monitoring of goals, which usually involves the readministration of assessment measures.

CASE STUDY

IDENTIFICATION

Brian is a 17-year-old Caucasian male from a moderate socioeconomic background. He lives with his mother, stepfather, and two male siblings in a metropolitan suburb in the southwestern United States. He is currently enrolled in his senior year of high school.

PRESENTING COMPLAINTS

Brian presented for assessment with his mother at an outpatient clinic specializing in substance abuse. He was referred for assessment by his probation officer after being arrested for driving while under the influence of alcohol and possession of alcohol by a minor. When asked what he hoped to achieve from the assessment process, Brian reported, "I just want to get my mother and this damn probation officer off my back." He acknowledged decreased academic performance subsequent to marijuana use and expressed concern about his motivation to attend work or school. He reported that he is being closely supervised by probation officers and his parents, which he reported is very troubling to him. He also reported frequent arguments with his stepfather, teachers, and peers and feels these arguments are founded on "disrespect." In addition he describes feeling anxious in social situations, which he identifies as a significant stressor. Brian's mother confirmed her son's heavy use of substances and poor academic performance at school. She indicated that she hoped Brian would "grow up and get along with his family and school teachers." She also reported that Brian has "always" been noncompliant to her directives and that she had hoped this could be addressed in therapy.

HISTORY

Brian's maternal family evidences a history of alcohol abuse and dependence (i.e., his mother and maternal grandfather), although his mother and grandmother discontinued their "heavy" use together subsequent to enrolling in a community drug-counseling program when Brian was approximately 5 years old. Brian's first use of alcohol occurred when he was approximately 15 years old. It was at this time that one of his friends became aware that access to alcohol in his home was unlikely to be noticed, and they "skimmed" alcohol from several liquor bottles in the liquor cabinet of his friend's house. He reported that he thought the resulting feeling was "great," and he began paying older adolescents and adults he did not know at the local convenience stores to buy beer for him. Later, he would get drunk with his "close" friends. He reportedly continued to get intoxicated with his friends approximately once or twice a week, usually weekends. He reportedly used marijuana for the first time three months after the onset of his alcohol use. He reported that he was at a "keg party" where marijuana was readily available. He admitted that he was initially nervous to smoke a joint that was passed to him but smoked it because "everyone else was doing it." He enjoyed the "high," and remembered laughing and having fun throughout the evening. At the party he met an older adolescent who became his drug supplier. Brian's use of alcohol and marijuana was limited to weekends for about a year (i.e., about 16 years old). However, he reported the amount of alcohol he consumed increased to over a case or more each weekend during this time. Indeed, he used alcohol rather exclusively for several months, with marijuana use occurring only when he "went out" with a couple of older adolescents he met outside a prominent urban adult dance club. Several months before he was arrested for driving while under the influence of alcohol, he initiated his first use of MDMA. His use of substances intensified to three to four days a week, and he began to "cut" school and to argue with his parents. Brian reported he decreased his drug use about two weeks prior to his arrest, in preparation for a new marking period at school.

DEVELOPMENT ISSUES

According to hospital records, Brian achieved all relevant developmental milestones during infancy and early childhood within normal limits, including gross and fine motor skills (i.e., sitting, crawling, grasping, walking, etc.), verbal abilities (i.e., onset of word and sentence construction), and social interactions (i.e., play, daily activities). His mother reported that as an infant he was "irritable" and that he "never really liked to be held." However, his middle childhood and early adolescence was described as a "good time" in their relationship. Accordingly she indicated that Brian received extensive reinforcement (i.e., praise, acknowledgment, and material goods) from his parents and extended family. As she reported, "My husband and I gave him anything he wanted. Well, maybe I should say I gave him everything. My husband often says I spoiled him."

Brian's presenting problems were reported to be associated with the onset of later adolescence. As is typical of adolescence, Brian reported, "I just wanted to be with my friends more often." However, his mother reported a different perspective: "He was hanging out with adult deadheads and kids who had pins in their noses and stuff." In response to his adolescent peer group, his stepfather reportedly became frequently irritated and attempted to disrupt his ability to spend time with "these idiots." In a separate interview, Brian reported that he would often sneak out of his room after his parents were sleeping and that when he was occasionally caught, his stepfather would "go crazy," yelling and throwing things in the house. His mother would cry and retreat to her room during these times. His mother reported that her husband was overly strict. This conflict in parenting led to an increase in both Brian's noncompliant behavior and coercive arguments at home among all three individuals. Thus, Brian experienced his home environment as aversive and began spending increasing amounts of time away from home in unsupervised environments. Concurrently, his peers were providing a level of emotional support, lack of structure and expectations, and access to exciting stimuli (including substances).

PEER AND SCHOOL ISSUES

Brian's peer network presently consists of seven male friends (established at the beginning of junior high school) and a girlfriend. His male friends use various illicit drugs and alcohol and have similar issues (i.e., arrests, poor school attendance, family conflict) to varying degrees. His girlfriend, however, does not use substances and has requested repeatedly that Brian cease his substance use. In a letter from his girlfriend, she indicated that he is a "loving and beautiful" person who is "out of control." When asked to describe his social skills, Brian reported, "I'm pretty good at parties and can make friends easily. I have a hard time handling my girlfriend when she starts complaining, and I probably yell at her too much." He is experiencing skill deficits in other aspects of peer interactions, such as problem solving, structuring activities, and declining offers of substance use. His deficits in this domain focus on impulsivity and social desirability, and he appears to be limited in his abilities to quickly assess potential negative consequences of his actions.

According to school reports, his academic strengths have been in quantitative and concrete subject areas, such as algebra, where his grades remain relatively high (i.e., B−). He is also more responsive to female instructors. In these settings he is more likely to attend the class and engage in adaptive behaviors (i.e., attentive, respectful, completes assignments). He is more challenged in verbal-based courses (English and history) or in courses taught by male instructors that necessitate assertive verbal responses in front of the class. The onset of his substance use was associated with school absences and the need for assistance to understand material, which Brian found uncomfortable to request. Inability to comprehend the material led to conflicts with teachers, resulting in Brian's feeling discouraged from attending school. His peers supported this negative perception of school.

BEHAVIORAL ASSESSMENT

Brian's medical records were unremarkable. His middle school records indicated an early history of academic success, with well-developed social relationships. His high school records revealed that his performance during the previous semester negatively impacted his overall academic record and provided specific details about this domain (i.e., course grades, attendance, extracurricular activities). He had no mental health treatment record prior to entering treatment at the present facility. Similarly, his probation officer's summary report indicated no previous arrests. His responses to the intake questionnaire provided information about his presenting problem, referral source and circumstances, family structure, drug use history, and Brian's initial goals for treatment, which helped the initial interview to progress smoothly.

During the initiation of a behavioral interview, Brian's affect was moderately expressive and his mood presented as calm and stable. He was alert and oriented to person, place, and time, and he was well spoken and well dressed in a T-shirt and jeans. He responded well to open-ended questions and empathic paraphrasing. His identified interests and strengths included enjoyment in playing guitar, playing baseball, and modeling. Brian perceived his strengths were determination once he sets goals, a sense of humor, and the respectful manner in which he treats his mom and girlfriend. He reported that his primary problems were school absences and legal probation due to substance use, and he reported that he was willing to eliminate use while in treatment and on probation and to reduce use on a permanent basis. He reported that his relationship with his stepfather was the second largest problem in his life at the time, and he indicated that he would like to improve this relationship. He identified occasional social anxiety as another area of concern, indicating that this anxiety is amplified in novel social situations (i.e., meeting new people, large gatherings, class presentations). As these problems were identified, their corresponding antecedents and consequences were also examined and outlined. He was also assessed for suicidal ideation and child maltreatment, both of which were denied, although he indicated that his stepfather did make occasional "cut-downs" and "swore a lot." His mother was then interviewed. Her reports coincided with Brian's primary areas of concern. She also added general information regarding the antecedents and consequences of Brian's behaviors. The ABCs of the functional analysis were reviewed with Brian, and he was asked to monitor several of the identified antecedent and consequent stimuli in response to a specific problem situation. For instance, he identified several antecedent stimuli related to anxiety at parties (e.g., fear of being the only one not using substances) as well as consequences to use at parties (e.g., feels relaxed, comfortable meeting new friends).

The next assessment session focused on objective, quantitative methods of gathering specific data related to these problems. Sections of a structured interview (SCID) specific to substance abuse and anxiety disorders were administered. The client met diagnostic criterion for a diagnosis of Alcohol and Poly-Substance Abuse. Although several of the criteria relevant to Social Phobia were met, he did not meet criteria for any anxiety disorders. The substance abuse diagnoses were confirmed through the administration of the SASSI-A2, which also established concurrent anxiety and a moderate level of treatment receptivity. Brian seemed to experience a tolerance for alcohol, for he reported a decreased response to prior levels of alcohol consumption, and was drinking five to six units of alcohol to reach intoxication. The results from youth and parent administration of the Alcohol Timeline Followback confirmed this pattern of alcohol use and revealed that marijuana use was approximately four nights a week (one to two units, or "joints"), with use of stimulant (i.e., amphetamines) or designer drugs (i.e., GHB, ecstasy) on weekends. His only symptoms of withdrawal were fatigue and extended periods of sleep after the use of illicit drugs. However, at times he also experienced decreased appetite and memory loss. He reported a decrease in previously enjoyable activities (i.e., guitar, baseball, and modeling). In addition, his use impacted his academic functioning, as evidenced by his declining grades during the prior academic year to mostly "Ds," some "Fs," and a "B–" in algebra. He had been unable to maintain a job in the retail sector (clothing and media stores). Prior to entering treatment, Brian reported that he had made a single effort at reducing the amount and frequency of his substance use, which he viewed as moderately successful. A broad-screen urinalysis was conducted during this session, and marijuana was present at a moderately high level, indicating recent use. This established a firm diagnosis and pattern of use from which to develop a conceptualization of substance use behavior.

In addition, measures related to general functioning and satisfaction in the family relationship were administered. The Child Behavior Checklist (CBCL), a measure of internalizing and externalizing problem behaviors in youth, was completed by Brian's mother. The results of this measure indicated a level of externalizing behaviors that was barely significant. An item analysis revealed that items related to school attendance and performance and to delinquency were elevated. The internalizing scales fell just short of significance, confirming the levels of anxiety that were present, but not at a clinical level. Brian declined the administration of the youth self-report version of the CBCL due to its length, but he subsequently agreed to take a shorter self-report measure. This measure confirmed substance use and school as the most problematic behaviors. The Parent Satisfaction with Youth Scale was also completed, and indicated that Brian's mother was most dissatisfied with his conduct in the following areas: curfew adherence, school performance, and response to discipline. Brian was particularly dissatisfied with his parents' methods of discipline and communication, according to his responses to the Youth Happiness with Parent Scale. To a lesser extent, he was dissatisfied with the rewards he receives from his parents. Thus, discipline, communication, and school performance appeared to be the areas of great concern. Brian also completed the Life Satisfaction Scale and rated substance use, school, work, and transportation as highly unsatisfactory. In all of the aforementioned satisfaction scales, the respondents were asked to disclose what would be different in their life in order to bring about 100% satisfaction with each of the lower-rated domains. For instance, relevant to the School Performance domain of the Parent Satisfaction with Youth Scale, Brian's mother reported that if her son simply attended his classes and did his homework every day she would be completely satisfied. This information was utilized to assist in developing the treatment plan and the monitoring process.

Brian's behavior was observed directly in the waiting room and tailored role-plays. Support staff reported that Brian and his mother were appropriate, warm, and respectful, laughing at times. The role-play scenarios were derived from problem areas identified during the behavioral interview and standardized questionnaires, and they included refusing offers of alcohol, requesting a later curfew from his stepfather, and asking an instructor for assistance with a late assignment. He had difficulty in generating a timely and effective refusal statement when offered alcohol, which revealed that his current strategy would be ineffective if attempted with peers during *in vivo* situations, i.e., parties. In the two subsequent role-plays he was unable to assert his position or needs. He became increasingly defensive in vocal intonation and volume as the brief scenarios progressed. These observations indicate that, though he is capable of positive social interactions during relatively pleasant interactions (i.e., positive assertion), his inability to confront opposition (i.e., negative assertion) is a relative deficit.

PROBLEM ANALYSIS

The information collected in the first two interviews was integrated with the data from the completed self-monitoring Brian was instructed to do between sessions to create a formal list of target behaviors. The primary presenting problem behaviors were grouped together, and these problem domains were labeled. For instance, the problem domain of "substance abuse" included the following related list of problem behaviors: use of alcohol, use of marijuana, use of hard drugs, driving while intoxicated. Other prominent problem domains included "interpersonal problems" and "poor academic functioning." Antecedent behaviors were placed to the left of each problem, and consequences were placed to the right of each problem. Some of the identified antecedents to marijuana use included boredom/inactivity, anxiety, thoughts regarding the reinforcing properties of marijuana, conflict with family members, and various friends that use marijuana. The consequences of marijuana use were pleasant conversations with peers, lack of motivation, arguments with parents and girlfriend, poor school grades, relaxation. Although these stimuli were consistent with the other target substances, use of alcohol additionally included antecedent stimuli associated with increased assertion, and consequent stimuli for this substance included physical fights, vomiting, and hangovers. In constructing the list, Brian spontaneously made several comments indicating he had gained insight regarding the causes and preventions of his substance use. Brian was informed that the problem lists would likely change as his repertoires improved, and he requested to review the ABCs in subsequent intervention sessions.

INTERVENTION

After the second session, the behavior inventory resulting from the functional analysis was utilized to assist in developing an initial treatment plan and further self-monitoring lists. Brian and his family were taught to utilize the functional analysis to conceptualize problem behavior and to generate solutions that were addressed during intervention sessions. Interventions addressed his substance abuse through behavioral interventions targeting environmental cues and the enhancement of social skills relevant to substance refusal and avoidance. Problem-solving techniques and social skills training related to assertiveness and communication were employed to resolve negative interactions and conflicts. Self-monitoring lists were employed to assist in monitoring progress and guiding intervention (see Table 14.2 for an example of a monitoring sheet for Brian's social anxiety).

TABLE 14.2 Example of Self-Monitoring Chart

Targets for Treatment	Mon.	Tues.	Wed.	Thur.	Fri.	Sat.	Sun.
Situation that led to anxious thought(s)	Oral report in speech class						
Anxious thought(s)	Everyone will laugh at me if I mess up; people may notice I'm nervous						
Highest level of anxiety (0 = none, 100 = completely)	85						
What did I do to reduce anxiety and still achieve my goal?	I practiced in front of a mirror and then with my mom						
Postanxiety rating	20						

PROGRESS ASSESSMENT

In addition to the continued functional analysis of behavior, Brian's progress was periodically assessed throughout the treatment process. This was done through readministration of the satisfaction scales and role-play scenarios approximately once a month, duc to ease of administration and direct applicability to treatment. However, the standardized questionnaires were administered only at the conclusion of treatment, to demonstrate Brian's scores on the behavioral inventories receded into the nonclinical range, as confirmed by school conduct reports, parent reports, self-monitoring sheets, and urinalysis. The attainment of satisfactory social skills in negative assertion was observed during Brian's role-play performance, and this was confirmed by both Brian and his mother.

ETHICAL AND LEGAL ISSUES

Two of the primary issues related to this case were both ethical and legal in nature. First, by law Brian's mother and probation officer needed to receive information about his progress. However, he is an older adolescent, and ethically he has an increasing right to confidentiality. Disclosure of information could be a treatment barrier if not addressed. This issue was dealt with at the initial intake session through the process of fully informing Brian of the potential consequences of providing his consent to be assessed and by obtaining his informed consent allowing the clinician to speak to his mother and probation officer openly about specific information. As a result of this process, he was aware that substance use (and other risk-related behaviors or situations) would be conveyed and that other assessment reports would be briefly summarized in a report, including his progress in treatment (i.e., therapy attendance, performance in school).

The second ethical and legal issue that arose was relevant to potential psychological abuse that may have accompanied his stepfather's derogatory statements during their arguments. Brian is still a minor, and the clinician is obligated to report "suspected" cases of child maltreatment. In this regard, a complete risk assessment was conducted as part of the initial assessment, and all participants were informed of the assessor's legal obligation to report child maltreatment before they provided informed consent and assent. In this risk assessment, Brian denied physical conflict, although he admitted they both exchanged derogatory statements about one another. Although reports of emotional or psychological abuse are rarely accepted, the assessor decided to report the incidents to the state's child protective services to determine his obligations to report. The hotline investigator reported that the incidents were not acceptable, and provided her identification number so the assessor could record the call in his case progress notes, to document his compliance with the law (i.e., report "suspected" child maltreatment).

SUMMARY

Alcohol and drug abuse is a widespread and significant problem among adolescents. Indeed, the identification and assessment of these disorders are complicated by unpredictable, and potentially fatal, physiological interactions resulting from overdose and simultaneous use of multiple substances, the presence of comorbid psychiatric and behavioral disorders that often mask or resemble symptoms of substance abuse, high risk of suicide due to the behavioral and chemical influences of substance use, and high potential for child maltreatment. Therefore, substance abuse must be assessed utilizing a comprehensive battery of empirically validated measures. In this chapter, various behavioral assessment procedures and strategies were examined within the context of a functional analysis. The importance of engaging the adolescent and the adolescent's family in therapy was emphasized, specific suggestions for improving initial session attendance were offered, and a structure for the assessment process was recommended. Assessment results should assist in guiding treatment plans and should be continued throughout the treatment process. A table containing some of the more validated measures of substance use and related problem behaviors was presented, and extensive details about a drug-abusing adolescent were provided to exemplify the assessment process.

REFERENCES AND RESOURCES

Aarons, G. A., Brown, S. A., Hough, R. L., Garland, A. F., & Wood, P. A. (2001). Prevalence of adolescent substance use disorders across five sectors of care. *Journal of the American Academy of Child and Adolescent Psychiatry, 40,* 419–426.

Alvarez, K. M., Donohue, B., Kenny, M. C., Cavanagh, N., & Romero, V. (2004). The process and consequences of reporting child maltreatment: A brief overview for professionals in the mental health field. *Aggression and Violent Behavior: A Review Journal, 9,* 563–578.

American Psychiatric Association. (2000). *Diagnostic and statistical manual of mental disorders* (4th ed. text revision). Washington, DC: Author.

Ary, D. V., Duncan, T. E., Duncan, S. C., & Hops, H. (1999). Adolescent problem behavior: The influence of parents and peers. *Behavioral Research Therapy, 37,* 217–230.

Ary, D. V., Tildesley, E., Hops, H., & Andrews, J. (1993). The influence of parent, sibling and peer modeling and attitudes on adolescent use of alcohol. *International Journal of Addiction, 28,* 853–880.

Azrin, N. H., Donohue, B., Besalel, V., Kogan, E., & Acierno, R. (1994). Youth drug abuse treatment: A controlled outcome study. *Journal of Child and Adolescent Substance Abuse, 3,* 1–16.

Azrin, N. H., Donohue, B., & Teichner, G. A. (2001). A controlled evaluation and description of individual-cognitive problem solving and family-behavior therapies in dually diagnosed conduct-disordered and substance-dependent youth. *Journal of Child and Adolescent Substance Abuse, 11,* 1–43.

Azrin, N. H., McMahon, P., Donohue, B., Besalel, V., Lapinski, K., Kogan, E., Acierno, R., & Galloway, E. (1994). Behavior therapy of drug abuse: A controlled outcome study. *Behaviour Research and Therapy, 32,* 857–866.

Baselt, R. C. (2002). *Disposition of toxic drugs and chemicals in man* (6th ed.) Foster City, CA: Biomedical Publications.

Bogenschnieder, K. (1997). Parental involvement in adolescent schooling: A proximal process with transcontextual validity. *Journal of Marriage and the Family, 59,* 718–733.

Brown, S. A., Christiansen, B. A., Goldman, M. S., & Inn, A. (1980). The development of alcohol-related expectancies in adolescents: Separating pharmacological from social learning influences. *Journal of Consulting Clinical Psychology, 50,* 336–344.

Brown, S. A., Myers, M. G., Lippke, L, Tapert, S. F., Stewart, D. G., & Vik, P. W. (1998). Psychometric evaluation of the Customary Drinking and Drug Use Record (CDDR): A measure of adolescent alcohol and drug involvement. *Journal of Studies on Alcohol, 59,* 427–438.

Centers for Disease Control. (2003). *Youth Risk Behavior Surveillance System.* Retrieved from http://www.cdc.gov/HealthyYouth/yrbs/index.htm, Retrieved 1/6/2005.

Chatoor, I., & Krupnick, J. (2001). The role of nonspecific factors in treatment outcome of psychotherapy studies. *European Child & Adolescent Psychiatry, 10,* 19–25.

Cull, J. G., & Gill, W. S. (1990). *Suicide Probability Scale Manual.* Los Angeles: Western Psychological Services.

Dacey, D., & Kenney, M. (1997). Cognitive development. *Adolescent development.* New York: McGraw-Hill.

Deas, D., Roberts, J., Randall, C. L., & Anton, R. (2001). Adolescent Obsessive-Compulsive Drinking Scale (A-OCDS): An assessment tool for problem drinking. *Journal of the National Medical Association, 93,* 92–103.

DeCato, L., Donohue, B., Azrin, N. H., & Teichner, G. (2001). Satisfaction of conduct-disordered and substance abusing youth with their parents. *Behavior Modification, 25,* 44–61.

De Leon, G., Melnick, G., Kressel, D., & Jainchill, N. (1994). Circumstances, Motivation, Readiness and Suitability (The CMRS Scales): Predicting retention in therapeutic community treatment. *American Journal of Drug and Alcohol Abuse, 20,* 495–515.

Dennis, M. L., & Stevens, S. J. (2003). Maltreatment issues and outcome of adolescents enrolled in substance abuse treatment. *Child Maltreatment: Journal of the American Professional Society on the Abuse of Children, 8,* 3–6.

Diego, A., Field, T., & Sanders, C. (2003). Academic performance, popularity, and depression predict adolescent substance use. *Adolescence, 38,* 35–42.

Donohue, B. (2004). Coexisting child neglect and drug abuse in adolescent mothers: Specific recommendations for treatment based on a review of the outcome literature. *Behavior Modification, 28,* 206–233.

Donohue, B., Carpin, K., & Alvarez, K. M. (2002). A standardized method of diplomatically and effectively reporting child abuse to state authorities: A controlled evaluation. *Behavior Modification, 25,* 684–699.

Donohue, B., DeCato, L. A., Azrin, N. H. (2001). Satisfaction of parents with their conduct-disordered and substance-abusing youth. *Behavior Modification, 25,* 21–43.

Donohue, B., Van Hasselt, V. B., Hersen, M., & Perrin, S. (1999). Substance refusal skills in a population of adolescents diagnosed with conduct disorder and substance abuse. *Addictive Behaviors, 24,* 37–46.

Donohue, B., Azrin, N. H., Lawson, H., Friedlander, J., Teichner, G., & Rindsberg, J. (1998). Improving initial session attendance of substance abusing and conduct disordered: A controlled study. *Journal of Child and Adolescent Substance Abuse, 8,* 1–13.

Donohue, B., Teichner, G., Azrin, N. H., Silver, N., Weintraub, N., Crum, T. A., & Decato, L. (2003). The initial reliability and validity of the Life Satisfaction Scale for Problem Youth in a sample of drug-abusing and conduct-disordered youth. *Journal of Child and Family Studies, 12,* 453–464.

Donohue, B., Azrin, N. H., Strada, M., Silver, C. S., Teichner, G., & Murphy, H. (2004). Psychometric evaluation of self and collateral Timeline Followback reports of drug and alcohol use in a sample of drug-abusing and conduct-disordered adolescents and their parents. *Psychology of Addictive Behaviors, 18,* 184–189.

Friedman, A. S., & Utada, A. (1989). A method for diagnosis and planning the treatment of adolescent drug abusers: The Adolescent Drug Abuse Diagnosis (ADAD). *Journal of Drug Education, 19,* 285–312.

Gariti, P., Alterman, A. I., Holub-Beyer, E., Volpicelli, J. R., Prentice, N., & O'Brien, C. (1995). Effects of an appointment reminder call on patient show rates. *Journal of Substance Abuse Treatment, 12,* 207–212.

Garland, A. F., Hough, R. L., McCabe, K. M., Yeh, M, Wood, P. A., & Aarons, G. A. (2001). Prevalence of psychiatric disorders in youths across five sectors of care. *Journal of the American Academy of Child and Adolescent Psychiatry, 40,* 409–418.

Giedd, J. N., Blumenthal, J., Jeffries, N. O., Castellanos, F. X., Liu, H., Zijdenbos, A., Paus, T., Evans, A. C., & Rapoport, J. L. (1999). Brain development during childhood and adolescence: A longitudinal MRI study. *National Neuroscience, 2,* 861–863.

Gorman-Smith, D., Tolan, P. H., Loeber, R., & Henry, D. B. (1998). Relation of family problems to patterns of delinquent involvement among urban youth. *Journal of Abnormal Child Psychology, 26,* 319–333.

Harrell, A. V., & Wirtz, P. W. (1999). *The Adolescent Drinking Index Professional manual.* Odessa, FL: Psychological Assessment Resources.

Hawkins, J. D., & Catalano, J. D. (1992). *Communities that care: Action for drug abuse prevention.* San Francisco: Jossey-Bass.

Haynes, S. N. (1998). The assessment–treatment relationship and functional analysis in behavior therapy. *European Journal of Psychological Assessment, 14,* 26–35.

Haynes, S. N., & Lench, H. C. (2003). Incremental validity of new clinical assessment measures. *Psychological Assessment, 15,* 456–466.

Johnston, L. D., O'Malley, P. M., Bachman, J. G., & Schulenberg, J. E. (2004). *Overall teen drug use continues gradual decline, but use of inhalants rises.* Ann Arbor, MI: University of Michigan News and Information Services. Retrieved December 21, 2005, from www.monitoringthefuture.org

Kaminer, Y., Bukstein, O., & Tarter, R. E. (1991). The Teen-Addiction Severity Index: Rationale and reliability. *International Journal of Addictions, 26,* 219–226.

Kendel, D. B., & Andrews, K. (1987). Processes of adolescent socialization by parents and peers. *International Journal of the Addictions, 22,* 319–342.

Kennedy, R. E. (1993). Depression as disorder of social relationships: Implications for school policy. In R. Learner (Ed.), *Early adolescence: Perspectives on research, policy, and intervention* (pp. 383–400). Hillsdale, N.Y: Erlbaum.

Kirisci, L., Mezzich, A., & Tarter, R. (1995). Norms and sensitivity of the adolescent version of the Drug Use Screening Inventory. *Addictive Behaviors, 20,* 149–157.

Lerner, J., & Vicary, J. (1984). Difficult temperament and drug use: Analysis from the New York Longitudinal Study. *Journal of Drug Education, 14,* 1–18.

Martin, C. S., Kaczynski, N. A., Maiso, S. A., Bukstein, O. M., & Moss, H. B. (1995). Patterns of DSM-IV alcohol abuse and dependence symptoms in adolescent drinkers. *Journal of Studies on Alcohol, 56,* 672–680.

Maskey, S., Crown, S., & Oyebode, F. (2004). Practical child and adolescent psychopharmacology. *British Journal of Psychiatry, 185,* 357.

Matas, M., Staley, D., & Griffin, W. (1992). A profile of the noncompliant patient: A thirty-month review of outpatient psychiatry referral. *General Hospital Psychiatry, 14,* 124–130.

Mayer, J., & Filstead, W. J. (1979). The Adolescent Alcohol Involvement Scale: An instrument for measuring adolescents' use and misuse of alcohol. *Journal of Studies on Alcohol, 40,* 291–300.

Maziade, M. (1989). Should adverse temperament matter to the clinician? An empirically based answer. In G. Kohnstrom, J. Bates, & M. Rothbart (Eds.), Temperament in childhood (pp. 421–435). New York: John Wiley & Sons.

Miller, G. A. (1985) *The Substance Abuse Subtle Screening Inventory (SASSI): Manual, second edition.* Springfield, IN: SASSI Institute.

Miller, W.R., & Rollnick, S. (2002). *Motivational interviewing: Preparing people for change* (2nd ed.). New York: Guilford Press.

Moberg, D. P., & Hahn, L. (1991). The Adolescent Drug Involvement Scale. *Journal of Adolescent Chemical Dependency, 2,* 75–88.

Moore, D. D. (1983). *Client Substance Index.* Olympia, WA: Olympic Counseling Services.

Nathan, P. E., Skinstad, A. H., & Dolan, S. (2001). Alcohol-related disorders: Psychopathology, diagnosis, etiology, and treatment. In P. B. Sutker & H. E. Adams (Eds.), *Comprehensive handbook of psychopathology* (3rd ed., pp. 295–622). New York: Kluwer Academic/Plenum Press.

Newcomer, L. L., & Lewis, T. J. (2004). Functional behavioral assessment: An investigation of assessment reliability and effectiveness of function-based interventions. *Journal of Emotional & Behavioral Disorders, 12,* 168–181.

Nigg, J. T., Glass, M., Wong, M. M., Poon, E., Jester, J. M., Fitzgerald, H. E., Puttler, L. I., Adams, K. M., & Zucker, R. A. (2004). Neuropsychological executive functioning in children at elevated risk for alcoholism. *Journal of Abnormal Psychology, 113,* 302–314.

Rahdert, E. (Ed.). (1991). *The Adolescent Assessment/Referral System manual.* Rockville, MD: U.S. Department of Health and Human Services, ADAMHA, National Institute on Drug Abuse, DHHS Pub. No. (ADM) 91-1735.

Rowan, A. B. (2001). Adolescent substance abuse and suicide. *Depression & Anxiety, 14,* 186–191.

Shaffer, D., Fisher, P., Lucas, P., Dulcan, M. K., & Schwab-Stone, M. E. (2000). NIMH Diagnostic Interview Schedule for Children Version IV (NIMH DISC-IV): Description, differences from previous versions, and reliability of some common diagnoses. *Journal of the American Academy of Child & Adolescent Psychiatry, 39,* 28–38.

Shedler, J., & Block, J. (1990). Adolescent drug use and psychological health: A longitudinal inquiry. *American Psychologist, 45,* 612–630.

Sobell, L. C., & Sobell, M. B. (1996). Timeline follow-back: A technique for assessing self-reported consumption. In R. Litten & J. Allen (Eds.), *Measuring alcohol consumption* (pp. 41–72). Totowa, N.J.: Humana Press.

Spitzer, R. L., Williams, J., & Gibbon, M. (1990). *User's guide for the structured clinical interview for DSM-III-R: SCID.* Washington, DC: American Psychiatric Association.

Tapert, S. F., Colby, S. M., & Barnett, N. P. (2003). Depressed mood, gender, and problem drinking in youth. *Journal of Child & Adolescent Substance Abuse, 12,* 55–68.

Tarter, R. E. (1990). Evaluation and treatment of adolescent substance abuse: A decision tree method. *American Journal of Drug and Alcohol Abuse, 16,* 1–46.

Tarter, R. E., Sambrano, S., & Dunn, M. G. (2002). Predictor variables by developmental stages: A Center for Substance Abuse Prevention multisite study. *Psychology of Addictive Behaviors, 16,* 3–10.

Thomas, D. W. (1990). *Substance abuse screening protocol for the juvenile courts.* Pittsburgh PA: National Center for Juvenile Justice.

U.S. Department of Health and Human Services. (2003). *About the Federal Child Abuse Prevention and Treatment Act.* Retrieved from http://nccanh.acf.hhs.gov/pubs/factsheets/about.cfm

White, H. R., & Labouvie, E. W. (1989). Towards the assessment of adolescent problem drinking. *Journal of Studies on Alcohol, 50,* 30–37.

Winters, K. C. (1992). Development of an adolescent alcohol and other drug abuse screening scale: Personal Experiences Screening Questionnaire. *Addictive Behavior, 17,* 479–490.

Winters, K. C., & Henly, G. A. (1989). *Personal Experience Inventory (PEI) test and manual.* Los Angeles: Western Psychological Services.

Winters, K. C., & Henly, G. A. (1993). *Adolescent Diagnostic Interview schedule and manual.* Los Angeles: Western Psychological Services.

Winters, K. C., Latimer, W. W., & Stinchfield, R. (2001). Assessing adolescent substance use. In E. F. Wagner & H. B. Waldron (Eds.), *Innovations in adolescent substance abuse interventions* (pp. 1–29). Amsterdam: Pergamon Press/Elsevier Science.

15

PEER RELATIONSHIP PROBLEMS

LINDA A. LEBLANC
RACHAEL A. SAUTTER
DAWN J. DORE

Department of Psychology
Western Michigan University
Kalamazoo, Michigan

INTRODUCTION

Children's interactions with their peers serve several critical developmental functions. A child's interactions with peers tend to be more egalitarian and free from constraint than their interactions with adults, providing opportunity to develop new skills for fair play and to explore the limits of social tolerance (Hetherington, Parke, & Locke, 1999). Peers serve as a source of information about social rules, a source of salient reinforcement, and as models for a variety of critical social behaviors (Bukowski, 2003). Finally, peers provide a standard against which children can compare themselves socially, playing a critical role in the children's developing self-image (Hetherington et al.).

As children mature, the nature and quality of their friendships change, based on expectations and activities (Hartup, 1999). Children typically have a friend by age 2 or 3 (Parker, Rubin, Price, & DeRosier, 1995), with that number increasing to an average of five friends by adolescence (Hartup). Most friendships in childhood last for about one year, and the ability to maintain friendships is relatively stable across childhood and adolescence (Hartup). With progressive development, the amounts of time children spend with their friends increases and the quality and basis for selection of childhood friendships changes (Parker et al.). In general, preschool children will often choose friends based on material qualities (e.g., types of toys in child's possession), while older children and adolescents select friends based on shared attitudes and values (Hetherington et al., 1999).

Unfortunately, not all children have uniformly effective peer relationships, and the development of peer relationship problems can have detrimental effects on the developing child (Kupersmidt & Dodge, 2004). Rejection by peers has been associated with a variety of negative outcomes, from poor academic results (e.g., poor performance, dropout status) to mental health issues (e.g., loneliness, depression, poor self-concept) and externalizing behavioral problems (e.g., aggression, delinquency, high-risk behaviors, and criminality) (McDougall, Hymel, Vaillancourt, & Mercer, 2001). In some instances, peer rejection occurs due to a disability or other characteristic outside of the control of the child. However, a significant body of research has focused on peer rejection resulting from behaviors that are amenable to change. These behaviors range from overt expressions of aggression to more subtle occurrences of social withdrawal (Parker et al., 1995), all of which are aversive to peers (Schwartz, McFayden-Ketchum, Dodge, Pettit, & Bates, 1999).

Research on peer relationship problems often focuses on the interactions of and the outcomes for bullies and victims (Kupersmidt & Dodge, 2004). The bully–victim interaction is not the only type of peer relationship problem but does account for the majority of peer rejection issues found in outpatient clinics and school settings. Descriptions of behaviors, considerations of parenting issues, and discussion of long-term consequences of bullies and victims follow.

BULLIES

Bullies are defined as children who engage in behavior that results in physical or emotional harm to another child in order to exert control over other children (Craig & Pepler, 2003; Smith, Bowers, Binney, & Cowie, 1993). Bullies are usually perceived as stronger than their victims (Smith et al.), are often seen as leaders by their peers, and may fall into the "controversial" or "rejected" sociometric category (Smith et al.). Contrary to popular opinion, most evidence suggests that bullies do not appear to have low self-esteem (Smith et al.), although there is still some debate in this area (Wolke, Woods, Bloomfield, & Karstadt, 2000). Some research indicates that bullies demonstrate lower levels of anxiety and increased self-esteem relative to nonbullies. In general, bullies do not acknowledge significant behavioral problems (Wolke et al.), though their parents, teachers, and peers report these problems about them.

Children who engage in bullying behavior often live in an environment that permits high levels of aggression as well as criticism (Stevens, DeBoudeaudhuij, & VanOost, 2002). Bullies perceive their families as less unified and more hostile (Stevens et al.) than do children who do not bully. In addition, children who bully may be reinforced in their home environment for using aggressive behavior to solve conflict (Stevens et al.).

The consequences of bullying are serious, and they affect the child and society for many years after the child has left school. In the long term, children identified as bullies are more likely to engage in delinquent behaviors and to abuse alcohol (Haynic et al., 2001). In addition, children who bully at early ages are at increased risk of criminal activity in young adulthood (Haynic et al.). They are also more apt to continue their victimization by engaging in acts of domestic or dating violence (Durlak, 2001).

VICTIMS

Victims are the recipients of hostile, repetitive physically or verbally aggressive acts (Craig & Pepler, 2003). Like bullies, victims have a higher probability of behavioral problems relative to children not involved in such interactions (Wolke et al., 2000). Recently, research has supported distinct subtypes of victims (Schwartz et al., 1999; Schwartz, 2000). The subtypes appear to break down into "innocent" and "provocative" victims (Smith et al., 1993). These two groups have different presentations, critical behaviors for intervention, and outcomes, so they will be reviewed separately.

INNOCENT VICTIMS

Innocent victims are also known as *passive/withdrawn* victims (Smith et al., 1993). Some evidence suggests that one precursor to victimization by bullies is the presence of shy or withdrawn behaviors, which may result in the child having fewer friends and less protection against bullies (Dill, Vernberg, Fonagy, Twemlow, & Gamm, 2004). Innocent victims tend to engage in developmentally inappropriate play and frequently withdraw from the social group (Parker et al., 1995). They may also have poor social and problem-solving skills and may develop a strong aversion to the school setting over time (Wolke et al., 2000). Some evidence suggests that shyness and social withdrawal may not result in peer rejection or victimization until middle childhood, leaving a window for possible interventions (Coplan, Prakash, O'Neil, & Armer, 2004). Shy, withdrawn children represent the "nonsqueaky wheel," until they become victims of predatory bullies. Therefore, it is critical that schools screen for peer relationship problems such as social withdrawal or shyness to prevent future negative outcomes.

Several lines of research support the relationship between overprotective parenting and subsequent shy behaviors in children. Overprotective parenting includes restricting the child's activities, being overly demonstrative with affection, and discouraging a child's attempts at independence (Coplan et al., 2004). Once victimized, children may demonstrate symptoms of internalizing disorders, such as depression and anxiety, and repeated victimization is linked to additional deleterious consequences, including anger, school avoidance, and increased social withdrawal (Dill et al., 2004; Wolke et al., 2000). Adults who report being bullied as children may be more vulnerable to depression and suffer from decreased self-esteem (Wolke et al.).

PROVOCATIVE VICTIMS

Provocative victims, also know as *bully/victims*, are typically the victims of certain children while actively engaging in bullying toward other children (Wolke et al., 2000). Relative to bullies and innocent victims, this group may demonstrate higher frequencies of both externalizing and internalizing symptoms. The behaviors of bully/victims may be particularly aversive to peers, and they are perceived as rarely cooperative and least liked (Smith et al., 1993). They often play alone and appear to be anxious and insecure (Smith et al.). They also exhibit excessive motor activity and are often viewed as impulsive (Schwartz et al., 1999; Wolke et al.). Provocative victims endorse higher levels of psychotic, neurotic, and depressive symptoms (Wolke et al.) and lower scores on measures of academic competence (Haynic et al., 2001) relative to those who do not bully.

Provocative victims may perceive their family as lacking warmth and being too protective (Stevens et al., 2002). Unlike children in the other categories, provocative victims report wielding a significant amount of power in the family. Similar to bullies, provocative victims may experience discipline that lacks consistency (Stevens et al.). Because the provocative victim category is new relative to the innocent victim and bully labels, little is known about the long-term consequences of being a bully/victim (Haynic et al., 2001). Wolke et al. (2000) describe the bully/victim as "the most behaviorally disturbed" relative to the bullies and innocent victims (p. 998). Research findings such as these predict dire long-term consequences.

Due to the immediate and long-term consequences of untreated peer relationship problems, practitioners must prioritize identification and intervention with bullies and victims and withdrawn children who may become victims. As with many childhood problems, the assessment process should sample as many relevant contexts as possible to fully understand the antecedents and consequences of the targeted behaviors. In addition, as bullies tend to underreport their problematic behaviors (Wolke et al., 2000) and victims may underreport their victimization due to fear, it is important to use multiple informants, such as involved adults (e.g., teachers, parents) and peers.

ASSESSMENT STRATEGIES

Children's peer relationship problems should be assessed using a multitrait, multimethod, multisource approach that focuses on problem identification and gathering information that directly guides intervention selection and implementation. The general aspects of peer relations that should be assessed are social status/peer acceptance, extent of peer networks (i.e., reciprocal friendships, friendship quality), and specific social behaviors related to peer relations (Furman, 1996). It is important to assess each of these aspects independently because social status or a limited peer network does not necessarily preclude having a high-quality friendship. Similarly, a child may exhibit social behaviors predictive of bullying while still having an extensive network, though the individuals in that network may socially reinforce bullying.

The most common sources of information about children's peer relationship problems are the target child, peers, parents, and teachers. Self-report of the target child can provide specific information about bullying and victimization events; however, these reports tend to be positively biased and unreliable (Pepler & Craig, 1998). That is, bullies seldom identify their bullying behavior with accuracy. Self-reports are valuable for evaluating a child's satisfaction with his or her own interpersonal relations and the valued features of relationships. Peer assessment measures provide an excellent way to assess the quality of the relationships among groups of children. Peer measures are usually completed by multiple informants, making them more accurate, reliable, and valid measures of friendships (Pepler & Craig). Peer assessments can also be used to provide information about mutual relationships (i.e., mutual best friends) and are the gold standard for information about social status in the form of sociometrics.

Adult informants provide information independent of the peer dynamic and may have unique insights into a child's social acceptance or the functions of his or her relations. Adults tend to be more sophisticated judges of social distinctions and are critical informants when the target child is younger (Ladd & Profilet, 1996). Parents provide valuable information because they have the unique opportunity to observe the child across social contexts for many hours each day. However, parent report may be impacted by social desirability bias if the parent was not the source of the referral. Teachers provide a valuable perspective based on substantial time spent with children in a variety of school social contexts and comparisons between children of the same age, perhaps resulting in a more developmentally accurate evaluation. Teacher reports also tend to be more time efficient and cost effective than peer assessments (Ladd & Profilet), but there is the potential for relationship bias and decreased accuracy in reporting frequency or rates of specific behaviors (Pepler & Craig, 1998).

The most commonly used methods of assessment are sociometric procedures, behavioral checklists (self, peer, teacher/parent), and direct observation (Pepler & Craig, 1998). A minimal description of sociometric procedures is provided here because of the extensive coverage in Chapter 10. In general, sociometric procedures include nominations of children with certain behavioral characteristics and identification and ranking of specific friendships within a class. Sociometrics can provide valuable information on social acceptance status and on the qualities of existing friendships. Several measures include an initial sociometric evaluation and subsequent assessment of the quality of the "mutual best friend" relationship identified via the nomination or ranking procedure (Parker & Asher, 1993).

Behavioral checklists are the most common self-report assessment measures of a child's friendship or peer network. These measures typically include a list of specific behaviors or characteristics to which the child should respond using a Likert-type rating scale. Checklists have been used to assess the quality or specific characteristics of a friendship, the frequency of specific behaviors or activities, or the applicability of certain situational descriptions to the target child's own friendships. Several self-report behavioral checklist measures are presented in Table 15.1, and a sample of the most promising ones are briefly described in the section on research basis.

Direct observations of peer interaction provide important information that is not subject to the same limitations and biases as other assessment measures (Howes & Matheson, 1992; Pepler & Craig, 1998). Naturalistic observations may reveal complex interpersonal dynamics between individuals or groups of children and may shed light on potential social functions of dysfunctional interpersonal behaviors. For example, aggressive behavior may be, in part, maintained by the social expectations and social reactions of the peer group of a bully. Several coding schemes are available for both younger and older children and for real-time and video-recorded observations (Bakeman & Gottman, 1986; Howes & Matheson, 1992; Craig, & Pepler, 1997). The primary concern about observation procedures is potential reactivity if the observers are too obtrusive. Other potential concerns for clinical utility are logistical issues, such as time and staff constraints and training of coders.

RESEARCH BASIS

A growing empirical literature on peer relationship problems includes several tools for assessing peer relationship problems. Table 15.1 provides details on assessment measures that children complete for their own behavior and the behaviors of their peers. A sample of these measures is described in greater detail here in the text.

Perhaps the most commonly used measure of quality of relationship in studies of peer relationships is the Friendship Quality Questionnaire (FQQ; Parker & Asher, 1993). The scale requires children to complete sociometric nominations of their best friend before answering 40 questions about different aspects of friendship using a 5-point Likert scale. Six features of the relationship are assessed: companionship and recreation, help and guidance, validation and caring, intimate exchange, conflict and betrayal, and conflict resolution.

There is evidence of satisfactory internal consistency for each subscale, with Chronbach's alpha coefficients ranging from .73 for the three-item subscale to .90 for two of the larger subscales (Parker & Asher, 1993). In addition, stability of scores over a two-week period is high ($r = .75$) (Furman, 1996). Parker and Asher assessed the qualities of a best-friend relationship in high-average and low-accepted children in grades three through six and an additional 153 children in grades three through five. Their findings indicate that even low-accepted children typically identified a best friend and reported satisfaction with that friendship. Satisfaction with a particular friendship was directly related to all six features;

TABLE 15.1 Student Report Checklists, Ratings Scales, and Nomination Inventories

Name of Measure	Author/Citation	Description	Psychometric Properties
Friendship Quality Questionnaire (FQQ)	Parker & Asher (1993)	• 40-item questionnaire that the child completes with reference to a specific friend (the child's best mutual friend) on a 5-point Likert scale • Assessed companionship and recreation, help and guidance, validation and caring, intimate exchange, conflict and betrayal, and conflict resolution	• Satisfactory alpha • Multiple validity investigation
Relationship Quality Questionnaire (Modified FQQ)	Meurling, Ray, & LoBello (1999)	• Measures companionship and recreation, conflict and betrayal, conflict resolution, help and guidance, intimate exchange, validation and caring, exclusivity on a 4-point scale	• No psychometric information provided
Friendship Satisfaction	Parker & Asher (1993)	• Two questions to assess friendship satisfaction (administered separately from FQQ): "How is the friendship going?" and "How happy are you with this friendship?" • For both questions, child responds on a 15-point continuum	• No psychometric information provided
McGill Friendship Questionnaires	Mendelson & Aboud (1999)	• Respondent's Affection Version: 9 items on positive feelings for a friend and 7 items on friendship satisfaction. Child responds on a 9-point scale • Friend's Function Versions: Assesses whether a friend fulfills the six friendship functions (5 items each). Child responds on a 9-point scale	• All subscales were reliable, with high internal consistency • Validity support
Loneliness Scale	Marcoen & Brumagne (1985)	• 28-item questionnaire consisting of statements with respect to parent-related and peer-related loneliness • Students judge items applicability personally on a 4-point Likert scale	• Alpha = .88 • Validity support
Loneliness & Social Dissatisfaction Scale (LSDS)	Asher & Wheeler (1985)	• 24-item self-report questionnaire (16 items on feelings of loneliness and social dissatisfaction in school) and child responds on a 5-point Likert scale • Addressed feelings of loneliness, appraisal of current peer relationships, degree to which important relationship needs are being met, and perception of social competence	• Alpha = .90

(continues)

TABLE 15.1 *(continued)*

Name of Measure	Author/Citation	Description	Psychometric Properties
Social Experience Questionnaire Self-Report (SEQ-S) Peer Report (SEQ-P)	Crick & Grotpeter (1996) Crick & Bigbee (1998)	• Children ages 9–11 self/peer-report of victimization on a 5-point Likert scale • Three subscales: relational victimization, overt victimization, and prosocial behaviors • Six questions added to original questionnaire to assess forms of overt and relational victimization	• 4-week test–retest = .90 • Internal consistencies ranging from .77 to .91
Berndt's assessment of friendship features	Berndt, Hawkins, & Hoyle (1986) Berndt & Keefe (1992)	• Examines positive and negative features of friendships: self-disclosure, prosocial behavior, self-esteem reports, and conflict and rivalry • Twelve positive items and eight negative items rated for each relationship on a 5-point scale	• Alphas high for subscales • Preliminary validity support
Friendship Questionnaire	Furman & Adler (1982)	• Assesses 16 features of warmth and closeness, conflict, exclusivity, and relative status and power • Children rate characteristics of a particular friendship on a 5-pt scale	• Satisfactory alphas • Preliminary validity findings
Network of relationships inventory	Furman & Buhrmester (1985)	• Twelve features of relationships with parents, siblings, boy/girlfriends, teachers, and close friends • The child rates how much each feature occurs in each relationship	• Satisfactory alphas • Validity support
Friendship Quality Scale	Bukowski, Hoza, & Boivin (1994)	• Assesses child's perception of his best friend on a 5-point scale • Completed with reference to a specific child • Twenty-three questions (closeness, security, help, companionship, and conflict)	• Acceptable but slightly low alphas • Concurrent validity evidence

Behavioral Systems Questionnaire (BSQ)	Furman & Wehner (1994)	• Conceptualizes romantic relationships, friendships, and parent–child relationships (mother–child and father–child) • Assessed generalized views of four different types of relationships, and students rate on a 5-point scale how much they agree or disagree with 92 statements about their friendships	• Satisfactory alphas • Reliable composite score • Convergent validity evidence
Participant Role Questionnaire	Salmivalli, Lagerspetz, Bjorkqvist, Osterman, & Kaukiainen (1996)	• Fifty-item questionnaire of self- and peer estimates of bullying behavior; 22- and 15-item versions (PRQ) also available • 10- to 14-year-olds evaluate self and peers against 50 behavioral descriptions • Bully scale, Assistant scale, Reinforcer Scale, Defender scale, Outsider scale, and Victim scale	• Alpha = .81–.93
Revised Olweus Bully/Victim Questionnaire	Olweus (1996)	• 40-item questionnaire for students 8–16 years old: Junior and Senior versions; they respond on a 5-point scale • Assessed children's perceptions of being bullied and about bullying others • Instrument and manual available from author	• Alpha = .80–.90
Measure of Adolescent Social Performance (MASP)	Cavell & Kelley (1992)	• Created to identify adolescents with social adjustment problems and to assess adolescent social performance • Fifty-four items for the adolescent to respond to, and each item describes a problematic social situation and asks them which of the four response options is most like what they would do or say (not what they should do or say) • Teachers rate adolescents' peer acceptance with a 5-point Likert scale	• Alpha coefficient of .87 • Adequate test–retest reliability • Initial support for concurrent validity

Alpha refers to Chronbach's alpha as a measure of internal consistency.

however, the qualities of the relationships of low-accepted children were substantially lower than those of accepted children on most dimensions.

The Social Experience Questionnaire (SEQ) is a 22-item inventory for elementary school–aged children that assesses self-report of victimization at the hands of peers and supportive acts by peers (Crick & Grotpeter, 1996). This inventory includes three subscales and uses a 5-point Likert rating. The test–retest reliability over four weeks is excellent, and the internal consistencies for subscales range from .82 to .97. In their study of third- to sixth-graders, most of the identified victims were the targets of either relational or overt aggression but not both forms of aggression. In addition, rejected children were more victimized than were well-accepted children. Finally, this study illustrated that victimization was significantly related to adjustment difficulties such as depression and loneliness.

The Loneliness and Social Dissatisfaction Scale (LSDS; Asher & Wheeler, 1985) is a 24-item measure that includes 16 items assessing feelings of loneliness, appraisal of peer relationships, the degree to which relationship needs are being met, and the child's perception of his or her own social competence. This scale has been used in several different studies involving elementary school children, and the results have shown that this questionnaire has excellent internal reliability and consistency (Cassidy & Asher, 1992; Parker & Asher, 1993). The psychometric properties of this scale have been directly supported in recent investigations with several non-Caucasian populations, including Hispanic American, African American, and Greek children (Bagner, Storch, & Roberti, 2004; Galanaki & Kalantzi-Azizi, 1999).

The Participant Role Questionnaire (PRQ) is a 50-item questionnaire that investigates self- and peer estimates of bullying behavior in specific situations (Salmivalli, Lagerspetz, Bjorkqvist, Osterman, & Kaukiainen, 1996). Students evaluate how well each child in their class fits the different bullying situations, and the instrument includes subscales, such as the bullying subscale, assistance scale, the reinforcer scale, defender scale, outsider scale, and victim scale. The PRQ has strong reported internal consistency for the six different subscales. Salmivalli et al. found support for identifiable roles within bullying situations and significant gender differences, with more female than male defenders and more male than female bullies and reinforcers. Students were moderately well aware of their own participant roles; however, they often underestimated their own active participation as a bully. Several other studies have used modified versions of this scale and have also reported sound psychometric properties (Sutton & Smith, 1999; Tani, Greenman, Schneider, & Fregoso, 2003).

Teacher reports are another beneficial way to gather information about a child's social acceptance and peer network. Typically, teachers are asked to rate the frequency of the target child's behavior in relation to the behaviors of the other children in the class. Teachers may rate the child on specific behaviors, such as shyness, aggression, bully behavior, antisocial behavior, hyperactivity, anxiety, irritability, and social competence. Teachers respond by providing the target child with a Likert scale rating for each of the behaviors identified on the assessment. Several teacher report measures are included in Table 15.2, and a subset of the most commonly used measures is detailed next.

The Teacher Rating Scale for Reactive and Proactive Aggression (TRSRPA; Price & Dodge, 1989) is a 24-item instrument that uses a 5-point Likert scale initially developed for use with kindergarten and first-grade students. Measures of reactive aggression assess a child's response to being teased, striking back against bullies, blaming others in fights, and overreacting to accidents. Items sampling proactive aggression focus on a child's use of physical force over others, ganging up on peers, and bullying others. The scale has evidence of high internal consistency (r = .95 and .94) and moderate construct validity (Dodge & Coie, 1987; Price & Dodge). Both proactive and reactive aggression are related to a child's classroom peer status, with reactive aggression toward peers in particular associated with social rejection. However, age variables mediate aggressiveness with kindergarteners rated higher on scales of both proactive and reactive aggression when compared with first-grade children.

The School Social Behavior Scales (SSBS; Merrell, 1993) is a 65-item teacher rating scale designed for use with elementary and high school–age children. Teachers rate children on social competence and antisocial behavior using a 5-point scale. The social competence scale consists of three primary subscales: interpersonal behavior, self-management skills, and academic performance. The scale measuring antisocial behavior also consists of three subscales: hostile-irritable behavior, antisocial-aggressive behavior, and disruptive-demanding behavior. The subscales have high internal consistency estimates, with coefficients ranging from r = .94 to r = .96. In addition, the overall scale has acceptable test–rest reliability (r = .76–.82) and interrater reliability (r = .72–.83) (Merrell).

The Child Behavior Scale (CBS; Ladd & Profilet, 1996) is a 59-item inventory that uses a 3-point Likert rating scale for teacher evaluation of aggressive behavior with peers, prosocial behavior with peers, and three different types of withdrawn behavior. Forty-four of the 59 items are grouped into six relevant subscales: aggressive with peers, prosocial with peers, asocial with peers, anxious-fearful, excluded by peers, and hyperactive-distractible. Nine of the remaining address nonaggressive problem behaviors, and six address general classroom behaviors. All six subscales have moderately high to high internal consistency estimates, with coefficients ranging from r = .77 to r = .96. In addition, the subscales are consistent across both samples and measurement occasions, with acceptable interrater reliability (r = .81–.88). Information exists for African American and Latino populations as well as Caucasian samples. Ladd and Profilet found that kindergarteners with higher aggression scores on the CBS were rated as dominating toward peers, less prosocial, and more distractible. Boys were rated significantly higher than girls on aggression with peers and hyperactivity-distractiblity subscales, while girls were generally rated as more prosocial than boys. Children rated as antisocial or anxious-fearful with peers were liked more

TABLE 15.2 Teacher Report Measures of Social Adjustment and Relationship Problems

Name of Measure	Author/Citation	Description	Psychometric Properties
Teacher Rating Scale for Reactive and Proactive Aggression (TRSRPA)	Price & Dodge (1989)	• Twenty-four items with subscales for reactive and proactive aggression • Teachers rate each item on a 5-point Likert scale	• Alpha coefficients of .95 and .94 for the two subscales • Validity support
Revised Teacher Rating Scale for Reactive and Proactive Aggression	K. Brown, Atkins, Osborne, & Milnamow (1996)	• Twenty-eight items measuring reactive aggression, proactive aggression, covert antisocial behavior, and prosocial behavior in 8- to 10-year-old children	• Alpha = .92–.94 • Test–retest .93 • Criterion validity acceptable
Teacher Assessment of Social Behavior Questionnaire	Cassidy & Asher (1992)	• Teacher rates the social behavior of a specific child in relation to other kids in the class on a 5-point scale • Looks at prosocial behavior, shyness, and aggression	• No psychometric information provided
Child Behavior Scale (CBS)	Ladd & Profilet (1996)	• Three-point teacher rating scale looking at aggressive behavior with peers, prosocial behavior with peers, and three types of withdrawn behavior (asocial with peers, excluded by peers, and anxious-fearful behavior) • Fifty-nine-item rating scale, with 44 of the items grouped into six subscales: aggressive with peers, prosocial with peers, asocial with peers, anxious-fearful, excluded by peers, and hyperactive-distractible • Nine items for problem behaviors and six for other classroom behaviors • Includes African American, Latino, and Caucasian children	• Alpha: .77–.96 • Test–retest: .54–.83 • Interrater: .81–.88 • Several studies support criterion validity

School Social Behavior Scales (SSBS)	Merrell (1993)	• Sixty-five-item teacher rating scale designed for use with grades K–12 • Teachers respond on a 5-point Likert scale • Scale A: social competence, with subscales interpersonal, self-management, and academic skills • Scale B: antisocial behavior, with subscales hostile-irritable, antisocial-aggressive, and disruptive-demanding • Available from Assessment-Intervention Resources, Eugene, OR • Includes African American, Native American, Latino, and Caucasian children	• Internal consistency: .94–.98 • Test–rest reliability: .60–.94 • Interrater reliability: .53–.83 • Criterion validity acceptable
Walker–McConnell Scale of Social Competence and School Adjustment (WMS)	Walker & McConnell (1988)	• Forty-three-item teacher rating scale to be used with grades K–6 • Teachers respond on a 5-point scale • Major scale: social competence • Three subscales: teacher-preferred social behavior, peer-preferred social behavior, and school adjustment • Previously available from Pro-Ed, Inc.; currently out of print	• Excellent alpha • Adequate-to-excellent test–retest reliability, adequate interrater reliability • Adequate content and criterion-related validity
School Social Skills Rating Scale (SSSRS)	L. J. Brown, Black, & Downs (1984)	• Forty-item teacher rating scale (6-point Likert scale) used for grades K–12 • Four subscales: adult relations, peer relations, school rules, and classroom behaviors • Designed to identify strengths and deficits in school social behaviors	• Adequate-to-excellent interrater reliability and test–retest reliability • Adequate content validity

by their classmates than children rated as aggressive with peers, hyperactive-distractible, and excluded by peers.

The Walker–McConnell Scale of Social Competence and School Adjustment (WMS; Walker & McConnell, 1988) is a 43-item teacher rating scale used with elementary school–aged children. Teachers rate a child's social competence along a 5-point continuum with respect to three primary subscales: teacher-preferred social behavior, peer-preferred social behavior, and school adjustment. Walker and McConnell reported excellent internal consistency and adequate-to-excellent test–retest reliabilities. In addition, they also reported adequate interrater reliability as well as adequate content and criterion-related validity.

CLINICAL UTILITY

In addition to research utility, many of the scales included in this chapter may provide valuable clinical information for identifying children suspected of experiencing peer relationship problems and for selecting specific targets for intervention. However, the clinical utility of these measures is limited by the overall lack of clinically designed measures that are commercially available and have norm-based clinical cutoff scores. Thus, an individual child's score on any of these measures will not tell you whether a given child is more aggressive toward her or his peers than most children of that child's age. These scales have been designed for comparisons with large groups of children rather than as individual clinical tools. Most scales are freely available as tables or appendices in research studies (Asher & Wheeler, 1985; Parker & Asher, 1993) and as unpublished manuscripts available from authors (Furman & Adler, 1982) rather than as published scales with technical manuals. Two notable exceptions are the School Social Behavior Scales (Merrell, 1993), available from Assessment-Intervention Resources, and the Revised Olweus Bully/Victim Questionnaire (Olweus, 1996), available from the author. The WMS (Walker & McConnell, 1988) has previously been available from Pro-Ed, Inc., but is now out of print.

Given the covert nature of peer relationship problems and the design of most of the tools, the most useful and efficient information might be obtained at a systems level by conducting screening of peer status and peer relationship problems for all children in classrooms or even specific grades. For example, school systems might conduct sociometric nominations and the PRQ for all children beginning in approximately first and second grade and use the results to target both bullies and victims or children at risk for these problems. These children might then undergo additional assessment and intervention.

Although most of the measures described in this chapter do not include clinical norms and cutoffs, they may provide excellent information about behavioral contributors to risk thereby providing specific information related to intervention planning. For example, the TRSRPA may assist in identifying those specific situations likely to provoke aggression for a given child, providing an approximation of a functional assessment of aggressive behavior. In addition, the PRQ identifies several roles other than bully and victim. Some identified roles facilitate and reinforce the bullying of other children, while other scales identify children whose primary role is that of defender of victimized children. This information may be critical for intervention development if the clinician wants to eliminate social reinforcement for bullying or wants to target peer mentors who may serve a protective role for a targeted victim.

DEVELOPMENTAL CONSIDERATIONS

The clinician should be mindful of several developmental considerations when assessing peer relationship problems. First, age is a critical factor when evaluating whether clinically important peer relationship problems exist. Kindergartners exhibit mildly aggressive behavior more frequently than older children (Price & Dodge, 1989), and it is developmentally normal for younger children to have fewer friends (Hartup, 1999). Thus, the clinician should not become alarmed if a child has only one to two close friends, because even one high-quality functional friendship can provide a buffering effect against some of the ill consequences of peer rejection (Schwartz et al., 1999; Vernberg, 1990). However, aggressiveness should be actively targeted, particularly if the child's rate of aggressive behavior is discrepant from that of other children in the social setting.

A second developmental consideration is the social function and reinforcement that may exist among peer networks. Peers are a powerful source of reinforcement for children and can play a critical role in increasing and maintaining the bullying behaviors of their friends. Clinicians should always examine functional reinforcers, such as peer attention, that may be contributing to bullying. A third developmental consideration is the impact of age on the utility of self-report measures. Self-report measures are typically not useful with young children because they often have relatively undifferentiated views of their behaviors in relation to peers and have limited language related to complex relations and interactions such as intimacy and conflict resolution (Pepler & Craig, 1998). For older children, however, self-report measures can provide valuable information on loneliness, friendship quality, and specific features of friendships unique to the respondent. Take caution, however, because older bullies will often present positively about their actions, so confirmatory evidence should be gathered from other class members (Pepler & Craig).

ASSESSMENT, CONCEPTUALIZATION, AND TREATMENT PLANNING

Many peer relationship issues will result directly in referral to a clinician, due to reported aggressiveness, victimization, or social isolation. However, other cases will initially present as a variety of potential mental health issues (e.g., anxiety, school refusal, depression, academic problems). The clinician should consider the possibility of peer relationship problems when assessing these other issues if there is any indication that peer relationships may not be strong for the client. Assessment should be approached using a multimethod, multi-informant approach.

Conceptualization of peer relationship problems should occur in a contextual and functional framework rather than in a pathological framework. That is, the clinician should consider aspects of the context and environment that may incite or maintain peer relationship problems rather than assuming that peer relationship problems always occur because of simple skills deficits. Peer networks may provide social support for bullying or avoidance behavior. Minor peer problems may be exacerbated by the occurrence of extended periods with minimal adult supervision or structured activities. Identification of these functional aspects and conceptualization of peer relationship problems from a functional perspective may directly inform treatment planning. For example, the clinician may identify ways to manipulate the environment to minimize opportunities for covert bullying or to facilitate minimally stressful social interactions for withdrawn or socially anxious children. When these contextual factors are combined with a specific social skills training program, interventions are more likely to produce maintenance and generalization of treatment effects. Additionally, structuring a schoolwide system that facilitates pro-social interactions and deters predatory or antisocial behavior has proven effective in prevention of antisocial behaviors in school settings (Sprague, Sugai, & Walker, 1998).

CASE STUDY I

IDENTIFICATION AND PRESENTING COMPLAINTS

Joey is a 12-year-old male referred to his school counselor in March. Joey has been suspended twice this year for fighting, and he will be expelled if another physical altercation occurs. Joey resides at home with his mother, stepfather, and 6-year-old stepsister. His family also reports problems with angry outbursts and noncompliance, and they are concerned about the possibility that more serious antisocial behavior will develop as Joey enters adolescence. Joey has a history of Oppositional Defiant Disorder and Attention-Deficit Hyperactivity Disorder, diagnosed at age 7, and academic problems beginning in third grade; however, no specific learning disabilities have been identified.

HISTORY, DEVELOPMENTAL ISSUES, AND SCHOOL ISSUES

Several developmental issues are worthy of note. Joey experienced adjustment problems when his mother remarried three years ago. He has not had contact with his biological father since age 2. Joey has few friends at school, but he is an excellent athlete. He is highly successful in his physical education classes and will likely play on his high school football and basketball teams if his skills continue to develop. However, his grades typically fall near the cutoff for academic eligibility.

BEHAVIORAL ASSESSMENT RESULTS

The counselor completed a comprehensive behavioral assessment of Joey's peer relationship problems, including an assessment of academic issues and a broad-based assessment of mental health issues. The Child Behavior Checklist (CBCL/6–18) and Teacher Report Form (TRF) indicate that Joey's previous diagnoses of ADHD and ODD remain pertinent and that Joey also experiences depressed mood (Achenbach & Rescorla, 2001). A follow-up assessment with the Children's Depression Inventory (CDI; Kovacs, 1992) substantiated the finding that Joey is depressed.

Results of the FQQ indicate that Joey has a "best friend" but that this relationship offers relatively little social support, validation, or caring. Joey reports that the primary strength of the relationship is recreational activities and that he and his friend have frequent conflicts. In a clinical interview, Joey's mother confirmed that Joey has conflicts with the children he refers to as friends and indicated that she does not think he benefits much from those relationships. The PRQ indicates that Joey acknowledges few behaviors indicative of bullying. Joey directly inquired whether his answers could be used against him with respect to expulsion. Although he was assured that the results would remain confidential, it is likely that a social bias affected his report. Peer responses on the PRQ conflict with Joey's perception, for they rank him high on the bully subscale. Information obtained from Joey's teacher confirmed the suspicion that Joey may bully other children. She completed the TRSRPA, indicating poor social problem solving and a mixture of reactive and proactive aggression. It appears that Joey targets certain children but is also a victim of bullying by other children.

CONCEPTUALIZATION AND TREATMENT RECOMMENDATIONS

A descriptive functional assessment indicates that Joey's aggressive behaviors are typically precipitated by a negative emotional experience during the prior 1–2 days (e.g., poor academic performance, athletic disappointment, an argument with his parents). He is most likely to aggress against other children during activities with a low level of monitoring, such as lunch, recess, and between-class transitions. Joey specifically targets children who are intelligent and small for their age. The PRQ indicates that three friends, including his best friend, typically provide social support for bullying but do not participate in physical altercations and have never been suspended.

The assessment results provide several important pieces of information for intervention planning. First, these results indicate a long-standing problem with externalizing behavior that has evolved into a pattern of bullying. Thus, treatment should focus on the overall pattern of behavior problems as well as specifically targeting bullying, to ensure broader therapeutic effect. Second, the functional assessment indicates that a group of children provide social reinforcement for his bullying while successfully avoiding consequences for their encouragement of antisocial behavior. These findings indicate that effective intervention will involve altering Joey's social environment to minimize contact with this peer group and to maximize contact with pro-social peers (e.g., Big Brothers of America, after-school YMCA mentoring program). Alternatively, an intervention might involve providing consequences for all children's encouragement of aggression as well as actual aggressive acts, in an effort to decrease social facilitation of bullying. The fact that other children may need to be targeted for intervention presents an ethical and practical consideration for the school, because these children have not been referred for services. The school personnel may choose to implement a classwide or schoolwide policy change to address this issue and may need to directly notify the parents of the other children of the potential future consequences. Finally, Joey's depression and status as both a bully and a victim of bullying indicate that psychological intervention services should be aimed at addressing his mood issues and teaching appropriate social skills.

CASE STUDY II

IDENTIFICATION AND PRESENTING COMPLAINTS

Dylan is an 8-year-old male presenting at his pediatrician's office for declining academic performance. His grades have been steadily declining from the beginning of the new academic year, 6 months prior to the evaluation. His physician referred him for psychological services to rule out a learning disability or other psychological condition.

HISTORY AND PEER ISSUES

Dylan lives with his mother and his maternal grandparents, his father is deceased. His mother is being treated for depression and resides with her parents due to financial and childcare constraints. Dylan reached all developmental milestones within age-appropriate norms, and his mother reports that he is a playful and loving child who spends much of his time in make-believe play, reading, or drawing. She reports that Dylan has had little contact with other children his age and did not attend preschool. He has been at the same elementary school since kindergarten.

BEHAVIORAL ASSESSMENT RESULTS

Prior to formal testing, a classroom observation was arranged. During the two-hour period, Dylan was observed in both structured and unstructured academic settings. There was no evidence of hyperactivity, impulsivity, or inattention. With structure, Dylan appeared to complete all tasks quietly. Dylan completes his work diligently, but many of the answers are incorrect. To assess academic achievement, the Wide Range Achievement Test—III (WRAT-III; Wilkonson, 1993) and the Peabody Picture Vocabulary Test—Third Edition (PPVT–III; Dunn, Dunn, Williams, & Wang, 1997) were administered. In addition, a Wechsler Intelligence Scale for Children—Fourth Edition (WISC-IV; Wechsler, 2003) was administered. Dylan scored at or above norms on all measures of achievement and aptitude.

The Childhood Anxiety Scale (CAS; Gillis, 1980) and the Children's Depression Inventory (CDI; Kovacs, 1992) were also administered, based on observations and parent concerns about withdrawal. His scores on the CAS and CDI were elevated above the clinically significant level, and Dylan was directly asked about his symptoms. Dylan reported that he was often sad and hated school because he was often teased specifically by one group of children in the fourth grade with a similar recess and lunch hour. Dylan reported few friends at school and stated that he was "very scared" of the older children. Based on this information, two relationship measures were administered to investigate peer relationship problems. The FQQ was completed for Dylan's reported best friend, and the PRQ was completed to assess his perceptions of being bullied. These measures indicated that Dylan is bullied and isolated and has no peer support during instances of victimization. Additionally, Dylan indicated that bullying typically involved physical and verbal aggression and that "was just the way it was," revealing his resignation to his status as a victim. He also reported that many children in his own class did not want to be his friend because of the teasing and bullying by the older kids.

CONCEPTUALIZATION AND TREATMENT RECOMMENDATIONS

The assessment results indicate that Dylan's academic performance is affected by symptoms of depression and anxiety related to bullying at school rather than a specific learning disability or mental retardation. Dylan has several social skills deficits due to infrequent contact with children his own age. Treatment should target not only the symptoms of depression and anxiety but also the social skills deficits, which may lead to the development of friendships that buffer the impact of the bullying.

SUMMARY

Healthy peer relations contribute greatly to a child's social and emotional development, and the influences of those peers become greater throughout childhood (Bukowski, 2003). When peer relationship problems exist, a child's risk increases for a variety of poor outcomes that can persist well into adulthood (Kupersmidt & Dodge, 2004). The most common peer relationship problems are bullying and being victimized by others, which are often accompanied by additional psychosocial problems, such as depression and conduct disorders. Because some of these problems are often covert, adults should look for subtle indications, such as isolation from peer groups and aggressive/dominant behavior toward others. Often, children who present with conditions of anxiety, depression, or academic difficulty and school refusal have some type of relationship problem as a functional contributing variable. Schools should consider conducting screening of all children for potential relationship problems, and clinicians should screen for relationship problems when assessing or treating other psychosocial conditions. A variety of measures of peer relationship functioning has been developed, primarily for research purposes; however, these scales might also be clinically useful in identifying children with peer relationship problems. In addition, these tools may be helpful in selecting target behaviors for treating relationship problems.

REFERENCES AND RESOURCES

Achenbach, T. M., & Rescorla, L. A. (2001). *Manual for ASEBA School-Age Forms and Profiles.* Burlington, VT: University of Vermont, Research Center for Children, Youth and Families.

Asher, S. R., & Wheeler, V. A. (1985). Children's loneliness: A comparison of rejected and neglected peer status. *Journal of Counseling and Clinical Psychology, 53,* 500–505.

Bagner, D. M., Storch, E. A., & Roberti, J. W. (2004). A factor analytic study of the Loneliness and Social Dissatisfaction Scale in a sample of African American and Hispanic American children. *Child Psychiatry & Human Development, 34,* 237–250.

Bakeman, R., & Gottman, J. (1986). *Observing interaction: An introduction to sequential analysis.* New York: Cambridge University Press.

Berndt, T. J., Hawkins, J. A., & Hoyle, S. G. (1986). Changes in friendship during a school year: Effects on children's and adolescents' impressions of friendship and sharing with friends. *Child Development, 57,* 1284–1297.

Berndt, T. J., & Keefe, K. (1992). Friends' influence on adolescents' perceptions of themselves at school. In D. H. Schunk & J. L. Meece (Eds.), *Student perceptions in the classroom* (pp. 51–73). Hillsdale, NJ: Englandiates.

Brown, K., Atkins, M. S., Osborne, M. L., & Milnamow, M. (1996). A revised teacher rating scale for reactive and proactive aggression. *Journal of Abnormal Child Psychology, 24,* 473–480.

Brown, L. J., Black, D. D., & Downs, J. C. (1984). *School Social Skills Rating Scale.* New York: Slosson Educational Publications.

Bukowski, W. M. (2003). Peer relationships. In M. H. Bornstein, L. Davidson, C. L. M. Keyes, & K. A. Moore (Eds.), *Well-being: Positive development across the life course* (pp. 221–233). Mahwah, NJ: Earlbaum.

Bukowski, W. M., Hoza, B., & Boivin, M. (1994). Measuring friendship quality during pre- and early adolescence: The development and psychometric properties of the Friendship Qualities Scale. *Journal of Social & Personal Relationships, 11,* 471–484.

Cassidy, J., & Asher, S. R. (1992). Loneliness and peer relations in young children. *Child Development, 63,* 350–365.

Cavell, T. A., & Kelley, M. L. (1992). The measure of adolescent social performance: Development and initial validation. *Journal of Clinical Child Psychology, 21,* 107–114.

Coplan, R. J., Prakash, K., O'Neil, K., & Armer, M. (2004). Do you "want" to play? Distinguishing between conflicted shyness and social disinterest in early childhood. *Developmental Psychology, 40,* 244–258.

Craig, W. M., & Pepler, D. J. (1997). Observations of bullying and victimization on the schoolyard. *Canadian Journal of School Psychology, 13,* 41–59.

Craig, W. M., & Pepler, D. J. (2003). Identifying and targeting risk for involvement in bullying and victimization. *Canadian Journal of Psychiatry, 48,* 577–582.

Crick, N. R., & Bigbee, M. A. (1998). Relational and overt forms of peer victimization: A multi-informant approach. *Journal of Consulting and Clinical Psychology, 66,* 337–347.

Crick, N. R., & Grotpeter, J. K. (1996). Children's treatment by peers: Victims of relational and overt aggression. *Development and Psychopathology, 8,* 367–380.

Dill, E. J., Vernberg, E. M., Fonagy, P., Twemlow, S. W., & Gamm, B. K. (2004). Negative affect in victimized children: The roles of social withdrawal, peer rejection and attitudes toward bullying. *Journal of Abnormal Child Psychology, 32,* 159–173.

Dodge, K. A., & Coie, J. D. (1987). Social information-processing factors in reactive and proactive aggression in children's peer groups. *Journal of Personality and Social Psychology, 53,* 1146–1158.

Dunn, L. M., Dunn, L. M., Williams, K. T., & Wang, J. J. (1997). *Peabody Picture Vocabulary Test: 3rd edition.* Circle Pines, MN: American Guidance Service.

Durlak, J. A. (2001). School problems of children. In C. E. Walker and M. C. Roberts (Eds.), *Handbook of clinical child psychology* (pp. 561–575). New York: John Wiley & Sons.

Furman, W. (1996). The measurement of friendship perceptions: Conceptual and methodological issues. In W. M. Bukowski, A. F. Newcomb, and W. W. Hartup (Eds.), *The company they keep: Friendship in childhood and adolescence* (pp. 41–65). New York: Cambridge University Press.

Furman, W., & Adler, T. (1982). *The Friendship Questionnaire.* Unpublished manuscript, University of Denver, Colorado.

Furman, W., & Buhrmester, D. (1985). Children's perceptions of the personal relationships in their social networks. *Developmental Psychology, 21,* 1016–1024.

Furman, W., & Wehner, E. A. (1994). Romantic views: Toward a theory of adolescent romantic relationships. In R. Montemayor (Ed.), *Advances in adolescent development, Vol. 6: Relationships in adolescence* (pp. 168–195). Newbury Park, CA: Sage Publications.

Galanaki, E. P., & Kalantzi-Azizi, A. (1999). Loneliness and social dissatisfaction: Its relation with children's self-efficacy for peer interaction. *Child Study Journal, 29,* 1–22.

Gillis, J. S. (1980). *Child Anxiety Scale.* Champaign, IL: Institute for Personality and Ability Testing.

Hartup, W. W. (1999). Peer experience and its developmental significance. In M. Bennett (Ed.), *Developmental psychology: Achievements and prospects* (pp. 106–125). New York: Psychology Press.

Haynic, D. L., Nansel, T., Eitel, P., Crump, A., Saylor, K., Yu, K., & Simons-Morton, B. (2001). Bullies, victims and bully/victims: Distinct groups of at-risk youth. *Journal of Early Adolescence, 21,* 29–49.

Hetherington, E. M., Parke, R. D., & Locke, V. O. (1999). *Child psychology: A contemporary viewpoint* (5th ed.). New York: McGraw-Hill.

Howes, C., & Matheson, C. C. (1992). Sequences in the development of competent play with peers: Social and social pretend play. *Developmental Psychology, 28,* 961–974.

Kovacs, M. (1992). *Children's Depression Inventory.* Wilmington, DE: Wide Range.

Kupersmidt, J. B., & Dodge, K. A. (2004). *Children's peer relations: From development to intervention.* Washington, DC: American Psychological Association.

Ladd, G. W., & Profilet, S. M. (1996). The Child Behavior Scale: A teacher-report measure of young children's aggressive, withdrawn, and prosocial behaviors. *Developmental Psychology, 32,* 1008–1024.

Marcoen, A., & Brumagne, M. (1985). Loneliness among children and young adolescents. *Developmental Psychology, 21,* 1025–1031.

McDougall, P., Hymel, S., Vaillancourt, T., & Mercer, L. (2001). The consequences of childhood peer rejection. In M. Leary (Ed.), *Interpersonal rejection* (pp. 213–247). London: University Press.

Mendelson, M. J., & Aboud, F. E. (1999). Measuring friendship quality in late adolescents and young adults: McGill Friendship Questionnaires. *Canadian Journal of Behavioural Science, 31,* 130–132.

Merrell, K. W. (1993). *School Social Behavior Scales.* Bradon, VT: Clinical Psychology Publishing.

Meurling, C. N., Ray, G. E., & LoBello, S. G. (1999). Children's evaluations of classroom friend and classroom best friend relationships. *Child Study Journal, 29,* 79–96.

Olweus, D. (1996). *Manual for the Revised Olweus Bully/Victim Questionnaire.* Available from author. Bergen, Norway: University of Bergen.

Parker, J. G., & Asher, S. R. (1993). Friendship and friendship quality in middle childhood: Links with peer group acceptance and feelings of loneliness and social dissatisfaction. *Developmental Psychology, 29,* 611–621.

Parker, J. G., Rubin, K. H., Price, J. M., & DeRosier, M. E. (1995). Peer relationships, child development and adjustment: A developmental psychopathology perspective. In D. Cicchetti and D. Cohen (Eds.), *Developmental psychopathology (Vol. 2): Risk, disorders and adaptation* (pp. 96–161). Oxford, UK: John Wiley & Sons.

Pepler, D. J., & Craig, W. M. (1998). Assessing children's peer relationships. *Child Psychology & Psychiatry Review, 3,* 176–182.

Pepler, D. J., Craig, W. M., & Roberts, W. L. (1998). Observations of aggressive and nonaggressive children on the school playground. *Merrill-Palmer Quarterly, 44,* 55–76.

Price, J. M., & Dodge, K. A. (1989). Reactive and proactive aggression in childhood: Relations to peer status and social context dimensions. *Journal of Abnormal Child Psychology, 17,* 455–471.

Salmivalli, C., Lagerspetz, K. M. J., Bjorkqvist, K., Osterman, K., & Kaukiainen, A. (1996). Bullying as a group process: Participant roles and their relations to social status within the class. *Aggressive Behavior, 22,* 1–15.

Schwartz, D. (2000). Subtypes of victims and aggressors in children's peer groups. *Journal of Abnormal Child Psycholgy, 28,* 181–192.

Schwartz, D., McFadyen-Ketchum, S., Dodge, K. A., Pettit, G. S., & Bates, J. E. (1999). Early behavior problems as a predictor of later peer group victimization: Moderators and mediators in the pathways of social risk. *Journal of Abnormal Child Psychology, 27,* 191–201.

Smith, P. K., Bowers, L., Binney, V., & Cowie, H. (1993). Relationships of children involved in bully/victim problems at school. In S. Duck (Ed.), *Learning about relationships* (pp. 184–204). Newbury Park, CA: Sage Publications.

Sprague, J., Sugai, G., & Walker, H. (1998). Antisocial behavior in schools. In T. S. Watson & F. M. Gresham (Eds.), *Handbook of child behavior therapy* (pp. 451–474). New York: Plenum Press.

Stevens, V., DeBourdeaudhuij, I., & VanOost, P. (2002). Relationship of the family environment to children's involvement in bully/victim problems at school. *Journal of Youth and Adolescence, 31,* 419–428.

Sutton, J., & Smith, P. K. (1999). Bullying as a group process: An adaptation of the participant role approach. *Aggressive Behavior, 25,* 97–111.

Tani, F., Greenman, P. S., Schneider, B. H., & Fregoso, M. (2003). Bullying and the big five: A study of childhood personality and participant roles in bullying incidents. *School Psychology International, 24,* 131–146.

Vernberg, E. M. (1990). Psychological adjustment and experiences with peers during early adolescence: Reciprocal, incidental or unidirectional relationships. *Journal of Abnormal Child Psychology, 18*(2), 187–198.

Walker, H. M., & McConnell, S. R. (1988). *The Walker–McConnell Scale of Social Competence and School Adjustment.* Austin, TX: Pro-Ed.

Wechsler, D. (2003). *Wechsler Intelligence Scales for Children* (4th ed.). San Antonio, TX: Harcourt Assessment.

Wilkonson, G. S. (1993). *Wide Range Achievement Test* (3rd ed.). Wilmington, DE: Wide Range.

Wolke, D., Woods, S., Bloomfield, L., & Karstadt, L. (2000). The association between direct and relational bullying and behaviour problems among primary school children. *Journal of Child Psychology and Psychiatry, 41,* 989–1002.

16

ATTENTION-DEFICIT/ HYPERACTIVITY DISORDER

MARK D. RAPPORT
THOMAS M. TIMKO, JR.
RACHEL WOLFE

Department of Psychology
University of Central Florida
Orlando, Florida

INTRODUCTION

Attention-Deficit/Hyperactivity Disorder (ADHD) is a complex and chronic disorder of brain, behavior, and development whose behavioral and cognitive consequences pervade multiple areas of functioning in an estimated 3% to 5% of school-age children. Accumulating evidence suggests that the core symptoms of ADHD—developmentally inappropriate and functionally impairing inattentiveness and hyperactivity-impulsivity—reflect dysfunction or dysregulation of cerebellar-striatal/adrenergic-prefrontal circuitry (Castellanos, 2001). The disorder is one of the most difficult and controversial disorders to diagnose because its core and secondary symptoms are (a) evident to some degree in most childhood disorders, (b) viewed by some as a variant of normal temperament, and (c) associated with different etiologies. As such, it presents unique challenges to clinicians.

The development of diagnostically valid instruments for assessing ADHD is in its inchoate stage, despite the plethora of rating scales and other measures made available over the past two decades. This predicament is attributable largely to two intertwined factors: the introduction of ADHD as a diagnostic category prior to developing appropriate tools to measure its core features, and the failure to scrutinize core deficits or features of the disorder and their underlying assumptions prior to designing assessment instruments. These issues are highlighted in the initial chapter section on current assessment strategies, followed by a more detailed discussion of theoretical and conceptual issues underlying the design of clinical assessment measures for ADHD in the research basis section. The clinical utility of modern-day assessment instruments and developmental considerations relevant to diagnosing ADHD are highlighted in the ensuing sections. The pivotal role of assessment in case conceptualization and treatment planning is described subsequently, highlighted by a case study.

DESCRIPTION OF ASSESSMENT STRATEGIES

Consummating a diagnosis of ADHD in children is a multifaceted, time-consuming endeavor that is complicated by multiple factors. Expert guidelines in psychiatry (McClelland & Werry, 2000) and psychology (Barkley, 1998) recommend that a qualified clinician conduct a comprehensive diagnostic evaluation utilizing multiple assessment instruments. These range from subjective measures such as ratings scales and clinical interviews to increasingly objective measures such as direct observation and sophisticated actigraphs. The process must also include careful review of psychoeducational test data and the child's social-developmental, medical, educational, psychiatric, familial, and treatment histories. These and other measures are reviewed herein.

OVERVIEW

A review of popularly used structured and semistructured clinical diagnostic interviews, behavioral rating scales, and checklists is presented in the first two parts of this section. Aside from the handful of small-*n* and uncontrolled case studies, the use of self-report and self-monitoring instruments has been confined to assessing treatment-emergent effects (i.e., side effect rating scales) and co-occurring symptomatology (e.g., self-report depression and anxiety inventories) in ADHD. Clinicians interested in these specialty instruments can find detailed discussions throughout this book and elsewhere (cf. Mash & Terdal, 1997).

HISTORICAL INFORMATION

Obtaining detailed and accurate historical information is essential to the assessment of ADHD. This is because information obtained concerning the onset, course, and duration of behavioral and/or emotional problems is one of the most valid means of separating ADHD from other childhood disorders. A child with a relatively benign history of behavioral and academic problems, for example, whose academic performance is compromised beginning in fifth grade, accompanied by an acute onset of behavioral and/or emotional difficulties, is unlikely to have ADHD, based on our knowledge of the disorder. Other candidates, such as Affective Disorder, Anxiety Disorder, Early Onset Schizophrenia, and abrupt environmental change, represent more likely alternatives to explain the difficulties.

Questions concerning pre-, peri-, and postnatal development, early or continued ingestion of alcohol, drugs, and other toxins, length and course of pregnancy, delivery and birth complications, Apgar scores, and other relevant information are outlined in the clinical intake form shown in Figure 16.1.

Detailed historical information must also be obtained concerning a child's medical, educational, and child/family psychiatric history, and social development (see Figure 16.1). Clinicians must be particularly attuned to asking about the onset, duration, and course of reported behavior and/or academic problems, following the early methods of defining clinical syndromes used by Hippocrates (i.e., recognized patterns or clusters of symptoms).

Obtained historical information contributes to the diagnostic process by providing converging evidence of occurrences common to children with ADHD. For example, slightly higher elevations of pregnancy or birth complications in ADHD relative to normal children are reported in some studies (Hartsough & Lambert, 1985). Relative to control children, children with ADHD tend to have more minor physical anomalies (i.e., slight deviations in appearance), more problems with general health (Hartsough & Lambert), more allergies (Trites, Tryphona, & Ferguson, 1980), more accidental injuries (Szatmari, Offord, & Boyle, 1989), and more poisonings (Stewart, Thach, & Friedin, 1970). Family psychiatric histories typically reflect a higher prevalence of ADHD in first-degree biological relatives of children with ADHD (25% to 37% average risk), particularly in fathers (44%) and brothers (39%) (Biederman, Faraone, Keenan, Knee, & Tsuang, 1990). Their educational history is usually characterized by an early onset and gradually worsening course of behavioral, emotional, and academic difficulties. Teachers invoke the term *immaturity* when describing 4- to 5-year-old children with ADHD. This adjective is soon replaced by a laundry list of pejorative characteristics that reflect gradually impairing levels of inattentiveness, impulsivity-hyperactivity, and general classroom disruptiveness between entry into the first grade and second grade. Intellectual development frequently lags behind same age peers by as much as 7–15 points on standardized intelligence tests; and academic functioning is nearly always impaired, except in high-IQ ADHD children. This constellation of chronic and worsening behavioral, cognitive, and emotional problems results in more failing grades and grades failed and culminates in a 10- to 30-point lag on standardized academic achievement tests (Barkley, DuPaul, & McMurray, 1990).

CLINICAL INTERVIEWS

The suggested practice of using a standardized interview format as a clinical diagnostic tool, and the recognition that parents and children frequently disagree regarding both the occurrence and severity of child dysfunction, is credited to the pioneering work of Rutter and Graham (1968). The development of these instruments also reflects the poor reliability and questionable validity of unaided clinical diagnosis.

Child's Name ____________________ DOB _____ Age ________

PREGNANCY

Prenatal History

Planned ______ Smoking ________ ETOH _________ Medications ______________

____

_________ Vitamins ______________________ Other substances ______________

[specify type, amount/dosage or number, and duration for each category]

Perinatal History

Full term/other _________ Medical Complications (e.g., Preeclampsia) ____________

____

Labor ______________________ Delivery (e.g., natural, induced, C-section) ________

Delivery Complications ____

Postnatal History

APGAR score ________ Height _____ Weight _______ Complications ____________

_________________________________ Hospital Stay ______________________

DEVELOPMENTAL HISTORY

Early temperament (describe child's reaction/interaction with caregivers and environment, including eye contact, ability to be comforted, use of and reaction to gestures, social bonding) ____

____

Early development problems (e.g., colic, eating difficulties, sleep problems) __________

____

Developmental Milestones (in months)

Roll over ________ Sit Up ________ Crawling ________ 1st Steps Unassisted ________
Independent walking ________ First words ________ 3-word sentences ________ Toilet training ________

MEDICAL HISTORY

Diseases/chronic infections/febrile illnesses _________________________________
[*Note:* Describe history, treatment, and outcome for each incident.]

Chronic ear infections (otitis media) _______________________________________
Hospitalizations/ER visits ____
Head injuries/loss of consciousness _______________________________________
Surgeries/sutures [event and number] ______________________________________
Broken bones/other medical problems ______________________________________
Allergies ______________________ Accidental poisonings ____________________
Medications (current/past) ____
Other medical problems (e.g., seizures, hearing loss, vision problems) _____________

____

FIGURE 16.1 M. D. Rapport CLC-IV Clinical Intake Form.

EDUCATIONAL HISTORY

Age [e.g., 4- to 5-Year-Old]
School/facility ______________________ Location ______________
Teacher ______________ Grades/comments ______________
Behavior ____
[*Note:* Complete above information for each grade/classroom placement.]

Previous testing/assessments/special education staffing/placements ______________
____

Suspensions/expulsions/school initiated punishments (include age/grade, event, outcome)
____

SOCIAL FUNCTIONING

Peer relationships (friends—younger/older preference, home/school) __________
____
Organized sports/activities (e.g., soccer, baseball, swimming, Scouts, karate) ________
____
Other preferred activities (e.g., hobbies, computer/video games, art, music, bicycling skateboarding, water sports) ______________________________
Family relationships (with parents, siblings, other family members) __________
____

FAMILY HISTORY

Paternal
Siblings ____
Parents ____
Grandparents ____

Maternal
Siblings ____
Parents ____
Grandparents ____

[*Note:* Describe all serious medical and psychiatric problems/diagnoses; include probes for school failure, learning problems, suicidal behavior/depression, anxiety, substance abuse, and treatments for unknown diagnoses.]

FIGURE 16.1 (*Continued*)

Clinical diagnosis relies primarily on recognized patterns or clusters of symptoms, due to a lack of understanding concerning the etiology of most childhood disorders. This information must be derived from adult informants (teachers, parents), because children with ADHD are particularly poor historians and unreliable reporters of both the presence and the severity of their difficulties (Barkley, 1998). The relative merits and specific advantages associated with clinical interviews have been reviewed (Weinstein, Stone, Noam, Grimes, & Schwab-Stone, 1989). Chief among them are their ability to reduce or minimize different sources of error variance that are internal (e.g., interviewer's behavior, training, and personal or professional biases) or external (e.g., informant and source discrepancies) to the interview. Structured and semistructured interviews also provide clinicians with a reliable method by which to probe, clarify, and facilitate the reporting of specific aspects of behavior and symptomatology (including history) that may be overlooked during the course of an unstructured clinical interview yet are relevant to treatment.

Popularly used structured and semistructured clinical interviews are listed in Table 16.1. Structured interviews are designed to elicit information from parents and children concerning various aspects of their functioning, including specific inquiries about the presence, absence, and severity of symptoms. The *structured* nature of inquiry reflects the degree to which an interviewer must follow an outlined script. *Semistructured* clinical interviews, in contrast, typically blend systematic screening inquiries with open-ended questions based on nonscripted verbal probes and/or other sources of information to assess and clarify symptoms. This amalgam of data reflects the fact that accurate information is optimized by incorporating a blend of structured systematic and open-ended questioning (Rutter, Cox, Egert, Holbrook, & Everitt, 1981).

All but one of the clinical interviews covers the full range of major DSM-IV diagnoses in children between 6 and 17 years of age. Administration time varies between 1 and 2 hours, depending on the informant, the interviewer's experience, and the range, severity, and duration of presenting problems. The Child and Adolescent Psychiatric Assessment (CAPA) is perhaps the most extensively developed of the available clinical interviews, but it requires up to 2 weeks of classroom work and an additional 1–2 weeks of practice to obtain the necessary certification (Angold & Costello, 2000). Training cost for the full CAPA is estimated at $600, in addition to $2000 fixed costs, which significantly limits its widespread use by clinicians. This diagnostic interview, however, may be peerless, due to a number of excellent features. Training and coding are based on a detailed glossary. The instrument provides for an intensity rating that varies by three symptom groupings—intrapsychic phenomenon such as worrying, qualitatively different symptoms such as psychosis, and conduct disturbances. Thoroughly investigated symptoms are matched to appropriate glossary definitions and levels of severity. Formal rules are provided for the use of screening, mandatory, and discretionary questions.

The Diagnostic Interview for Children and Adolescents (DICA) is one of the most popularly used structured interviews for assessing information about the psychiatric status of children based on DSM-III-R or DSM-IV criteria. Separate versions are available for children (6–12 years) and adolescents (13–18 years), following extensive field testing of interview questions with different gender, age, and racial groups. Although typically classified as a structured interview, the DICA provides for specific methods for follow-up questioning (probes) to enhance interviewer reliability. Extensive training—2–4 weeks, depending on rater experience—is necessary to achieve a desired degree of clinical competence; this includes learning how to maintain a child's interest, use age-specific probes, speak in an animated tone of voice, and employ gestures appropriately. Reliability estimates vary by disorder and are consistent with other research findings that children are poorer reporters of externalizing behavior problems but better reporters of internalizing symptoms relative to their parents (Reich, 2000). Test–retest reliability estimates for interviewing ADHD children (.32) and adolescents (.59) are lower relative to all other diagnostic groups, suggesting that adult informants must be relied on to obtain a valid assessment of ADHD behavior problems. Computer versions for children, adolescents, and adults are available and can be administered by an interviewer or self-administered for interviewees without reading difficulties. Preliminary research, however, indicates that reliability is compromised, relative to the traditional format administration, when adolescents independently complete the interview. Computerized versions may best serve as screening instruments until acceptable reliability is demonstrated.

The Schedule for Affective Disorders and Schizophrenia for School-Age Children (K-SADS) is currently the most widely used semistructured clinical interview; it utilizes a flexible yet systematic approach to assess symptomatology. Several versions are available, but the recently developed K-SADS-P/L (present and lifetime version) is the instrument of choice for most clinical interviewing purposes. Information is gathered concerning both lifetime and current diagnostic status, focusing on disorder chronology, treatment, impairment, and severity. An 82-item screen interview rates key symptoms for current and past episodes and shortens administration time by allowing the interviewer to omit nonsignificant symptoms following negative endorsement of key symptoms. Extensive training is required to become proficient with the K-SADS, due to its semistructured nature. The interviewer must be familiar with diagnostic and symptom subtleties and proficient in using noncued verbal probes to elicit examples and clarify behavioral and emotional problems. The parent is interviewed initially and rates the persistence and severity of symptoms when they were at their worst over a specific time period and during the current episode or previous week. A separate interview is conducted with the child alone, and a third pair of ratings is generated based on a summary of all information available (e.g., parent–child interviews, historical records, rating scales). Additional interviewing is recommended to address discrepancies in obtained information. Rater reliability for the K-SADS-PL for six diagnoses is excellent, and obtained kappa values of .80 for ADHD are among the highest for all clinical interviews.

CHECKLISTS AND RATING SCALES

Behavior checklists and rating scales play a prominent role in assessing children with ADHD. They serve as an important source of information concerning a child's behavior in different settings, how it is judged by significant others, and the extent to which it deviates from age- and gender-related norms. The information obtained contributes to the diagnostic process, and some instruments are used to assess treatment efficacy. Popularly used instruments for assessing children with ADHD are listed in Tables 16.2 and 16.3. Descriptions and critiques of these instruments are provided in numerous sources (cf. Barkley, 1998; Mash

TABLE 16.1 Clinical Child Diagnostic Interviews

Measures	Symptom History	Age Range	Time (min)	Test–Retest (Kappa)	Disorders Considered	Scoring Format	Instrument Cost	Training Required
Parent Version								
Structured Interviews								
Diagnostic Interview Schedule for Children—IV (DISC-IV)	4 weeks 12 months	6–17	90–120	.79	All major Dx	Y/N	$150– $2000	2- to 3-day training module
Diagnostic Interview for Children and Adolescents—IV (DICA-IV)	4 weeks 12 months	6–17	60–120	NR	All major Dx	Y/N	$1000	2–4 weeks
Children's Interview for Psychiatric Syndromes (ChIPS)	Current episode 12 months	6–18	40	.4	All major Dx	Y/N	$115	NDR
Semistructured Interviews								
Schedule for Affective Disorders and Schizophrenia for School-Age Children (K-SADS)	6 months Lifetime	6–17	30–90	.63	All major Dx	0–3	Free online	CTR
Semistructured Clinical Interview for Children and Adolescents (SCICA)	NR	13–18	60–90	.57 (Atten. Prob. Scale)	Does not correspond with DSM-IV	0–3	$110–$295 $25 for 50	NDR
Child and Adolescent Psychiatric Assessment (CAPA)	3 months	9–17	20–210 $M = 66$	NR for ADHD .55 for CD	All major Dx	0–3	$600 + $2000 fixed costs	BA
Interview Schedule for Children and Adolescents (ISCA)	6 months	8–17	120–150	Between .64 and 1.0	All major Dx	0–3	Free— Author	CTR

Child and Adolescent Version								
Structured Interviews								
Diagnostic Interview Schedule for Children—IV (DISC-IV)	4 weeks 12 months	9–17	45–90	.42	All major Dx	Y/N	$150–$2000	2- to 3-day training module
Diagnostic Interview for Children and Adolescents—IV (DICA-IV)	4 weeks 12 months	6–17	60–120	.32 C .59 A	All major Dx	Y/N	$1000	2–4 weeks
Children's Interview for Psychiatric Syndromes (ChIPS)	Current episode 12 months	6–18	40	.40	All major Dx	Y/N	$115	NDR
Semistructured Interviews								
Schedule for Affective Disorders and Schizophrenia for School-Age Children (K-SADS)	6 months Lifetime	6–17	30–90	.63	All major Dx	0–3	Free online	CTR
Semistructured Clinical Interview for Children and Adolescents (SCICA)	NR	13–18	60–90	.57 (Atten. Prob. Scale)	Does not correspond with DSM-IV	0–3	$110–$295 $25 for 50	NDR
Child and Adolescent Psychiatric Assessment (CAPA)	3 months	9–17	22–150 $M = 59$	NR for ADHD .55 for CD	All major Dx	0–3	$600 + $2000 fixed costs	BA
Interview Schedule for Children and Adolescents (ISCA)	6 months	8–17	45–90	Between .64–1.0	All major Dx	0–3	Free—Author	CTR

A = adolescent; BA = Bachelor's-level training; C = child; CTR = clinical training required; Dx = Diagnosis; NDR = no degree requirements; NR = not reported.

& Terdal, 1997). Checklists and rating scales are listed under *broadband* and *narrow-band* categories. This distinction illustrates differences in scale development and the breadth of behavioral-emotional problems assessed by the instruments.

Broadband Rating Scales and Checklists

The usefulness of scales that assess both broad- and narrow-band dimensions of child psychopathology is their ability to provide a means by which to compare children with expected, normative levels of developmentally and gender-appropriate behavior. When present, the severity or deviance of ADHD symptomatology can be assessed in particular and the presence or pattern of more generalized psychopathological dysfunction documented. This has become increasingly important in recent years because of the shared symptom pattern of several childhood disorders, relatively high comorbidity of ADHD with other disorders (e.g., CD, ODD, and LD), and converging evidence that ADHD alone may be associated with a different longitudinal course and outcome relative to other disorders alone or in combination with ADHD (e.g., Fergusson, Lynskey, and Horwood, 1997; Rapport, Scanlan, & Denney, 1999).

Characteristics of the most popularly used parent and teacher broadband instruments are shown in Table 16.2. Most instruments are suitable for assessing children between 6 and 18 years of age, and a few extend downward to as young as 2.5 years of age. All six of the broadband scales provide age and gender norms, but they vary in their estimated administration time (5–30 minutes). Test–retest kappa coefficients and internal consistency estimates for most scales are within an acceptable range. Some instruments provide both dimensional and categorical (DSM-IV) scales related to child psychopathology, whereas others contain general behavior indices (e.g., attention) based on factor analysis (see Table 16.2).

The Achenbach scales (Child Behavior Checklist, Teacher Report Form) are currently the most widely used of the broadband instruments. The Child Behavior Checklist (CBCL) assesses two higher-order dimensions (Internalizing, Externalizing) and eight narrow-band clinical domains that reflect the emotional and behavioral functioning of children. Internalizing problems reflect depression, anxiety, and somatic complaints, whereas externalizing problems reflect rule-breaking behavior, aggressive behavior, oppositional problems, and attention/hyperactivity problems. The instrument also assesses three areas of children's competence (personal activities, social activities, school functioning) and provides scores for DSM-IV–oriented scales that correlate with clinical disorders frequently observed in children and adolescents as described in the DSM-IV (American Psychiatric Association, 1994). CBCL scale scores convert to T-scores for interpretative purposes, with a mean of 50 and standard deviation of 10. T-scores between 65 and 69 (93rd to 97th percentiles) and at 70 or above fall within the borderline and clinical range, respectively. Scores within the clinical range are typical of children receiving mental health services based on the national standardization sample.

TABLE 16.2 Broadband Rating Scales

Measure	Age Range[1]	Norms [Age/Gender]	Time (min)	Test–Retest (kappa)	Internal Consistency	Syndromes/ Disorders	Scale Format (Items)	Estimated Cost
Broadband Parent Rating Scales								
Behavioral Assessment System for Children (BASC): Parent Rating Scale (PRS)	2.5–5 6–11 12–18	[Y/Y]	10–20	.85–.95	.70–.80	10 cat, including Hyperactivity & Atten Prob	4-point (126–138)	\$330–\$450 \$39 for 25 forms
Child Behavior Checklist (CBCL): Parent Report Form (PRF)	1.5–5 6–18	[Y/N]	20–30	.80–.94	.63–.97	8 cat, including Atten Prob & 6 DSM Scales	3-point (118)	\$325 \$25 for 50 forms
Child Symptom Inventory—IV Parent Version (CSI-IV-P)	3–5 5–12 12–18	[Y/Y]	10–15	.66–.88	.74–.94	All major Dx	4-point (77)	\$98–\$358 \$13 for 50 forms
Conners' Rating Scales—Revised (CRS-S): Conners' Parent Rating Scale—Revised (CPRS-R)	3–17	[Y/Y]	Long, 15–20 Short, 5–10	.47–.85	.73–.94	10 subscales, including Hyper Cog Prob/inatten and ADHD index	4-point (80) (28)	\$180–\$425 \$26 for 25 forms
Devereux Scales of Mental Disorders (DSMD)	5–18	[Y/Y]	15	.80–.90	.90–.95	10 behaviors Internal, External, Total Score	5-point (111)	\$239 \$79 for 25 forms
Revised Behavioral Problems Checklist (RBPC)	5–18	[Y/N]	15–20	.73–.94	.63–.97	6 cat Including Atten Prob	4-point (89)	\$172 \$55 for 25 forms

(*continues*)

TABLE 16.2 *(continued)*

Measure	Age Range[1]	Norms [Age/Gender]	Time (min)	Test–Retest (kappa)	Internal Consistency	Syndromes/ Disorders	Scale Format (Items)	Estimated Cost
Broadband Teacher Rating Scales								
Behavioral Assessment System for Children (BASC): Teacher Rating Scale (TRS)	2.5–5 6–11 12–18	[Y/Y]	10–20	.85–.95	.70–.90	10 cat, including Hyperactivity and Atten Prob	4-point (126–138)	$330–$450 $39 for 25 forms
Child Behavioral Checklist (CBCL): Teacher Report Form (TRF)	1.5–5 6–18	[Y/N]	20–30	.60–.96	.72–.95	8 cat, including Atten Prob & 6 DSM scales	3-point (118)	$325 $25 for 50 forms
Child Symptom Inventory—IV: Teacher Version (CSI-IV-T)	3–5 5–12 12–18	[Y/Y]	10–15	.66–.88	.74–.94	All major Dx	4-point (99)	$98–$358 $13 for 50 forms
Conners' Rating Scales—Revised (CRS-R): Conners' Teacher Rating Scale—Revised (CTRS-R)	3–17	[Y/Y]	Long, 15–20 Short, 5–10	.47–.88 .72–.92	.77–.96 .88–.95	10 subscales, including Hyper Cog prob/inatten and ADHD index	4-point (59) (27)	$180–$425 $26 for 25 forms
Devereux Scales of Mental Disorders (DSMD)	5–18	[Y/Y]	15	.80–.90	.90–.95	10 behaviors Internal, External, Total Score	5-point (111)	$239 $79 for 25 forms
Revised Behavioral Problems Checklist (RBPC)	5–18	[Y/N]	15–20	.63–.83	.70–.95	6 cat, including Atten Prob	4-point (89)	$172 $55 for 25 forms

[1]Multiple age ranges in this column indicate that separate scales are available for each age range listed; Atten = attention; cat = categories; CD = Conduct Disorder; Cog = cognitive; Dx = diagnosis; Hyper = hyperactive; Impulse = impulsivity; inatten = inattention; min = minutes; ODD = Oppositional Defiant Disorder; Prob = problem; Y/N = indicates whether norms are available (Yes, No) based on age and gender.

The Teacher Report Form (TRF) of the CBCL is nearly identical to the CBCL just described, but it contains five scales that assess children's adaptive functioning (i.e., Academic Performance, Working Hard, Behaving, Learning, and Happy) and a total score, rather than the three competency scales in the parent version. The instrument is designed to obtain classroom teachers' perceptions of possible emotional and behavioral problems commonly experienced by children, relative to nationally established age and gender norms. TRF scale scores are converted to T-scores for interpretative purposes, and borderline and clinical ranges are identical to the parent version. The newer version of the TRF also provides norm-based attention problem subscales for differentiating inattention and hyperactivity-impulsivity problems. This is useful for identifying ADHD subtypes—inattentive only, hyperactive-impulsive only, and combined subtype. An office assistant, using available scoring software, can input obtained parent and teacher information with minimal instruction.

The Child Symptom Inventory (CSI) stands in contrast to the CBCL and TRF scales—the latter two are based on a multivariate approach for investigating clinical syndrome and higher-order (internalizing-externalizing) behavioral and emotional problems, whereas CSI scale items reflect DSM-IV criteria for ADHD and other frequently diagnosed childhood disorders. Parent and teacher versions are normed separately, and the companion scoring sheet provides clinical cutoff scores for each disorder with adjacent columns that facilitate parent–teacher rating contrasts. The CSI is particularly useful for quantifying the pervasiveness of ADHD symptoms across settings, as required by current diagnostic standards, and as a screening measure for other commonly occurring childhood disorders.

Narrow-Band Rating Scales and Checklists

Broadband rating scales and checklists are used primarily during the initial screening or diagnostic process, whereas the strength of the narrow-band scales lies in their quantification of specific types of dysfunction that are usually more relevant to setting or situational characteristics associated with ADHD. Most instruments were created for somewhat different purposes, and each has its particular strengths and limitations (for a review, see Barkley, 1998). Age and gender norms are available for some, but not all, scales—a serious limitation in light of the well-documented gender and developmental differences in children's activity level and attention (see Table 16.3). Administration time for most narrow-band scales is between 5 and 15 minutes. Basic reading ability is required for all scales; however, items can be read to and recorded for the interviewee. Several of the scales are worded to reflect DSM diagnostic criteria for ADHD (e.g., AD/HD and SNAP scales), whereas scales such as the Barkley Home Situations Questionnaire (HSQ) provide a quantitative index of more general behavior problems characteristic of children with ADHD in particular settings. The HSQ can also be used to identify areas in need of targeted intervention (e.g., mealtime behavior problems) and as an outcome measure for initiated therapies.

TABLE 16.3 Narrow-Band Rating Scales

Measure	Age Range	Norms [Age/Gender]	Time (min)	Test–Retest (kappa)	Internal Consistency	Syndromes/ Disorders	Scale Format (Items)	Estimated Cost
Narrow-Band Parent Rating Scales								
AD/HD Comprehensive Teacher's Rating Scale (ACTeRS-2)	5–13	[N/Y]	10–15	.68–.78	.92–.97	ADHD	5-point (25)	$54 $37 for 50 forms
ADHD Symptom Rating Scale (ADHD-SRS)	5–18	[Y/Y]	10–15	.93–.98	.92–.99	ADHD	5-point (56)	$85–$149 $38 for 25 forms
Attention Deficit Disorders Evaluation Scale—Second Edition (ADDES-2)	4–18	[Y/Y]	10–15	.88–.93	.96–.98	ADHD	5-point (46)	$206 $31 for 50 forms
Attention Deficit Hyperactivity Rating Scale—IV (AD/HD-RS–IV)	5–18	[Y/Y]	5–10	.86	.86–.92	ADHD	4-point (18)	$42
Barkley Home Situation Questionnaire—Revised (HSQ-R)	4–18	[N/N]	5–10	.60–.89	.64–.66	ADHD	9-point (20)	$33
Brown Attention Deficit Disorder Scale (BADDS)	3–12	[Y/Y]	10–20	.61–.93	.73–.89	ADHD	4-point (50)	$270
Strengths and Weakness of ADHD Symptoms and Normal Behavior (SWAN)	5–11	[N/N]	5	NR	NR	ADHD	7-point (30)	Free online
Swanson, Kotkin, Agler, Mylnn, and Pelham Rating Scale (SKAMP)	7–12	[N/N]	5	.78	NR	ADHD	7-point (13)	Free online
Swanson, Nolan, and Pelham Rating Scale (SNAP-IV)	5–11	[Y/Y]	20–30	.70–.90	.90	ADHD, ODD, CD	4-point (90)	Free online

Narrow-Band Teacher Rating Scales								
AD/HD Comprehensive Teacher's Rating Scale (ACTeRS-2)	5–13	[N/Y]	10–15	.68–.78	.78–.96	ADHD	5-point (25)	$54 $37 for 50 forms
ADHD Symptom Rating Scale (ADHD-SRS)	5–18	[Y/Y]	10–15	.93–.98	.92–.99	ADHD	5-point (56)	$85–$149 $38 for 25 forms
Attention Deficit Disorders Evaluation Scale—Second Edition (ADDES-2)	4–18	[Y/Y]	10–15	.88–.97	.98–.99	ADHD	5-point (46)	$206 $31 for 50 forms
Attention Deficit Hyperactivity Rating Scale—IV (AD/HD-RS–IV)	5–18	[Y/Y]	5–10	.88–.90	.88–.96	ADHD	4-point (18)	$42
Barkley Home Situation Questionnaire—Revised (HSQ-R)	4–18	[N/N]	5–10	.64–.77	.65–.74	ADHD	9-point (20)	$33
Brown Attention Deficit Disorder Scale (BADDS)	3–12	[Y/Y]	10–20	.61–.93	.73–.89	ADHD	4-point (50)	$270
Strengths and Weakness of ADHD Symptoms and Normal Behavior (SWAN)	5–11	[N/N]	5	NR	NR	ADHD	7-point (30)	Free online
Swanson, Kotkin, Agler, Mylnn, and Pelham Rating Scale (SKAMP)	7–12	[N/N]	5	.78	NR	ADHD	7-point (13)	Free online
Swanson, Nolan, and Pelham Rating Scale (SNAP-IV)	5–11	[Y/Y]	20–30	.70–.90	.90	ADHD, ODD, CD	4-point (90)	Free online

[1] Atten = attention; cat = categories; CD = Conduct Disorder; Cog = cognitive; Dx = diagnosis; Hyper = hyperactive; Impulse = impulsivity; inatten = inattention; min = minutes; ODD = Oppositional Defiant Disorder; Prob = problem; Y/N = indicates whether norms are available (Yes, No) based on age and gender.

PSYCHOEDUCATIONAL TEST DATA AND PATTERNS

Psychoeducational assessment is an integral and necessary part of a diagnostic evaluation for children presenting with ADHD-like behavior problems, owing to the high percentage who have corresponding learning problems and disabilities. Information relevant to the child's overall intellectual functioning and academic achievement are used to discern both the general level of cognitive functioning and specific strengths and weaknesses that may contribute to an understanding of the child's academic functioning. Comparisons between ability and achievement are also essential to ascertain whether learning disabilities are apparent to a significant degree to warrant special placement and/or accommodations.

Children with ADHD—as a *group*—lag in their intellectual development, relative to unaffected peers, on standardized intelligence tests by an estimated 7–15 points, placing them in the lower part of the average range or the upper part of the below-average range. These differences may be partially attributable to direct and indirect effects of underlying core deficits. For example, working memory deficits may adversely affect several IQ subtests (arithmetic, digit span), and the underlying inattentive-impulsive response style characteristic of ADHD contributes to lower scores on subtests requiring careful analysis, planning, and sustained effort. Many children with ADHD assessed at the University of Central Florida (UCF) Children's Learning Clinic-IV (CLC-IV), for example, emit quick verbal responses on Wechsler Intelligence Scale for Children (WISC) similarities subtest items, earning them a suboptimal score. *Testing the limit* procedures frequently reveals that they are able to generate 2-point item verbal responses. This nonreflective response style likely contributes to less-than-optimal performance estimates on many standardized tests.

Psychoeducational assessment is also needed to explore higher-order deficiencies (e.g., working memory) and specific patterns of intellectual functioning that have direct bearing on understanding special needs and recommendations for services. High percentages of children with ADHD are comorbid for learning disability, with estimates ranging from 8% to 39%, depending on the criteria used to define LD and the area of disability (Barkley, 1998). Academic achievement on standardized tests is usually significantly below normal, with math, reading, and spelling test scores typically falling toward the lower end of the normal range. Increasingly greater numbers of children with ADHD meet LD criteria over time, following years of impaired attention, hyperactivity-impulsivity, and lack of intervention. Longitudinal studies document the effects of making more failing grades, failing more grades, and struggling through the academic environment year after year—an estimated 23% of children with ADHD fail to complete high school, and significantly fewer go on to college or complete professional degrees, relative to peers (Mannuzza, Gitteman-Klein, Bessler, Malloy, & LaPadula, 1993).

Clinical lore frequently implicates the *Freedom From Distractibility* (FFD) factor score derived from the *Wechsler Intelligence Scale for Children*—3rd edition (WISC-III; Wechsler, 1991) as an index of inattention that can be used to diagnose children with ADHD. Empirical comparisons of FFD scores among children with ADHD, normal, and psychiatric controls yield equivocal between-group results (e.g., Riccio, Cohen, Hall, & Ross, 1997). FFD scores also fail to correlate with commonly used measures of attention in some studies (Kostura, 1993) and cannot be considered a useful assessment instrument for diagnosing ADHD without clear evidence of positive and negative predictive power—that is, convincing evidence that factor scores can reliably identify individual children with ADHD (not groups) from other children.

DIRECT OBSERVATION

In school and without treatment, most children with ADHD experience problems in at least four primary areas—staying on task, consistently completing academic assignments correctly, peer and interpersonal relationships, and learning/memory. Learning and memory difficulties are especially handicapping under conditions involving complex tasks that require the use and generation of careful, logical search strategies and perceptual analysis (Douglas, 1988).

The impulsivity component of the disorder tends to interact with and pervade other areas of functioning. For example, children with ADHD frequently pay attention, but to what *other* children are doing in the classroom. They speak out of turn and initiate actions that are inconsistent with and disruptive to ongoing classroom activities. They begin academic assignments before receiving or fully understanding instructions. They vacillate between not attempting assignments and rushing through them without regard for correctness. Most children with ADHD are quite sociable, but they tend to overwhelm their peers with their unbridled enthusiasm and intrusiveness. They experience particular difficulty paying attention during what they perceive to be *nonstimulating* activities that require waiting, taking turns, and reflection, preferring activities that are limited to small groups of children and that are relatively *active* by comparison.

A recent meta-analytic review confirms that children with ADHD are significantly less attentive and complete fewer academic assignments relative to same-age and -gender classmates (Kofler, Timko, Rapport, Weiss, & Begolli, 2004). They are also more motorically active relative to same-gender, same-age peers—a finding that inveigles even experienced clinicians to weigh observations of activity level during an office or clinic visit in their diagnostic formulation. This practice, however, is fraught with pitfalls. A past study illustrates this point—approximately 80% of children meeting ADHD diagnostic criteria were misdiagnosed by their primary pediatrician because they failed to exhibit a higher-than-normal level of motor activity during the office examination. At three-year follow-up, these children were no different from obviously hyperactive children with respect to their continuing behavior problems, poor grades, and medication status (Sleator & Ullmann, 1981). There are also no published norms for judging whether children exceed developmentally appropriate levels of activity, with the exception of rating scales, and their validity is uncertain when scale scores are compared directly to objective measures of activity level such as the actigraph (cf. Rapport, Kofler, & Himmerich, Chapter 6).

Direct observations of children with ADHD have focused traditionally on two central aspects of their behavior—school functioning and personal or interpersonal interactions and relationships. Information derived from rating and direct observation instruments range from straightforward data regarding time spent on task and academic efficiency (Rapport, Denney, DuPaul, & Gardner, 1994) to relatively complex information obtained using multicategory ratings of conduct (Abikoff, Gittelman-Klein, & Klein, 1977). The former are used primarily as outcome measures and to study treatment effects, whereas the complex, multifaceted coding instruments are used more for heuristic purposes. Children with ADHD are off-task more frequently and complete fewer academic assignments correctly on a daily basis (Rapport et al., 1994). Scrutiny of minute-to-minute interval data reveals that classroom peers attend to their academic assignments for an average of 3 min, 20 sec before taking a brief 40-sec respite, whereas children with ADHD cycle significantly more frequently between attentive and off-task states—1 min, 40 sec on-task, followed by 1 min, 20 sec off-task (Rapport, Timko, Kofler, Sims, & DuPaul, under review). There are currently no absolute cutoff scores, however, that reliably distinguish children with ADHD from classroom peers with acceptable accuracy. Normed rating instruments, such as the Academic Performance Rating Scales (APRS: DuPaul, Rapport, & Perriello, 1991), however, are useful for determining a child's standing relative to same-age peers with respect to classroom attention and academic performance.

ACTIVITY MEASURES

A variety of objective instruments for measuring children's activity level are commercially available. These include pedometers, actometers, and actigraphs as well as measures used exclusively in research settings, such as stabilimeters, photoelectric cells, ultrasound, and infrared motion analysis. A detailed discussion of these instruments and their clinical utility for assessing children with ADHD is presented in Chapter 6, on children's activity level.

RESEARCH BASIS

THEORETICAL AND CONCEPTUAL ISSUES

The appropriate design of assessment instruments for diagnosing children with ADHD and assessing treatment outcome rests on whether underlying assumptions concerning core deficits associated with the disorder are correctly specified. Elucidation of core deficits, central processes, and the means by which they cause ADHD behavior problems informs us about the types of instruments (and their

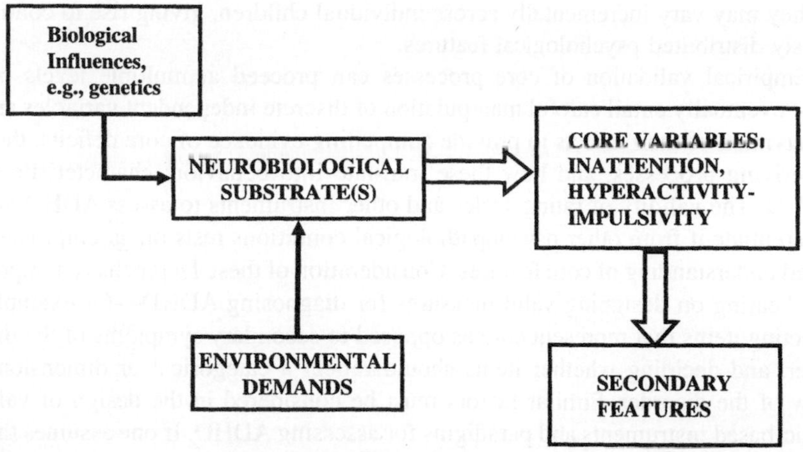

FIGURE 16.2 Conceptual model of ADHD, which presumes that biological influences give rise to individual differences in the functional properties of neurobiological systems that are etiologically responsible for core psychological features (inattention, hyperactivity-impulsivity) of ADHD. Secondary features (e.g., academic underachievement, poor peer relations) are hypothesized causal by-products of core features.

content) to develop that will enable valid measurement or, in the case of neurocognitive instruments, provide adequate challenge to suspected systems by careful design and manipulation of task parameters. A conceptual model based on the extant literature, illustrated in Figure 16.2, elucidates the implicit and explicit causal assumptions underlying current conceptualizations of ADHD. It suggests that biological influences (e.g., genetics, prenatal insults) give rise to individual differences in the functional properties of neurobiological systems (e.g., dopaminergic-noradrenergic neurotransmission) that are etiologically responsible for the core psychological (i.e., cognitive and behavioral) features of ADHD. Core features of the disorder are currently conceptualized as involving attention and hyperactivity-impulsivity. Peripheral, or secondary, features of ADHD (e.g., those listed as associated features in the *Diagnostic and Statistical Manual of Mental Disorders* [4th edition]; American Psychiatric Association, 1994) are conceptualized as causal by-products of the core features. For example, the academic underachievement observed in many children with ADHD is presumed to be a causal consequence of broader, more primary features of the disorder, such as chronic inattention to and lack of persistence on classroom tasks. Other peripheral features common to ADHD, such as inadequate social skills and peer relationships, low frustration tolerance, and strained family relationships, are similarly presumed to be due to core behavioral and cognitive influences. This conceptual framework can accommodate either categorical or dimensional views of psychopathology. Thus, neurobiological substrates may be either present or absent and give rise to correspondingly categorical symptomatic presentations, or they may vary incrementally across individual children, giving rise to continuously distributed psychological features.

Empirical validation of core processes can proceed at multiple levels but must eventually entail careful manipulation of discrete independent variables and observation of their effects to provide compelling evidence of core deficits, their underlying processes, and how these translate into behaviors characteristic of ADHD. The validity of rating scales and other instruments to assess ADHD and differentiate it from other psychopathological conditions rests on an empirically based understanding of core features. Consideration of these factors has an important bearing on designing valid measures for diagnosing ADHD—for example, selecting items that represent core as opposed to secondary symptoms of the disorder, and deciding whether items should reflect a categorical or dimensional view of the disorder. Similar factors must be considered in the design of valid clinic-based instruments and paradigms for assessing ADHD. If one assumes that individual differences associated with underlying affected substrates are always present and relatively constant, these differences should be expressed on outcome measures designed to assess core psychological (cognitive and behavioral) features of the disorder and should vary both within and across children, depending on demands imposed on the underlying substrate. Creative design of clinic-based instruments will succeed to the extent that tasks are designed to impose demands on suspected systems and concomitantly permit assessment of children's tolerance for challenge at both individual and normative levels of functioning.

Variation of scores within and across diagnostic groups and the general population on paradigms, rating scales, and other instruments designed to assess ADHD is also desirable and should be in accord with theoretical expectations. Instruments designed to permit a wide distribution of scores (versus the use of artificial cutoffs) are preferred, to permit consideration of both categorical and dimensional views of ADHD. Conversely, minimal intraindividual and interindividual variation on measures precludes ascertainment of reliable diagnostic judgments.

EMPIRICAL SUPPORT FOR ADHD ASSESSMENT MEASURES

A pivotal issue relevant to nearly all ADHD diagnostic assessment instruments is their egregious lack of construct validity, the *sine qua non* of assessment. Most available instruments have acceptable reliability and internal consistency—necessary but not sufficient psychometric properties of construct-valid instruments. Confidence that an instrument measures a particular target construct, such as attention or hyperactivity-impulsivity, rests on establishing diagnostic validity. This is traditionally accomplished using one of several approaches—by (a) comparing experienced clinicians' diagnosis with diagnosis elicited from a clinical interview; (b) examining construct validity—a type of inferential validity wherein a measure is compared with other measures that are known to be associated with the disorder or associated features of the disorder; and (c) establishing predictive validity, the precision by which a diagnostic category predicts developmental or treatment outcome.

Most commonly used interviews, rating scale, and clinic-based instruments estimate validity based on how well they correlate with other rating scales and instruments or, in the case of clinical interviews, with clinician (i.e., sometimes termed "expert") diagnosis. This approach is woefully inadequate for demonstrating convergent validity, because most available rating scales use near identically worded symptom descriptions of behavior problems (e.g., based on DSM-IV criteria). Essential to construct validation is the requirement that scale or interview items be evaluated against independent measures of the construct. The same holds for comparisons between clinical interviews and expert judges' opinions. Clinicians are not particularly reliable at assessing diagnosis, and the validity of a diagnostic instrument must be independent of the diagnostic criteria it assesses—that is, research must distinguish between the validity of a disorder and the criteria used to define it. Extant research also reveals that even when scales scores are significantly correlated, they may be unrelated to objective measures (Rapoport, Abramson, Alexander, & Lott, 1971; Stevens, Kupst, Suran, & Schulman, 1978). When assessing activity level in particular, past studies demonstrate that children receiving higher teacher activity ratings than other children in the same classroom may actually be less motorically active according to precision counters used concurrently to measure motor movement. For example, nearly 64% of children rated as clinically hyperactive were less active than the most active child rated as being normal by the teacher (Tryon & Pinto, 1994). Collectively, these shortcomings limit the interpretability and usefulness of most available ADHD rating scales when used in isolation.

Overreliance on clinical interviews or direct observation is equally problematic. Both structured and semistructured clinical interviews overdiagnose clinical psychopathology in general and ADHD specifically. Children are likely to end up with multiple diagnoses based solely on information obtained from a clinical interview. Heeding this caution, coupled with careful probing concerning the onset, course, and duration of symptoms, will reduce the tendency to overdiagnose caseness.

Many clinicians weigh a child's activity level during the diagnostic evaluation as converging evidence of ADHD. This practice may result in a high number of missed diagnoses, owing to two spurious assumptions. The first is that children with ADHD exhibit higher-than-normal levels of activity during a clinical evaluation. Its companion assumption is that clinicians are able to accurately estimate developmentally appropriate activity level in structured settings in the absence of available norms. As noted earlier, approximately 80% percent of children meeting ADHD diagnostic criteria are misdiagnosed because they fail to exhibit a higher-than-normal level of motor activity during the office examination (Sleator & Ullmann, 1981), and there are no published norms available that establish a clear linkage between activity level and clinical diagnosis in clinic or office settings.

The information contained in this section implies that extant measures of ADHD cannot be used in isolation and that informed clinical judgment must be based on multiple sources, settings, and measures, coupled with a sound knowledge of temporal behavioral patterns characteristic of different clinical disorders and normal development for accurate clinical diagnosis.

CLINICAL UTILITY

Little is known concerning the convergence of clinical child diagnosis and behavior problems quantified by checklist and rating scales; for this reason, none of the existing scales can be used as a stand-alone diagnostic instrument. They also fail to provide necessary information concerning the onset, duration, and course of behavioral-emotional problems and whether these problems are better accounted for by other factors or clinical disorders. Information must be obtained from both the parent and the teacher and from other settings and sources whenever possible. Discrepancies between settings and raters require additional inquiry and may provide information critical to case conceptualization.

DIAGNOSTIC UTILITY

The diagnostic utility of most activity rating scales is unknown. Four metrics address this concern: sensitivity, specificity, positive predictive power (PPP), and negative predictive power (NPP). Sensitivity and specificity indicate the proportion of the group with and without a target diagnosis who test positive and negative on a measure, respectively. These two indices are useful for examining the overall classification accuracy of rating scales and other instruments, but they are not particularly valuable to clinicians unaware of a child's diagnostic standing prior to referral. PPP and NPP are the statistics most relevant for this purpose. PPP, as it applies to rating scale utility, indicates the conditional probability that a child exceeding a rating scale cutoff score meets criteria for a particular diagnosis, such as ADHD (i.e., the ratio of true positive cases to all test positives). NPP, in contrast, indicates the conditional probability that a child who doesn't exceed an established cutoff score will not meet criteria for a particular clinical diagnosis (i.e., the ratio of true negative cases to all test negatives). High values (e.g., >.80) for all four indices are desirable.

Sensitivity, specificity, PPP, and NPP are also used to examine individual scale items and specific clinical diagnostic criteria, such as those contained in structured and semistructured clinical interviews. The diagnostic utility of DSM-III (APA, 1980) activity level descriptions—many of which are identical to DSM-IV items—was investigated in a study of seventy-six 6- to 12-year-old boys referred to a child psychiatry outpatient clinic (Milich, Widiger, & Landau, 1987). Children met diagnostic criteria for ADHD, Conduct Disorder (CD), both diagnoses, some other diagnosis, or an unspecified deferred diagnosis based on a comprehensive clinical assessment. Base rates for DSM-III items "shifts activities," "runs/climbs," "can't sit still," "runs around," and "on the go" ranged from .25 to .51 in the children with ADHD. As such, these descriptions occurred with relatively low frequency, and only two ("shifts activities," "on the go") identified a reasonably large proportion of the children (i.e., sensitivity rates of .70, .40, .38, .38, .68, respectively). The items were fairly specific to the disorder (specificity rates of .69, .78, .89, .86, .67, respectively) and served as moderately strong inclusion criteria (PPP rates of .72, .67, .79, .75, .69, respectively). NPP rates ranged from .54 to .68 and indicate that none of the items are particularly useful as exclusion criteria—that is, absence of the symptoms does not necessarily mean that ADHD can be ruled out. Collectively, these findings support current clinical practice parameters that recommend conducting a comprehensive clinical assessment, as opposed to relying on particular symptom counts or endorsements for identifying caseness.

TREATMENT OUTCOME UTILITY

Gauging treatment success by obtaining measures before, during, and after behavioral or psychopharmacological treatment is an additional common use of activity rating scales. Rating scales used for assessing treatment outcome must have high test–retest reliability over brief periods of time and with repeated administration (>.70), demonstrate sensitivity to treatment-related activity level change, and be constructed to minimize floor and ceiling effects. Instruments such as the Conners' Teacher Rating Scale (CTRS; Conners, Sitarenios, Parker, & Epstein, 1998), SNAP-IV (Swanson, 1992), ACTeRS (Ullman et al., 1997), ADHD-IV (DuPaul, Powers, Anastopoulos, & Reid, 1998), and Academic Performance Rating Scale (APRS; DuPaul et al., 1991) are useful for this purpose because of their proven sensitivity to overall and between-dose psychostimulant effects (Rapport, 1990). These and other scales are also useful for monitoring changes in activity level that accompany behavioral interventions (e.g., Rapport, Murphy, & Bailey, 1982; MTA Multimodal Treatment Study of Children with ADHD Cooperative Group, 1999); however, only the APRS has factor scores that permit evaluation of children's adaptive function (e.g., improved academic performance). This may be particularly important because a reduction in activity level and behavior problems does not necessarily correlate with improved adaptive functioning (Rapport et al., 1994).

DIFFERENTIAL DIAGNOSIS

Nearly all clinical disorders common to children must be considered and ruled out as part of the diagnostic evaluation. None of the ADHD diagnostic criteria have sufficient levels of sensitivity, specificity, and positive and negative predictive power to confidently render a clinical diagnosis. This is because several of the central features (inattention, higher-than-normal activity level) and secondary features (compromised academic performance, difficult peer and parent–child relationships) of ADHD are common to other clinical disorders. Table 16.4 details the typical onset, course, and duration of the most common child and adolescent clinical disorders.

High percentages of children with ADHD exhibit sufficient behavioral and emotional problems to warrant an additional diagnosis of Oppositional Defiant Disorder (ODD), and more moderate numbers exhibit an increasing disregard for societal norms and unacceptable conduct. ODD problems emerge later than ADHD problems, usually around 8 years of age, whereas conduct problems (CD) emerge between 10 and 16 years of age and show an escalating pattern of severity. Both ODD and CD are typically associated with an insidious onset of behavior problems. ADHD with co-occurring Conduct Disorder places children at high risk for adolescence substance use; however, this risk appears to be carried almost entirely by the development of CD symptoms.

Bipolar Disorder shares considerable similarity to ADHD in symptom manifestation, particularly for ADHD children comorbid for ODD. Similarities between the two disorders include concentration difficulties, higher-than-normal gross motor activity, labile emotion, irritability, disruptive behavior, impulsivity, low frustration tolerance, poor or inconsistent academic achievement, decreased need for sleep, restlessness, talkativeness, psychopathology in family members (alcoholism, CD, antisocial personality), denial of problems, and poor judgment. Differential diagnosis must center on the known presentation and historical differences between the two disorders.

The onset of ADHD, although believed present from birth (genetic), is typically reported by parents to occur during the preschool years (mean = 3.5 years), whereas Early-Onset Bipolar Disorder is more commonly reported between 5 and 11 years of age. ADHD symptoms are almost always chronic and unremitting—early-onset bipolar illness, in contrast, tends to be variable. Mood disturbance is nearly always present in mania, with approximately 50% reporting a primarily elated mood and 50% primarily an irritable mood. In ADHD, mood disturbance may co-occur but is more typically seen during later childhood and adolescent years. Decreased need for sleep is a continual and chronic problem for children with ADHD. In mania, sleep disturbance occurs episodically and corresponds with a manic or hypomanic episode. Persecutory delusions (70%) as well as visual (70%) and auditory (50%) hallucinations are relatively common in children with early-onset mania. These symptoms are rarely reported by children with ADHD. Pressured speech and racing thoughts, as classically described, are common in children with mania and may be difficult to distinguish from the verbal intrusiveness and disorganization characteristic of ADHD. Talkativeness and distractibility are common to both disorders, but occur regularly in ADHD and episodically in mania. Grandiose delusions are not reported in children with ADHD but may occur in upwards of 20% of mania cases; and upwards of 50% of children with mania present with a positive family history of depression, whereas no such relationship exists for children with ADHD.

TABLE 16.4 Onset, Course, and Duration of Major Clinical Disorders of Childhood

Clinical Disorders	Onset[a,b,c]	Course	Duration
Disruptive Behavior Disorders			
Attention-Deficit/ Hyperactivity Disorder (ADHD)	3.5[b]	Chronic	Adoles—lifelong
Conduct Disorder (CD)[d]	<10[c]	Variable	Adulthood
	<16[c]	Variable	Early adult
Oppositional Defiant Disorder (ODD)	<8[c]	Variable	Remits or antecedent to CD
Pervasive Developmental Disorders			
Asperger's Disorder	3–6[c]	Chronic	Lifelong
Autistic Disorder[e]	<3[b]	Chronic	Lifelong
Childhood Disintegrative Disorder[e]	3–4[b] or[c]	Chronic	Lifelong
Rett's Disorder[e]	1–2 and <4[c]	Chronic	Lifelong or fatal
Mood Disorders			
Major Depressive Disorder[f]	5–19[b] or[c]	Variable	Remits or variable
Dysthymic Disorder[g]	8.5[c]	Variable	Remits or variable
Mania Episode (in context of Bipolar Disorder)	5–14	Variable	Lifelong
Anxiety Disorders			
Acute Stress Disorder	Any age[i]	1 month	2 days to 1 month
Obsessive-Compulsive Disorder[j]	6–15 (m)[c]	Chronic	Lifelong
	20–29 (f)[c]	Chronic	Lifelong
Post-traumatic Stress Disorder	Acute or	Variable	2 months to
	delayed[i]	Variable	2 years
Separation Anxiety Disorder[m]	9–13[b] or[c]	Variable	2 years—Adoles
Social Phobia[m]	Mid-teens[b] or[c]	Chronic	Remits by adulthood
Specific Phobia[k,m]	7–12[b] or[c]	Variable	Remits by Adoles
Other Clinical Disorders			
Tourette's Disorder	7[c]	Variable	Lifelong
Early-Onset Schizophrenia	5–11[b] or[c]	Variable	Lifelong

[a]Age of onset indicates age in years at which symptoms are most frequently first reported in children; [b]acute onset; [c]insidious onset; [d]at risk for Antisocial Personality Disorder and Substance Abuse Disorder as adults; [e]typically associated with an anxiety disorder; [g]frequently associated with Conduct Disorder; [i]onset immediately following a traumatic event; [j]commonly associated with depression, other anxiety disorders, and/or Tourette's; [k]slightly higher rates in females and dependent on the type of phobia; [l]significantly higher number of males versus females prior to age 10; [m]frequently continuous with Adult Anxiety Disorder; Adoles = adolescence; (f) = females; (m) = males.

Collectively, the chronic (ADHD) versus episodic (mania) course, relative absence of abnormally expansive or elevated mood, psychotic features, and family history are the most distinguishing features differentiating ADHD from mania. Children with mania also tend to respond poorly to psychostimulants and antidepressants; the onset of the disorder usually represents a distinct change in the child's behavior; there are frequently signs of strong (and early) sexual interest and behavior and explosive anger (rages) and vindictiveness, bullying, and a focus on emotions rather than novelty. Long-lasting tantrums as a toddler are reported in some studies.

Some anxiety disorders, such as PTSD and abrupt environmental change (e.g., parent divorce, relocation, school change), can also result in behavior patterns reminiscent of ADHD. Characterizing the onset, duration, and course of behavioral and emotional problems is required to differentiate ADHD-like symptoms in these children from those with ADHD. Some children with mild forms of Pervasive Developmental Disorder and Early-Onset Schizophrenia present with ADHD-like symptoms, but their qualitatively different symptom picture generally enables a rapid rule-out.

DEVELOPMENTAL CONSIDERATIONS

A normative-developmental framework is required to understand what is atypical and potentially pathological at different stages of development. This understanding, in turn, governs our ability to identify the emergence of abnormal behavior patterns in children. Knowledge of children's speech and language development is also necessary if children are queried about their behavioral and emotional difficulties, temporal events, and experiences.

More than half of all children with ADHD begin to manifest behavior problems by 3 years of age. Noncompliance, impulsiveness, and higher-than-normal activity level are commonplace. Attendance at preschool is marked by teacher complaints of hyperactivity, peer relationship problems, and the inability to settle down and stay with one task for a developmentally appropriate period of time. Behavioral difficulties remain relatively stable between preschool and entry into formal schooling but are typically exacerbated in first grade because of the increasing demands associated with sustained attention, effort, and working memory. The activity level of children with ADHD is relatively unchanged during these years, whereas normal children exhibit a *decrease* in overall activity level. The increasing cognitive challenges that accompany grade advancement is typically associated with more serious behavior problems—particularly around the fourth grade and entry into middle school—due to the organizational requirements (e.g., written reports, increasingly complex assignments, frequent moves to different classes), larger class sizes, and reduced structure associated with these grades.

Consideration of this early emerging behavior pattern requires understanding how attention, impulse control, activity level, and cognitive characteristics change over time in normally developing children. Other than the isolated outcome or direct observation studies comparing small numbers of children at particular ages, most available information concerning developmental changes in these areas is derived from rating scale data or large-scale normative studies of neurocognitive instruments, such as the Continuous Performance Test (CPT) and Matching Familiar Figures Test (MFFT). Rating scale studies are highly consistent and reveal a clear developmental trend in children's attention, impulse control, and activity level with increasing age—that is, typical children are able to pay attention for longer time periods, become more reflective, and show lower rates of gross motor activity with increasing age. This developmental trend is consistent with cross-sectional, longitudinal findings that reveal an initial diminution in attentional problems between the first and second assessment years but continuing problems thereafter. Hyperactivity-impulsivity problems, in contrast, show a gradual decline with increasing age (Hart, Lahey, Loeber, Applegate, & Frick, 1995).

Developmental changes in language development have a direct bearing on children's ability to conceptualize and to verbally respond to structured and semi-structured clinical interview questions. Very young children are generally unable to understand and respond to symptom-related questions and probes, and parents and other informants must be relied on to provide essential information. Even older children experience difficulty describing emotional states (e.g., mood) and thought processes (racing or unusual thoughts, hallucinations), and children with ADHD appear to have little or no insight concerning their behavioral difficulties or how they disrupt the environment. A wide range of age-appropriate examples and probes, coupled with gestures and visual stimuli (e.g., pictures of emotional states), are recommended to facilitate clinician–child interviews.

ASSESSMENT, CONCEPTUALIZATION, AND TREATMENT PLANNING

A chief role of behavioral assessment is the identification of prominent behavioral or social, cognitive, affective, and physical signs and symptoms in the individual. Information obtained may be used subsequently to formulate initial diagnosis, select and evaluate response to treatment, and in some cases portend long-term outcome. The complexity and multifaceted nature of ADHD eludes facile efforts at clarification and measurement. Broad-based behavioral and sensory domains are affected in the disorder. Many areas of dysfunction are apparent only under certain environmental conditions or situations (Douglas, 1988; Whalen & Henker, 1985). To complicate matters, children with ADHD frequently exhibit an inconsistent pattern of deficits from day to day, even when tasks and other parameters are held constant. This phenomenon has been observed in both field and highly controlled laboratory settings, to the dismay of researchers and clinicians alike (for a review, see Rapport, 1990).

Eliciting information from single sources and limiting or relying exclusively on certain types of information to determine a diagnosis of ADHD results in a high rate of misidentified cases. A careful, thorough evaluation that assesses multiple modalities, relies on multiple informants, and incorporates a variety of instruments and methods is preferred. It is equally important to gain an experienced clinical appreciation of ADHD phenomenology and its *consistently inconsistent* behavioral and cognitive manifestations.

A desirable evaluation for children suspected of ADHD includes comprehensive history taking, parent (and, when appropriate, child) clinical interview, review of teacher and parent broad- and narrow-band rating scale data, psychoeducational test data, and behavioral observation. Direct observation of children while functioning in an academic setting can be extraordinarily helpful, but it is usually not feasible owing to time and cost constraints. Auxiliary neurocognitive assessment coupled with behavioral observation during testing can provide valuable converging or diverging clinical evidence. Currently, this includes some versions of the CPT, the MUFTy (see below), select experimental paradigms, and objective measures of activity level and behavior.

CASE STUDY

IDENTIFICATION

Kamana was an 8-year-old male referred by a rural school system for a comprehensive clinical diagnostic evaluation and second opinion. He was previously seen by a licensed clinical psychologist, who concluded that he met diagnostic criteria for ADHD based on parent and teacher rating scales, a 30-minute parent interview, a brief interview with the child, and the absence of anxiety based on a normed child anxiety rating scale. Kamana's parents requested special accommodations by the school to address his disabilities, and the school system sought to ensure that the ADHD diagnosis was accurate before scheduling an Individualized Educational Assessment Plan (IEP) meeting to determine appropriate educational goals, interventions to accomplish these goals, and assessment procedures.

PRESENTING COMPLAINTS

Kamana's parents sought an initial evaluation through the school system, owing to their son's chronic and worsening difficulties at school, questions concerning their son's diagnostic status, and the appropriateness of his current educational placement.

HISTORY

A historical review of records indicated long-standing difficulties at home and in school, despite above-average intelligence. School problems included attentional difficulties, impulsivity, and sporadic hyperactivity. Records also indicated difficulties with peer relationships, poor organization skills, difficulties completing academic assignments on a routine basis, and a growing dislike for school.

PEER AND SCHOOL ISSUES

Kamana had no close friends in school and only one or two in his neighborhood, despite the availability of children his age in both settings. He frequently came to school late and ate lunch by himself in the school cafeteria. His peer relationships were mixed. He got along with other children, but characteristically elected to avoid companionship. The parent–school personnel relationship was acrimonious at best. Kamana's parents were frustrated concerning the school's failure to properly educate their son despite having obtained a formal diagnosis of ADHD from a qualified professional; school system personnel were unconvinced of the ADHD diagnosis and did not wish to begin the IEP process without the benefit of a second opinion.

BEHAVIORAL ASSESSMENT RESULTS

School Observations

Kamana was observed in his classroom to obtain information concerning his ability to pay attention, complete academic assignments, and participate in classroom discussions and peer interactions. This part of the evaluation was scheduled as a first step to minimize reactivity, because he was unacquainted with the clinician. The 2-day, 6-hour observation revealed that Kamana could read at his desk for 30 contiguous minutes, complete a reading assignment without difficulty, and occasionally volunteer to answer questions posed by the classroom teacher. On other occasions, the teacher prompted him to pay attention to the ongoing instruction or academic exercise being discussed. During small-group work, Kamana worked cooperatively with other children. He requested to go to the bathroom on several occasions, which the teacher attributed to water consumption throughout the day due to the high elevation–low humidity climate. Kamana sat near other children, but distanced himself from them by several feet in the cafeteria while eating lunch. He ate slowly, picked at his food, and appeared deep in thought throughout the lunch period.

Psychoeducational Assessment

Results revealed that Kamana's intellectual abilities were within the very superior range, with no significant discrepancies noted in higher-order factor scores or individual subtests, except for coding and digit span, which were moderately lower. Kaufman Test of Educational Achievement (K-TEA) results revealed above-grade and -age expectancy achievement in mathematical applications (98th percentile) and computation (77th percentile), reading comprehension (99th percentile), and decoding (63rd percentile). Spelling achievement was average but below expectancy based on assessed intelligence. Behavioral observation of Kamana during the psychoeducational evaluation indicated that he exhibited excellent concentration and reflection during several of the subtests but became visibly fidgety, motorically overactive (sitting on edge of chair, increased leg and foot movement), and impulsive (e.g., blurting out answers, heavy and hurried pencil marks) during other subtests. A common denominator of the latter subtests was their timed nature. Collectively, psychoeducational results indicated superior intellectual functioning and a corresponding high level of academic achievement, with the exception of spelling. These findings are not typical of children with ADHD, but they may reflect his intellectual abilities.

Teacher and Parent Rating Scales

Broadband (CBCL, TRF, CSI) and narrow-band (ADHD Rating Scale, SNAP checklist) rating scales completed by the classroom teacher and parents revealed a mixed pattern of results. Teacher ratings were all within 1 standard deviation of the mean, based on age norms. TRF adaptive functioning indices indicated above-average learning and school performance but below-average functioning in areas related to happiness, mood/affect, and effort. Internalizing dimension TRF scores were moderately but not significantly elevated, indicating possible anxiety and social withdrawal. Externalizing dimension scores indicated mild-to-moderate inattentiveness and nervousness/overactivity. Parent endorsements were between 1.5 and 2 standard deviations above the mean for ADHD-related symptoms (inattention, hyperactivity-impulsivity) and moderately elevated for anxiety symptoms, based on age and gender norms. The externalizing broadband scale was significantly elevated, due to endorsement of ADHD, ODD, and CD behavior problems. The CSI was elevated for symptoms related to ADHD, Overanxious Disorder, Generalized Anxiety Disorder, Separation Anxiety Disorder, and specific phobias. Multiple elevations on broadband scales frequently indicate a more severe yet untapped form of psychopathology, rater psychopathology, or a plea for help. Collectively, parent and teacher ratings present a mixed picture of ADHD-like symptoms (primarily by parent endorsement) and anxiety symptoms.

Neurocognitive Assessment

Kamana was administered a 9-minute AX version of the CPT, a Paired Associate Learning Test (PAL-T), and the MUFTy to assess attention, working memory, and cognitive tempo (reflectivity-impulsivity), respectively.

CPT results revealed age-appropriate ability to sustain attention but an initially high rate (20%) of commission errors (CEs) during the initial 3-minute time block. Performance during the remainder of the test was flawless, with no drop off in performance accuracy. Verbal comments during the initial 3 minutes suggested frustration related to making impulsive responses (CEs) and the speeded nature of the test. Children with ADHD tend to make more omission and commission errors throughout the test, and some studies suggest they show a greater vigilance decrement with time on task.

The PAL-T requires children to learn five pairs of previously unlearned pairs of letter bi-grams and numbers across six trials, with each trial followed by a recall test. PAL-T results revealed superior working memory ability during the first four trials, followed by a significant performance drop-off during the last four trials. Kamana expressed clear frustration during the final two trials—he thought the test was supposed to be over after four test trials. Children with ADHD typically show lower overall levels of performance and a pattern of increasing errors over time.

The MUFTy provides an index of children's cognitive tempo while engaged in visual problem solving. A single visual stimulus (i.e., complex visual design) is presented on a computer screen and surrounded by eight similar visual designs, with only one being exactly identical to the center stimulus. The child must locate the sole identical match during 20 trials. MUFTy results revealed a low error rate coupled with long response latencies characteristic of a reflective (slow-accurate) cognitive tempo. Children with ADHD typically show a fast-inaccurate or impulsive response pattern, characterized by a high error rate (particularly during the last 10 trials) and short response latencies.

Collectively, Kamana's performance on the neurocognitive assessment instruments was inconsistent with a diagnosis of ADHD and more suggestive of an anxiety disorder.

Semistructured Clinical Interview

The K-SADS was completed separately with Kamana and his parents. Parents endorsed all items relevant to ADHD, with early onset and continuing, worsening course. ODD items were also endorsed with high frequency, with onset at 7 years and a progressive, worsening course. Separation anxiety criteria were fully met, but follow-up probes indicated that Kamana did not experience the classical symptoms while attending school or somatic complaints prior to schooldays. Several Panic Attack symptoms were endorsed (shortness of breath, accelerated heart rate, occasional trembling and shakiness, feelings of unreality), but a negative history of discrete episodes of spontaneous panic attacks was reported. Evidence for Simple and Social Phobia was negative, except for airplanes (related to a fear of dying). Review of Generalized Anxiety symptoms yielded endorsements of nearly every item. No evidence of other disorders, including mood and thought disturbance, was revealed. Overall, Kamana's parents describe him as a "worrier" with multiple fears and concerns.

The child interview was remarkable. Kamana admitted some difficulties with concentration and completing academic assignments, but he denied other symptoms characteristic of ADHD, mood disorders, thought disorders, CD, ODD (except for arguing with and disobeying parents), PTSD, and other anxiety disorders until reviewing Obsessive-Compulsive symptoms. Kamana described a chronic and worsening history of obsessional thinking, particularly thoughts concerning contamination and, to a lesser extent, "getting things right." Onset was established as 7–7.5 years of age and may have coincided with an outbreak of body warts, which necessitated careful hygiene and regular washing. Kamana currently washes his hands between 20 and 30 times daily after touching various objects or if his washing rituals have not been successfully concluded. Morning and nighttime rituals are laborious and complex and accompanied by excessive worry concerning whether the ritual was performed correctly, particularly morning bathing. Myriad other rituals were described in detail, such as not permitting his silverware to touch anything off of his plate, having his parents wrap his lunch in a prescribed manner to avoid contamination, checking under tables at restaurants for gum, and touching one hand or foot an equal number of times while avoiding sidewalk cracks.

His symptoms were particularly disabling at school. Trips to the bathroom were for the purpose of hand washing—he feels clean for approximately 0.5 hours before having to repeat the ritual. He frequently counts the assigned math problems, checking and rechecking for accuracy to the point that he is either unable to turn in his assignment or has to suspend the ritual and rush its completion. Similar rituals were reported while reading—checking and rechecking words on pages to ensure every word is read properly. Many OCD symptoms accounted for parent-endorsed behavioral difficulties—for example, his inability to stay at a friend's house overnight was related to the need to engage in daily rituals and possible embarrassment rather than separation fears.

Collectively, the parent and child K-SADS resulted in an overendorsement of clinical diagnoses, as is frequently the case. Epidemiological evidence indicates a low to nearly nonexistent probability for three or more diagnoses in one child—symptom overlap, poorly defined symptom boundaries, and a failure to appreciate the importance of diagnostic phenomena (e.g., onset, course, duration) contribute to the overdiagnosis of caseness. This case also supports past findings that children are often the most knowledgeable source for examining internalizing problems—Kamana's parents had limited knowledge concerning the intrusive nature or impairing extent of his illness.

ETHICAL AND LEGAL ISSUES OR COMPLICATIONS

Case complications and legal issues arose owing to multiple factors. None of the professionals in the rural community (psychiatrists, psychologists) were experienced treating children with OCD, even though all the psychiatrists were knowledgeable about appropriate pharmacological treatment. Kamana's parents believed that the school system was legally and morally responsible for providing an appropriate educational program for their son, which could not be accomplished because of his impairing OCD symptoms. The school system believed that the parents were responsible for obtaining necessary clinical intervention and offered to design an IEP to complement treatment. The case was eventually resolved at a formal hearing. The school system agreed to pay for out-of-district treatment.

SUMMARY

Millions of children are misdiagnosed with ADHD every year because of truncated diagnostic evaluations. Attentional problems are endemic to most childhood disorders, and hyperactivity remains a poorly defined construct whose primary measurement index (rating scales) correlates poorly with objective measures of motor activity. There are no stand-alone instruments, diagnostic tests, or experimental paradigms that can reliably yield a diagnosis. Epidemiological and developmental studies inform us that ADHD-related behavior problems typically emerge by 3–3.5 years of age and worsen significantly when children enter a structured environment that requires them to pay attention to and complete academic tasks for age-appropriate time intervals. Socialization processes are also strained at this time. Parents are placed in the uncomfortable position as controller-managers, and same-age peers reject the intrusive but well-intentioned nature of children with ADHD. A psychoeducational assessment, comprehensive clinical evaluation, intensive historical review, and advanced knowledge concerning differences between and among common clinical child disorders with overlapping symptom presentations is needed to accurately distinguish ADHD from other clinical disorders. Renewed efforts to challenge and explore potential underlying core deficits associated with ADHD, such as working memory, will stimulate the creation of valid assessment instruments for diagnosing ADHD.

REFERENCES AND RESOURCES

Abikoff, H., Gittelman-Klein, R., & Klein, D. F. (1977). A replication of validity. *Journal of Consulting and Clinical Psychology, 48,* 555–565.

American Psychiatric Association. (1980). *Diagnostic and statistical manual of mental disorders* (3rd ed.). Washington, DC: Author.

American Psychiatric Association. (1994). *Diagnostic and statistical manual of mental disorders* (4th ed.). Washington, DC: Author.

Angold, A., & Costello, E. J. (2000). The Child and Adolescent Psychiatric Assessment (CAPA). *Journal of the American Academy of Child and Adolescent Psychiatry, 39,* 39–48.

Barkley, R. A. (1998). *Attention-Deficit hyperactivity disorder: A handbook for diagnosis and treatment* (2nd ed.). NY: Guilford Press.

Barkley, R. A., DuPaul, G. J., & McMurray, M. B. (1990). A comprehensive evaluation of attention deficit disorder with and without hyperactivity. *Journal of Consulting and Clinical Psychology, 58,* 775–789.

Biederman, J., Faraone, S. V., Keenan, K., Knee, D., & Tsuang, M. T. (1990). Family-genetic and psychosocial risk factors in DSM-III attention deficit disorder. *Journal of the American Academy of Child and Adolescent Psychiatry, 29,* 526–533.

Castellanos, F. X. (2001). Neuroimaging studies of ADHD. In M. V. Solanto, A. F. T. Arnsten, & F. X. Castellanos (Eds.), *Stimulant drugs and ADHD: Basic and clinical neuroscience* (pp. 243–258). New York: Oxford University Press.

Conners, C. K., Sitarenios, G., Parker, J. D. A., & Epstein, J. N. (1998). Revision and restandardization of the Conners' Teacher Rating Scale (CTRS-R): Factor structure, reliability, and criterion validity. *Journal of Abnormal Child Psychology, 26,* 279–291.

Douglas, V. I. (1988). Cognitive deficits in children with attention deficit disorder with hyperactivity. In L. M. Bloomingdale & J. A. Sergeant (Eds.), *Attention deficit disorder: Criteria, cognition, intervention* (pp. 65–81). New York: Pergamon Press.

DuPaul, G. J., Powers, T. J., Anastopoulos, A. D., & Reid, R. (1998). *ADHD Rating Scale-IV: Checklists, norms, and clinical interpretation.* New York: Guilford Press.

DuPaul, G. J., Rapport, M. D., & Perriello, L. M. (1991). Teacher ratings of academic skills: The development of the Academic Performance Rating Scale. *School Psychology Review, 20,* 284–300.

Fergusson, D. M., Lynskey, M. T., & Horwood, L. J. (1997). Attentional difficulties in middle childhood and psychosocial outcomes in young adulthood. *Journal of Child Psychology and Psychiatry, 38,* 633–644.

Hart, E. L., Lahey, B. B., Loeber, R., Applegate, B., & Frick, P. J. (1995). Developmental change in attention-deficit hyperactivity disorder in boys: A four-year longitudinal study. *Journal of Abnormal Child Psychology, 23,* 729–749.

Hartsough, C. S., & Lambert, N. M. (1985). Medical factors in hyperactive and normal children: Prenatal, developmental, and health history findings. *American Journal of Orthopsychiatry, 55,* 190–210.

Kofler, M. J., Timko, T. M., Rapport, M. D., Weiss, K., & Begolli, G. (2004). *Direct observations of ADHD children in the classroom: A review.* Paper presented at the 16th annual conference of the American Psychological Society, Chicago, IL.

Kostura, D. D. (1993). Using the WISC-R Freedom from Distractibility factor to identify attention deficit hyperactivity disorder in children referred for psychoeducational assessment. *Canadian Journal of Special Education, 9,* 91–99.

Mannuzza, S., Gitteman-Klein, R. G., Bessler, A. A., Malloy, P., & LaPadula, M. (1993). Adult outcome of hyperactive boys: Education achievement, occupational rank, and psychiatric status. *Archives of General Psychiatry, 50,* 565–576.

Mash, E. J., & Terdal, L. G. (1997). *Assessment of childhood disorders* (3rd ed.). New York: Guilford Press.

McClellan, J. M., & Werry, J. S. (2000). Research psychiatric diagnostic interviews for children and adolescents. *Journal of the American Academy of Child and Adolescent Psychiatry, 39,* 19–27.

Milich, R., Widiger, T. A., & Landau, S. (1987). Differential diagnosis of attention deficit and conduct disorders using conditional probabilities. *Journal of Consulting and Clinical Psychology, 55,* 762–767.

Multimodal Treatment Study of Children with ADHD Cooperative Group (US). (1999). A 14-month randomized clinical trial of treatment strategies for attention-deficit/hyperactivity disorder. *Archives of General Psychiatry, 56,* 1073–1086.

Rapoport, J., Abramson, A., Alexander, D., & Lott, I. (1971). Playroom observations of hyperactive children on medication. *Journal of the American Academy of Child Psychiatry, 10,* 524–534.

Rapport, M. D. (1990). Controlled studies of the effects of psychostimulants on children's functioning in clinic and classroom settings. In C. K. Conners & M. Kinsbourne (Eds.), *Attention deficit hyperactivity disorder* (pp. 77–111) Munich, Germany: Medizin Verlag Munchen.

Rapport, M. D., Denney, C., DuPaul, G. J., & Gardner, M. J. (1994). Attention deficit disorder and methylphenidate: Normalization rates, clinical effectiveness, and response prediction in 76 children. *Journal of the American Academy of Child and Adolescent Psychiatry, 33,* 882–893.

Rapport, M. D., Murphy, A., & Bailey, J. S. (1982). Ritalin versus response cost in the control of hyperactive children: A within-subject comparison. *Journal of Applied Behavior Analysis, 15,* 20–31.

Rapport, M. D., Scanlan, S. W., & Denney, C. B. (1999). Attention-deficit/hyperactivity disorder and scholastic achievement: A model of dual developmental pathways. *Journal of Child Psychology and Psychiatry, 40,* 1169–1183.

Rapport, M. D., Timko, T., Kofler, M., Sims, V., & DuPaul, G. (under review). Attention processes in ADHD: Observations from the classroom.

Reich, W. (2000). Diagnostic interview for children and adolescents (DICA). *Journal of the American Academy of Child and Adolescent Psychiatry, 39,* 59–66.

Riccio, C. A., Cohen, M. J., Hall, J., & Ross, C. M. (1997). The third and fourth factors of the WISC-III: What they don't measure. *Journal of Psychoeducational Assessment, 15,* 27–39.

Rutter, M., Cox, A., Egert, S., Holbrook, D., & Everitt, B. (1981). Psychiatric interviewing techniques, IV: Experimental study: Four contrasting styles. In *British Journal of Psychiatry, 138,* 456–465.

Rutter, M., & Graham, P. (1968). The reliability and validity of the psychiatric assessment of the child: I. Interview with the child. *British Journal of Psychiatry, 114,* 563–579.

Sleator, E. K., & Ullmann, R. K. (1981). Can the physician diagnose hyperactivity in the office? *Pediatrics, 67,* 13–17.

Stevens, T. M., Kupst, M. J., Suran, B. G., & Schulman, J. L. (1978). Activity level: A comparison between actometer scores and observer ratings. *Journal of Abnormal Child Psychology, 6,* 163–173.

Stewart, M. A., Thach, B. T., & Friedin, M. R. (1970). Accidental poisoning and the hyperactive child syndrome. *Disease of the Nervous System, 31,* 403–407.

Swanson, J. M. (1992). *School-based assessments and interventions for ADD students.* Irvine, CA: K. C. Publications.

Szatmari, P., Offord, D. R., & Boyle, M. H. (1989). Correlates, associated impairments, and patterns of service utilization of children with attention deficit disorders: Findings from the Ontario Child Health Study. *Journal of Child Psychology and Psychiatry, 30,* 205–217.

Trites, R. L., Tryphonas, H., & Ferguson, H. B. (1980). Diet treatment of hyperactive children with food allergies. In R. M. Knight & D. Bakker (Eds.), *Treatment of hyperactive and learning-disordered children* (pp. 151–166). Baltimore: University Park Press.

Tryon, W. W., & Pinto, L. P. (1994). Comparing activity measurements and ratings. *Behavior Modification, 18,* 251–261.

Ullmann, R. K., Sleator, E. K., & Sprague, R. L. (1997). *ACTeRS teacher and parent forms manual.* Champaign, IL: MetriTech, Inc.

Wechsler, D. (1991). *Manual for the Wechsler Intelligence Scale for Children* (3rd ed.). New York: Psychological Corporation.

Weinstein, S. R., Stone, K., Noam, G. G., Grimes, K., & Schwab-Stone, M. (1989). Comparison of DISC with clinicians' DSM-III diagnoses in psychiatric inpatients. *Journal of the American Academy of Child and Adolescent Psychiatry, 28,* 53–60.

Whalen, C. K., & Henker, B. (1985). The social worlds of hyperactivity (ADDH) children. *Clinical Psychology Review, 5,* 447–478.

17

EATING DISORDERS

MICHELLE HEFFNER MACERA

Center for Hope of the Sierras
Reno, Nevada

J. SCOTT MIZES

Department of Behavioral Medicine and Psychiatry
West Virginia University School of Medicine
Morgantown, West Virginia

INTRODUCTION

"Mary Kate Olsen's Eating Disorder Crisis" was the cover headline on the July 5, 2004, cover of *People* magazine. Mary Kate and her fraternal twin sister, Ashley, were child stars on the television sitcom *Full House*, making their show business debut on the program at just 9 months old. Since then, they have capitalized on their clean, cute, girl-next-door image to create their own multimillion-dollar entertainment and marketing company. The risk of describing Mary Kate's story is that of perpetuating the myth that eating disorders afflict mainly affluent, high-achieving white females, even though current research suggests that eating disorders occur across socioeconomic and educational levels. Nonetheless, media reports of Mary Kate's case illustrate many features of the development and clinical aspects of the eating disorder anorexia nervosa.

Mary Kate was hospitalized at an exclusive residential treatment facility shortly after her high school graduation and just before she would turn 18 on June 13, 2004. Reports were that the 5-foot 2-inch actress's weight was as low as 86 pounds, representing a body mass index (BMI) of 15.6. Based on medical weight charts, her expected weight for height and age is approximately 119 lb. Thus, her reported weight was 72% of expected weight. As discussed later, both her BMI and expected weight met current diagnostic criteria for anorexia nervosa.

By most accounts, Mary Kate's eating disorder became evident to others about 2 years earlier, when she was 15–16. She initially hid her eating disorder, which reportedly angered those close to her. In an interview in 2003 on CBS's *48 Hours*, Mary Kate compared herself to her sister, Ashley, commenting, "I'm, like, 'Why do you look pretty and I look ugly?'" She was initially treated via outpatient therapy, including meals supervised by adults. However, her condition did not improve enough to prevent the need for hospitalization. As is true of many patients with eating disorders, Mary Kate's symptoms reportedly worsened during stressful periods in her life, such as when taking her SATs for college admission. Although reports differed on how willingly she entered residential treatment, there was speculation on whether the timing of her hospitalization was influenced by the fact that her parents had the legal right to hospitalize her prior to her turning 18, a right they would lose when she reached the age of majority.

Like Mary Kate, who entered residential treatment at age 18, most clients with eating disorders are adolescents or young adults. However, development of eating disorders can begin in childhood, for body image problems and dietary restraint among elementary-school-aged children are a predictor of eating disorder onset in later years (Marchi & Cohen, 1990). Among 7- to 12-year-old children, 55% of girls and 45% of boys desired an ideal body mass index that ranks at less than the 10th percentile, an extremely thin, biologically impossible body size for many children (Truby & Paxton, 2002). In other research, 21% of first-grade children report having tried to lose weight, with an increase to 25% of girls one year later (Halvarsson, Lunner, & Sjoden, 2000). Another study also found that 27.5% of normal-weight second-grade girls have dieted (Thelen, Powell, Lawrence, & Kuhnert, 1992).

Psychological assessment of eating-disordered behaviors in children and adolescents can lead to early detection of a potentially life-threatening problem. The purpose of this chapter is to describe assessment measures commonly used to assess for eating disorder symptoms and associated features in children and adolescents. Before presenting available measures, we briefly review the diagnostic criteria for the eating disorders listed in the *Diagnostic and Statistical Manual for Mental Disorders* (*DSM*; American Psychiatric Association, 2000a).

DIAGNOSTIC CRITERIA

ANOREXIA NERVOSA

Symptoms of Anorexia Nervosa (AN) include extremely low body weight, caloric restriction, fear of weight gain, body-image disturbance, and amenorrhea for at least three consecutive menstrual cycles in postmenarchal females (APA, 2000a). Of the two subtypes of AN, restricting type is characterized by caloric restriction, whereas binge-purge type is characterized by caloric restriction plus overeating and engagement in compensatory behaviors such as self-induced vomiting, laxatives abuse, diet pills use, and/or diuretics. According to the *DSM*, the prevalence of AN is 1% among female teenagers. The average age of first onset of AN is 17 years, with 68% of cases beginning between the ages of 14 and 20 (Willi, Giacometti, & Limbacher, 1990). Although most cases of anorexia are diagnosed in adolescents, approximately 5% occur in children under age 12 (Atkins, 1993).

BULIMIA NERVOSA

The *DSM* (APA, 2000a) defines symptoms of Bulimia Nervosa (BN) as body-image disturbance plus binge eating with compensatory behavior. Purging-type bulimia is diagnosed if compensatory behaviors include vomiting, laxatives, enema use, and/or diuretics. Nonpurging type is assigned if compensatory behaviors include fasting or excessive exercise. Purging type is more common and is associated with an earlier age of onset as compared to nonpurging type (Garfinkel et al., 1996). Onset of BN occurs later in adolescence than anorexia, at an average age of 21 (Kendler et al., 1991); however, 68% of first cases of BN start between the ages of 15 and 27. Although only 2% of female and 0.3% of male adolescents (point prevalence) meet full criteria for a BN diagnosis, as many as 15% of adolescents binge eat and purge (Schneider, 2003). Cases of bulimia in preadolescent children are extremely rare. One study (Kent, Lacey, & McCluskey, 1992) found that only three of 323 (<1%) eating disorder clinic clients report premenarchal onset of bulimia.

EATING DISORDER

Cluster analysis results indicate two categories of eating disorder Not Otherwise Specified (NOS): Binge Eating Disorder (BED) and subthreshold anorexia or bulimia that do not meet the full DSM diagnostic criteria (Mizes & Sloan, 1998).

The *DSM* (APA, 2000a) defines BED as recurrent binge eating without engagement in compensatory behavior. Binge eating symptoms also include rapid eating, eating alone to avoid embarrassment, eating until uncomfortably full, and guilt. BED is currently listed as an example of Eating Disorder (ED) NOS and not as a separate diagnosis. Full criteria for BED are listed in category of diagnoses requiring further study. Among a sample of nearly 5000 adolescents, 3% of girls and 1% of boys met full criteria for binge eating and 17% of girls and 8% of boys report overeating problems (Ackard, Neumark-Sztainer, Story, & Perry, 2003). Binge eating can lead to obesity, and overweight children who experience out-of-control eating episodes are more obese and report more psychological distress than overweight children who deny loss of control over eating (Morgan et al., 2002).

ED NOS cases, as a subthreshold AN or BN diagnosis, may demand as much clinical attention as cases of AN or BN that meet full diagnostic criteria. For example, adolescents with subthreshold bulimia symptoms are likely to have

TABLE 17.1 Suggested Measures to Assess Eating Disorders in Children and Adolescents

Name of Measure	Type of Measure
Eating Disorders Inventory for Children (EDI-C)	Questionnaire
Children's Eating Attitudes Test (ChEAT)	Questionnaire
Questionnaire for Eating and Weight Patterns (QEWP-A)	Questionnaire
McKnight Risk Factors Survey (MRSF-IV)	Questionnaire
Kid's Eating Disorder Survey	Questionnaire
Body Esteem Scale	Questionnaire
MSCARED	Stage-of-change questionnaire
Perceived Body Image Scale	Silhouette body-image scale
Children's Body Image Scale	Pictorial body-image scale
Eating Disorders Examination for Children	Interview
Diagnostic Interview Schedule for Children	Interview
Kiddie Schedule for Affective Disorders and Schizophrenia	Interview
Diagnostic Interview for Children and Adolescents	Interview
Forbidden Food Questionnaire	Behavioral rating scale
Body Image Avoidance Questionnaire	Behavioral rating scale

similar levels of self-esteem, depression, dietary restraint, and body dissatisfaction as those who meet full BN criteria, with the only difference between subthreshold and BN groups being frequency of binge-purge episodes (Le Grange, Loeb, Van Orman, & Jellar, 2004). Therefore, even if a child does not meet full criteria for a specific eating disorder diagnosis (i.e, AN or BN), treatment may be necessary.

ASSESSMENT STRATEGIES

A thorough eating disorder assessment integrates self-report, interview, and functional assessment data to detect eating disorder symptoms, self-harm, family functioning, and other comorbid diagnoses in children and adolescents. Table 17.1 summarizes commonly used measures.

SELF-REPORT

Crowther and Sherwood (1997) describe self-report questionnaires as useful for initial screening, evaluation of progress over the course of treatment, selection of symptoms to target for treatment planning, and assessment of general distress and other issues that affect eating behavior (e.g, family functioning, self-harm).

The Eating Disorders Inventory (EDI; Garner, 1991; Garner, Olmsted, & Polivy, 1983) is a 64-item self-report measure of eating disorder symptoms that was normed on college-aged females, with questionable validity with children and adolescents due to lack of normative data for younger age groups, problems with reading level, and item wordings that are more applicable to adults (Franko et al., 2004). An adaptation of the EDI was recently developed for use with children (Eating Disorders Inventory for Children; EDI-C; Franko et al.). This preliminary version of the 64-item EDI-C includes 16 original EDI items, 29 items with slight wording changes, and 19 items with significant changes. EDI-C items are based on a four-point Likert scale, rather than a six-point scale used in the adult version. Additional research is needed to determine the psychometric properties of this measure.

The Children's Eating Attitudes Test (ChEAT; Maloney, McGuire, & Daniels, 1988) is a 26-item measure of eating attitudes and behavior among 8- to 15-year-old children. The ChEAT is an adaption of a 26-item adult self-report measure (Eating Attitudes Test; Garner, Olmsted, Bohr, & Garfinkel, 1982) that was modified with simplified language for children. ChEAT items, rated on a six-point Likert scale, assess dieting, compensatory behavior, food preoccupation, and oral control (Smolak & Levine, 1994). Psychometric data show that the ChEAT is moderately correlated with other eating disorder measures and demonstrates adequate test–retest reliability and adequate internal consistency, with more reliable data obtained from older children (Maloney et al.; Smolak & Levine). Better reliability and validity data were obtained from a 23-item ChEAT, which drops three items (Smolak & Levine).

The Questionnaire for Eating and Weight Patterns—Adolescent Version (QEWP-A; Johnson, Grieve, Adams & Sandy, 1999) is a modification of an adult measure, the 13-item QEWP, used to identify BED in adults (Spitzer et al., 1992). QEWP-A includes simplified language and combines two items on the adult version into one, simpler item. The QEWP-A is a 12-item BED measure that was normed on 367 10- to 18-year-old children in grades six to twelve. The QEWP-A can be administered with a parent version, the QEWP-P, in which QEWP-A items are reworded from "you" to "your child." QEWP-A and QEWP-P items reflect *DSM* criteria for BED to identify individuals with no diagnosis, subclinical BED, and BED symptoms. Psychometric data on the QEWP-A show that adolescents identified with BED, compared to subclinical BED and no BED diagnosis, had higher levels of depression, as measured by the Children's Depression Inventory (CDI; Sitarenios & Kovacs, 1999) and higher scores on the ChEAT-26 (Johnson et al., 1999). Morgan et al. (2002) administered the QEWP-A to 112 6- to 10-year-old children. Children who endorsed loss of control weighed more, had more body fat and more body dissatisfaction, and experienced higher levels of anxiety and depression, compared to children who reported no loss of control over eating on the QEWP-A. Test–retest reliability data at 3 weeks shows that male responding is more stable, for females' responses were likely to change from subclinical to no diagnosis (Johnson, Kirk, & Reed, 2000). Due to the poor test–retest reliability of QEWP-A for females, this measure may not yield valid data for reassessment of treatment progress. Interrater reliability is also questionable. On the QEWP-A and QEWP-P, parents and children agreed in 87% of no-diagnosis cases (Johnson et al., 1999), but parents were less likely to report

BED symptoms in children whose QEWP-A results suggest BED (25% parent–child agreement) or subclincal BED (15% parent–child agreement).

The Mizes Anorectic Cognitions (MAC) questionnaire (Mizes & Klesges, 1989) is a 33-item Likert-format instrument designed to assess core cognitions in eating disorders. The MAC, which assesses cognitions relevant to bulimia and anorexia nervosa, has three subscales measuring the following factors: rigid weight regulation and fear of weight gain, excess self-control of eating and weight as a basis of self-esteem, and beliefs that body weight is an important factor in approval from others. A review of studies of the MAC found that it has favorable reliability and validity characteristics (Mizes & Christiano, 1995). The MAC has recently been revised, resulting in a 24-item questionnaire (MAC-R; Mizes et al., 2000). Initial evidence suggests that the MAC-R has improved internal consistency of the subscales. As opposed to the original MAC, significant differences were found between anorectics and bulimics on the self-control and weight and approval subscales. The MAC-R has been studied in a sample of high school and technical school students, age range of 14–20 (Guillard, 2002). The majority of the participants (91%) were within the age range of 15–18. A modification of the MAC-R used in this study was found to have good concurrent validity.

Body-image disturbance is one specific symptom of an eating disorder, and several assessment measures have been developed to assess for body-image disturbance in children and adolescents. These measures include questionnaires (e.g., Body Esteem Scale; Mendelson & White, 1982) and silhouette body figure rating scales (e.g., Perceived Body Image Scale; Manley, Tonkin, & Hammond, 1988). Sihouette rating scales involve asking a child to select a silhouette figure to match his/her own body size (i.e., perceived body image) and a figure to represent his/her desired or ideal body size.

One of the most recent body-image assessment measures is the Children's Body Image Scale (CBIS; Truby & Paxton, 2002). CBIS is a pictoral scale to assess perceived and ideal body image in children. The CBIS is unique because it contains actual photographs of the bodies of seven boys (male version) or seven girls (female versions) facing frontward in their underwear, with a standard computer-generated male or female face inserted above each body. To represent the range of body mass index (BMI), the BMI represented in each photograph fits into one of seven categories, ranging from 0 to 97th percentiles of 1979 National Center for Health Statistics norms for each gender. The authors contend that photographic body shapes, rather than silhouettes or drawings, may help young children identify body shapes. The CBIS was tested on 312 children, ages 7–12. Each child was weighed and measured, and his or her BMI was categorized into one of the seven categories. Each child was instructed to point out the body figure most like his or her own (perceived body image) and the body figure he or she most want to have (ideal body image). Body dissatisfaction was determined by substracting ideal from perceived. Positive scores represent a desire to be thinner, whereas negative scores represent a desire to be heavier. The absolute value of the perceived–ideal discrepancy determines the extent of body dissatisfaction, with higher numbers indicating more body dissatisfaction. Construct validity was adequate for girls only. One limitation of this measure is the need for a verbal explanation of instructions, which requires clinical time, because children's ability to comprehend written instructions for this measure has not been examined.

In addition to the measures just described, instruments have been developed to assess children and adolescents potentially at risk for an eating disorder. The McKnight Risk Factors Survey—IV (MRFS-IV; Shisslak et al., 1999) can be administered to assess for eating disorder risk and protective factors among children in grades six to twelve, with another version for children in grades four and five. Likewise, the Kid's Eating Disorder Survey (KEDS; Childress, Jarrell, & Brewerton, 1993) is a 14-item self-report measure to assess body dissatisfaction and purging in middle school children (grades five to eight) to identify children at risk for developing an eating disorder.

CLINICAL INTERVIEWS

Although self-reports provide supplemental data about symptoms, they do not yield diagnostic information. The most commonly used semistructured interview for diagnosis of eating disorders in children is the Eating Disorder Examination adapted for Children (ChEDE; Bryant-Waugh, Cooper, Taylor, & Lask, 1996), a child version of the Eating Disorder Examination interview for adults (Cooper & Fairburn, 1987). In addition to wording modifications, the ChEDE has a sorting task in which the child rank-orders values, including the value of weight and shape. The ChEDE requires one hour of administration. In addition, the Diagnostic Interview Schedule for Children (DISC: Shaffer & Fisher, 2000), the Kiddie version of the Schedule for Affective Disorders and Schizophrenia Present and Lifetime version (K-SADS-PL; Kaufman et al., 1997), and Diagnostic Interview for Children and Adolescents (DICA; Reich, 2000) all include eating disorder sections, and these interviews may be useful in the diagnosis of eating disorders as well as the assessment of other childhood disorders.

FUNCTIONAL ANALYSIS AND AVOIDANCE MEASURES

Possible functions of eating disorder behavior may include emotional regulation or escape from aversive emotional states. For example, reduction of negative affect is a consequence of purging (Mizes & Arbitell, 1991). A functional analysis can aid in differential diagnosis by identifying if weight loss and food refusal are acquired or maintained due to depression or opposition-defiance. If, however, the results of a functional assessment indicate that eating disorder behaviors are functionally related to weight-gain fears or body-image disturbance, the functional assessment can guide treatment planning by identifying feared or avoided stimuli to construct a hierarchy for exposure treatment.

Identification of target behaviors can begin with direct observation. With eating disorders, direct observation may include observation of the child looking in the mirror or eating meals. Rosen, Leitenberg, Gross, and Willmuth (1985) developed the test meal as a direct observation procedure. Clients with bulimia are instructed to eat as much high-calorie food as they comfortably can without vomiting. Rosen et al. found that normal-weight bulimic women (mean age 24) ate less than nonclinical control participants. The authors concluded that women with bulimia, when they believe they are unable to vomit, experience anxiety, negative food-related thoughts, and avoidance of high-calorie food. Although no studies were found using the test meal approach in adolescents, it would appear possible to adapt it for use in a younger population.

In some cases, direct observation is not possible, and indirect methods, such as self-report measures, can provide a more practical alternative. For example, instead of directly observing a client's reaction to various types of food, the Forbidden Food Survey can be administered (FSS; Ruggiero, Williamson, Davis, Schlundt, & Carey, 1988). The FSS is a questionnaire that lists 45 specific foods and beverages, including nine items for each of the five food groups and foods with low, medium, and high calorie content. Clients rate how each food item makes them feel about themselves using a five-point Likert scale, ranging from "I would feel very good about myself after eating this food" to "I would feel very badly about myself after eating this food." Psychometric data show that the FSS is a reliable measure with high internal consistency. Validity data show that eating-disordered clients experienced more negative reactions to medium- or high-calorie foods than normal eaters (Ruggiero et al.). Of the eating-disordered clients, those with bulimia reported the strongest negative reactions to high-calorie foods, carbohydrates, and fats. The FSS questionnaire was developed on a sample of women that included eating-disordered clients as young as 15.

While the FSS can be used in planning exposure to forbidden food, the Body Image Avoidance Questionnaire can be used to construct a hierarchy for exposure to body-image avoidance (BIA; Rosen, Srebnik, Saltzberg, & Wendt, 1991). The BIA is a 19-item self-report measure in which clients rate how often they engage in specific body-image avoidance behavior, such as wearing darker clothing or avoiding physical intimacy. BIA was developed on a sample of undergraduate women. Although there is no child version of the BIA, it can be used successfully with younger clients to identify a hierarchy of avoidance behavior within the individual. Research has shown that BIA is a reliable and valid measure, and high scores on this measure are associated with higher body dissatisfaction, fear of fat, and desire to lose weight (Rosen et al.).

In addition to the self-report measures just described, indirect observation includes self-monitoring of antecedents, behaviors, and consequences (ABCs). Lee and Miltenberger (1997) describe three variations of self-monitoring: description, checklists, and interval recording. Using the descriptive method, the client writes narrative comments to describe ABCs on a three-column data sheet. The checklist method involves providing the client with a checklist of potential antecedents, behaviors, and consequences and requiring the client to check off each ABC when it occurs. The interval recording method involves having the client record ABCs that occur during predetermined time intervals (Lee & Miltenberger).

Self-monitoring data can lead to a useful functional assessment of variables maintaining eating-disordered behavior. In addition to overt behavior, private events associated with eating disordered behavior should be self-monitored, for cognitive variables often play a prominent role in the disorder. For example, women with bulimia, including participants as young as age 17, report more negative affective thoughts and more eating/weight-related thoughts than non-eating-disordered controls (Zotter & Crowther, 1991).

To monitor thoughts, a thought-sampling procedure requires clients to wear an alarm wristwatch that sounds at regular intervals throughout the day as a prompt to record current thoughts. Thought sampling can be used in conjunction with test meals, a direct observation method described earlier. Clients can write or speak aloud into a tape recorder, word-for-word, the content of thoughts, along with situational antecedents and emotional or behavioral consequences of the thought. In other cases, the client can endorse thoughts listed on a thought inventory to indicate if she is experiencing one or more of the thoughts commonly experienced by eating-disordered clients. In one study (Bonifazi, Crowther, & Mizes, 2000), participants were prompted every 30 minutes to complete the Bulimia Cognition Inventory (BCI), which consists of 12 statements about food and eating, such as "I should not have eaten that." The BCI was normed on college undergraduates, and further research is needed to assess its validity with younger clients (Bonifazi & Crowther, 1996). Although thought sampling and self-monitoring provide a practical alternative to direct observation, younger children may have trouble completing them, or they may be selective about what they record due to embarrassment, fatigue, or other reasons (Crowther & Sherwood, 1997).

COMORBID DIAGNOSES

Eating disorders have been shown to have a high comorbidity with both anxiety and depression (Bulik, 2002). Persons with AN show elevated rates of Generalized Anxiety Disorder, phobias, and Panic Disorder, while those with BN show elevated rates of Social Phobia and Generalized Anxiety Disorder. Depression is the most commonly found comorbid condition for both AN and BN.

It is necessary to make a differential diagnosis as to whether depression symptoms represent a comorbid condition or the effect of the eating disorder. Depression should only be diagnosed if the depressed mood is not directly related to the eating disorder or the consequences of malnutrition. Depression should not be diagnosed if there is much overlap between depression symptoms and the effects of semistarvation, including sleep disturbance, low energy, and concentration problems. It may be helpful to inquire if the loss of interest in activities is solely due to body-image concerns in social situations, or if feelings of guilt stem from the child's shame about engagement in compensatory behaviors.

The comorbidity of eating disorders with post-traumatic stress (Fallon & Wonderlich, 1997) and substance abuse (Wilson, 2002) has been well documented, and a thorough eating disorder evaluation should include assessment of trauma and substance use history.

RESEARCH BASIS

The assessment strategies discussed thus far address aspects of eating disorders that are part of their diagnostic criteria (i.e, binge eating, purging, food restriction, eating disorder cognitions, and body-image disturbance). In this section we briefly review research relative to two important clinical issues in eating disorders: family functioning and risk of suicide.

Because children and adolescents, as opposed to adults, continue to live with their family of origin, family functioning takes on greater significance in the treatment of these patients. Additionally, research suggests that family functioning has a role in the etiology of eating disorders. Families of eating-disordered clients tend to be unsupportive and overinvolved and have difficulty resolving conflict (Vandereycken, Kog, & Vanderlinden, 1989; Mizes, 1995). Parents, especially mothers more than fathers, who express dissatisfaction with their own weight, use extreme weight loss techniques, and comment on their daughter's weight are likely to have a daughter who diets (Keel, Heatherton, Harnden, & Hornig, 1997; Benedikt, Wertheim, & Love, 1998; Smolak, Levine, & Schermer, 1999). Pike and Rodin (1991) found that mothers of eating-disordered girls want their daughters to lose weight, whereas mothers of non-eating-disordered girls wanted their daughters to gain weight. Additionally, mothers of eating-disordered daughters were more likely than mothers of non-eating-disordered daughters to rate their daughter as less attractive than the daughter rated herself. A related study found that mothers of bulimic students were more likely than mothers of nonbulimics to encourage weight loss, dieting, and exercise (Moreno & Thelen, 1993). However, it is also important to keep in mind that pathology seen in the families of persons with eating disorders may be an effect of the stress of the disorder on the family. Moreover, many families show no more pathology than "normal" families (Mizes).

Research has suggested an association between eating disorders and suicidal behavior. Both male and female adolescents who reported suicidal ideation scored higher on eating disorder measures than nonsuicidal teens (Miotto, de Coppi, Frezza, & Preti, 2003). For girls, 28% of binge eaters, compared to 10% of nonbingers, have attempted suicide, and 28% of male binge eaters attempted suicide, compared to 5% of nonbingers (Ackard et al., 2003). Also, anorexia nervosa has the highest death rate of all the psychiatric disorders. While a substantial proportion of these deaths are due to the medical complications of the disorder, suicide is also a frequent cause of death (Sullivan, 2002).

CLINICAL UTILITY

Recommendations on which assessment strategies have the most clinical utility can consider ease of administration and the usefulness of the measure in diagnosis and treatment planning. Also, some measures have been developed more for research applications.

For routine clinical practice, we do not recommend use of the available diagnostic interviews, for two reasons. First, structured interviews are time consuming and therefore are less efficient. Second, clinicians familiar with and skilled in the assessment and treatment of eating disorders can diagnose an eating disorder using clinical interview alone. We have not found any particular questionnaire that provides significant additional information for diagnosing an eating disorder beyond that obtained in a quality clinical interview. For example, we do not use the Eating Disorders Inventory routinely for diagnostic purposes. We have found the EDI and other measures useful for adolescents who deny that they have an eating disorder. The purpose here is to provide the adolescent "data" that their body-image concerns and drive for thinness are consistent with an eating disorder and that they are in excess of the dieting and weight concerns of their peers. This also serves to make the diagnosis not just a matter of the clinician's opinion, but makes it based on objective data that the clinician and adolescent can evaluate together.

In terms of treatment planning, we have found it useful to assess readiness to change (see later), because this will determine the extent to which it will be necessary to engage the adolescent in treatment before addressing actual change of relevant eating-disordered thoughts and behavior. In order to assess core eating-disordered cognitions from a cognitive behavioral perspective, we utilize the Mizes Anorectic Cognitions questionnaire. Feedback to patients on the MAC is a useful way to introduce them to an important aspect of a cognitive behavioral conceptualization of their disorder. Additionally, changes in core eating-disordered cognitions are an important indicator of clinical improvement.

In terms of planning and monitoring specific behavior change, self-monitoring has a central role in cognitive behavioral treatments for eating disorders and may be the most useful behavioral assessment strategy. Self-monitoring is at the heart of all existing manualized cognitive behavioral treatments (CBT) for eating disorders. There are many treatment targets in CBT for eating disorders, including reducing avoidance of feared foods so that they are routinely included in the diet and reducing negative body image, especially avoidance of situations that are associated with high levels of negative body image. Thus, the

Forbidden Food Questionnaire and the Body Image Avoidance Questionnaire are useful for identifying individualized treatment targets for patients.

DEVELOPMENTAL CONSIDERATIONS

Eating-disordered behaviors can hinder a child's physical development and lead to growth retardation, sexual problems (e.g., infertility), and osteoporosis (Robin, Gilroy, & Dennis, 1998). A thorough medical evaluation should be a routine part of every eating disorder evaluation, and a medical hospitalization should be required if severe physical problems are detected.

Developmental issues may complicate diagnostic assessments. Due to developmental considerations, *DSM* criteria for eating disorders are not always applicable to children. For example, amenorrhea is a diagnostic criterion for anorexia, and up to 50% of women with bulimic symptoms experience menstrual irregularity (Le Grange et al., 2004). However, menstrual abnormalities in children and prepubertal adolescents can be difficult to assess because menstrual cycles may not be established (Robin et al., 1998). In addition, the amenorrhea criterion is not applicable if the adolescent is using a hormonal birth control method regulating the menstrual cycle (Walsh & Garner, 1997).

For anorexia, the *DSM* criteria include weight loss resulting in body weight that is less than 85% of expected weight; however, what constitutes "expected weight" is not defined and therefore is unclear. To avoid this issue, some clinicians rely on the *International Classification of Mental and Behavioral Disorders: Clinical Descriptions and Diagnostic Guidelines* (*ICD-10*; World Health Organization, 1992), which in addition to weight loss of at least 15% of expected weight, uses a body mass index (BMI) of 17.5. The criterion of a BMI of 17.5 is appropriate only for those 18 and older, due to differences between the stature of preteens and adolescents versus adults. BMI values representing the 5th percentile for age (1–19) and sex, presented on tables developed by Hammer, Kraemer, Wilson, Ritter, and Dornbusch (1991), can be used as an age- and sex-adjusted weight criterion for adolescent AN. However, these methods may not be appropriate for children and adolescents because normative growth charts do not account for individual puberty changes and BMI only corrects for height (Drewnowski & Garn, 1987; Robin et al., 1998). In addition to body-weight assessment, it may be more valid to consider lean body mass, body fat percentage, and maturational status (Drewnoski & Garn).

Finally, puberty and psychosexual change during adolescence can interact with other risk factors to lead to the development of an eating disorder. Developmental factors, such as early menarche for females, early or late onset of ejaculation for males, and early age of sexual activity for both genders, have been associated with the development of bulimia (Kaltiala-Heino, Rimpela, Rissanen, & Rantanen, 2001).

ASSESSMENT, CONCEPTUALIZATION, AND TREATMENT PLANNING

One goal of assessment is to determine treatment. Eating disorders treatment may include self-help (Heffner & Eifert, 2004), individual psychotherapy, family therapy, psychotropic medication, intensive outpatient treatment, day treatment, group psychotherapy, inpatient psychiatric hospitalization, or some combination of all of these.

STAGE OF CHANGE

A client's response to treatment is often related to the client's willingness to change and participate in treatment. In some cases, an adolescent client is ambivalent or resistant to making changes and will attend sessions only because a parent "forces" her to have treatment. Such treatment resistance is one indicator of poor prognosis (Groth-Marnat, 1997). Assessment of a client's readiness to change can help plan treatment, because clients with high resistance benefit most from a supportive, nondirective treatment approach, and clients with a low resistance are more receptive to a structured, directive approach (Groth-Marnat).

The Motivational Stages of Change for Adolescents Recovering from an Eating Disorder (MSCARED; Gusella, Butler, Nichols, & Bird, 2002) was developed on a sample of female adolescent eating-disordered clients at an average age of 15. On the questionnaire, participants selected one of six descriptions to indicate which of the six Prochaska and Diclemente stages of change (precontemplation, contemplation, preparation, action, maintenance, and recovery) best describes her current situation. If the action or maintenance stage was endorsed, the participant also indicated action-oriented changes she was currently making.

FAMILY THERAPY

As result of the growing research on familial influences on eating-disordered behavior, family therapy is considered the treatment of choice for adolescent eating-disordered clients (Garner & Needleman, 1997). Family functioning can be assessed using the Family Adjustment Device General Functioning Scale (FAD-GFS) is a 12–item sub-scale of the FAD, a self-report measure (Epstein, Baldwin, & Bishop, 1983). McDermott, Batik, Roberts, and Gibbon (2002) administered the FAD-GFS to 66 eating-disorder clinic clients, ages 9–18, and 75 of their parents. There was a moderate correlation between child and parent ratings of the family relationship ($r = .51$). Compared to scores obtained from nonclinical participants, scores obtained from the eating-disordered sample were higher, suggesting more family dysfunction. However, the FAD-GFS did not discriminate between the functioning of families of anorexic and bulimic children. Additional self-report measures of family functioning include the Issues Checklist (Robin & Foster, 1989), Family Environment Scale (Moos & Moos, 1981), and Parent–Adolescent Relationship Questionnaire (Robin, Koepke, & Moye, 1990). Self-report measures of family functioning can be used as outcome measures or as a means of identifying specific family problems to target in treatment.

HOSPITALIZATION

Psychiatric hospitalization is necessary if a client engages in self-harm or plans to commit suicide (or homicide, in rare cases). Suicide assessment should be included in an eating disorder evaluation, for research has documented a relationship between eating disorder symptoms and suicidal behaviors. Despite the risk of self-harm, none of the commonly used eating disorder measures contains self-harm items (Sansone & Sansone, 2002). Therefore, suicide assessment needs to be conducted as part of the routine mental status examination or through administration of an adolescent-normed measure of self-harm, such as the Life Attitudes Schedule—Short Form (Rohde, Seeley, Langhinrichsen-Rohling, & Rohling, 2003).

Hospitalization is needed much more commonly for AN than for BN, due to the semistarvation and associated medical problems accompanying the former. The APA's practice guidelines for eating disorders (APA, 2000b) delineate medical criteria for inpatient hospitalization. For children and adolescents, these include bradycardia (i.e., heart rate 40–49 bpm), tachycardia (heart rate over 110 bpm), blood pressure less than 80/50 mm Hg, core body temperature of less than 97°F, hypokalemia (potassium less than 3.0 meq/liter), dehydration, and orthostatic hypotension. Weight of less than 75% of expected weight merits inpatient hospitalization for patients of all ages. However, children and adolescents who are not less than 75% of expected weight but who have acute and rapid weight loss and significant food refusal should be hospitalized.

Other factors leading to consideration of hospitalization include poor motivation for treatment and being uncooperative on an outpatient basis, inability to eat enough food to gain weight, and inability to refrain from purging or compulsive exercise without close supervision. APA practice guidelines also provide criteria for selecting various levels of care, including outpatient, intensive outpatient, partial hospitalization, residential treatment center, and inpatient hospitalization.

CASE STUDY

In this section, we describe an adolescent eating disorder case. This fictional case is based on actual eating clients we have assessed. Adolescents are often resistant to acknowledging that they have an eating disorder, which can be problematic since most of the eating disorder assessment approaches have a great deal of face and content validity. Thus, it is easy for the adolescent not to endorse indicators of eating disorder pathology. In fact, clinically we have observed that assessment scores from a patient that are less pathological than what are observed in a normal population is a clue that the assessment results may not be accurate. The following case illustrates one approach to determining that a clinical eating disorder is present despite the lack of scores in the clinical range on commonly used eating disorder assessments.

IDENTIFICATION

Anna Rexia is a 15-year-old Caucasian female who resides in rural West Virginia with her biological parents and 9-year-old brother.

PRESENTING COMPLAINTS

Anna is 5 feet 7 inches and weighs 94lb. During an annual medical exam, Anna's heart rate was 44 beats per minute, and she was diagnosed with bradycardia, an abnormally low heart rate. She was immediately hospitalized on the pediatric unit at West Virginia University Hospitals, and an eating disorder consult was ordered.

HISTORY

This is Anna's first hospitalization for medical reasons. Anna has never been hospitalized for psychiatric reasons, and she has never participated in outpatient counseling.

DEVELOPMENTAL ISSUES

Anna's medical records indicate that she met developmental milestones on time throughout early childhood, with no indication of developmental delays.

Anna has never had a menstrual period. The average age of menarche for Caucasian females is 12.6 years, with nearly all girls reaching menarche by age 15 (Anderson, Dallal, & Must, 2003). As discussed earlier, it is likely, but not certain, that Anna's delayed menarche is a symptom of an eating disorder. It is also possible that Anna is experiencing a statistically deviant age of menarche.

Anna's body mass index is 14.7. As discussed earlier, the BMI criterion of 17.5 must be adjusted to account for the differences in stature between preteens and adolescents versus adults (i.e., age 18 and over). The 5th percentile for a 15-year-old girl is a BMI of 16.1 (Hammer et al., 1991). Thus, Anna's BMI is well below the adjusted BMI anorexia cutoff for an adolescent.

PEER AND SCHOOL ISSUES

Anna is an attractive young woman who is concerned about her appearance. She wore makeup daily during her hospitalization. She reported that she is popular in school. She has several close female friends, but she has never dated.

Anna is a high school freshman who maintains a 3.72 grade point average and participates on the track team. Due to Anna's low body weight, the track coach recently benched Anna and prevented her from participating in practices.

Teachers and classmates often make comments about Anna's low weight and express concern for her. The attention that Anna is receiving from coaches, teachers, and peers may serve to reinforce her dietary restrictions. It would be helpful to assign self-monitoring homework in which Anna records the attention she receives and her reactions (including dietary restriction) to these comments. If comments about Anna's weight and eating behavior function as an antecedent or consequent of her dietary restriction, a behavioral treatment plan may need to be developed to eliminate attention to weight and eating behavior. This plan can be implemented by working with the school system to provide instructions directly to staff/students and/or helping Anna to be more assertive so that she can inform others to stop making comments about her weight and appearance.

BEHAVIORAL ASSESSMENT RESULTS

Assessment began with an unstructured interview with Anna. Anna denied a history of trauma, including child abuse and neglect. She denied substance use. Last year, Anna began to diet, and she has since lost 20 pounds. She said she needs to follow a strict diet for health reasons. Specifically, she feels that she needs to eliminate carbohydrates and fats from her diet to avoid developing medical problems, such as high cholesterol, high blood pressure, and diabetes. Although Anna restricts her dietary intake, she denied engagement in compensatory behaviors.

She denied body-image problems and stated that she needs to follow a no-fat, no-carbohydrate diet for health reasons. She was adamant that she did not have an eating disorder. Anna completed three self-report measures: EDI, MAC, and MSCARED. On the EDI, Anna's symptoms of perfectionism were elevated, but all other eating disorder symptoms were in the nonclinical range. The MAC questionnaire, using adolescent norms, showed no evidence of eating disorder symptoms. On the MSCARED, Anna's score was in the precontemplative range.

The self-report questionnaires that Anna completed were face-valid measures of eating disorder symptoms. One of the limitations of eating disorder self-report measures is the potential for respondents to downplay symptoms, particularly if they are precontemplative or resistant to change. Therefore, we administered the MMPI-A. Although no MMPI-A scales assess for eating disorders, we were mainly interested in Anna's response to the validity scales. Anna's profile was invalid due to extremely high elevation on the L scale, suggesting that she is either naive about her psychological problems or intentionally downplaying her symptoms.

Based on the interview, self-report measures, and MMPI-A results, we concluded that follow-up eating disorder treatment was necessary. Anna was scheduled to participate in one-hour weekly individual therapy, and her parents were scheduled for separate family therapy sessions.

ETHICAL AND LEGAL ISSUES

In cases such as Anna's, the client is not a willing participant in treatment. She may be "forced" into treatment by concerned parents or health care providers. Parents have the right and the responsibility to consent to treatment, and to hospitalization if needed, until the adolescent reaches the age of 18. Once the adolescent turns 18, she is legally an adult; then only she can consent to treatment. Of course, this also includes the right to *refuse* treatment. At that point, the only option for parents is to initiate an involuntary psychiatric commitment. As may have been the case with Mary Kate Olsen, parents may often hospitalize their daughter before the age of 18, while they still have the right to do so.

A particularly difficult situation exists when it is apparent to health care providers that a child or adolescent has a serious eating disorder and that both the patient and the parents are resistant to treatment. There appears to be little clinical or research literature on this topic, so the professional experiences of one of the authors (JSM) will be briefly discussed here. Parents can be resistant to treatment in a variety of ways, including, but not limited to, refusing to seek treatment altogether, disagreeing with or resisting the goals or methods of treatment (such as disagreeing with making weight gain contingent on privileges, or the weight gain goal itself), or refusing a recommended level of care (such as hospitalization). This can create significant ethical dilemmas for health professionals, who try to engage the parents while at the same time recognizing that the patient may not get the treatment she needs. This dilemma becomes even more pronounced when the patient is experiencing significant, dangerous medical complications. One of the authors (JSM) has been involved in a few cases where a physician has reported the parents for child neglect for failing to obtain adequate treatment for the patient. Even with the state mandating treatment, the limited experience of only a few cases is discouraging. These cases have been fraught with conflict between the parents and the treatment team (even when the treatment team members are not the ones who reported the presumed neglect). As would be expected under these circumstances, the clinical outcome has been poor. There may be no good answers in such difficult situations.

SUMMARY

Several assessment devices are available for eating disorders in children and adolescents. Many, however, are adaptations of measures developed for adults. Few have been developed from inception specifically to assess eating disorders in children and adolescents. Those assessments that have been developed for children and adolescents are relatively new; thus these assessment approaches have not had extensive evaluation of their psychometric soundness. In developing assessment strategies for children and adolescent eating disorders, it will likely be useful to develop different measures for childhood onset (before the age of 14) versus adolescent onset due to the significant cognitive, emotional, and developmental differences of these two age groups.

REFERENCES AND RESOURCES

Ackard, D. M., Neumark-Sztainer, D., Story, M., & Perry, C. (2003). Overeating among adolescents: Prevalence and associations with weight-related characteristics and psychological health. *Pediatrics, 111,* 67–74.

American Psychiatric Association. (2000a). *Diagnostic and statistical manual of mental disorders* (4th ed. text revision). Washington, DC: Author.

American Psychiatric Association. (2000b). *Practice guideline for the treatment of patients with eating disorders* (2nd ed.). Washington, DC: Author.

Anderson, S. E., Dallal, G. E., & Must, A. (2003). Relative weight and race influence average age of menarche: Results from two nationally representative surveys of U.S. girls studied 25 years apart. *Pediatrics, 111,* 844–850.

Atkins, D. M. (1993). Clinical spectrum of anorexia nervosa in children. *Journal of Developmental and Behavioral Pediatrics, 14,* 211–216.

Benedikt, R., Wertheim, E. H., & Love, A. (1998). Eating attitudes and weight-loss attempts in female adolescents and their mothers. *Journal of Youth & Adolescence, 27,* 43–57.

Bonifazi, D. Z., & Crowther, J. H. (1996). *In vivo* cognitive assessment in bulimia nervosa and restrained eating. *Behavior Therapy, 27,* 139–158.

Bonifazi, D. Z., Crowther, J. H., & Mizes, J. S. (2000). Validity of questionnaires for assessing dysfunctional cognitions in bulimia nervosa. *International Journal of Eating Disorders, 27,* 464–470.

Bryant-Waugh, R. J., Cooper, P. J., Taylor, C. L., & Lask, B. D. (1996). The use of the eating disorder examination with children: A pilot study. *International Journal of Eating Disorders, 19,* 391–397.

Bulik, C. M. (2002). Anxiety, depression, and eating disorders. In C. G. Fairburn & K. D. Brownell (Eds.), *Eating disorders and obesity: A comprehensive handbook* (2nd ed.). New York: Guilford Press.

Childress, A. C., Jarrell, M. P., & Brewerton, T. D. (1993). The Kids' Eating Disorders Survey (KEDS): Internal consistency, component analysis, and reliability. *Eating Disorders: Journal of Treatment & Prevention, 1,* 123–133.

Cooper, Z., & Fairburn, C. (1987). The Eating Disorders Examination: A semistructured interview for the assessment of specific psychopathology of eating disorders. *International Journal of Eating Disorders, 6,* 1–8.

Crowther, J. H., & Sherwood, N. E. (1997). Assessment. In D. M. Garner & P. E. Garfinkel (Eds.), *Handbook for treatment for eating disorders.* New York: Guilford Press.

Drewnowski, A., & Garn, S. M. (1987). Concerning the use of weight tables to categorize patients with eating disorders. *International Journal of Eating Disorders, 6,* 639–646.

Epstein, N. B., Baldwin, L. M., & Bishop, D. S. (1983). The McMaster Family Assessment Device. *Journal of Marital and Family Therapy, 9,* 171–180.

Fallon, P., & Wonderlich, S. A. (1997). Sexual abuse and other forms of trauma. In D. M. Garner & P. E. Garfinkel (Eds.), *Handbook for treatment for eating disorders.* New York: Guilford Press.

Franko, D. L., Striegel-Moore, R. H., Barton, B. A., Schumann, B. C., Garner, D. M., Daniels, S. R., et al. (2004). Measuring eating concerns in black and white adolescent girls. *International Journal of Eating Disorders, 35,* 179–189.

Garfinkel, P. E., Lin, E., Goering, P., Spegg, C., Goldbloom, D. S., Kennedy, S., et al. (1996). Purging and nonpurging forms of bulimia nervosa in a community sample. *International Journal of Eating Disorders, 20,* 231–238.

Garner, D. M. (1991). *Eating Disorder Inventory—2, professional manual.* Odessa, FL: Psychological Assessment Resources.

Garner, D. M., & Needleman, L. D. (1997). Sequencing and integration of treatments. In D. M. Garner & P. E. Garfinkel (Eds.), *Handbook for treatment for eating disorders.* New York: Guilford Press.

Garner, D. M., Olmsted, M. P., Bohr, Y., & Garfinkel, P. (1982). The Eating Attitudes Test: Psychometic features and clinical correlates. *Psychological Medicine, 12,* 871–878.

Garner, D. M., Olmsted, M. P., & Polivy, J. (1983). Development and validation of a multidimensional eating disorder inventory for anorexia nervosa and bulimia. *International Journal of Eating Disorders, 2,* 15–34.

Groth-Marnat, G. (1997). *Handbook of psychological assessment.* New York: John Wiley & Sons.

Guillard, Jr., R. P. (2002). *The validity of the Mizes Anorectic Cognitions Questionnaire—Revised, with a racially mixed, nonclinical population of 14- to 19-year-old adolescents.* Unpublished doctoral dissertation, Philadelphia College of Osteopathic Medicine, Philadelphia.

Gusella, J., Butler, G., Nichols, L., & Bird, D. (2002). A brief questionnaire to assess readiness to change in adolescents with eating disorders: Its application to group therapy. *European Eating Disorders Review, 11,* 58–71.

Halvarsson, K., Lunner, K., & Sjoden, P. O. (2000). Assessment of eating behaviours and attitudes to eating, dieting, and body image in preadolescent Swedish girls: A one-year follow-up. *Acta Paediatr, 89,* 996–1000.

Hammer, L. D., Kraemer, H. C., Wilson, D. M., Ritter, P. L., & Dornbusch, S. M. (1991). Standardized percentile curves of body-mass-index for children and adolescents. *American Journal of Diseases of Children, 145,* 259–263.

Heffner, M., & Eifert, G. H. (2004). *The anorexia workbook.* Oakland, CA: New Harbinger Publications.

Johnson, W. G., Grieve, F. G., Adams, C. D., & Sandy, J. (1999). Measuring binge eating in adolescents: Adolescent and parent version of the questionnaire of eating and weight patterns. *International Journal of Eating Disorders, 26,* 301–314.

Johnson, W. G., Kirk, A. A., & Reed, A. E. (2000). Adolescent version of the questionnaire of eating and weight patterns: Reliability and gender differences. *International Journal of Eating Disorders, 29,* 94–96.

Kaltiala-Heino, R., Rimpela, M., Rissanen, A., & Rantanen, P. (2001). Early puberty and early sexual activity are associated with bulimic-type eating pathology in middle adolescence. *Journal of Adolescent Health, 28,* 346–352.

Kaufman, J., Birmaher, B., Brent, D., Rao, U., Flynn, C., Moreci, P., Williamson, D., & Ryan, N. (1997). Schedule for Affective Disorders and Schizophrenia for School-Age Children—Present and Lifetime version (K-SADS-PL): Initial reliability and validity data. *Journal of the American Academy of Child and Adolescent Psychiatry, 36,* 980–988.

Keel, P. K., Heatherton, T. F., Harnden, J. L., & Hornig, C. D. (1997). Mothers, fathers, and daughters: Dieting and disordered eating. *Eating Disorders: The Journal of Treatment & Prevention, 5,* 216–228.

Kendler, K. S., MacLean, C., Neale, B. A., Kessler, R., Heath, A., & Eaves, L. (1991). The genetic epidemiology of bulimia nervosa. *American Journal of Psychiatry, 148,* 1627–1637.

Kent, A., Lacey, J. H., & McCluskey, S. E. (1992). Premenarchal bulimia nervosa. *Journal of Psychosomatic Research, 36,* 205–210.

Le Grange, D., Loeb, K. L., Van Orman, S., & Jellar, C. C. (2004). Bulimia nervosa in adolescents. *Archives of Pediatrics & Adolescent Medicine, 158,* 478–482.

Lee, M. I., & Miltenberger, R. G. (1997). Functional assessment of binge eating. *Behavior Modification, 21,* 159–171.

Maloney, M. J., McGuire, J. B., & Daniels, S. R. (1988). Reliability testing of the children's version of the eating attitudes test. *Journal of the American Academy of Child and Adolescent Psychiatry, 27,* 541–543.

Manley, R. S., Tonkin, R., & Hammond, C. (1988). A method for the assessment of body-image disturbance in patients with eating disorders. *Journal of Adolescent Health Care, 9,* 384–388.

Marchi, M., & Cohen, P. (1990). Early childhood eating behaviors and adolescent eating disorders. *Journal of the American Academy of Child & Adolescent Psychiatry, 29,* 112–117.

McDermott, B. M., Batik, M., Roberts, L., & Gibbon, P. (2002). Parent and child report of family functioning in a clinical child and adolescent eating disorders sample. *Australian and New Zealand Journal of Psychiatry, 36,* 509–514.

Mendelson, B. K., & White, D. R. (1982). Relation between body esteem and self-esteem of obese and normal children. *Perceptual & Motor Skills, 54,* 899–905.

Miotto, P., de Coppi, M., Frezza, M., & Preti, A. (2003). Eating disorders and suicide risk factors in adolescents: An Italian community–based study. *Journal of Nervous and Mental Disorders, 191,* 437–443.

Mizes, J. S. (1995). Eating disorders. In M. Hersen & R. Ammerman (Eds.), *Advanced abnormal child psychology* (pp. 375–391). Hillsdale, NJ: Erlbaum.

Mizes, J. S., & Arbitell, M. R. (1991). Bulimic's perceptions of emotional responding during binge–purge episodes. *Psychological Reports, 69,* 527–532.

Mizes, J. S., & Christiano, B. A. (1995). Assessment of cognitive variables relevant to cognitive behavioral perspectives on anorexia nervosa and bulimia nervosa. *Behavior Research and Therapy, 33,* 95–105.

Mizes, J. S., & Klesges, R. C. (1989). Validity, reliability, and factor structure of the Mizes Anorectic Cognitions Questionnaire. *Addictive Behaviors, 14,* 589–594.

Mizes, J. S., & Sloan, D. M. (1998). An empirical analysis of eating disorder, not otherwise specified: Preliminary support for a distinct subgroup. *International Journal of Eating Disorders, 23,* 233–242.

Mizes, J. S., Christiano, B. A., Madison, J., Post, G., Seime, R., & Varnado, P. (2000). Development of the Mizes Anorectic Cognitions Questionnarie—Revised: Psychometric properties and factor structure in a large sample of eating-disorder patients. *International Journal of Eating Disorders, 28,* 415–421.

Moos, R. H., & Moos, B. S. (1981). *Family Environment Scale manual.* Palo Alto, CA: Consulting Psychologists Press.

Moreno, A., & Thelen, M. H. (1993). Parental factors related to bulimia nervosa. *Addictive Behaviors, 18,* 681–689.

Morgan, C. M., Yanovski, S. Z., Nguyen, T. T., McDuffle, J., Sebring, N. G., Jorge, M. R., Keil, M., & Yanovski, J. A. (2002). Loss of control over eating, adiposity, and psychopathology in overweight children. *International Journal of Eating Disorders, 31,* 430–441.

Pike, K. M., & Rodin, J. (1991). Mothers, daughters, and disordered eating. *Journal of Abnormal Psychology, 100,* 198–204.

Reich, W. (2000). Diagnostic Interview for Children and Adolescents (DICA). *Journal of the American Academy of Child and Adolescent Psychiatry, 39,* 59–66.

Robin, A. L., & Foster, S. L. (1989). *Negotiating parent–adolescent conflict: A behavioral-family systems approach.* New York: Guilford Press.

Robin, A. L., Gilroy, M., & Dennis, A. B. (1998). Treatment of eating disorders in children and adolescents. *Clinical Psychology Review, 18,* 421–446.

Robin, A. L., Koepke, T., & Moye, A. (1990). Multidimensional assessment of parent–adolescent relations. *Psychological Assessment, 2,* 451–459.

Rohde, P., Seeley, J. R., Langhinrichsen-Rohling, J., & Rohling, M. L. (2003). The Life Attitudes Schedule—Short Form: Psychometric properties and correlates of adolescent suicide proneness. *Suicide and Life-Threatening Behavior, 33,* 249–260.

Rosen, J. C., Leitenberg, H., Gross, J., & Willmuth, M. (1985). Standardized test meals in the assessment of bulimia nervosa. *Advances in Behavior Research and Therapy, 7,* 181–197.

Rosen, J. C., Srbenik, D., Saltzberg, E., & Wendt, S. (1991). Development of a body image avoidance questionnaire. *Psychological Assessment, 3,* 32–37.

Ruggiero, L., Williamson, D., Davis, C. J., Schlundt, D. G., & Carey, M. P. (1988). Forbidden Food Survey: Measure of bulimic's anticipated emotional reactions to specific foods. *Addictive Behaviors, 13,* 267–274.

Sansone, R. A., & Sansone, L. A. (2002). Assessment tools for self-harm behavior among those with eating disorders. *Eating Disorders, 10,* 193–203.

Schneider, M. (2003). Bulimia nervosa and binge eating disorder in adolescents. *Adolescent Medicine, 14,* 119–131.

Shaffer, D., & Fisher, P. (2000). NIMH Diagnostic Interview Schedule for Children—Version IV (NIMH DISC-IV): Description. *Journal of the American Academy of Child and Adolescent Psychiatry, 39,* 28–38.

Shisslak, C. M., Renger, R., Sharpe, T., Crago, M., McKnight, K. M., Gray, N., et al. (1999). Development and evaluation of the McKnight Risk Factor Survey for assessing potential risk and protective factors for disordered eating in preadolescent and adolescent girls. *International Journal of Eating Disorders, 25,* 195–214.

Sitarenios, G., & Kovacs, M. (1999). Use of the Children's Depression Inventory. In M. E. Maruish (Ed.), *Use of psychological testing for treatment planning and outcomes assessment* (2nd ed.). Mahwaw, NJ: Erlbaum.

Smolak, L., & Levine, M. P. (1994). Psychometric properties of the Children's Eating Attitudes Test. *International Journal of Eating Disorders, 16,* 275–282.

Smolak, L., Levine, M. P., & Schermer, F. (1999). Parental input and weight concerns among elementary school children. *International Journal of Eating Disorders, 25,* 263–271.

Spitzer, R. L., Devlin, M. J., Walsh, B. T., Hasin, D., et al. (1992). Binge eating disorder: A multisite field trial of the diagnostic criteria. *International Journal of Eating Disorders, 11,* 191–203.

Sullivan, P. F. (2002). Course and outcome of anorexia nervosa and bulimia nervosa. In C. G. Fairburn & K. D. Brownell (Eds.), *Eating disorders and obesity: A comprehensive handbook* (2nd ed.). New York: Guilford Press.

Thelen, M. H., Powell, A. L., Lawrence, C., & Kuhnert, M. E. (1992). Eating and body image concerns among children. *Journal of Clinical Child Psychology, 21,* 41–47.

Truby, H., & Paxton, S. J. (2002). Development of the children's body image scale. *British Journal of Clinical Psychology, 41,* 185–203.

Vandereycken, W., Kog, E., & Vanderlinden, J. (1989). *The family approach to eating disorders: Assessment and treatment of anorexia nervosa and bulimia.* New York: PMA.

Walsh, B. T., & Garner, D. M. (1997). Diagnostic issues. In D. M. Garner & P. E. Garfinkel (Eds.), *Handbook for treatment for eating disorders.* New York: Guilford Press.

Willi, J., Giacometti, G., & Limacher, B. (1990). Update on the epidemiology of anorexia nervosa in a defined region of Switzerland. *American Journal of Psychiatry, 147,* 1514–1517.

Wilson, G. T. (2002). Eating disorders and addictive disorders. In C. G. Fairburn & K. D. Brownell (Eds.), *Eating disorders and obesity: A comprehensive handbook* (2nd ed.). New York: Guilford Press.

World Health Organization. (1992). *ICD-10 classification of mental and behavioral disorders: Clinical descriptions and diagnostic guidelines.* Geneva, Switzerland: Author.

Zotter, D. L., & Crowther, J. H. (1991). The role of cognitions in bulimia nervosa. *Cognitive Therapy and Research, 15,* 413–426.

18

MENTAL RETARDATION

V. MARK DURAND

University of South Florida, St. Petersburg
St. Petersburg, Florida

KRISTIN V. CHRISTODULU

Department of Psychology
State University of New York, Albany

INTRODUCTION

Mental retardation is a disorder characterized by significant limitations in cognitive functioning and adaptive behavior (Luckasson et al., 1992). Individuals with mental retardation experience difficulties with day-to-day activities, to an extent that reflects both the severity of their cognitive deficits and the type and amount of assistance they receive. Manifestations of mental retardation are varied. Some individuals function quite well, even independently, in society. Others with mental retardation have significant cognitive and physical impairments and require considerable assistance to carry on day-to-day activities. Because many cognitive processes are adversely affected, individuals with mental retardation have difficulty learning, the level of challenge depending on the extent of the cognitive disability.

Two primary diagnostic systems have outlined criteria for mental retardation and include the *Diagnostic and Statistical Manual of Mental Disorders*, 4th edition, Text Revision (DSM-IV-TR; American Psychiatric Association, 2000) and *Mental Retardation: Definition, Classification, and Systems of Support*, 10th edition (American Association on Mental Retardation, 2002). Both classification systems highlight below-average intellectual functioning as the core component of mental retardation and indicate that impairment in adaptive functioning (i.e., communication, self-care, social skills, leisure and work, and personal safety) is also required for a diagnosis. Both systems also agree on the onset of mental retardation before age 18.

People with mental retardation differ significantly in their degree of disability. Almost all classification systems have differentiated these individuals in terms of their ability or on the etiology of mental retardation (Hodapp & Dykens, 1994). *DSM-IV-TR* (APA, 2000) uses four degrees of mental retardation to designate severity of impairment. A corresponding IQ range is assigned for each level: *mild mental retardation* (IQ level of 50–55 to approximately 70), *moderate mental retardation* (IQ level of 35–40 to 50–55), *severe mental retardation* (IQ level of 20–25 to 35–40), and *profound mental retardation* (IQ level below 20 or 25). Rather than using the traditional IQ-based levels of impairment, the American Association on Mental Retardation (AAMR; 2002) categorizes people with mental retardation according to the level of support needed. *Intermittent* (support on an "as needed" basis), *limited* (support that is more consistent over time), *extensive* (support characterized by regular [daily] involvement), and *pervasive* (support that is constant and of high intensity).

DSM-IV-TR criteria for mental retardation are in three groups. First, a person must have significantly below-average intellectual functioning, a determination made with one of several IQ tests, with the cutoff score set by *DSM-IV-TR* at approximately 70 or below. Roughly 2% to 3% of the population score at 70 or below on these tests. The AAMR, which has its own, very similar definition of mental retardation, has a cutoff score of approximately 70–75 or below (Popper, Gammon, West, & Bailey, 2003).

The second criterion of both the *DSM-IV-TR* and AAMR definitions for mental retardation calls for concurrent deficits or impairments in adaptive functioning. In other words, scoring "approximately 70 or below" on an IQ test is not sufficient for a diagnosis of mental retardation; a person must also have significant difficulty in at least two of the following areas: communication, self-care, home living, social and interpersonal skills, use of community resources, self-direction, functional academic skills, work, leisure, health, and safety. This aspect of the definition is important because it excludes people who can function quite well in society but for various reasons do poorly on IQ tests. For instance, someone whose primary language is not English may do poorly on an IQ test but still function at a level comparable to his or her peers. This person would not be considered to have mental retardation even if he or she scored below 70 on the IQ test.

The final criterion for mental retardation is age of onset. The characteristic below-average intellectual and adaptive abilities must be evident before the person is 18. This cutoff is designed to identify affected individuals during the developmental period, when the brain is developing and therefore when any problems should become evident. The age criterion rules out the diagnosis of mental retardation for adults who suffer from brain trauma or forms of dementia that impair their abilities. The age of 18 is somewhat arbitrary, but it is the age at which most children leave school, when our society considers a person an adult.

The imprecise definition of mental retardation points up an important issue: Mental retardation, perhaps more than any of the other disorders, is defined by society. The cutoff score of 70 or 75 is based on a statistical concept (two or more standard deviations from the mean) and not on qualities inherent in people who supposedly have mental retardation. There is little disagreement about the diagnosis for people with the most severe disabilities; however, most people diagnosed with mental retardation are in the mild range of cognitive impairment. About 90% of individuals with mental retardation fall within the category of mild mental retardation (IQ of 50–70) (Popper & West, 1999), and when individuals with moderate, severe, and profound mental retardation (IQ below 50) are added they represent 1% to 3% of the general population (Larson et al., 2001). Those individuals at the mild end of the cognitive impairment continuum need some support and assistance, but the criteria for using the label of "mental retardation" are based partly on a somewhat arbitrary cutoff score for IQ that can (and does) change with changing social expectations.

Recent analyses showing that IQ scores increase by a few points every few years illustrate the somewhat arbitrary nature of using a fixed cutoff score. To adapt to this increase in scores, IQ tests are modified periodically to reset the average to 100. For most individuals, these increasingly difficult IQ tests have no practical impact. However, for those hovering at the cutoff point (70–75), this may mean the difference between receiving a diagnosis of mental retardation and not receiving one. In one study, the number of students scoring just below 70 tripled when they were administered a revised test (Kanaya, Scullin, & Ceci, 2003). These results further emphasize the importance of assessing adaptive behavior as a supplement to a diagnosis of mental retardation.

ASSESSMENT STRATEGIES AND RESEARCH BASIS

Conducting a thorough assessment is essential to providing effective services for individuals with mental retardation (Matson, Mayville, & Laud, 2003). Reliable and valid assessment protocols incorporate multiple methods and multiple sources in order to obtain the information needed to make an accurate diagnosis of mental retardation as well as to guide intervention efforts.

Assessing general intellectual functioning is crucial to a diagnosis of mental retardation and is defined by an intelligence quotient (IQ or equivalent) based on assessment with one or more standardized, individually administered intelligence tests. Commonly used intelligence tests include the *Wechsler Preschool and Primary Scale of Intelligence—Revised* (Wechsler, 1989); the *Wechsler Intelligence Scale for Children* (3rd ed.) (WISC-III; Wechsler, 1991); the *Stanford-Bine* (4th ed.) (Stanford–Binet IV; Thorndike, Hagen, & Sattler, 1986); the *Kaufman Assessment Battery for Children* (2nd ed.) (KABC-II; Kaufman and Kaufman, 2003); the *Bayley Scales of Infant Development* (2nd ed.) (Bayley II; Bayley, 1993). A variety of other assessment tools are used to determine general adaptive functioning. We review assessment strategies in three areas essential for identification and intervention: cognitive assessments, overall adaptive behavior assessment, and individual skills assessment.

ASSESSMENT OF COGNITIVE ABILITY

Cognitive assessment for the purpose of determining IQ levels is necessary (but not sufficient) for obtaining a diagnosis of mental retardation. The most widely used standardized tests typically contain verbal scales (which measure vocabulary, knowledge of facts, short-term memory, and verbal reasoning skills) and performance scales (which assess psychomotor abilities, nonverbal reasoning, and ability to learn new relationships) (Tulsky, Zhu, & Prifitera, 2000).

Initially, IQ scores were calculated by using the child's mental age (MA). For example, a child who passed all the questions on the 7-year-old level and none of the questions on the 8-year-old level was said to have a mental age of 7. This mental age was then divided by the child's chronological age (CA) and multiplied by 100 to get the IQ score. However, there were problems with using this type of formula for calculating an IQ score. For example, a 4-year-old needed to score only 1 year below his or her chronological age to be given an IQ score of 75, although an 8-year-old had to score 2 years below his or her chronological age to be given the same score (Bjorklund, 1989). Current tests use a deviation IQ such that a person's score is compared only to scores of others of the same age. The IQ score, then, is really an estimate of how much a child's performance in school will deviate from the average performance of others of the same age.

The revised version of the Stanford–Binet (Stanford–Binet IV) and the Wechsler tests have been the focus of most of the normative research on cognitive ability (Sattler, 2002). The Stanford–Binet IV is appropriate for use on individuals from 2 to 23 years of age. It has 15 subtests (Vocabulary, Comprehension, Pattern Analysis, Quantitative, Bead Memory, and Memory for Sentences, Picture Absurdities, Paper Folding and Cutting, Copying, Repeating Digits, Similarities, Form-Board Items, Memory for Objects, Number Series, and Equation Building). The Wechsler tests include versions for adults (Wechsler Adult Intelligence Scale—III [WAIS-III], for the age range of 16 years, 0 months, to 74 years, 11 months), children (Wechsler Intelligence Scale for Children (3rd ed.) [WISC-III], for children ranging in age from 6 years through 16 years of age), and for young children (Wechsler Preschool and Primary Scale of Intelligence—Revised [WPPSI-R], for children ranging in age from 3 years to 7 years, 3 months). Unfortunately, neither of these tests is appropriate for assessing cognitive ability in persons at the severe-profound end of cognitive impairment.

A variety of other cognitive assessment tools are used for younger children and for those at the more extreme end of the cognitive continuum. For example, the *Kaufman Assessment Battery for Children* (2nd ed.) (KABC-II; Kaufman and Kaufman, 2003) is an intelligence and achievement test for children ages 2½ to 12½. It consists of 16 subtests, not all of which are used for every age group. Unlike other cognitive assessments, underlying the KABC is a conceptual definition of intelligence as a problem-solving ability rather than knowledge of facts. Test scores may be converted to competitive rankings (percentiles and age or grade equivalents). The KABC is often used to assess learning disabilities and mental retardation.

The *Bayley Scales of Infant Development* (2nd ed.) (Bayley, 1993) assesses the development of infants and very young children. It is designed for children from 2 months to 3½ years and includes three scales (the Mental Scale, the Motor Scale, and the Behavior Rating Scale). The Bayley Scales represent one of the more popular infant assessment tools and can be used to determine the IQ scores of children older than 3½ years who have very significant delays and cannot be evaluated using more age-appropriate cognitive measures. The *Differential Ability Scales* (*DAS*) (Elliott, 1990) comprise a battery of individually administered cognitive and achievement tests subdivided into three age brackets: lower preschool (2½ years to 3 years, 5 months), upper preschool (3½ years to 5 years, 11 months), and school age (6 years to 17 years, 11 months). The DAS is very well standardized and correlates highly with other cognitive measures (i.e., the Wechsler Scales) and can be used to assess significantly delayed children who are over the age of 3½ years.

The *Peabody Picture Vocabulary Test—Revised* (*PPVT-R*) (Dunn & Dunn, 1981) is an easily administered and commonly used assessment appropriate for individuals between the ages of 2½ and adulthood. Because it requires only a pointing response and no reading ability, the PPVT-R is appropriate for individuals with a wide range of abilities. Taken alone, the results of the PPVT-R are not interchangeable with IQ scores obtained with more traditional assessments. However, some clinicians combine the results of the PPVT-R with the *Columbia Mental Maturity Scale* (Burgemeister, Blum, & Lorge, 1972)—a test of general reasoning ability that can be used with children who have significant physical limitations. Taken together, the results of these two tests can provide reasonably accurate cognitive status information. Finally, the *Leiter International Performance Scale* (Leiter, 1948) is a nonverbal assessment of intelligence that provides information about the cognitive status of children with hearing impairments or severe language disabilities. It can be used with children ages 2 through adulthood.

When assessing cognitive ability, it is important to ensure that testing procedures are sensitive to the child's ethnic, cultural, or linguistic background. Using tests in which the child's relevant characteristics are represented in the standardization sample of the test or employing an examiner who is familiar with aspects of the child's ethnic or cultural background will help accomplish this.

Providing a standardized administration of cognitive assessments is essential for achieving reliable and valid results from these tests. However, at times, behaviors exhibited by some individuals with mental retardation may interfere with a valid administration. For example, if a student refuses to comply with the assessor's instructions or actively resists participation through aggression, the resulting IQ score may seriously underestimate the student's cognitive abilities. Some researchers are evaluating motivational interventions to be used during cognitive assessments in order to ensure optimal student performance. For example, one group assessed the functions of student problem behaviors and adapted the testing situation to minimize disruption and maximize participation (Koegel, Koegel, & Smith, 1997). An argument can be made that by improving compliance but not changing the task demands, a more accurate estimate of cognitive abilities can be determined.

The criterion for a diagnosis of mental retardation is approximately two standard deviations below the mean (IQ of about 70 or below), taking into consideration the standard error of measurement for the specific assessment instrument used and the instrument's strengths and limitations. Selection of assessment procedures and interpretation of results should take into account factors that may limit test performance (e.g., the child's sociocultural background, native language, and associated communicative, motor, and sensory difficulties). When significant scatter in subtest scores is present, the profile of strengths and weaknesses, instead of the mathematically derived full-scale IQ, will more accurately reflect the child's learning abilities. Averaging to obtain a full-scale IQ can be misleading when there is a marked discrepancy across verbal and performance scores (APA, 2000).

ASSESSMENT OF ADAPTIVE BEHAVIOR

In addition to measuring cognitive development, it is also necessary to administer a measure of adaptive functioning to determine the diagnosis of mental retardation. *Adaptive functioning* refers to how effectively individuals cope with common life demands and how well they meet the standards of personal independence expected of someone in their age group, sociocultural background, and community setting (APA, 2000). Unlike the concept of cognitive ability, adaptive functioning can vary substantially depending on the situation (e.g., home or at school) and the background of the individual. In fact, this is part of the argument raised by the American Association on Mental Retardation (AAMR) to use level of needed support rather than an ability-based definition of mental retardation. A variety of tools can be used to assess adaptive behavior (Sattler, 2002).

The *Vineland Adaptive Behavior Scales* (*VABS*) (Sparrow, Balla, & Cicchetti, 1984)—as with the other adaptive behavior assessments—is an informant-based tool that involves either the completion of a questionnaire or an interview with persons familiar with the subject. Scales of the VABS include Communication, Daily Living Skills, Socialization, Motor Skills, and Maladaptive Behavior. Subdomains within these scales assess a variety of adaptive skills (e.g., receptive and expressive language, domestic task performance, use of free time, gross motor skills). The VABS can be used with persons from birth to adulthood and a Classroom Edition can be used for persons from 3 years to 12 years, 11 months.

The *Battelle Developmental Inventory* (*BDI*) (Newborg, Stock, & Wnek, 1984) assesses developmental skills and is used with only young children (birth to 8 years of age). Skills are measured in five domains (Personal-Social, Adaptive, Motor, Communication, and Cognitive).

The *AAMR Adaptive Behavior Scale—School: 2nd ed.* (*ABS-S:2*) (Nihira, Leland & Lambert, 1993) is an adaptive behavior assessment appropriate for persons from 3 to 21 years of age. The ABS-S:2 includes a total of 16 domains (Independent Functioning, Physical Development, Economic Activity, Language Development, Numbers and Time, Prevocational/Vocational Activity, Self-Direction, Responsibility, Socialization, Social Behavior, Conformity, Trustworthiness, Stereotyped and Hyperactive Behavior, Self-Abusive Behavior, Social Engagement, and Disturbing Interpersonal Behavior). A second version (the *AAMR Adaptive Behavior Scale—Residential and Community: 2nd ed.* (*ABS-RC:2*) (Nihira, Leland, & Lambert, 1993)) extends the age range of this assessment to persons from 18 to 79 years of age. In addition to the domains included in the ABS-S:2 it adds a consideration of Domestic Activity and Sexual Behavior.

The *Scales of Independent Behavior—Revised* (*SIB-R*) (Bruininks, Woodcock, Weatherman, & Hill, 1996) is an adaptive skills assessment covering the full range of skills across the life span (from infancy to 80 years and older). Several forms of the SIB-R are available for varying needs: the Full Scale (includes assessment of Motor Skills, Social Interaction and Communication Skills, Personal Living Skills, and Community Living Skills), the Problem Behavior Scale (Internalized Maladaptive Behavior, Asocial Maladaptive Behavior, Externalized Maladaptive Behavior), the Short Form, and the Early Developmental Scale (infancy through 8 years).

The *Adaptive Behavior Assessment System* (2nd ed.) (*ABAS:2*) (Harrison & Oakland, 2000, 2003) also measures adaptive skills in persons across a broad age range (ages 5 to 89 years). Three forms of this assessment are designed to assess both home and school (the Teacher Form, the Parent Form, and the Adult Form). The ABAS:2 is the only adaptive behavior assessment system designed to directly assess the 10 adaptive skill areas proposed in the AAMR definition of mental retardation (Communication, Community Use, Functional Academics, Home/School Living, Health and Safety, Leisure, Self-Care, Self-Direction, Social, and Work).

It is important to make mention of the *Supports Intensity Scale* (*SIS*), a new scale published by American Association on Mental Retardation (Tassé, Schalock, Thompson, & Wehmeyer, 2005; Thompson et al., 2004). The SIS is not an adaptive behavior assessment device per se but a semi-structured interview the outcome of which is to determine the level of types of supports needed for an individual—in line with the AAMR definition of mental retardation. The SIS is intended to be a support needs assessment and planning approach that includes (a) identifying a person's desired life experiences and goals, (b) determining an individual's intensity of support needs across a wide range of environments and activities, (c) developing an individualized support plan, and (d) monitoring outcomes and assessing the effectiveness of the plan (Tassé et al.,

2005). The SIS is used with a person-centered planning process to assist teams to design individualized support plans that are responsive to the needs and choices of persons with disabilities.

In general, each of the adaptive behavior assessments provides useful information for determining an overall level of functioning. Only the Adaptive Behavior Assessment System (2nd ed.) is specifically designed to assess the 10 adaptive skill areas proposed in the AAMR definition of mental retardation; therefore it can be used more directly in determining a diagnosis of mental retardation. It is important to note that additional instruments, such as measures of academic achievement, are often administered when conducting a comprehensive battery in the assessment of children to formulate a diagnosis of mental retardation.

ASSESSMENT OF EMOTIONAL/BEHAVIOR PROBLEMS

Individuals with mental retardation have a higher prevalence of comorbid disorders and behavior problems than do those in the general population (Borthwick-Duffy, 1994; Matson & Barrett, 1993). Assessment procedures for specific emotional and behavioral problems are generally placed into the following categories: interviews, behavior rating scales, self-report measures, and direct observation procedures (AAMR, 2000; Johnson, 1998; Paclawskyj, Kurtz, & O'Connor, 2004).

Interviews

A history of how difficulties develop helps determine the nature of the presenting problem. To make an accurate diagnosis, it is essential to gather information on the course and context of how symptoms developed. This is especially important for individuals with mental retardation (Silka & Hauser, 1997). However, because many individuals with mental retardation have difficulties with language, relevant information is generally gathered from interviews with family members and/or caregivers. Levitas and Silka (2001) outline two different, but equally valid, approaches to gathering information: a more traditional approach, which begins with the presenting problem and proceeds to a developmental history, and an alternative approach, which starts with gathering a complete developmental history and progresses to the current concern. A clear advantage of conducting interviews is the ability to gather a significant amount of information in a short period of time (Rush, Bowman, Eidman, Toole, & Mortenson, 2004).

Behavior Rating Scales

Administering rating scales to caregivers can be a cost-effective method for obtaining reliable and valid assessment information (Matson, Mayville, & Laud, 2003). Although behavior scales created for typically developing children, such as the *Child Behavior Checklist* (CBCL; Achenbach & Edelbrock, 1991), the *Preschool Behavior Questionnaire* (Behar & Stringfield, 1974), and the *Conners' Rating Scales—Revised* (CRS-R; Conners, 1997), have been used with children and adolescents with mild mental retardation, the measures may be insensitive and inappropriate for assessment of children with more severe levels of mental retardation (Johnson, 1998). The *Developmental Behavior Checklist* (DBC; Einfeld & Tonge, 1989), an adaptation to the CBCL, includes items more specific to children with mental retardation and other developmental disabilities. Two scales developed specifically for use with individuals with mental retardation are the *Behavior Problem Inventory* (Rojahn, 1989) and the *Aberrant Behavior Checklist* (ABC; Aman & Singh, 1986). An additional scale developed for the behavioral assessment of children and adolescents with mental retardation is the *Nisonger Child Behavior Rating Form* (CBRF; Aman, Tassé, Rojahn, & Hammer, 1996). Rating scales typically have better psychometric properties than interviews and can recognize low-frequency behaviors. On the other hand, rating scales rely on recollections, which are subjective in nature and subject to bias (Rush, Bowman, Eidman, Toole, & Mortenson, 2004).

Self-Report Measures

Self-report instruments are commonly used with children and adolescents with mild mental retardation. The *Child Depression Inventory* (Kovacs, 1981), the *Revised Children's Manifest Anxiety Scale* (Reynolds & Richmond, 1978), and the *Self-Report Depression Questionnaire* (Reynolds, 1989) can be used with children and adolescents with mental retardation, especially if there is a concern about a coexisting mood or anxiety disorder. The *Psychopathology Instrument for Mentally Retarded Adults* (PIMRA; Matson, 1988) is the most widely administered and researched instrument for assessing psychopathology in individuals with developmental disabilities. The PIRMA, available in two versions (self-report and informant), can be administered to adolescents with mild (and perhaps moderate) mental retardation.

Direct Observation Procedures

Behavioral observation is an instrumental part of assessment when working with individuals who may not have the ability to verbally report symptoms, such as children and adolescents with mental retardation. Direct observation can occur in either *naturalistic* (e.g., observing the child in his/her classroom) or *analogue* conditions (e.g., observing the child in a setting similar to his/her classroom) (Bielecki & Swender, 2004). Assessment in the natural environment is preferable because results of the observation may generalize better across setting and time (Gettinger & Kratochwill, 1987). Although structured observations yield more objective and reliable data than subjective measures (e.g., interviews and rating scales), conducting interviews is generally more costly and time consuming. In addition, the presence of an observer can cause reactivity with the individual being observed.

Important considerations for direct observation procedures are identifying and operationally defining the target behaviors, determining the duration of the observation session (e.g., frequently occurring behaviors may be assessed in short observations, while infrequently occurring behaviors require longer periods of observation), and selecting the observation schedule (e.g., continuous vs. sampling) (Rush et al., 2004). If there is uncertainty as to when a behavior occurs or under what conditions, other assessments can be useful.

A scatter plot is practical for assessing low-frequency behaviors or behaviors that occur in bursts, and it assists with identifying patterns of responding (Touchette, MacDonald, & Langer, 1985). Scatter plots are also useful for recognizing changes in behavior patterns. Another technique useful when dealing with low-frequency and burst behaviors is an ABC assessment. In this assessment, the events that immediately precede a behavior (A), the target behavior (B), and the events that immediately follow a behavior (C) are recorded. With this method it can be determined if there are particular circumstances in which the behavior is more likely to occur.

Since many problem behaviors are related to behavioral function (e.g., escape from the demands of others, seek attention from others), a comprehensive assessment of maladaptive behavior should include a functional assessment of behavior. Measures of behavioral function, such as the *Questions About Behavioral Function* (QABF; Paclawskyj, Matson, Rush, Smalls, & Vollmer, 2000), the *Motivation Assessment Scale* (MAS; Durand & Crimmins, 1988), and the *Functional Analysis Interview Form* (FAIF; O'Neill, Horner, Albin, Storey, & Sprague, 1990), are useful alternatives to conducting analogue functional analyses. More research is needed, however, for these tools in order to demonstrate and improve their psychometric properties (e.g., reliability, validity).

Assessment of Psychiatric Disorders

Because mental illness is prevalent among individuals with disabilities (MacLean, 1993), screening for coexisting psychiatric disorders is an essential component of a comprehensive assessment (Rush et al., 2004). For individuals with mild or moderate mental retardation, the *Assessment of Dual Diagnosis* (ADD; Matson & Bamburg, 1998) can be used to assess for psychopathology. The *Diagnostic Assessment for the Severely Handicapped—II* (DASH-II; Matson, 1994) is recommended for use with individuals in the severe-and-profound range of impairment. The *Reiss Screen for Maladaptive Behavior* (RASMB; Reiss, 1988) is a rating scale used to identify symptoms of psychopathology in adults and adolescents diagnosed with mental retardation. The *Reiss Scales for Children's Dual Diagnosis* (Reiss & Valenti-Hein, 1994) is a psychopathology rating scale for children with mental retardation. Particular care must be taken when using such assessments, since some behavioral characteristics of persons with mental retardation may mimic symptoms of other psychiatric problems.

Assessment of Social Skills

Social skills deficits (e.g., poor eye contact) and excesses (e.g., holding on to others and not letting go) are common features of mental retardation (Duncan, Matson, Bamburg, Cherry, & Buckley, 1999). Matson, Helsel, Bellack, and

Senatore (1983) revised the *Social Performance Survey Schedule* (SPSS) for use with individuals with mild and moderate mental retardation, and the *Matson Evaluation of Social Skills in Individuals with Severe Retardation* (MESSISR; Matson, 1995) is indicated for persons with severe and profound cognitive impairments. Conducting an accurate assessment of social functioning is important for designing an intervention procedure that will help these individuals better integrate into typical settings.

Assessment of Feeding Problems

Since difficulties associated with feeding behavior are common in children with developmental disabilities (Gravestock, 2000; Kuhn & Matson, 2004), a comprehensive assessment of mealtime behavior and feeding problems should be completed. The *Screening Tool of Feeding Problems* (STFP; Matson & Kuhn, 2001) is a behavior rating scale designed to identify feeding problems (e.g., food-type selectivity, food-texture selectivity, vomiting, rumination, pica, food refusal, and insufficient feeding skills) in individuals with mental retardation. Feeding problems are often confounded by other deficits common in individuals with mental retardation, such as communication difficulties (Poulton & Algozzine, 1980), poor motor skills/abilities (Newell, 1997), physical abnormalities (Pulsifer, 1996), and nutritional imbalances (Lofts, Schroeder, & Maier, 1979; Pace & Toyer, 2000). Dehydration from vomiting, poisoning from pica, and malnutrition due to inadequate food intake (Kern & Marder, 1996; Pueschel, Cullen, Howard, & Cullinane, 1977–78; Rogers, Stratton, Msall, & Andres, 1994) are all severe health problems that can result from persistent difficulty at mealtime.

ASSESSMENT, CONCEPTUALIZATION, AND TREATMENT PLANNING

Mental retardation is a multifaceted diagnosis that requires assessment across a range of domains. Once a diagnosis is determined, however, there is not yet sufficient information to begin treatment planning. Generally, treatment of individuals with mental retardation involves attempting to teach them the skills they need to become more productive and independent. For individuals with mild mental retardation, intervention is similar to that for people with learning disorders. Specific learning deficits are identified and addressed to help the person improve such skills as reading and writing. At the same time, these individuals often need additional support to live in the community. For people with more severe disabilities, the general goals are the same; however, the level of assistance they need is frequently more extensive. The expectation for all people with mental retardation is that they will in some way participate in community life, attend school and later hold a job, and have the opportunity for meaningful social relationships.

Conceptualization of an individual's circumstance, therefore, must involve a view that incorporates skill strengths and deficits as well as a consideration of family/friends, school, and community supports. A treatment–environment fit is particularly important for persons with mental retardation since opinions about a person's ability to be successful may differ dramatically across settings. The following case of Peter illustrates these concerns.

CASE STUDY[1]

IDENTIFICATION AND PRESENTING COMPLAINTS

Peter's mother contacted us because he was disruptive at school and at work. Peter was 17 and attended the local high school. He had Down syndrome and was described as very likable and, at times, mischievous. He enjoyed skiing, bike riding, and many other activities common among teenage boys. In fact, his desire to participate in a variety of more age-appropriate activities was a source of some conflict between him and his mother: He wanted to take the driver's education course at school, which his mother felt would set him up for failure; and he had a girlfriend he wanted to date, a prospect that also caused his mother concern.

Peter received a battery of formal and informal tests over the years. Assessment of his overall cognitive abilities (primarily using the Wechsler tests) placed him in the moderate range of mental retardation (with scores ranging from 40 to 50). Formal assessment of his adaptive functioning using the Vineland Adaptive Behavior Scales showed strengths in Daily Living Skills and Socialization but significant deficits in Communication and Maladaptive Behavior. His overall adaptive functioning was consistent with his cognitive assessments.

PEER AND SCHOOL ISSUES

School administrators were concerned because Peter didn't participate in activities such as physical education. And at the work site that was part of his school program, he was often sullen, sometimes lashing out at the supervisors. They were considering moving him to a program with more supervision and less independence.

Peter's family had moved frequently during his youth, and they experienced striking differences in the way each community responded to him and his mental retardation. In some school districts, he was immediately placed in classes with other children his age and his teachers were provided with additional assistance and consultation. In others, it was just as quickly recommended that he be taught separately. Sometimes the school district had a special classroom in the local school for children with mental retardation. Other districts had programs in other towns, and Peter would have to travel an hour to and from school each day. Every time he was assessed in a new school, the evaluation was similar to earlier ones.

[1] Adapted with permission from Barlow, D. H., & Durand, V. M. (2005). *Abnormal psychology: An integrative approach* (4th ed.). Belmont, CA: Wadsworth/Thomson Learning.

He received scores on his IQ tests and on measures of adaptive behavior that placed him in the moderate range of mental retardation. Each school gave him the same diagnosis: Down syndrome with moderate mental retardation. At each school, the teachers and other professionals were competent and caring individuals who wanted the best for Peter and his mother. Yet some believed that in order to learn skills, Peter needed a separate program with specialized staff. Others felt they could provide a program with specialized staff. Still others felt they could provide a comparable education in a regular classroom and that to have peers without disabilities would be an added benefit.

In high school, Peter had several academic classes in a separate classroom for children with learning problems, but he participated in some classes, such as gym, with students who did not have mental retardation. His current difficulties in gym (not participating) and at work (being oppositional) were jeopardizing his placement in both programs. When I spoke with Peter's mother, she expressed frustration that the work program was beneath him because he was asked to do boring, repetitious work such as folding paper. Peter expressed a similar frustration, saying that he was treated like a baby. He could communicate fairly well when he wanted to, although he sometimes would get confused about what he wanted to say, and it was difficult to understand everything he tried to articulate.

BEHAVIORAL ASSESSMENT RESULTS

We conducted both direct observations and had his teachers complete the Motivation Assessment Scale. Information from these assessments indicated that his disruptive behavior seemed to function as an effort to escape from unpleasant situations—primarily when he was not being challenged. These results indicated that a common paradox had developed. Peter resisted work he thought was too easy. His teachers interpreted his resistance to mean that the work was too hard for him, and they gave him even simpler tasks. He resisted or protested more vigorously, and they responded with even more supervision and structure.

This conceptualization of his challenging behaviors led us to design an intervention plan. Among the more important components of the plan was a negotiation with his teachers to attempt a trial letting him be more independent (rather than increasing structure, which had been their previous reaction to his disruption) and providing him with more challenging work. These changes, in addition to teaching him how to appropriately respond when he was bored (saying things such as "I'm finished. Can I go on to a new job?"), resulted in significant improvements in his behavior at the work site. Following the success of this approach at work, we designed a similar plan for his classroom teachers and observed comparable success there as well.

The functional assessment of his behavior proved invaluable for case conceptualization and treatment planning. This information, along with guidance from his cognitive and adaptive assessments (particularly his need for assistance in communication), allowed us to design a highly successful plan.

SUMMARY

Assessment of persons with mental retardation involves first a determination of the diagnosis and the level of ability. The current cognitive and adaptive behavior assessment instruments have good psychometric properties and are available for persons of any age and ability. Skills assessment, including the functional assessment of behavior, is an essential next step for proper development of treatment plans. Fortunately, assessment of particular skill areas has a growing base of tools that can assist clinicians with the information needed to design effective interventions. More work is still needed, however, to increase the sophistication of behavioral assessments to include a closer consideration of their psychometric properties (reliability, validity, standardization), especially in terms of population-based concerns (i.e., larger-*N* studies).

REFERENCES AND RESOURCES

Achenbach, T. M., & Edelbrock, C. S. (1991). *The Child Behavior Checklist.* Burlington: University of Vermont, Department of Psychiatry.

Aman, M. G., & Singh, N. N. (1986). *Aberrant Behavior Checklist: Manual.* East Aurora, NY: Slosson Educational Publications.

Aman, M. G., Tassé, M. J., Rojahn, J., & Hammer, D. (1996). The Nisonger CBRF: A child behavior rating form for children and adolescents with developmental disabilities. *Research in Developmental Disabilities, 17,* 41–57.

American Association on Mental Retardation. (2000). Guideline 1: Diagnosis and assessment. *American Journal on Mental Retardation, 3,* 165–168.

American Association on Mental Retardation. (2002). *Mental retardation: Definition, classification, and systems of supports* (10th ed.). Washington, DC: Author.

American Psychiatric Association. (2000). *Diagnostic and statistical manual of mental disorders* (4th ed., text revision). Washington, DC: Author.

Bayley, N. (1993). *Bayley Scales of Infant Development* (2nd ed.). San Antonio, TX: Psychological Corporation.

Behar, L., & Stringfield, S. (1974). *Preschool Behavior Questionnaire.* Durham, NC: LINC Press.

Bielecki, J., & Swender, S. L. (2004). The assessment of social functioning in individuals with mental retardation: A review. *Behavior Modification, 28*(5), 694–708.

Bjorklund, D. F. (1989). *Children's thinking: Developmental function and individual differences.* Belmont, CA: Brooks/Cole.

Borthwick-Duffy, S. A. (1994). Epidemiology and prevalence of psychopathology in people with mental retardation. *Journal of Consulting and Clinical Psychology, 62,* 17–27.

Bruininks, R. H., Woodcock, R. W., Weatherman, R. F., & Hill, B. K. (1996). *Scales of Independent Behavior—Revised.* Itasca, IL: Riverside.

Burgemeister, B. B., Blum, L. H., & Lorge, I. (1972). *Colombia Mental Maturity Scale* (3rd ed.). New York: Harcourt Brace.

Conners, C. K. (1997). *Conners' Rating Scales—Revised.* Toronto, Ontario, Canada: Multi-Health Systems.

Duncan, D., Matson, J. L., Bamburg, J. W., Cherry, K. E., & Buckley, T. (1999). The relationship of self-injurious behavior and aggression to social skills in persons with severe and profound learning disability. *Research in Developmental Disabilities, 20,* 441–448.

Dunn, L. M., & Dunn, L. M. (1981). *Peabody picture vocabulary test—revised: Manual for forms L and M*. Circle Pines, MN: American Guidance Service.

Durand, V. M., & Crimmins, D. B. (1988). Identifying variables maintaining self-injurious behavior. *Journal of Autism and Developmental Disabilities, 18,* 99–117.

Einfeld, S., & Tonge, B. J. (1989). *Developmental Behavior Checklist (DBC)*. Sydney, Australia: University of Sydney.

Elliott, C. D. (1990). *Differential ability scales*. San Antonio, TX: Psychological Corporation.

Gettinger, M., & Kratochwill, T. R. (1987). Behavioral assessment. In C. L. Frame & J. L. Matson (Eds.), *Handbook of assessment in childhood psychopathology: Applied issues in differential diagnosis and treatment evaluations* (pp. 131–161). New York: Plenum Press.

Gravestock, S. (2000). Eating disorders in adults with intellectual disability. *Journal of Intellectual Disability Research, 44,* 625–637.

Harrison, P. L., & Oakland, T. (2000). *Adaptive Behavior Assessment System*. San Antonio, TX: Psychological Corporation.

Harrison, P. L., & Oakland, T. (2003). *Adaptive Behavior Assessment System* (2nd ed.). San Antonio, TX: Psychological Corporation.

Hodapp, R. M., & Dykens, E. M. (1994). Mental retardation's two cultures of behavioral research. *American Journal of Mental Retardation, 98,* 675–687.

Johnson, C. R. (1998). Mental retardation. In V. B. Van Hasselt & M. Hersen (Eds.), *Handbook of psychological treatment protocols for children and adolescents* (pp. 17–46). Mahwah, NJ: Erlbaum.

Kanaya, T., Scullin, M. H., & Ceci, S. J. (2003). The Flynn effect and U.S. policies: The impact of rising IQ scores on American society via mental retardation diagnoses. *American Psychologist, 58,* 778–790.

Kaufman, A. S., & Kaufman, N. L. (2003). *Kaufman Assessment Battery for Children* (2nd ed.). Circle Pines, MN: American Guidance Service.

Kern, L., & Marder, T. J. (1996). A comparison of simultaneous and delayed reinforcement as treatments for food selectivity. *Journal of Applied Behavior Analysis, 29,* 243–246.

Koegel, L. K., Koegel, R. L., & Smith, A. (1997). Variables related to differences in standardized test outcomes for children with ASD. *Journal of Autism and Developmental Disorders, 27,* 233–243.

Kovacs, M. (1981). Rating scales to assess depression in school-age children. *Acta Paedopsychiatry, 46,* 305–315.

Kuhn, D. E., & Matson, J. L. (2004). Assessment of feeding and mealtime behavior problems in persons with mental retardation. *Behavior Modification, 28*(5), 638–648.

Larson, S. A., Lakin, K. C., Anderson, L., Kwak, N., Lee, J. H., & Anderson, D. (2001). Prevalence of mental retardation and developmental disabilities: Estimates from the 1994/1995 National Health Survey Disability Supplements. *American Journal on Mental Retardation, 106,* 231–252.

Leiter, R. G. (1948). *Leiter International Performance Scale*. Chicago: Stoelting.

Levitas, A. S., & Silka, V. R. (2001). Mental health clinical assessment of persons with mental retardation and developmental disabilities: History. *Mental Health Aspects of Developmental Disabilities, 4*(1), 31–42.

Lofts, R. H., Schroeder, S. R., & Maier, R. H. (1979). Effects of serum zinc supplementation on pica behavior of persons with mental retardation. *American Journal on Mental Retardation, 95,* 103–109.

Luckasson, R., Coulter, D. L., Polloway, E. A., Reiss, S., Schalock, R. L., Snell, M. E., Spitalnik, D. M., & Stark, J. A. (1992). *Mental retardation: Definition, classification, and systems of supports* (9th ed.). Washington, DC: American Association on Mental Retardation.

MacLean, W. E. (1993). Overview. In J. L. Matson & R. P. Barrett (Eds.), *Psychopathology in the mentally retarded* (2nd ed., pp. 1–16). Needham Heights, MA: Allyn & Bacon.

Matson, J. L. (1988). *The PIMRA manual*. Orland Park, IL: International Diagnostic Systems.

Matson, J. L. (1994). *The Diagnostic Assessment for the Severely Handicapped—II (DASH-II). User's guide*. Baton Rouge, LA: Scientific Publishers.

Matson, J. L. (1995). *Manual for the Matson Evaluation of Social Skills for Individuals with Severe Retardation*. Baton Rouge, LA: Scientific Publishers.

Matson, J. L., & Bamburg, J. W. (1998). Reliability of the Assessment of Dual Diagnosis (ADD). *Research in Developmental Disabilities, 19,* 89–95.

Matson, J. L., & Barrett, R. P. (1993). *Psychopathology in the mentally retarded* (2nd ed.). Boston: Allyn and Bacon.

Matson, J. L., Helsel, W. J., Bellack, A. S., & Senatore, V. (1983). Development of a rating scale to assess social skills deficits in mentally retarded adults. *Applied Research in Mental Retardation, 4,* 399–407.

Matson, J. L., Mayville, S. B., & Laud, R. B. (2003). A system for adaptive behavior, social skills, behavioral function, medication side effects, and psychiatric disorders. *Research in Developmental Disabilities, 24,* 75–81.

Newborg, J., Stock, J., & Wnek, L. (1984). *Battelle Developmental Inventory Screening Test.* Allen, TX: LINC Associates.

Newell, K. M. (1997). Motor skills and mental retardation. In E. W. MacLean Jr. (Ed.), *Ellis' handbook of mental deficiency, psychological theory and research* (3rd ed.). Mahwah, NJ: Erlbaum.

Nihira, K., Leland, H., & Lambert, N. M. (1993). *Adaptive Behavior Scale—Residential and Community: 2nd ed. (ABS-RC:2).* Austin, TX: Pro-Ed.

O'Neill, R. E., Horner, R. H., Albin, R. W., Storey, K., & Sprague, J. R. (1990). *Functional analysis: A practical assessment guide*. Sycamore, IL: Sycamore.

Pace, G. M., & Toyer, E. A. (2000). The effects of vitamin supplement on the pica of a child with severe mental retardation. *Journal of Applied Behavior Analysis, 33,* 619–622.

Paclawskyj, T. T., Kurtz, P. F., & O'Connor, J. T. (2004). Functional assessment of problem behaviors in adults with mental retardation. *Behavior Modification, 28,* 649–667.

Paclawskyj, T. R., Matson, J. L., Rush, K. S., Smalls, Y., & Vollmer, T. R. (2000). Questions About Behavioral Function (QABF): A behavioral checklist for functional assessment of aberrant behavior. *Research in Developmental Disabilities, 21,* 223–229.

Popper, C. W., Gammon, G. D., West, S. A., & Bailey, C. E. (2003). Disorders usually first diagnosed in infancy, childhood, or adolescence. In R. E. Hales & S. C. Yudofsky (Eds.), *Textbook of clinical psychiatry* (4th ed., pp. 833–974). Washington, DC: American Psychiatric Association Press.

Popper, C. W., & West, S. A. (1999). Disorders usually first diagnosed in infancy, childhood, or adolescence. In R. E. Hales, S. C. Yudofsky, & J. A. Talboot (Eds.), *Textbook of psychiatry* (3rd ed., pp. 825–954). Washington, DC: American Psychiatric Association Press.

Poulton, K. T., & Algozzine, B. (1980). Manual communication and mental retardation: A review of research and implications. *American Journal of Mental Deficiency, 85,* 145–152.

Pueschel, S. M., Cullen, S. M., Howard, R. B., & Cullinane, M. M. (1977–78). Pathogenic considerations of pica in lead poisoning. *International Journal of Psychiatry in Medicine, 8,* 13–24.

Pulsifer, M. B. (1996). The neuropsychology of mental retardation. *Journal of the International Neuropsychological Society, 2,* 159–176.

Reiss, S. (1988). *Test manual for the Reiss Screen for maladaptive behavior*. Orland Park, IL: International Diagnostic Systems.

Reiss, S., & Valenti-Hein, D. (1994). Development of a psychopathology rating scale for children with mental retardation. *Journal of Consulting and Clinical Psychology, 62,* 28–33.

Reynolds, W. M. (1989). *Self-Report Depression Questionnaire (SRDQ).* University of Wisconsin, Madison.

Reynolds, W. M., & Richmond, B. O. (1978). What I think and feel: A revised measure of children's manifest anxiety. *Journal of Abnormal Child Psychology, 6,* 271–280.

Rogers, B. T., Stratton, P., Msall, M., & Andres, M. (1994). Long-term morbidity and management strategies of tracheal aspiration in adults with severe developmental disabilities. *American Journal on Mental Retardation, 98,* 490–498.

Rojahn, J. (1989). *The Behavior Problem Inventory.* Nisonger Center for Mental Retardation and Developmental Disabilities, Ohio State University.

Rush, K. S., Bowman, L. G., Eidman, S. L., Toole, L. M., & Mortenson, B. P. (2004). Assessing psychopathology in individuals with developmental disabilities. *Behavior Modification, 28,* 621–637.

Sattler, J. M. (2002). *Assessment of children: Behavioral and clinical applications* (4th ed.). San Diego, CA: Sattler.

Silka, V. R., & Hauser, M. J. (1997). Psychiatric assessment of the person with mental retardation. *Psychiatric Annals, 27*(3), 162–169.

Sparrow, S. S., Balla, D. A., & Cicchetti, D. V. (1984). *Vineland Adaptive Behavior Scales.* Circle Pines, MN: American Guidance Service.

Tassé, M. J., Schalock, R., Thompson, J. R., & Wehmeyer, M. (2005). *Guidelines for interviewing people with disabilities: Supports Intensity Scale.* Washington, DC: American Association on Mental Retardation.

Thompson, J. R., Bryant, B., Campbell, E. M., Craig, E. M., Hughes, C., Rothholz, D. A., et al. (2004). *The Supports Intensity Scale (SIS): Users manual.* Washington, DC: American Association on Mental Retardation.

Thorndike, R. L., Hagen, E. P., & Sattler, J. M. (1986). *Stanford–Binet Intelligence Scale* (4th ed.). San Antonio, TX: Psychological Corporation.

Touchette, P. E., MacDonald, R. F., & Langer, S. N. (1985). A scatterplot for identifying stimulus control of problem behavior. *Journal of Applied Behavior Analysis, 18,* 343–351.

Tulsky, D. S., Zhu, J., & Prifitera, A. (2000). Assessing adult intelligence with the WAIS—III. In G. Goldstein & M. Hersen (Eds.), *Handbook of psychological assessment* (3rd ed., pp. 97–129). Amsterdam: Pergamon Press.

Wechsler, D. (1989). *Wechsler Preschool and Primary Scale of Intelligence—Revised.* San Antonio, TX: Psychological Corporation.

Wechsler, D. (1991). *Wechsler Intelligence Scale for Children* (3rd ed.). San Antonio, TX: Psychological Corporation.

19

CONDUCT DISORDERS

KURT A. FREEMAN
Child Development and Rehabilitation Center
Oregon Health and Science University
Portland, Oregon

JENNIFER M. HOGANSEN
Child Development and Rehabilitation Center
Oregon Health and Science University
Eugene, Oregon

INTRODUCTION

Conduct problems (CP) are the most common treatment referrals for child mental health clinics (Keenan & Wakschlag, 2002), making up 30% to 50% of all referrals (Bassarath, 2001). Further, conduct disorders are the most frequently occurring behavior disorders in children, with a prevalence of clinically significant problems between 2% and 10% in nonclinical samples (see Costello, 1990). CP range from mild misbehavior (e.g., sassing parents) to dangerous externalizing behaviors (e.g., stealing and physical aggression). Research suggests that oppositional and defiant behaviors (e.g., noncompliance, sassiness) may serve as precursors to more serious forms of antisocial behavior (Beiderman et al., 1996; Loeber, Green, Keenan, & Lahey, 1995). Current conceptualizations suggest that CP can be considered within a multidimensional framework consisting of two bipolar continuums (i.e., overt–covert and nondestructive–destructive; Frick et al., 1993). Using such an approach, CP has been categorized into four quadrants: (a) oppositional behavior (e.g., stubborn, angry, touchy), (b) aggression (e.g., bullies, fights, blames others), (c) property violations (e.g., vandalism, fire setting, cruelty to animals), and (d) status violations (e.g., substance use, truancy).

Clinically significant CP often occur as part of a constellation of misbehavior. When sufficient numbers of problems co-occur, they can be categorized within diagnostic systems. Typical diagnoses that incorporate CP include Oppositional Defiant Disorder (ODD), Conduct Disorder (CD), and Disruptive Behavior Disorder, Not Otherwise Specified (American Psychiatric Association [APA], 2000). ODD is characterized by a pervasive tendency to demonstrate negativistic, argumentative, defiant, and hostile behavior, persisting for more than 6 months. CD is diagnosed when persistent and pervasive patterns of misbehavior are present in which the basic rights of others and/or societal norms and rules are violated. Finally, Disruptive Behavior Disorder, Not Otherwise Specified is used to categorize a child's CP that are not captured within the criteria for CD or ODD but that are resulting in clinically significant impairment.

Age and gender differences have been noted in CP. Research shows that children who are more behaviorally impaired at younger ages are more likely to have significant and persistent difficulties than those who develop CP during adolescence (see Bassarath, 2001). As for gender, males are two to four times more likely to be diagnosed with a behavioral disorder than females (Loeber, Burke, Lahey, Winters, & Zera, 2000). Further, differences in forms of CP exist across genders. Specifically, males tend to engage in confrontational misbehaviors (e.g., physical violence, vandalism), whereas females tend to engage in nonconfrontational CP (e.g., lying and running away; Frick, 1998). More frequent covert CP in females than males may account for lower rates of identification (O'Keefe, Carr, & McQuaid, 1998).

CP are often comorbid with a variety of other psychiatric conditions, particularly for girls (McMahon & Wells, 1998). In fact, approximately 46% of youth with CP will develop an additional secondary psychiatric diagnosis (Loeber et al., 2000). Most notably, research consistently shows a high co-occurrence of CP and ADHD (e.g., Waschbusch, 2002), with some suggesting that the essential features of ADHD (i.e., impulsivity or hyperactivity) may facilitate the development of early-onset CP (see McMahon & Wells, 1998). In addition to being comorbid with ADHD, CP have been associated with internalizing disorders such as anxiety and affective disorders (Hinden, Compas, Howell, & Achenbach, 1997), academic underachievement (Hinshaw, 1992), suicidal behavior (Renaud, Brent, Birmaher, Chiappetta, & Bridge, 1999), and substance use disorders during adolescence (Hawkins, Cataldo, & Miller, 1992).

The goal of the current chapter is to integrate information from the research on CP with the application of this information in clinical practice. We review available behavioral assessment strategies for CP, considerations when selecting assessment methods (i.e., clinical utility), developmental factors to consider in behavioral assessment of CP, and the relationship between behavioral assessment data and case conceptualization and treatment. Finally, we provide a case example of the application of behavioral assessment methods to CP.

ASSESSMENT STRATEGIES

When assessing children with concerns of CP, gathering information from multiple sources and across environments is beneficial (McMahon & Wells, 1998), for children often behave differently across settings and caregivers. Further, caregivers often have difficulty accurately reporting specific information relating to situational factors contributing to CP. Thus, a comprehensive understanding of CP (e.g., topography, severity, contributing factors) is more likely when information is gathered using a multimethod, multi-informant approach. Various methods of completing such an assessment are available, which are reviewed herein. Please note that this review is not exhaustive of all available assessment methods, but instead focuses on those that are well researched and/or used frequently in clinical practice and research on CP.

INTERVIEWS

Completion of a thorough clinical interview is ubiquitous when conducting behavioral assessment services for children with CP. Quite often clinicians rely on unstructured interview formats (Barlow & Durand, 2005). Increasingly, semi-structured and structured diagnostic interviews are used in clinical and research settings so as to improve the reliability and validity of diagnostic processes and outcomes (Shaffer, Fisher, & Lucas, 1999). Available semistructured clinical interviews containing sections on CP include the Child Assessment Schedule (CAS; Hodges, Kline, Stern, Cytryn, & McKnew, 1982) and the Schedule for Affective Disorders and Schizophrenia for School-Aged children (K-SADS; Spitzer, Endicott, Loth, McDonald-Scott, & Wasek, 1998). Each provides prompts for gathering information about the presence or absence of diagnostic symptoms and allows clinicians to formulate additional follow-up probes as needed. Currently, there are child (7–12), adolescent, and parent versions of the CAS available. Multiple versions of the K-SADS exist, all having in common that they allow for determination of diagnosis and are administered by a clinician (Angold & Fisher, 1999). Across versions, different rating options are available to document current, lifetime, and/or "worst episode" impressions.

Structured diagnostic interviews that contain sections for CP include the Diagnostic Interview Schedule for Children (DISC-IV; Shaffer, Fisher, Lucas, Dulcan, & Schwab-Stone, 2000) and the Diagnostic Interview for Children and Adolescents (DICA-IV; Reich, Welner, & Herjanic, 1997). These instruments are considered structured because they do not allow for any additional follow-up probes or clinical decision making on behalf of the interviewer. The DISC covers over 30 diagnoses listed in the *DSM-IV*. Separate parent (for ages 6–17) and youth (for ages 9–17) interview versions exist. Multiple administration versions are available, including computerized (i.e., interviewer administered) and voice versions. Multiple versions of the DICA are available, including a computerized version, as well as versions for multiple informants. Self-report versions are available for children ages 6–12 and 13–17 (Angold & Fisher, 1999).

Research Basis of Interviews

Multiple studies have been conducted investigating the reliability and validity of semistructured and structured interviews. Such research is challenging, given that each interview contains multiple sections relevant to specific diagnoses and that psychometric properties of specific sections may differ. Thus, many studies focus on particular diagnostic categories, including those related to CP. Available research is promising, but certainly limitations exist. For example, CAS scores discriminate between inpatient, outpatient, and normal groups (Hodges et al., 1982), and scores on the CAS and common broadband behavior rating scales are positively correlated (Verhulst, Berden, & Sanders-Woudstra, 1985). Additionally, diagnostic concordance between the CAS and K-SADS-Present was found to be moderate (Hodges, McKnew, Burbach, & Roebuck, 1987). Ambrosini's (2000) recent review of various versions of the K-SADS suggests promising findings on reliability and validity of the measures, although significant gaps in psychometric evaluation were noted for some versions and certain diagnostic categories. The DISC appears to be a reliable measure (e.g., Shaffer et al., 1996; Lewczyk, Garland, Hurlburt, Gearity, & Hough, 2003). Further, external validity of the DISC-IV has been found for behavioral disorders (Friman et al., 2000). Although limited studies of reliability and validity of the DICA have been conducted, those completed are generally favorable (Reich, 2000), particularly for externalizing disorders. Please see Chapter 7 (by Orvaschel) for more details about psychometric evaluations of semistructured and structured interviews used with children and adolescents.

BEHAVIOR RATING SCALES

Behavior rating scales are used to complete a relatively quick, normative-based assessment of child behavior. Multiple scales are available for the assessment of CP in children and adolescents (see Hinshaw & Nigg, 1999; McMahon & Estes, 1997; McMahon & Wells, 1998), including those that assess CP and other emotional and behavioral symptoms (i.e., broadband) and those that are CP specific (i.e., narrowband).

Several broadband instruments are used frequently to assess CP. The Child Behavior Checklist (CBCL; Achenbach, 2001a, 2001b) is perhaps one of the best known and widely used multi-informant, multiversion rating systems for the assessment of children, including those with CP. Currently, versions of the CBCL are available for children ranging from 1.5 to 18 years of age. Further, parent, teacher, and self-report forms, as well as a direct observation system, are available, although the ages for which these different versions are appropriate vary. Common syndrome categories exist across versions (divided into "externalizing," "internalizing," and "other problems" categories), as well as several that are unique to particular forms. Additionally, CBCL versions for children ages 6–18 (including the teacher and self-report versions) allow for an assessment of competence (i.e., social and academic). The CBCL system was updated in 2001 (Achenbach, 2001a, 2001b), resulting in more recent norms, slightly different factor structures, and separate syndrome-specific and *DSM*-specific analyses.

The Conners' Rating Scales (Conners, Sitarenios, Parker, & Epstein, 1998a, 1998b), another broadband tool, include both parent and teacher versions. There are long and short versions of both, which were revised in 1997 (Conners et al., 1998a, 1998b). Research on the revised versions resulted in factors that signify both internalizing (e.g., psychosomatic complaints) and externalizing (e.g., oppositional behavior, hyperactivity) behavioral/emotional problems. Previous reviewers (e.g., Kamphaus & Frick, 1996) cautioned against the use of these scales because of the confusion regarding the multiple versions available, inconsistently demonstrated psychometric properties, and the availability of other instruments (e.g., CBCL). However, revised versions do not necessarily suffer from the same problems (Conners et al., 1998a, 1998b).

Several additional broadband assessment tools are available for use with youth with CP. The Behavior Assessment System for Children (BASC; Reynolds & Kamphaus, 1992) is a questionnaire with parent, teacher, and self-report versions available. Versions exist for children ages 2–18, with consistent subscales across genders, ages of child, and informants (parent and teacher only). The Revised Behavioral Problems Checklist (RBPC; Quay & Peterson, 1983, as cited in Hart & Lahey, 1999) is an 89-item checklist for parents and/or teachers that yields six factors, two relevant to CP (i.e., Conduct Disorder and Socialized Aggression).

Narrowband behavior rating scales exist to assess CP exclusively, including the Eyberg Child Behavior Inventory (ECBI) and its companion, the Sutter–Eyberg Student Behavior Inventory (SESBI; Eyberg, 1992; Eyberg & Pincus, 1999). The ECBI is a 36-item parent report form used to assess the frequency and difficulty of externalizing CP displayed by children ages 2–16. Parents rate each behavior on a 7-point Likert scale while also indicating whether they consider each behavior problematic. Analysis of results allows for a determination of the severity of behavior difficulties as well as hypothesis development regarding parental expectations and attitudes toward their child's behavioral presentation. The SESBI, a teacher-report form, was developed by modifying the ECBI to be applicable to school settings. Specifically, 13 items from the ECBI were removed and replaced with items pertinent to educational settings. As with the ECBI, results allow for an analysis of the intensity of behavioral difficulties as well as teacher attitudes about the child's behavior problems.

Research Basis of Behavior Rating Scales

An extensive amount of research has been conducted on the psychometric properties of the broadband and narrowband measures just discussed, which will only be briefly reviewed here. While there are some differences in findings, the reliability and validity of the CBCL are adequate overall (Achenbach, 2001a,

2001b). Further, although initially developed and normed in the United States, adequate psychometric properties and robust factor structures are obtained with translated versions used in other cultures and nationalities (e.g., Carter, Grigorenko, & Pauls, 1995; Koot, Van Den Oord, Verhulst, & Boomsma, 1997). Regarding the Conners' Rating Scales, research conducted on the revised versions demonstrates good internal reliability coefficients, high test–retest reliability, and effective discriminatory power (Conners et al., 1998a, 1998b). More recently developed, the BASC has demonstrated adequate psychometric properties as well (Reynolds & Kamphaus, 1992). For example, temporal stability and convergent validity have been demonstrated (Merydith, 2001). Further, the BASC discriminates ADHD from non-ADHD children, with better success than the CBCL (Ostrander, Weinfurt, Yarnold, & August, 1998). Good internal consistency, test–retest reliability, and interrater reliability have been found for the ECBI (Eisenstadt, McElreath, Eyberg & McNeil, 1994; Eyberg & Pincus, 1999). The ECBI demonstrates adequate discriminate (Eyberg & Pincus) and concurrent (Boggs, Eyberg, & Reynolds, 1990) validity. Although less well researched, current evidence on the SESBI suggests adequate reliability and discriminate, incremental, predictive, and concurrent validity (Eyberg & Pincus; Querido & Eyberg, 2003). Finally, changes in scores on the ECBI and SESBI are positively correlated (McNeil, Eyberg, Eisenstadt, Newcomb, & Funderburk, 1991).

OBSERVATIONAL ASSESSMENTS

To assess interaction patterns between youth with CP and care providers (e.g., parents, teachers), use of behavioral observation is encouraged (Loney & Lima, 2003). While interviewing care providers, opportunities often naturally arise to observe child misbehavior and careprovider reactions. Further, when appropriate and possible, clinicians may choose to conduct unstructured observations in school and/or home environments. Doing so allows one to learn about the general structure of those settings as well as about interaction patterns with people other than care providers (e.g., peers).

Structured observations may be conducted to ensure opportunity to learn about the influence of particular situations on child behavior and the reactions that parents have to behavior problems. Multiple approaches are available for conducting structured behavioral observations of children with CP in clinic-based assessments (Roberts, 2001). While variations in specific procedures exist, several general approaches are described in the literature.

Parent–Child Interaction Observations

Three common approaches to conducting structured parent–child interaction observations with younger children include the free-play analogue, parent-directed-play analogue, and parent-directed-chore or -cleanup analogue situations (Roberts, 2001). Necessary requirements include several age-appropriate toys, a parent and one or more children, a therapy room, and a coding system. Although beneficial, the ability to observe parent–child interactions behind a one-way mirror is not essential.

Free-play analogue observations, the two most common types being the "Child's Game" (e.g., Forehand & McMahon, 1981) and "Child-Directed Interactions" (Hebree-Kigin & McNeil, 1995), involve allowing the parent and child to play together with enjoyable toys while instructing the parent to (a) allow the child to pick what s/he wants to play with and (b) simply follow along with the play. The goal of free-play analogue situations is to assess a parent's ability to allow the child to direct the play (Hebree-Kigin & McNeil), to assess a parent's misguided attention (e.g., ignoring appropriate behavior, responding to misbehavior), and to evaluate the frequency of commands and negative verbalizations made by the parent when instructed to allow the child to lead the play (Roberts, 2001).

Parent-directed-play analogue observations involve instructing the parent to select activities in which to engage and attempt to have the child play along (Hebree-Kigin & McNeil, 1995; Roberts, 2001). The goal is to assess child compliance with parental expectations as well as the parenting strategies used in order to gain compliance. Typical behaviors targeted for assessment include the type (e.g., indirect versus direct) and frequency of parental commands, frequency of child compliance and misbehavior, and frequency/probability of parental attention contingent on compliance or noncompliance.

Finally, cleanup or parent-directed-chore analogues may be conducted. Most commonly, the parent is instructed to have the child clean up the session room by putting toys away without assistance. No other instructions are given regarding how the parents should obtain compliance. Roberts and Powers (1988) developed a variation of this approach called the Compliance Test. This approach eliminates the confound of instructional quality on compliance by standardizing the types and methods of instructions given by parents (Roberts, 2001). With this approach, the parent issues 30 two-step commands, one at a time, with a 5-second pause between instructions. The parent is instructed to remain silent otherwise. In cleanup/parent-directed-chore analogues, parent and child behaviors coded are identical to those assessed during the parent-directed-play analogue. Assessment is limited to child behavior codes in the Compliance Test (Roberts).

Observational Strategies with Older Children and Adolescents

When working with older children and adolescents, conducting certain structured observations described previously may be developmentally inappropriate. However, other approaches may be potentially beneficial. For instance, clinicians may ask parents and adolescents to discuss topics that typically produce arguments, allowing for an evaluation of interaction patterns. Alternatively, parents and adolescents may be asked to solve a problem, resulting in the ability of the clinician to evaluate several important parent (e.g., limit setting, negotiation) and child (e.g., appropriate language, acceptance of limits) behaviors as well as general interaction patterns (e.g., frequent interruptions, raising of one's voice).

One example of a structured system for observing and coding interactions between older children/adolescents and parents is the Interpersonal Process Code (IPC; Rubsy, Estes, & Dishion, 1991). The IPC system can be used to analyze various types of interactions (e.g., problem solving in the clinic between adolescents and family members, family therapy processes in session). Three behavioral dimensions are coded (i.e., *activity*, or global context of interaction; *content*, or type of interaction and whether it is positive, negative, or neutral; and *affect*, or codes that describe the affective quality of the content of the interaction), resulting in a sequential analysis of the focus person's interactions with others.

Research Basis of Observational Assessments

When evaluating research on observational strategies, assessment of both the strategies themselves and how they assist with making clinical decisions and coding methods used to collect data from the observations is important. Research demonstrates that both parent and child behavior can be reliably coded during parent–child interactions (e.g., Niec, 2004; Roberts, 2001). Regarding observational situations, critical review of the literature suggests that some standardized parent–child interaction situations lack adequate theoretical rationale or adequate psychometric properties (Roberts). For example, clinical utility of child-directed free-play situations has not been established, because positive parenting behavior typically does not differentiate comparison groups (Forehand, 1987) and enhancements in parental responsiveness to child play may not relate to reductions in child misbehavior (Eisenstad, Eyberg, McNeil, Newcomb, & Funderburk, 1993). However, others, such as parent-directed-chore situations, demonstrate clinical utility (Roberts), because they predict child behavior in home situations (Roberts & Powers, 1988).

FUNCTIONAL ASSESSMENT

Functional assessment refers to systematically gathering information to identify the setting events, antecedents, and consequences related to the occurrence of particular behaviors (O'Neill et al., 1997). Functional assessment methods include interviews, questionnaires, and observational procedures (i.e., analogue functional analysis).

Interviews

Although completing an unstructured functional assessment interview is feasible and common, specific interview formats are described in the literature. The Functional Assessment Interview (FAI; O'Neill et al., 1997) is used to interview parents/care providers of individuals with CP and developmental disabilities. It covers areas such as general health and living arrangements, ecological variables that may impact aberrant behavior (e.g., medical conditions, sleep patterns, social involvement opportunities), and specific antecedents and consequences that may be functionally related to those behaviors. Further, it assists one in gathering information about functional communication skills. Another example is the Student Guided Functional Assessment Interview (Reed, Thomas, Sprague, & Horner, 1997), which is used to interview children with CP and covers information similar to the FAI.

Questionnaires

Questionnaires useful as indirect methods of functional assessment also exist. Examples of such measures include the Motivation Assessment Scale (MAS; Durand & Crimmins, 1992), a 16-item care-provider report form, and the Questions About Behavioral Functioning (QABF; Matson & Vollmer, 1995), a 25-item measure. On both forms, caregivers choose an answer for each question, which relates to a particular situation in which CP may occur, using a Likert scale format. Responses are categorized into factors (e.g., attention, escape), and raw scores are converted to rank orders. Factors ranked higher are hypothesized to be more important in understanding variables affecting CP.

Analogue Functional Analysis

The goal of conducting an analogue functional analysis is to empirically evaluate which variables (e.g., parental reaction, escape from tasks) reinforce or maintain problematic behavior (Iwata, Dorsey, Slifer, Bauman, & Richman, 1982/1994). The strategy involves exposing the child to several conditions designed to mimic naturally occurring situations (i.e., analogues). For example, one might create a condition during which the child is only able to gain parental reaction by misbehaving, so as to test whether access to attention is the primary motivating variable. Traditionally, the child is exposed to each condition multiple times (e.g., Iwata et al., 1982/1994), although brief versions have been investigated (e.g., Northup et al., 1991). Then rates of behavior across conditions are compared. The condition during which the child exhibited the most frequent CP is said to contain the maintaining variables, and treatment is then designed to address those variables.

Research on Functional Assessment Strategies

Extant literature on the psychometric properties of functional assessment interviews is quite limited. Available information demonstrates adequate interinterviewee agreement between teachers and students (Kinch, Lewis-Palmer, Hagan-Burke, & Sugai, 2001; Reed et al., 1997) and between student and teacher report and direct observation (Lewis-Palmer, Sugai, & Horner, 1999, as cited in Kinch et al., 2001; Nippe, Lewis-Palmer, & Sprague, 1998, as cited in Kinch et al., 2001).

Regarding functional assessment questionnaires, both original (Durand & Crimmins, 1988) and more recent (Shogren & Rojahn, 2003) research suggests that the MAS has adequate psychometric properties. However, other studies have shown poor reliability and poor-to-moderate internal consistency (Conroy, Fox, Bucklin, & Good, 1996; Duker, Sigafoos, Barron, & Coleman, 1998). In addition, some studies have found that factor analyses did not support the four factors of the MAS (Duker et al.). Initial research on the QABF is promising, showing that the instrument has good test–retest and interrater reliability and adequate internal consistency (Paclawskyj, Matson, Rush, Smalls, & Vollmer, 2001), although some research suggests poor interrater reliability (Shogren & Rojhan, 2003). Paclawskyj et al. also showed that the QABF and MAS were highly correlated and that the QABF demonstrated stronger correlation than the MAS to concomitant analogue functional analyses.

Finally, there is a long tradition of using analogue functional analysis with individuals with developmental disabilities and CP (Iwata, Vollmer, & Zarcone, 1990), with research establishing test–retest reliability (Anderson, Freeman, & Scotti, 1999) and predictive validity (e.g., Iwata, Pace, Kalsher, Cowdery, & Cataldo, 1990; Northup et al., 1991). Further, meta-analyses and experimental summaries indicate that preintervention analogue functional analysis leads to effective treatment development (e.g., Iwata et al., 1994; Scotti, Evans, Meyer, & Walker, 1991). However, use of this technology with typically developing children with CP is relatively new, and the applicability to this population is not well understood (Sasso, Conroy, Peck Stichter, & Fox, 2001). Current findings (e.g., Reimers et al., 1993; Foster, Field, & Handwerk, 2004) suggest that such an approach can be useful with this population as well, although its relative benefit beyond other methods of assessment is unknown.

CLINICAL UTILITY

As should be evident, various strategies are available for assessing children with CP and their families. Because all measures have their own strengths and weaknesses, clinicians must decide which measure(s) to use with each client. The decision to choose a particular measure or set of measures is a serious, thoughtful endeavor for most practitioners, and this decision involves consideration of certain pragmatic issues. We concentrate on four specific clinical matters: (1) purpose, (2) time, (3) available resources, and (4) reimbursement. Although presented individually, these matters are interrelated and often need to be considered in sum.

PURPOSE OF THE ASSESSMENT

Decisions regarding the appropriateness of assessment strategies are most often considered in light of the purpose, or goal, of the assessment. While assessments are conducted for many common purposes, Mash and Terdal (1997) broadly conceived of the following four: (1) *diagnosis*, focusing on classifying the presenting problems; (2) *prognosis*, generating predictions regarding future behavior; (3) *treatment design*, to develop and implement effective interventions;

and (4) *evaluation*, assessing treatment efficacy. Multiple goals may be involved in the assessment of one child.

The intent of assessment is often a function of the setting in which the client presents. For instance, a parent may bring a child to an outpatient psychology clinic to procure treatment services. Or school personnel may request a behavioral evaluation for a particular student so that an education plan can be formulated. In another example, the juvenile justice system may insist on a risk assessment for a youth about to be released from a detention center. In each of these cases, the clinician is asked to provide assessment services that meet the needs of the setting in which they are working. In the case of the outpatient clinic, the assessments of choice will often incorporate diagnosis, prognosis, and treatment design. In contrast, at the juvenile detention center, the focus is likely to be evaluation and prognosis.

TIME ALLOTTED FOR THE ASSESSMENT

Ideally, a clinician would administer whatever measures necessary, no matter how much time it takes, to address the purpose, or goal, of the assessment. In reality, however, time allotted for assessment places constraints on the choices available. Therefore, a balance between these two issues must be achieved. Clinic settings, for example, may dictate a 1.5-hour time limit on face-to-face contact with a patient. In this situation, there may not be enough time to conduct a diagnostic interview with parents, complete an observational measure of child with family, and gather collateral information. Rather, an approach that utilizes at least one broadband interview and one behavior rating scale may be best (McMahon & Estes, 1997). In schools, where budgets are often limited and personnel are frequently stretched across many schools and children, clinicians may have even less time to devote to one child. Thus, combining observation with completion of a behavior rating scale (by the teacher) may maximize resources.

RESOURCES AVAILABLE FOR THE ASSESSMENT

In addition to time, other resources are of limited availability to practitioners and must therefore influence one's assessment strategy. For instance, many researchers in the field recommend the use of a *multiagent, multimethod* strategy (e.g., Patterson, Reid, & Dishion, 1992), such that data about a child's behavior problems are gathered from parents, teachers, and objective observers through multiple formats (e.g., interview, direct observation, questionnaires). The reality of clinical practice, however, often prohibits access to the resources necessary to accomplish this ambitious agenda.

Of particular concern, the accessibility of reporting agents influences the selection of assessments. For example, access to a child's primary caregiver(s) is more likely in a clinic setting, making it possible to acquire information from assessment tools such as structured clinical interview and broadband behavior rating scales. A disadvantage of the clinic setting, though, is the difficulty in gathering information about a child's CP in other settings, such as school. To circumvent this obstacle, some clinics send questionnaires to teachers prior to the clinic appointment and/or interview them by telephone. An advantage of a school or residential setting is the accessibility of nonfamilial reporting agents; however, the availability of an informant with historical data about the youth necessary for diagnostic determination may be limited. In this latter case, reliance on other-report instruments and direct observation may be necessary.

Access to particular methods of behavioral assessment must also factor into a clinician's assessment strategy. A good illustration for discussion is direct observation, which is increasingly recommended to aid both diagnosis and treatment of CP (Loney & Lima, 2003). Recall that behavioral observations can vary in structure, from a basic description of child's behavior (e.g., in the clinic or classroom) to a structured format accompanied by a standardized coding system (e.g., dyadic parent–child interactions as prescribed in Parent Child Interaction Therapy; Hebree-Kigin & McNeil, 1995). Whereas clinic-based observations may be easier to accomplish than school- or home-based observations, ideally a clinician would observe a child's behavior (with family) through a one-way mirror; however, access to such a resource is not always available. In such cases, observation requires the presence of the clinician, which should be considered when analyzing results. Further, certain CP symptoms occur with low frequency and are covert (e.g., mugging, truancy, running away), particularly in older children and adolescents (Frick, 1998); thus, they may not arise during observation. Therefore, one should not rely solely on this method of assessment for diagnosis and treatment planning in any situation.

REIMBURSEMENT FOR SERVICES

Last, but certainly not least, the issue of reimbursement for clinical services is an increasing concern for many practitioners. In the current health care environment, practitioners are being asked to provide services for reduced rates within shorter time frames (Austad & Berman, 1991). Variations in coverage for mental health services exist, making the task of securing reimbursement even more difficult. Some health care plans may require clinicians to submit a priori requests and justification for certain services. Other plans may differentiate between clinic- and community-based assessment, not willing to pay for services rendered outside the clinic (e.g., school, home).

DEVELOPMENTAL CONSIDERATIONS

In the past, a distinction has been drawn between behavioral and developmental approaches to child psychopathology (Edelbrock, 1984). Whereas behavioral assessment was considered primarily idiographic, the developmental approach was said to be nomothetic. These approaches, however, are not incompatible; indeed, integration is realized in the *developmental psychopathology* (*DP*) perspective. DP has been defined as a broadly conceptualized approach to understanding human development (Cummings, Davies, & Campbell, 2000), providing a systematic framework to approach the investigation of developmental phenomena. It crosses disciplines (e.g., clinical child psychology, psychiatry, developmental psychology), concerns itself with multiple rather than single outcomes (e.g., normal, at-risk, and abnormal), and conceptualizes psychopathology as a dynamic, as opposed to static, entity.

Inherent in its name, DP combines both developmental psychology (i.e., study of group averages in normal populations) with that of clinical child psychology (i.e., focus on abnormal psychology in individuals; Cummings et al., 2000). Prior to this combination, developmental psychology often ignored the role of individual differences in developmental functioning (Hinde, 1992), and clinical child psychology relatively neglected group-level information about normal, healthy individuals (Sroufe & Rutter, 1984). The simultaneous focus on normal and abnormal functioning over time, then, not only bridges fields of study but, more importantly, aims to articulate the actual processes that underlie human development.

The DP perspective affects behavioral assessment in three primary ways. First, it argues for establishment of normative baselines, where evaluation of behavior occurs within a normative context. Thus, standardized measures like the CBCL, with its behavioral norms, facilitate direct comparison of an individual child's behavior with that of normal and abnormal populations. In this way, one can determine whether a certain child's behavior problems resemble typical (normal) problem behaviors or, rather, warrant clinical significance in their similarity to children diagnosed with CP.

Second, the DP approach highlights the importance of examining age differences in patterns of behavior. Here, the term *development* must truly be accounted for, because symptoms of CP are known to vary with age. Again, the CBCL provides a good illustration of this issue. The 2/3 version of the CBCL, for children ages 2 and 3 (Achenbach, Edelbrock, & Howell, 1987), contains empirically derived CP that differ with that of the version for ages 4–16. Indeed, Owens and Shaw (2003) documented that the two forms only contain 10 identical items for CP. In this example, the same assessment tool contains different forms to account for the fact that younger children are more likely to manifest overt behavior problems (e.g., noncompliance, oppositionality), while older children and adolescents are more likely to engage in covert behavior problems (e.g., lying or cheating, stealing, vandalism). In DP terminology, this is the concept of *homotypic continuity*, or the expression of similar behaviors or attributes in individuals at different periods of development.

Third, the DP perspective influences behavioral assessment by increasing attention to stability and change in behavior over time. The DP approach appreciates the concept of change over time, paying close attention to developmental pathways and trajectories. Thus, a clinician should examine not only present CP, but also issues such as age of onset and stability in symptoms over time. For instance, a distinction has drawn between those with an early versus late onset of first symptoms of CP, with early onset proving to be more suggestive of persistent CP problems over time (Burke, Loeber, & Lahey, 2003). The "early-starter" pathway (Patterson, Capaldi, & Bank, 1991) is characterized by onset of CP in the preschool and early school-age years, followed by continuity throughout childhood and adulthood. Over time, these children seem to progress from relatively less serious CP-like frequent tantrums to more serious behavior, such as physical aggression. Thus, while there is a high degree of continuity across the developmental period in this pathway to CP, the constellation of problem behaviors changes as a function of the child's developmental stage and environment (Moffitt, 1993). The second major pathway of CP, in contrast, is thought to begin later in development (i.e., adolescence). While more children seem to be involved in this late- versus early-starter trajectory, the result is thought to be less serious and to portend better rates of recovery (McMahon & Estes, 1997).

ASSESSMENT, CONCEPTUALIZATION, AND TREATMENT PLANNING

A GENERAL FRAMEWORK

Beyond documenting the presence and severity of clinically significant CP, assessment data are integral to case conceptualization and treatment planning. In this section, we outline a general framework for a dynamic interplay between assessment and treatment of CP described by Barrios (1988), which encompasses four phases. These phases resemble a funnel, beginning with a broad scope and progressively narrowing to a particular focus. The four phases represent attempts to address specific requests for particular types of information (Barrios). In the first phase, *screening*, the need is simply to determine if the child is suitable for treatment services; information gathered from this initial phase yields a broad view of the child's current functioning. In the next phase, *problem identification and analysis*, finer discriminations in the collection of data need to be made. The clinician must identify problematic aspects of the child's functioning, the order in which these areas should be addressed in treatment, and the factors that maintain problematic behavior. Indeed, this is the phase in which the information necessary for case conceptualization is gathered. *Treatment selection* is the third phase, where assessment data provide information on the variables mediating the efficacious treatment of the child's behavior problems. The focus of data collection is to determine the prerequisites of the available treatment alternatives that satisfy the child, the child's environment, and the skills and training of the practitioner. The final phase, *treatment evaluation*, occurs after treatment has been selected and implementation has begun; the concern now is with treatment fidelity and efficacy. Thus, assessment of the integrity of treatment application is completed, and care is taken to identify the changes that have occurred in the child's problem behaviors.

CONCEPTUALIZATION

Now that a general framework for integrating assessment and treatment of CP has been outlined, we expand on the phase of *problem identification and analysis* to provide information on the ways in which assessment data can inform the clinician's conceptualization of the treatment of children with CP. Specifically, we discuss major research findings of children with CP and their families and their implications for case conceptualization. We focus on data related to the assessment of familial factors and child characteristics, with the goal being the identification of potential targets of intervention.

There is a large body of research linking aspects of a child's environment with CP (Frick, 1998); in light of the consistency of these findings, appropriate case conceptualization must address these factors. Parental socialization practices, in particular, have been linked to CP, including ineffective and inconsistent discipline strategies, lack of parental involvement, and poor parental supervision (Frick). Interventions that target these parenting factors have been found to be some of the most successful interventions for CP (Kazdin, 1987). The clinician's conceptualization of the treatment case, then, must determine the role these factors play in the treatment process, and information on such aspects of familial functioning should be collected during the assessment of a child presenting with CP (e.g., observation of parent–child interaction; measurement of parental discipline practices). Additional environmental factors that warrant attention include parental psychopathology (Connell & Goodman, 2002), the child's peer group (Patterson et al., 1992), and the parental marital relationship (Amato & Keith, 1991).

CP has also been linked to certain child characteristics. Factors such as a child's developmental and medical history may be relevant to case conceptualization, especially with respect to medical and neuropsychological factors that have been associated with either the development or the maintenance of CP. For instance, higher rates of CP are found in youth with mental retardation in comparison to control groups (Benson & Aman, 1999). Studies have also linked CP with intellectual and academic underachievement (Hinshaw, 1992) and social information–processing deficits (Dodge, Bates, & Pettit, 1990). These areas can be evaluated briefly during an initial interview with parents or more thoroughly with extended assessment (e.g., intelligence tests). Children with CP may also present with comorbid disorders, in particular depressive disorders and ADHD (Angold, Costello, & Erkanli, 1999), that should be accounted for in case conceptualization. The presence of additional disorders could alter the manifestation and course of CP and, moreover, likely affect treatment.

TREATMENT PLANNING AND EVALUATION

Once case conceptualization of the child presenting for treatment of CP has occurred, it is incumbent upon the clinician to create a treatment plan. Typically, this involves the selection of a particular treatment strategy. Because of the heterogeneity of CP, a plethora of interventions has been developed to treat its various manifestations (see McMahon & Wells, 1998, for review). Case conceptualization, then, greatly influences the selection of a particular treatment. For instance, behavioral assessment may reveal that certain parenting practices maintain or even increase CP for a particular child. Such a result would suggest the need for parent management training, given research findings that link the reduction of CP with changes in maladaptive and negative parent–child interactions (Kazdin, 2003).

In addition to influencing conceptualization, behavioral assessment should continue throughout treatment. Therapists may have parents fill out the same questionnaire periodically (e.g., the ECBI) to monitor change in CP. Between treatment sessions, families may be asked to keep quantitative records of frequency and duration of CP at home, which can then be reviewed in session with the therapist. Direct observations by the clinician can occur in natural settings (e.g., home, school) or the clinic at regular intervals. This latter strategy in particular can be used to determine treatment fidelity (e.g., examine the degree to which the parent utilizes skills appropriately). Thus, a variety of measures can be successfully used throughout the treatment process to evaluate the effectiveness of the selected treatment strategy.

It is also important to use behavioral assessment to evaluate treatment program success at the conclusion of services. The most frequently used evaluation of treatment outcome in the clinical setting is the A-B design (where A stands for baseline and B stands for intervention; Nelson & Hayes, 1981). For example, a reduction on the CBCL subscale for aggressive behavior at treatment termination may document changes in CP since treatment services began. While not as rigorous as other experimental designs, such an approach satisfactorily documents whether change has occurred.

CASE STUDY

IDENTIFICATION

"Ned" was a 6-year, 4-month-old Caucasian male presenting with a history of significant behavior problems. He resided with his biological parents, Mr. and Ms. Q, as well as an older sister and brother.

PRESENTING COMPLAINTS

Ned presented with a variety of difficult CP. Of primary concern were his frequent temper tantrums, which consisted of throwing himself to the floor, hitting others, head butting others, and yelling and screaming. Several tantrums occurred daily and often lasted for extended periods of time (e.g., greater than 20 minutes). In addition, Mr. and Ms. Q raised concerns about Ned's compliance, indicating that they were able to achieve a 50% compliance ratio, but only with significant effort. Noncompliance was both passive (e.g., simply not responding to requests) and active (e.g., defiantly saying "No.").

MEDICAL HISTORY AND DEVELOPMENTAL ISSUES

Ned presented with a significant medical history. He was born at approximately 24 weeks gestational age and weighed 1 pound 8 ounces, experienced postnatal breathing difficulties requiring ventilation, and had a hernia that was repaired postnatally while he was in the hospital. He also experienced a Grade III intraventricular hemorrhage, which resulted in the placement of a shunt to drain fluid from his brain. At approximately 2 years of age, Ned developed seizures, which were managed using valproic acid. He also had had multiple surgeries, including several to repair his shunt, one for circumcision, and one to have tubes placed in his ears.

Formal developmental and intellectual testing through his educational school district and an interdisciplinary clinic had been completed prior to receiving psychological services. Intelligence testing indicated functioning in the mild-to-high-moderate range of mental retardation. Additionally, his adaptive behavior, fine and gross motor skills, and language abilities were significantly delayed.

PEER AND SCHOOL ISSUES

Ned was in a regular education kindergarten classroom, receiving assistance from a one-on-one aide. Parental report indicated that CP were present in that setting as well, although they historically were less intense than at home/with family members. However, reportedly school personnel were concerned that Ned's behavioral problems might interfere with educational and social progress. He was interested in friendships and had several classmates whom he referred to as his friends. However, parental report indicated that Ned's teachers had commented that some children were leery of him due to his temper tantrums.

BEHAVIORAL ASSESSMENT RESULTS

A variety of formal behavioral assessment strategies was used to better understand Ned's behavioral difficulties and the factors contributing to their continued occurrence, including the ECBI, the Parenting Scale (Arnold, O'Leary, Wolff, & Acker, 1993), and functional assessment strategies.

Mr. and Ms. Q completed the ECBI separately. Mr. Q's responses resulted in Intensity and Problem standard scores well above the cutoff, indicating the presence of clinically significant behavior problems. A similar result was obtained on the ECBI based on Ms. Q's responses. Further, ratings on the ECBI were similar across parents, suggesting that they had consistent views of their son's CP. Together, these results confirmed that Ned displayed CP that were significantly greater than most children and that intensive intervention was needed.

To better understand how parenting practices might contribute to Ned's continued difficulties, Mr. and Ms. Q completed the Parenting Scale (Arnold et al., 1993), which is a 30-item parent-report form designed to assess dysfunctional discipline use. Mr. and Ms. Q reported using multiple ineffective parenting strategies, including talking a significant amount as a means of correcting misbehavior, threatening consequences that are not followed through on, not addressing misbehavior immediately when it occurs, having a difficult time ignoring pestering, and issuing multiple reminders or warnings before issuing a consequence.

Specific functional assessment strategies completed included an interview and a brief analogue functional analysis (Northup et al., 1991). The functional assessment interview revealed that behavioral difficulties were significantly worse when Ned was ill, even with a minor illness, and later in the daytime. Further, the presence of people other than family members seemed to increase the likelihood of defiant noncompliance. Finally, it was learned during the course of treatment that Ned's behavioral difficulties fluctuated significantly in relation to metabolic state of seizure medications (i.e., subtherapeutic blood levels) and that behavior improved or worsened when seizure medications were changed.

Antecedents for temper tantrums included being denied access to preferred activities or being asked to complete a nonpreferred task. In response to tantrums, Ms. Q frequently rationalized with Ned about the inappropriateness of his misbehavior. Further, both parents attempted to utilize time out, but often spent a significant amount of time interacting with him to keep him in the time-out area. This information suggested that temper tantrums functioned either to gain attention or to gain access to preferred activities. Noncompliance occurred in response to multiple instructions, particularly those that involved being required to sit and complete a task. Consequences for noncompliance included threats to remove access to a preferred toy/activity and doing the task for him. Such information suggested that noncompliance functioned to escape/avoid tasks.

To confirm hypotheses generated through the functional assessment interview, a brief functional analysis was completed. This involved exposing Ned to four specific analogue conditions (i.e., attention, tangible, demand, free play/control) and comparing rates of behavior across conditions. For all conditions, his mother served as the "therapist" in the room, and she was coached via a bug-in-the-ear device on how to implement specific tasks in each condition. Behavior problems were high in all conditions, with the exception of the free-play/control condition. This suggested that Ned's CP were multiply maintained, such that temper tantrums and noncompliance function to gain attention, escape tasks/demands, and/or gain/sustain involvement in preferred activities.

ETHICAL AND LEGAL ISSUES OR COMPLICATIONS

Any time one conducts a behavioral assessment with a patient with CP, there are a variety of ethical and legal issues to consider (e.g., informed consent, involvement of a minor, parental rights to access information). The behavioral assessment procedures completed with Ned also presented unique ethical considerations. Specifically, analogue functional analysis procedures are designed to evoke CP in children, and thus the potential for distress or harm during such an assessment exists. Consequently, it is incumbent on clinicians completing such assessments to ensure that patients (or their legal guardians) are fully informed of risks and benefits. Further, specifying a plan for terminating assessment sessions if intolerable distress or harm is evident is advised. If parents are involved in the analogue assessment or at the least are observing, then they can be advised they are free to terminate an observation session if they become uncomfortable with their child's behavior or distress. In fact, Ned's mother terminated the escape condition session because Ned's tantrum escalated such that it was no longer possible to keep him safe (i.e., he began banging his head forcefully on the walls and floor).

SUMMARY

Various behavioral assessment methods are available to assist the clinician working with youth with CP and their families. While historically behavioral assessment relied primarily on idiographic methods of assessment, modern behavioral assessment involves a blend of idiographic and nomothetic approaches (Haynes, 1998). Such an approach is consistent with the developmental psychopathology approach to understanding childhood difficulties (Sroufe, 1997), which is increasingly permeating thinking about child psychopathology.

In the current chapter, five main issues were discussed: (a) characteristics, prevalence, and comorbidity of CP, (b) instruments available to assess CP, (c) considerations when selecting assessment methods (e.g., goals of assessment, time allotted for assessment), (d) developmental factors and considerations in behavioral assessment of CP, and (e) case presentation. Methods described to assess this clinical problem, the main focus of the chapter, included both broadband and narrow-band measures involving multiple assessment types (e.g., interviews, rating scales, observations). While information presented is not exhaustive, a review of well-researched, commonly used instruments available was provided.

The process of assessing CP can be interesting and challenging. Given that multi-informant, multimethod assessment is often recommended when dealing with CP (McMahon & Estes, 1997; Patterson et al., 1992), clinicians are encouraged to utilize various strategies to better understand the severity of, and contextual variables influencing, CP. Further, a stepwise approach may be the most efficient and cost-effective strategy (Barrios, 1988; McMahon & Estes). In other words, less costly procedures (e.g., interviews, behavior rating scales) can be used to screen all children referred for CP. Clinicians can then follow up with more costly procedures (e.g., observations) for those children for whom the initial screening suggested a need for further detail. A similar approach is also recommended for assessment of comorbid conditions, family variables, and other contextual influences (McMahon & Estes).

As research continues to provide information about the presentation of CP and the variables impacting their development and maintenance, researchers also continue to focus on psychometrically sound, clinically relevant assessment instruments and practices. For example, some researchers (e.g., Kolko & Kazdin, 1989) have focused on assessment strategies applicable to covert CP, whereas others (e.g., Walker, Severson, & Feil, 1995) have focused on utilization of assessment tools to screen and identify young children at risk for developing CP. Additionally, others have investigated methods and practices of screening for CP in pediatric primary care settings (e.g., Simonian & Tarnowski, 2001; Stancin & Palermo, 1997), attempting to increase identification and appropriate referral for further services. Finally, researchers are increasingly evaluating technology transfer by examining the utility of analogue functional analysis procedures with typically developing children with CP (e.g., Reimers et al., 1993; Foster et al., 2004). These and other research efforts help inform clinicians of best practices in the behavioral assessment of CP.

REFERENCES AND RESOURCES

Achenbach, T. M. (2001a). *Manual for the Achenbach System of Empirically Based Assessment School-Age Forms & Profiles*. Burlington: University of Vermont, Department of Psychiatry.

Achenbach, T. M. (2001b). *Manual for the Achenbach System of Empirically Based Assessment Preschool Forms & Profile*. Burlington: University of Vermont, Department of Psychiatry.

Achenbach, T. M., Edelbrock, C., & Howell, C. T. (1987). Empirically based assessment of the behavioral/emotional problems of 2- and 3-year-old children. *Journal of Abnormal Child Psychology, 15,* 629–650.

Amato, P. R., & Keith, B. (1991). Parental divorce and the well-being of children: A meta-analysis. *Psychological Bulletin, 110,* 26–46.

Ambrosini, P. J. (2000). Historical development and present status of the Schedule for Affective Disorders and Schizophrenia for School-Aged Children (K-SADS). *Journal of the American Academy of Child and Adolescent Psychiatry, 39,* 49–51.

American Psychiatric Association. (2000). *Diagnostic and statistical manual* (4th ed., text revision). Washington, DC: Author.

Anderson, C. M., Freeman, K. A., & Scotti, J. R. (1999). Evaluation of the generalizability (reliability and validity) of analog functional assessment methodology. *Behavior Therapy, 30,* 31–50.

Angold, A., Costello, E. J., & Erkanli, A. (1999). Comorbidity. *Journal of Child Psychology & Psychiatry, 40,* 57–87.

Angold, A., & Fisher, P. W. (1999). Interviewer-based interviews. In D. Shaffer, C. P. Lucas, & J. E. Richters (Eds.), *Diagnostic assessment in child and adolescent psychopathology* (pp. 34–64). New York: Guilford Press.

Arnold, D., O'Leary, S., Wolff, L., & Acker, M. (1993). The Parenting Scale: A measure of dysfunctional parenting in discipline situations. *Psychological Assessment, 5,* 137–144.

Austad, C. S., & Berman, W. H. (1991). Managed health care and the evolution of psychotherapy. In C. S. Austad & W. H. Berman (Eds.), *Psychotherapy in managed health care: The optimal use of time and resources* (pp. 3–18). Washington, DC: American Psychological Association.

Barlow, D., & Durand, V. (2005). *Abnormal Psychology: An integrative approach* (4th ed.). Belmont, CA: Wadsworth.

Barrios, B. A. (1988). On the changing nature of behavioral assessment. In A. S. Bellack & M. Hersen (Eds.), *Behavioral assessment: A practical handbook* (pp. 3–41). New York: Pergamon Press.

Bassarath, L. (2001). Conduct Disorder: A biopsychosocial review. *Canadian Journal of Psychiatry, 46,* 609–616.

Beiderman, J., Faraone, S. V., Milberger, S., Jetton, J. G., Chen, L., Mick, E., et al. (1996). Is childhood Oppositional Defiant Disorder a precursor to adolescent Conduct Disorder? Findings from a four-year follow-up study of children with ADHD. *Journal of the American Academy of Child & Adolescent Psychiatry, 35,* 1192–1204.

Benson, B. A., & Aman, M. G. (1999). Disruptive behavior disorders in children with mental retardation. In H. C. Quay & A. E. Hogan (Eds.), *Handbook of disruptive behavior disorders* (pp. 559–578). New York: Kluwer Academic/Plenum.

Boggs, S. R., Eyberg, S., & Reynolds, L. A. (1990) Concurrent validity of the Eyberg Child Behavior Inventory. *Journal of Clinical Child Psychology, 19,* 75–78.

Burke, J. D., Loeber, R., & Lahey, B. B. (2003). Course and outcomes. In C. A. Essau (Ed.), *Conduct and oppositional defiant disorders: Epidemiology, risk factors, and treatment* (pp. 61–94). Mahwah, NJ: Erlbaum.

Carter, A. S., Grigorenko, E. L., & Pauls, D. L. (1995). A Russian adaptation of the Child Behavior Checklist: Psychometric properties and associations with child and maternal affective symptomotology and family functioning. *Journal of Abnormal Child Psychology, 23,* 661–684.

Connell, A. M., & Goodman, S. H. (2002). The association between psychopathology in fathers versus mothers and children's internalizing and externalizing behavior problems: A meta-analysis. *Psychological Bulletin, 128,* 746–773.

Conners, C. K., Sitarenios, G., Parker, J. D. A., & Epstein, J. N. (1998a). Revision and restandardization of the Conners Parent Rating Scale (CPRS-R): Factor structure, reliability, and criterion validity. *Journal of Abnormal Child Psychology, 26,* 257–268.

Conners, C. K., Sitarenios, G., Parker, J. D. A., & Epstein, J. N. (1998b). Revision and restandardization of the Conners Teacher Rating Scale (CTRS-R): Factor structure, reliability, and criterion validity. *Journal of Abnormal Child Psychology, 26,* 279–291.

Conroy, M., Fox., J., Bucklin, A., & Good, W. (1996). An analysis of the reliability and stability of the Motivation Assessment Scale in assessing the challenging behaviors of persons with developmental disabilities. *Education & Training in Mental Retardation & Developmental Disabilities, 31,* 243–250.

Costello, E. J. (1990). Child psychiatric epidemiology: Implications for clinical research and practice. In B. B. Lahey & A. E. Kazdin (Eds.), *Advances in clinical child psychology* (Vol. 13, pp. 53–90). New York: Plenum Press.

Cummings, E. M., Davies, P. T., & Campbell, S. B. (2000). *Developmental psychopathology and family process: Theory, research, and clinical implications.* New York: Guilford Press.

Dodge, K. A., Bates, J. E., & Pettit, G. S. (1990). Mechanisms in the cycle of violence. *Science, 250,* 1678–1683.

Duker, P., Sigafoos, J., Barron, J., & Coleman, F. (1998). The Motivation Assessment Scale: Reliability and construct validity across three topographies of behavior. *Research in Developmental Disabilities, 19,* 131–141.

Durand, V. M., & Crimmins, D. B. (1988). Identifying the variables maintaining self-injurious behavior. *Journal of Autism & Developmental Disorders, 18,* 99–117.

Durand, V. M., & Crimmins, D. B. (1992). *The Motivation Assessment Scale (MAS) administration guide.* Topeka, KS: Monaco and Associates.

Edelbrock, C. (1984). Developmental considerations. In T. H. Ollendick & M. Hersen (Eds.), *Child behavioral assessment: Principles and procedures* (pp. 20–37). New York: Pergamon Press.

Eisenstadst, T. H., Eyberg, S. M., McNeil, C. B., Newcomb, K., & Funderburk, B. (1993). Parent–Child interaction therapy with behavior problem children: Relative effectiveness of two stages and overall treatment outcome. *Journal of Clinical Child Psychology, 22,* 42–51.

Eisenstadt, T. H., McElreath, L. H., Eyberg, S. M, & McNeil, C. B. (1994). Interparent agreement on the Eyberg Child Behavior Inventory. *Child & Family Behavior Therapy, 16,* 21–27.

Eyberg, S. M. (1992). Parent and teacher behavior inventories for the assessment of conduct problem behaviors in children. In L. VandeCreek, S. Knapp, & T. L. Jackson (Eds.), *Innovations in clinical practice: A sourcebook* (Vol. 11, pp. 261–270). Sarasota, FL: Professional Resources Exchange.

Eyberg, S. M., & Pincus, D. (1999). *Eyberg Child Behavior Inventory & Sutter–Eyberg Student Behavior Inventory: Professional manual.* Lutz, FL: Psychological Assessment Resources.

Forehand, R. (1987). Parental roles in childhood psychopathology. In C. L. Frame & J. L. Matson (Eds.), *Handbook of assessment in childhood psychopathology: Applied issues in differential diagnosis and treatment evaluation. Applied clinical psychology* (pp. 489–507). New York: Plenum Press.

Forehand, R., & McMahon, R. J. (1981). *Helping the noncompliant child: A clinician's guide to parent training.* New York: Guilford Press.

Foster, N., Field, C. E., & Handwerk, M. L. (2004, November). *The effectiveness of time out with escape maintained behaviors of typically developing children.* Presented at the annual convention for the Association for the Advancement of Behavior Therapy, New Orleans, LA.

Frick, P. (1998). Conduct disorders. In T. H. Ollendick & M. Hersen (Eds.), *Handbook of Child Psychopathology* (3rd ed., pp. 213–237). New York: Plenum Press.

Frick, P. J., Van Horn, Y., Lahey, B. B., Christ, M. A. G., Loeber, R., Hart, E. A., et al. (1993). Oppositional Defiant Disorder and Conduct Disorder: A meta-analytic review of factor analyses and cross-validation in a clinical sample. *Clinical Psychology Review, 13,* 319–340.

Friman, P. C., Handwerk, M. L., Smith, G. L., Larzelere, R. E., Lucas, C. P., & Shaffer, D. M. (2000). External validity of conduct and oppositional defiant disorders determined by the NIMH Diagnostic Interview Schedule for Children. *Journal of Abnormal Child Psychology, 28,* 277–286.

Hart, E. L., & Lahey, B. B. (1999). General child behavior rating scales. In D. Shaffer, C. P. Lucas, & J. E. Richters (Eds.), *Diagnostic assessment in child and adolescent psychopathology* (pp. 65–87). New York: Guilford Press.

Hawkins, J. D., Cataldo, R. F., & Miller, J. Y. (1992). Risk and protective factors for alcohol and other drug problems in adolescence and early adulthood: Implications for substance abuse prevention. *Psychological Bulletin, 112,* 64–105.

Haynes, S. N. (1998). On the changing nature of behavioral assessment. In A. S. Bellack & M. Hersen (Eds.), *Behavioral assessment: A practical handbook* (4th ed., pp. 1–21). Boston: Allyn & Bacon.

Hebree-Kigin, T. L., & McNeil, C. B. (1995). *Parent–child interaction therapy.* New York: Plenum Press.

Hinde, R. A. (1992). Developmental psychology in the context of other behavioral sciences. *Developmental Psychology, 28,* 1018–1029.

Hinden, B. R., Compas, B. E., Howell, D. C., & Achenbach, T. M. (1997). Covariation of the anxious-depressed syndrome during adolescence: Separating fact from artifact. *Journal of Consulting & Clinical Psychology, 65,* 6–14.

Hinshaw, S. P. (1992). Externalizing behavior problems and academic underachievement in childhood and adolescence: Causal relationships and underlying mechanisms. *Psychological Bulletin, 111,* 127–155.

Hinshaw, S. P., & Nigg, J. T. (1999). Behavior rating scales in the assessment of disruptive behavior problems in childhood. In D. Shaffer, C. P. Lucas, & J. E. Richters (Eds.), *Diagnostic assessment in child and adolescent psychopathology* (pp. 91–126). New York: Guilford Press.

Hodges, K., Kline, J., Stern, L., Cytryn, L., & McKnew, D. (1982). The development of a child assessment interview for research and clinical use. *Journal of Abnormal Child Psychology, 10,* 173–189.

Hodges, K., McKnew, D., Burbach, D. J., & Roebuck, L. (1987). Diagnostic concordance between the Child Assessment Schedule (CAS) and the Schedule for Affective Disorders and Schizophrenia for School-Aged Children (K-SADS) in an outpatient sample using lay interviewers. *Journal of the American Academy of Child and Adolescent Psychiatry, 26,* 654–661.

Iwata, B. A., Dorsey, M. F., Slifer, K. J., Bauman, K. E., & Richman, G. S. (1994). Toward a functional analysis of self-injury. *Journal of Applied Behavior Analysis, 27,* 197–209. (Reprinted from *Analysis and Intervention in Developmental Disabilities, 2,* 3–20, 1982.)

Iwata, B. A., Pace, G. M., Kalsher, J. J., Cowdery, J. E., & Cataldo, M. F. (1990). Experimental analysis and extinction of self-injurious escape behavior. *Journal of Applied Behavior Analysis, 23,* 11–27.

Iwata, B. A., Vollmer, T. R., & Zarcone, J. R. (1990). The experimental (functional) analysis of behavior disorders: Methodology, applications and limitations. In A. C. Repp & N. N. Singh (Eds.), *Perspectives on the use of nonaversive and aversive interventions for persons with developmental disabilities* (pp. 301–330). Sycamore, IL: Sycamore.

Iwata, B. A., Pace, G. M., Dorsey, M. F., Zarcone, J. R., Vollmer, T. R., Smith, R. G., et al. (1994). The functions of self-injurious behavior: An experimental-epidemiological analysis. *Journal of Applied Behavior Analysis, 27,* 215–240.

Kamphaus, R. W., & Frick, P. J. (1996). *Clinical assessment of child and adolescent personality and behavior.* Needham Heights, MA: Allyn & Bacon.

Kazdin, A. E. (1987). Treatment of antisocial behavior in children: Current status and future directions. *Psychological Bulletin, 102,* 187–203.

Kazdin, A. E. (2003). Problem-solving skills training and parent management training for Conduct Disorder. In A. E. Kazdin & J. R. Weisz (Eds.), *Evidence-based psychotherapies for children and adolescents* (pp. 241–262). New York: Guilford Press.

Keenan, K., & Wakschlag, L. S. (2002). Can a valid diagnosis of disruptive behavior disorder be made in preschool children? *American Journal of Psychiatry, 159,* 351–358.

Kinch, C., Lewis-Palmer, T., Hagan-Burke, S., & Sugai, G. (2001). A comparison of teacher and student functional behavior assessment interview information from low-risk and high-risk classrooms. *Education & Treatment of Children, 24,* 480–494.

Kolko, D. J., & Kazdin, A. E. (1989). Assessment of dimensions of childhood firesetting among patients and nonpatients: The Firesetting Risk Interview. *Journal of Abnormal Child Psychology, 17,* 157–176.

Koot, H. M., Van Den Oord, E. J. C. G., Verhulst, F. C., & Boomsma, D. I. (1997). Behavioral and emotional problems in young preschoolers: Cross-cultural testing of the validity of the Child Behavior Checklist/2–3. *Journal of Abnormal Psychology, 25,* 183–196.

Lewczyk, C. M., Garland, A. F., Hurlburt, M. S., Gearity, J., & Hough, R. L. (2003). Comparing the DISC-IV and clinician diagnoses among youths receiving public mental health services. *Journal of the American Academy of Child and Adolescent Psychiatry, 42,* 349–367.

Loeber, R., Burke, J., Lahey, B., Winters, A., & Zera, M. (2000). Oppositional Defiant Disorder and Conduct Disorder: A review of the past 10 years, Part I. *Journal of the America Academy of Child and Adolescent Psychiatry, 39,* 1468–1484.

Loeber, R., Green, S. M., Keenan, K., & Lahey, B. B. (1995). Which boys will fare worse? Early predictors of the onset of conduct disorder in a six-year longitudinal study. *Journal of the American Academy of Child & Adolescent Psychiatry, 34,* 499–509.

Loney, B. R., & Lima, E. N. (2003). Classification and assessment. In C. A. Essau (Ed.), *Conduct and Oppositional Defiant Disorders: Epidemiology, risk factors, and treatment* (pp. 3–31). Mahwah, NJ: Erlbaum.

Mash, E. J., & Terdal, L. G. (1997). Assessment of child and family disturbance: A behavioral-systems approach. In E. J. Mash & L. G. Terdal (Eds.), *Assessment of childhood disorders* (3rd ed., pp. 3–68). New York: Guilford Press.

Matson, J. L., & Vollmer, T. R. (1995). *User's guide: Questions About Behavioral Function (QABF).* Baton Rouge, LA: Scientific Publishers.

McMahon, R. J., & Estes, A. M. (1997). Conduct problems. In E. J. Mash & L. G. Terdal (Eds.), *Assessment of Childhood Disorders* (3rd ed., pp. 130–193). New York: Guilford Press.

McMahon, R. J., & Wells, K. C. (1998). Conduct problems. In E. J. Mash & R. A. Barkley (Eds.). *Treatment of childhood disorders* (pp. 111–207). New York: Guilford Press.

McNeil, C. B., Eyberg, S., Eisendstat, T. H., Newcomb, K., & Funderburk, B. (1991). Parent–child interaction therapy with behavior problem children: Generalization of treatment effects to the school setting. *Journal of Clinical Child Psychology, 20,* 140–151.

Merydith, S. P. (2001). Temporal stability and convergent validity of the Behavior Assessment System for Children. *Journal of School Psychology, 39,* 253–265.

Moffitt, T. E. (1993). "Adolescence-limited" and "life-course persistent" antisocial behavior: A developmental taxonomy. *Psychological Review, 100,* 674–701.

Nelson, R. O., & Hayes, S. C. (1981). Nature of behavioral assessment. In M. Hersen & A. S. Bellack (Eds.), *Behavioral assessment: A practical handbook* (2nd ed., pp. 3–37). New York: Pergamon Press.

Niec, L. N. (2004, November). Chair. *Assessing parent–child interactions across diagnoses: Validity of the Dyadic Parent–Child Coding System.* Symposium presented at the annual convention for the Association for the Advancement of Behavior Therapy, New Orleans, LA.

Northup, J., Wacker, D., Sasso, G., Steege, M., Cigrand, K., Cook, J., & DeRaad, A. (1991). A brief functional analysis of aggression and alternative behavior in an outpatient clinic setting. *Journal of Applied Behavior Analysis, 24,* 509–522.

O'Keefe, J. J., Carr, A., & McQuaid, P. (1998). Conduct disorder in girls and boys: The identification of distinct psychological profiles. *Irish Journal of Psychology, 19,* 368–385.

O'Neill, R. E., Horner, R. H., Albin, R. W., Sprague, J. R., Storey, K., & Newton, J. S. (1997). *Functional assessment and program development for problem behavior: A practical handbook.* Pacific Grove, CA: Brooks/Cole.

Ostrander, R., Weinfurt, K. P., Yarnold, P. R., & August, G. J. (1998). Diagnosing attention deficit disorders with the Behavioral Assessment System for Children and the Child Behavior Checklist: Test and construct validity analyses using optimal discriminant classification trees. *Journal of Consulting & Clinical Psychology, 66,* 660–672.

Owens, E. B., & Shaw, D. S. (2003). Predicting growth curves of externalizing behavior across the preschool years. *Journal of Abnormal Child Psychology, 31,* 575–590.

Paclawskyj, T., Matson, J., Rush, K., Smalls, Y., & Vollmer, T. (2001). Assessment of the convergent validity of the Questions About Behavioral Function scale with analogue functional analysis and the Motivation Assessment Scale. *Journal of Intellectual Disability Research, 45,* 484–494.

Patterson, G. R., Capaldi, D., & Bank, L. (1991). An early-starter model for predicting delinquency. In D. J. Pepler & K. H. Rubin (Eds.), *The development and treatment of childhood aggression* (pp. 139–168). Hillsdale, NJ: Erlbaum.

Patterson, G. R., Reid, J. B., & Dishon, T. J. (1992). *Antisocial boys.* Eugene, OR: Castalia.

Querido, J., & Eyberg, M. (2003). Psychometric properties of the Sutter–Eyberg Student Behavior Inventory—Revised with preschool children. *Behavior Therapy, 34,* 1–15.

Reed, H., Thomas, E., Sprague, J. R., & Horner, R. H. (1997). The Student Guided Functional Assessment Interview: An analysis of student and teacher agreement. *Journal of Behavioral Education, 7,* 33–49.

Reich, W. (2000). Diagnostic Interview for Children and Adolescents (DICA). *Journal of the American Academy of Child and Adolescent Psychiatry, 39,* 59–71.

Reich, W., Welner, Z., & Herjanic, B. (1997). *Diagnostic Interview for Children and Adolescents—IV (DICA-IV): Software manual for the child/adolescent and parent version.* North Tonawanda, NY: Multi-Health Systems.

Reimers, T. M., Wacker, D. P., Cooper, L. J., Sasso, G. M., Berg, W. K., & Steege, M. W. (1993). Assessing the functional properties of noncompliant behavior in an outpatient setting. *Child and Family Behavior Therapy, 15,* 1–15.

Renaud, J., Brent, D. A., Birmaher, B., Chiappetta, L., & Bridge, J. (1999). Suicide in adolescents with disruptive disorders. *Journal of the American Academy of Child & Adolescent Psychiatry, 38,* 846–851.

Reynolds, C. R., & Kamphaus, R. W. (1992). *Behavioral Assessment System for Children.* Circle Pines, MN: AGS.

Roberts, M. W. (2001). Clinic observations of structured parent–child interactions designed to evaluate externalizing disorders. *Psychological Assessment, 13,* 46–58.

Roberts, M. W., & Powers, S. W. (1988). The Compliance Test. *Behavioral Assessment, 10,* 375–398.

Rubsy, J. C., Estes, A., & Dishion, A. (1991). *The Interpersonal Process Code (IPC).* Unpublished manuscript. Eugene, OR: Oregon Social Learning Center.

Sasso, G. M., Conroy, M. A., Peck Stichter, J., & Fox, J. J. (2001). Slowing down the bandwagon: The misapplication of functional assessment for students with emotional or behavioral disorders. *Behavioral Disorders, 26,* 282–296.

Scotti, J. R., Evans, I. M., Meyer, L. H., & Walker, P. (1991). A meta-analysis of intervention research with problem behavior: Treatment validity and standards of practice. *American Journal of Mental Retardation, 96,* 233–256.

Shaffer, D., Fisher, P. W., & Lucas, C. P. (1999). Respondent-based interviews. In D. Shaffer, C. P. Lucas, & J. E. Richters (Eds.), *Diagnostic assessment in child and adolescent psychopathology* (pp. 3–33). New York: Guilford Press.

Shaffer, D., Fisher, P., Lucas, C., Dulcan, M. K., & Schwab-Stone, M. (2000). NIMH Diagnostic Interview Schedule for Children, Version IV (NIMH DISC-IV): Description, differences from previous versions and reliability of some common diagnoses. *Journal of the American Academy of Child and Adolescent Psychiatry, 39,* 28–38.

Shaffer, D., Fisher, P., Dulcan, M., Davies, M., Piacentini, J., Schwab-Stone, et al. (1996). The NIMH Diagnostic Interview Schedule for Children version 2.3 (DISC-2.3): Description, acceptability, prevalence rates, and performance in the MECA study. *Journal of the American Academy of Child and Adolescent Psychiatry, 35,* 865–886.

Shogren, K., & Rojahn, J. (2003). Convergent reliability and validity of the Questions About Behavioral Function and the Motivation Assessment Scale: A replication study. *Journal of Developmental & Physical Disabilities, 15,* 367–375.

Simonian, S. J., & Tarnowski, K. J. (2001). Utility of the Pediatric Symptom Checklist for behavioral screening of disadvantaged children. *Child Psychiatry & Human Development, 31,* 269–278.

Spitzer, R., Endicott, J., Loth, J., McDonald-Scott, P., & Wasek, P. (1998). *Kiddie Schedule for Affective Disorders and Schizophrenia.* New York: Department of Research Assessment and Training.

Sroufe, A. (1997). Psychopathology as an outcome of development. *Development and Psychopathology, 9,* 251–268.

Sroufe, L. A., & Rutter, M. (1984). The domain of developmental psychopathology. *Child Development, 55,* 17–29.

Stancin, T., & Palermo, T. M. (1997). A review of behavioral screening practices in pediatric settings: Do they pass the test? *Journal of Developmental & Behavioral Pediatrics, 18,* 183–194.

Verhulst, F. C., Berden, G. F., & Sanders-Woudstra, J. A. (1985). Mental health in Dutch children: II. The prevalence of psychiatric disorder and relationship between measures. *Acta Psychiatrica Scandinavica, 72*(Suppl. 324), 45.

Walker, H. M., Severson, H. H., & Feil, E. G. (1995). *The Early Screening Project: A proven child-find process.* Longmont, CO: Sopris West.

Waschbusch, D. A. (2002). A meta-analytic examination of comorbid hyperactive-impulsive-attention problems and conduct problems. *Psychological Bulletin, 128,* 118–150.

20

PERVASIVE DEVELOPMENTAL DISORDERS

LAURA SCHREIBMAN

Psychology Department
University of California, San Diego
La Jolla, California

AUBYN C. STAHMER

Child and Adolescent Services Research Center
Children's Hospital and Health Center of San Diego
San Diego, California

NATACHA AKSHOOMOFF

Department of Psychiatry
School of Medicine
University of California, San Diego
San Diego, California

INTRODUCTION

The Pervasive Developmental Disorders represent a diagnostic category of severe psychopathology in childhood. The *Diagnostic and Statistical Manual of Mental Disorders*, 4th ed. (*DSM-IV*; American Psychiatric Association [APA], 1994), differentiates five disorders under this category, of which Autistic Disorder is the most severe. Other disorders include Asperger's Disorder (often not differentiated from "high-functioning" autism), Pervasive Developmental Disorder, Not Otherwise Specified (PDD-NOS), Rett's Disorder, and Childhood Disintegrative Disorder. This chapter is primarily concerned with assessment issues for Autistic Disorder (autism), PDD-NOS, and, to some extent, Asperger's Disorder.

Though the assessment of autistic symptoms in Rett's Disorder and Childhood Disintegrative Disorder follows the same general guidelines discussed here, these disorders will not be discussed due to their relative rarity and the differences in onset and course from those of the other pervasive developmental disorders.

Autism is a neurodevelopmental disorder characterized by core impairments in social interaction and communication and the presence of repetitive behaviors and restricted interests. In the social domain, these children are characterized by a failure to interact appropriately with peers, social avoidance and detachment, and general nonresponsiveness to the social environment. These children also either fail to develop functional communication or are severely delayed and/or deviant in communicative behavior. Typically they fail to use instrumental gestures such as pointing and waving bye-bye and do not use eye gaze to share experiences ("joint attention"). If vocal language develops it is likely characterized by specific speech anomalies, including echolalia, neologisms, idiosyncratic language, and dysprosody. Repetitive behaviors may include stereotyped body movements (e.g., body rocking, hand or arm flapping) and repetitive vocalizations. Restricted interests are noted when the child lines up objects in a ritualistic manner, speaks about only one narrow subject, or otherwise is inflexible about his behavior or the environment.

As with any disorder, assessment is critical and serves many purposes. Autistic Disorder, Asperger's Disorder, and PDD-NOS are now more commonly seen as a "spectrum" of disorders, which vary in the severity of social/communication difficulties and language outcome (Lord & Bailey, 2002). Diagnostic accuracy has been an important area of investigation for autism researchers for a number of years. Diagnostic precision is critical for research aimed at uncovering the underlying biological causes, but the heterogeneity and overlap of the behavioral phenotype make characterization within the autism spectrum difficult (Akshoomoff et al., 2004; Akshoomoff, Pierce, & Courchesne, 2002; Lord, Leventhal, & Cook, 2001). Proper diagnosis is critical for epidemiological research to accurately report the prevalence of pervasive developmental disorders and also to address issues related to diagnostic distinctions within the autism spectrum. An accurate diagnosis is also crucial for access to appropriate intervention, treatment planning, information regarding the developmental course of the disorder, and caregiver understanding of the disorder as well as providing a common language for researchers. Good assessment is also necessary for the identification, design, and implementation of appropriate, effective treatment strategies.

ASSESSMENT STRATEGIES

Use of the *DSM-IV* criteria to make a diagnosis of a pervasive developmental disorder requires an experienced clinician as well as extensive information about a child's history, developmental level, behavior in a variety of settings, and medical status (Gillberg et al., 1990; Lord, Storoschuk, Rutter, & Pickles, 1993). Impairments in social interaction and communication and a restricted repertoire of interests, behaviors, and activities are the core domains required for diagnosis, but several additional domains can be affected and influence manifestation of symptoms. It is therefore often recommended that an evaluation for a pervasive developmental disorder be conducted by a team of professionals experienced with these disorders and include a formal multidisciplinary evaluation of social behavior, language and nonverbal communication, adaptive behavior, motor skills, atypical behaviors, and cognitive status (Charman & Baird, 2002; Filipek et al., 2000; National Research Council, 2001; Shriver, Allen, & Matthews, 1999). The evaluation team will typically include an experienced clinical psychologist or school psychologist, a speech/language pathologist, and an occupational therapist. Many children with an Autism Spectrum Disorder (ASD) experience difficulties with fine motor coordination, low muscle tone, difficulties with behavior control and aggression, and/or the presence of a seizure disorder, warranting a consultation with an experienced pediatric neurologist or child psychiatrist.

Several detailed guidelines for diagnosis of ASD have been developed. The most comprehensive of these is the Practice Parameter for the Screening and Diagnosis of Autism (Filipek et al., 1999, 2000). These guidelines were developed by a team that included members from nine professional organizations, four parent organizations, and liaisons from the National Institutes of Health. The multidisciplinary team's comprehensive examination of the scientific literature on autism resulted in a multitiered approach to diagnosis that includes developmental surveillance, screening, and varied levels of assessment, depending on specific symptomatology. Recommendations for assessment procedures for a variety of fields, expanded medical tests, and referrals were provided. The California Department of Developmental Services (2002) also developed guidelines for the evaluation process for young children suspected of having an ASD in order to provide appropriate intervention planning.

The five areas of evaluation recommended in these two guidelines will be used here to outline our general discussion of appropriate assessment in autism. An evaluation for an ASD should include (at minimum) a parent/caregiver interview, a medical evaluation, direct behavioral observation, a cognitive assessment, and an assessment of adaptive functioning. No assessment instruments are available that can be used in isolation to make a diagnosis of autism, but the combined use of evidence-based, standardized, objective measures is recommended for providing information relevant to making an appropriate diagnosis. Formal clinical measures (e.g., the Autism Diagnostic Interview—Revised) are often best for determining risk for autism rather than determining which specific pervasive developmental disorder most accurately describes the child (Stone et al., 1999). Clinical judgment by an experienced diagnostician using the *DSM-IV* is necessary for determining the specific diagnosis.

The first step in making a diagnosis is *the parent/caregiver interview*, which should include information about a child's medical and developmental history, a description of past and current functioning, behavioral and social issues, and a family history. This can be conducted using informal interview techniques and/or a structured interview. Several standardized interviews are available for assisting with diagnosing an ASD.

The *Autism Diagnostic Interview—Revised* (ADI-R; Lord, Rutter, & Le Couteur, 1994; Rutter, Le Couteur, & Lord, 2003) is a standardized instrument administered via a semistructured interview with the parent or caregiver, with questions in each of the diagnostic areas of social relatedness, communication, and ritualistic or perseverative behaviors. The respondent is asked about the child's current behavior and, for older individuals, probed for behavior at ages 4–5, when autistic symptoms tend to be most prominent. Assessed individuals can be of any age, as long as their mental abilities are at a developmental level of at least 18–24 months. Diagnostic decisions are based on algorithm items and correspond with both *DSM-IV* and *ICD-10* diagnoses. While the use of this instrument is considered part of the current "gold standard" for diagnosis in the research arena (Filipek et al., 1999), its length (approximately 2 hours) and the level of training needed to reliably conduct the assessment may limit its use in clinical settings.

The *Social Communication Questionnaire* (SCQ; Rutter, Bailey, & Lord, 2003) is a brief instrument that helps evaluate communication skills and social functioning in children who may have autism. This instrument, formerly known as the Autism Screening Questionnaire, has good discriminate validity with respect to the separation of ASD from non-ASD diagnoses at all IQ levels (Berument, Rutter, Lord, Pickles, & Bailey, 1999; Bishop & Norbury, 2002). It can be used with any individual over 4 (with a mental age exceeding 24 months). The form can be given to the parent or caregiver and is available in Spanish as well as English.

The *Gilliam Autism Rating Scale* (GARS; Gilliam, 1995) and the *Gilliam Asperger's Disorder Scale* (GADS; Gilliam, 2001) are questionnaires completed by parents, teachers, or professionals. These instruments were normed on individuals with autism and Asperger's disorder, respectively. The items, based on *DSM-IV* criteria for each disorder, also offer an optional subtest describing development during the first three years of life. These tools are appropriate for individuals ages 3–22 and provide a global rating of the probability that an individual has the disorder. The GARS appears to have limited use for diagnostic purposes and to be better used as a screening device (California Department of Developmental Services, 2002; South et al., 2002).

Other interviews or questionnaires include the *Autism Behavior Checklist* (ABC; Krug, Arick, & Almond, 1980), which is completed by a parent or teacher and includes questions in the areas of sensory, relating, body and object use, language and social/self-help skills. It can be used with children age 3 years and above. The *Pervasive Developmental Disorders Screening Test—Stage 2* (PDDST; Siegel, 2004) is part of a three-stage assessment, which begins with an initial short screening for autistic symptoms. This tool can be used with children as young as 18 months of age and has cutoffs for further consideration of a diagnosis of an ASD.

A *medical evaluation* is recommended in order to rule out other specific conditions that may cause symptoms similar to autism (e.g., fragile X syndrome; fetal alcohol syndrome; tuberous sclerosis; and congenital infections) as well as comorbid medical conditions, such as seizures. Genetic testing may be needed if there is a family history of autism, mental retardation, fragile X syndrome, or tuberous sclerosis (Filipek et al., 1999). Additionally, Rett's Disorder is now identifiable through genetic testing. The American Academy of Pediatrics recommends that assessment of every child with autism include laboratory tests such as audiologic and vision assessments, a lead screening, genetic testing, and a neurological evaluation. Additional testing can be conducted based on symptomatology, for example, allergy testing or gastrointestinal testing.

A direct *behavioral observation* is paramount to an appropriate diagnosis because it provides the opportunity for the clinician to observe the child directly and to obtain information that may not be readily reported by parents or caregivers. Parents may also compensate for behavioral deficits that can be more easily identified when a child interacts with a clinician. The behavioral observation can be an informal play-based assessment or can include more formal, standardized behavior assessment. Behavioral observations of social behaviors, communicative skills, and stereotyped behaviors should be included. Ideally, observation should take place in more than one setting, including observing the child interacting with peers.

Some professionals contend that naturalistic behavioral observations provide the best source of information for a diagnosis for very young children with autism, above and beyond what can be obtained with standardized assessments. Several assessments are not specific to diagnosing autism, such as the *Transdisciplinary Play-Based Assessment* (Linder, 1993) and the *Communication and Symbolic Behavior Scales* (CSBS; Wetherby, 1993), which allow coding of a variety of functioning areas (e.g., play, communication, reciprocity, symbolic behavior, social-emotional development) through structured- and unstructured-play observations. Although these assessments do not provide information regarding a specific diagnosis, they can be used to examine characteristics useful for determining a child's functioning in a variety of areas helpful to determining a diagnosis.

There are also standardized observational scales specific to autism. For example, The *Childhood Autism Rating Scale* (CARS; Schopler, Reichler, & Rochen Renner, 1988) is used by experienced professionals to rate a child's behavior. The CARS consists of 15 four-point scales, based on *DSM-III-R* criteria. It requires direct observation of the child and an interview of the child's caregiver, but it does not provide guidelines on a standardized method of observation. The CARS has fair agreement with the ADI-R (Saemundsen, Magnusson, Smari, & Sigurdardottir, 2003). Some argue that the CARS may be best used as a screening measure (Shriver et al., 1999). The CARS is useful for children over the age of 2 years and is widely used in the clinical diagnosis of autism.

The *Autism Diagnostic Observation Schedule* (ADOS) is a standardized observation of social behavior in naturalistic and communicative contexts. It has four different modules, with corresponding tasks for individuals of different ages and language levels (DiLavore, Lord, & Rutter, 1995; Lord et al., 2000; Lord, Rutter, DiLavore, & Risi, 2001; Lord et al., 1989). Each module includes standardized activities, or "presses," that allow the evaluator to assess communication, social interaction, play, repetitive behaviors, and other autistic features in individuals with autism from 24 months through adulthood. The ADOS yields scores that fall within a range from autism to autism spectrum disorder, and so may be particularly helpful with difficult-to-diagnose cases. The ADOS can be used with children with cognitive skills as young as 18–24 months through adulthood. The assessment takes between 30 and 60 minutes to complete.

The ADI-R (described earlier) and the ADOS are complementary diagnostic instruments originally created for research studies but now available for clinical purposes. Both the ADI-R and the ADOS operationally define current *DSM-IV* and *ICD-10* criteria in the three domains that define autism spectrum disorders: social reciprocity, communication, and restricted, repetitive behaviors and interests. This can be very helpful in increasing parents' understanding of their children's disabilities and in setting goals. Training and practice in observation, administration, and scoring is necessary. Interrater reliability within a clinic or through the use of videotapes (available from the test publisher) is desirable. Individuals using the ADOS and/or the ADI-R in research studies should attend specific research training workshops and obtain reliability with workshop leaders and with researchers from other sites.

Most children with an ASD are mentally retarded. A *cognitive assessment* is essential to understanding a child's behavior in the context of his or her functioning level and is crucial to the differential diagnosis of ASD from other developmental disabilities. Information about functioning level can also provide an understanding of prognosis. Standardized cognitive assessments can be used to determine a child's ability level in a structured setting, but they should be interpreted with caution, particularly before intervention has been attempted. Motivation can affect test results, so it is important to enhance motivation as much as possible without affecting standardized procedures of the assessment (Koegel, Koegel, & Smith, 1997).

Children with ASD tend to perform better on rote, mechanical, or perceptual tasks and more poorly on complex, abstract tasks. While it was assumed that children with autism were more likely to have higher nonverbal than verbal skills (e.g., Lincoln, Courchesne, Kilman, Elmasian, & Allen, 1988), recent studies with larger and more diverse samples suggest that it is more common for cognitive development to be uneven in children with ASD rather than following a "typical profile" (Joseph, Tager-Flusberg, & Lord, 2002; Siegel, Minshew, & Goldstein, 1996). Assessing intelligence levels in younger children with ASD can be particularly challenging (Akshoomoff, submitted). The Mullen Scales of Early Learning (Mullen, 1995) and the Bayley Scales of Infant Development—II

(Bayley, 1993) can provide an estimate of the child's current developmental level. Higher-functioning children can be tested using the Differential Ability Scales (DAS; Elliott, 1990) or the Stanford–Binet IV (Thorndike, Hagen, & Sattler, 1986). The Wechsler Intelligence Scale for Children (WISC-IV; Wechsler, 2003) is typically reserved for higher-functioning ohildren with good verbal skills (Filipek et al., 1999). Neuropsychological, behavioral, and academic assessments should be performed as needed, particularly in conjunction with the child's IEP team.

In addition to information provided about the child's receptive and expressive language skills from a standardized intelligence test, it is important to obtain more in-depth information about the child's language and communication skills using the most appropriate standardized test. Typical instruments include the Peabody Picture Vocabulary Test—III (Dunn & Dunn, 1997), the Reynell Developmental Language Scale (Reynell & Grueber, 1990), the Clinical Evaluation of Language Fundamentals—4th Edition (Semel, Wiig, & Secord, 2003), or the CELF-Preschool (Wiig, Secord, & Semel, 1992). For young children with minimal functional language, the caregiver can be asked to complete the MacArthur Communicative Development Inventory (Fenson et al., 1993).

Finally, assessment of *adaptive functioning* can provide information about how a child is functioning in his or her environment and may be used to augment cognitive assessments. Such information is critical for determining whether an individual has mental retardation and assists in treatment planning. The *Vineland Adaptive Behavior Scales* (Sparrow, Balla, & Cicchetti, 1984) are typically a preferred measure for children with autism (e.g., Volkmar, Klin, Marans, & Cohen, 1996). This is a caregiver interview that provides standard scores and age equivalents for four domains, including communication, social skills, daily living skills, and, for children under age 6, motor skills. Caregivers are asked to describe what their child actually does in each of these areas. The assessment can be used for individuals of any age.

RESEARCH BASIS

Although a biological marker for autism has not yet been identified, autism is one of the most reliably diagnosed behavioral disorders (Bristol-Power & Spinella, 1999). As already discussed, several standardized measures can be used to assist in making an autism diagnosis. However, at all ages, experienced clinical judgment using information from a variety of sources is more reliable for determination of diagnosis than the use of standard assessment instruments alone (Chakrabarti & Fombonne, 2001; Charman & Baird, 2002; Lord, 1995). Currently, the most controversial topic in autism is the accuracy of early diagnosis, especially at very early ages.

In the past few years, progress has been made in the early identification of children with autism, so most children are identified in the preschool period

(Baird et al., 2001; Charman & Baird, 2002; Filipek et al., 2000; Rogers, 2001). Part of this is due to improvements in the recognition of the early features of autism among primary health care providers and other professionals who interact with very young children, the development of appropriate screening tools, and the availability of early intervention services (Baird et al., 2000; Robins, Fein, Barton, & Green, 2001; Siegel, 1999). Research has demonstrated that the use of standardized test instruments by experienced clinicians results in a relatively stable early diagnosis in children as young as 2 (Lord, 1995). Recent research also suggests that identification of the disorder may be made as early as 8–12 months (Mars, Mauk, & Dowrick, 1998; Teitelbaum, Teitelbaum, Nye, Fryman, & Maurer, 1998; Werner, Dawson, Osterling, & Dinno, 2000), although the clinical implications of these findings are not yet clear.

The National Research Council's Committee on Educational Interventions for Children with Autism (NRCA) recommended that early diagnosis be emphasized; however, children under the age of 4 who appear to have an ASD should be given a "provisional diagnosis" (Lord & Risi, 1998; National Research Council, 2001). A proportion of the children identified with possible autism before age 3 may not meet criteria for *DSM-IV* Autistic Disorder at later follow-up but are highly likely to meet criteria for PDD-NOS, a less severe form of autism (Cox et al., 1999; Lord, 1995; Stone et al., 1999). Alternatively, a proportion of children under the age of 3 who do not meet criteria for autism on a standardized parent report measure, such as the ADI-R, may nonetheless receive a clinical diagnosis of Autistic Disorder at a later follow-up. Therefore, a clinical diagnosis of autism is often sensitive and stable over time, and stability increases when an autism spectrum approach is used. It is clear that behavior-based diagnostic distinctions and long-term outcome for children with ASD are more reliable and predictable when diagnostic and functional outcomes are ascertained after age 5 (Coplan, 2000; Lord & Risi, 2000; Venter, Lord, & Schopler, 1992).

Longitudinal research studies of young children also have demonstrated that the use of a standardized observation of social and communicative behavior and play, such as the ADOS, may be more sensitive and stable over time than results from a standardized parent report measure alone. Children under age 4 may not show significant evidence of repetitive and stereotyped behaviors and restricted patterns of interest, as required to meet the cutoff for autism on the ADI-R or according to *DSM-IV* criteria. In one study of 2-year-olds suspected of having autism, use of one of two instruments that rely on the clinician's ratings of the child, the ADOS or CARS, instead of the ADI-R alone, identified children who appeared to meet the social and communication criteria for autism but did not yet show significant evidence of restricted or repetitive behaviors (Lord & Risi, 2000). A follow-up assessment confirmed the diagnosis of autism in the vast majority of these children. It is not known how these research findings translate into everyday clinical practice or clinical practice in the schools, where the mix of developmental problems is wide compared to specialty clinics or research studies targeted toward children with ASD. Additional research is needed to examine the reliability of diagnoses made in community settings outside of research programs.

One major area of difficulty in autism research is the inconsistent use of assessment tools across different intervention programs. When looking at many of the model programs for young children with autism, Handleman and Harris (2001) found that while all of the programs assessed children in the multiple areas discussed earlier, the specific tests used often varied across the programs, thus making comparisons difficult. A majority of programs reported using the Vineland Adaptive Behavior Scales to measure adaptive behavior. A wide variety of communication and cognitive assessments were used and often varied, depending on the age and functioning level of the child. For diagnostic purposes, the CARS was used most often, followed by the ADOS and then the ADI-R (programs using the ADI-R always used the ADOS as well). Many programs used idiosyncratic behavioral measures to examine changes in social, sensory, play, and communicative behavior as well. It is clear from this examination of model programs, which often include a research component, that no battery of specific assessments established for providing a diagnosis or examining program progress is yet preferred. This is very important for future understanding of the effects of different interventions and consistent diagnosis of this population (e.g., Lord et al., in press).

CLINICAL UTILITY

In addition to beginning intervention as soon as possible, it appears that the outcome of children with ASD is dependent, to some degree, on the type of intervention prescribed. Therefore in order for assessment to lead to appropriate clinical treatment, what is required are both careful early diagnosis and accurate determination of which intervention methods are effective for the various needs of children with ASD. The progress of the children needs to be monitored carefully, both across time for an individual child and across children in different intervention programs. This requires comparable assessment protocols (California Departments of Education and Developmental Services, 1997; Martin, Bibby, Midford, & Eikeseth, 2003). An appropriately written, individualized family service plan (ages 0–3 years), individualized education program (ages 3–21 years) or intervention plan (all ages) needs to be based on knowledge of current, relevant research, effective practices, and recognition of the wide range of characteristics that are classified as symptoms of various ASDs (California Departments of Education and Developmental Services). This means that professionals responsible for assessment need to be knowledgeable in the area of autism and that appropriate assessments need to be utilized. As is true for other best-practices guidelines, two "best practices" guidelines from California present a list of instruments for diagnostic and educational assessment (California Department of Developmental Services, 2002; California Departments of Education and

Developmental Services). Limited specific information is provided about reliability, validity, and training requirements for each instrument. It is also important to note that information is limited about the utility of these instruments in educational or community mental health settings (Shriver et al., 1999). This type of "best practices" guide therefore has limited practical value for professionals responsible for assessment in the schools or clinicians who are asked to provide assessment information and recommendations for the child that will be utilized by the school.

CLINICAL UTILITY IN EARLY SCREENING

As already mentioned, we are now seeing children with autism accurately diagnosed as early as 18 months of age (e.g., Lord, 1995; Stone et al., 1999). However, in order to obtain a diagnosis, a child must first be identified as being in need of an evaluation. Because pediatricians and other health care professionals maintain the earliest contact with the children, they are the most likely to detect and refer young children with developmental delays. However, a recent survey of pediatric physicians found that while they agreed that primary care providers should inquire about a child's development, two-thirds did not feel adequately trained to conduct developmental assessments (American Academy of Pediatrics, 2000; Halfon, Regaldo, McLearn, Kuo, & Wright, 2003). A majority of these doctors (70%) identified children without formal screening tools, and 62% did not use any form of parent interview.

The practice parameters developed by Filipek et al. (1999) specify clear criteria for ASD screening, which begins with routine developmental surveillance at all well-child visits. Failure at this stage would lead to audiological assessment and lead screening and a specific screening for autism. Several screening tools are recommended in the practice parameters. The Checklist for Autism in Toddlers (CHAT; Baron-Cohen, Allen, & Gillberg, 1992; Baron-Cohen et al., 1996) was developed for use in the primary care setting at 18–24 months and consists of a short interview with the parents as well as five items to be observed or administered by the provider. It is easy to administer; however, it will fail to identify children who are higher functioning or who have milder symptoms, such as those associated with PDD-NOS. The PDDST—Stage 1 (Siegel, 2004) is the first part of a staged screening assessment designed for use in primary care settings. This assessment has a wider range of questions than the CHAT and rates both positive and negative symptoms of autism. The Modified Checklist for Autism in Toddlers (M-CHAT; Robins et al., 2001) is a 23-item parent questionnaire with no behavioral component. Preliminary findings indicate that the M-CHAT evinces improved sensitivity from the original CHAT without significantly compromising specificity (Robins, 2003); however, further studies with larger samples are currently under way.

The literature indicates that rather than using screening and/or assessment tools, most primary care providers use their clinical judgment when evaluating a child for developmental problems. This may seriously reduce the number of children who are appropriately identified (Glascoe, 2000). Reasons for not screening may include lack of time, limited staffing, and poor reimbursement as well as lack of clinical expertise in the area of autism and developmental delay (American Academy of Pediatrics, 2000). Education of primary care providers in the use of screening tools as well as policy changes that would allow for appropriate reimbursement are essential to early identification and treatment of this disorder.

CLINICAL UTILITY IN EDUCATIONAL SYSTEMS

There can be significant differences between the school and mental health agencies in their practices related to identification, assessment, diagnosis, and treatment of children with ASD. The role of the school psychologist is exponentially expanding as reform movements in education, health care, and developmental services converge on providing services in the schools. Assessments conducted by school psychologists may include testing in the areas of cognition, academic achievement, learning modalities, and socio-behavioral functioning. Tools used are both norm referenced and idiographic in nature (e.g., direct observation, achievement tests, functional assessment, curriculum-based measurement) and focus on educational variables relating to school performance. The purpose of the assessment is to provide reliable and valid information to assist in classification for special education services, placement decisions, and intervention planning (Shriver et al., 1999). The educational classification system used by the schools is derived from the federal guidelines of IDEA, most recently amended in 2002. Based on assessment data, schools can classify students into one of 13 federal handicapping categories. Autism was not recognized as a disability under the IDEA until 1990. Congress found that before the introduction of this category, children with autism were typically classified as "other health impaired" or "multihandicapped." The federal handicapping code for autism states, "A child is classified as having autism when the child has a developmental disability that significantly affects verbal and nonverbal communication and social interaction, that is generally evident before age 3, and that adversely affects educational performance." This definition is fairly broad, in comparison to the specific criteria in the *DSM-IV* (APA, 1994). One may assume that the majority of children would either meet criteria for Autistic Disorder, PDD-NOS, or Asperger's Disorder. However, it is possible that differential diagnoses may not be adequately taken into consideration, leading to misclassification (e.g., inclusion of children with severe-to-profound mental retardation, emotional disturbance, ADHD, or specific learning disability). Other factors may also result in false positives, such as parental desire for the more intensive and specialized services associated with autism programs.

While many schools or school districts may have "resident ASD experts," the majority of educators and professionals have a limited understanding of ASD. Many researchers and clinicians agree that optimal diagnosis of an ASD requires that experienced professionals utilize a clinical best-estimate approach using evidence-based standardized test instruments (Ozonoff, Rogers, & Hendren, 2003). Noland and Gabriels (2004) suggested a model process for ASD diagnosis in schools that included training in screening for ASD as well as the development of a team with increased knowledge and experience with ASD to perform evaluations. Although this is a start, research is needed to determine what the "best practices" approach for school districts should be, given personnel and budgetary limitations.

CLINICAL DIAGNOSIS IN COMMUNITY MENTAL HEALTH PROGRAMS

The *DSM-IV* (APA, 1994) remains the most frequently utilized diagnostic system by mental health professionals for diagnosis of developmental disorders, including autism. However, methods used by even experienced community mental health professionals for assessment of ASD vary a great deal. For example, interviews and observations are typically unstructured, particularly among experienced clinicians, and the format can vary according to theoretical orientation and training. While written reports include information obtained through the use of standardized tests, the context surrounding the test results may not be explicitly stated. It is typically unclear how to determine the accuracy of an assessment conducted with a child suspected to have autism. The autistic symptoms and developmental delays associated with ASD are more commonly identified at age 3 by mental health professionals and developmental service agencies, while fewer children with mild delays are identified before kindergarten.

Differences in assessment methods, experience, and philosophy appear sometimes to lead to different conclusions about the needs of the child and how they should be served among the various professionals who have evaluated the child. Differences in classification/diagnosis guidelines and resources also appear to lead to differences in decisions about eligibility for services. A multidisciplinary approach, where mental health, medical, and school professionals integrate assessment findings and design a comprehensive plan, along with the use of standardized autism assessments, is often a more optimal approach. But practical, economical, and political barriers make this approach difficult to implement.

DEVELOPMENTAL CONSIDERATIONS

The importance of understanding a child's developmental level when making a diagnosis of autism cannot be overestimated. Many of the characteristics of autism include delayed rather than deviant development, and no single characteristic can be used to identify a child with autism. Some behaviors seen in autism, such as echolalia, tantrums, and repetitive play, may be observed in typically developing children as well as children with other disorders, including developmental delay. Therefore, when assessing a child suspected of having autism, the diagnostician must often determine whether the frequency of a certain behavior is unusual or the intensity or quality of a specific behavior is distinct from what a typical child at the same developmental level might exhibit (Campbell, 1990).

In order to obtain an estimate of developmental level in young children with autism, both a standardized cognitive assessment and behavioral observations are necessary. Because many children with autism have behavioral issues, such as difficulty adjusting to new environments and tantrum behavior, they may be uncooperative during standard cognitive assessment. While this in itself may be somewhat diagnostic, obtaining estimates of developmental skills from caregiver interview and observations of naturalistic skills will assist in providing baseline expectations for social and communicative skills.

There is no standard for presence or absence of any specific behavior in the *DSM-IV* criteria for autism, so all of the behaviors must be examined developmentally. For example, impaired peer interaction will be very different for a 5-year-old child functioning at the 4-year-old level and a 5-year-old child functioning at the 18-month level. For the former, we would expect to hear reports of peer interaction involving symbolic play, the ability to perform basic adaptive skills such as potty training and dressing, etc. For the latter child, lack of symbolic play or continence would not be diagnostic of autism, but poor eye contact, sensory sensitivities, and unusual affect might be. That is, the diagnostician must determine whether the child's social skills are delayed even further than the child's cognitive level. In addition, children with intellectual and adaptive abilities in the severe-to-profound level of mental retardation (IQ < 35 or MA < 18 months) are not appropriately assessed by the diagnostic measures for autism. Therefore a primary diagnosis of autism must be made with caution in these individuals.

It is important to note that there are significant developmental changes in autistic symptoms that may be independent of age or IQ level (Fecteau, Mottron, & Burack, 2003). For example, recall that repetitive behaviors may not be evident in very young children with autism (Lord & Risi, 2000) and may decrease at older ages in individuals with higher IQs (Collacott, Cooper, Brandford, & McGrother, 1998; Murphy, Hall, Oliver, & Kissi-Debra, 1999). In a comparison of verbal children with Autistic Disorder using the ADI-R, Fecteau et al. found improvement in all three domains (social, communicative, and restricted and repetitive behaviors) with age for children with a range of IQ levels. They posit that these improvements may be part of the natural progression of autism and that symptoms of autism are dependent on developmental age.

ASSESSMENT, CONCEPTUALIZATION, AND TREATMENT PLANNING

Assessment data need to be in place for determining treatment strategies. The various standardized assessments described earlier are necessary to determine cognitive, language, social, and adaptive functioning and to provide specific information for deciding on treatment targets and thus the curriculum of an intervention. However, other forms of assessments are available and important in the design of treatment interventions.

We know that the only form of treatment empirically validated as effective for children with autism is treatment based on a behavioral model (e.g., National Research Council, 2001). Specifically, we know that the systematic application of the principles of learning (particularly when the child is very young) can lead to substantial gains in many of these children. Highly structured discrete trial training (DTT, sometimes referred to as *applied behavior analysis*) and naturalistic behavioral strategies are most often utilized. Both of these forms of treatment are based on the behavioral model. Additionally, augmentative teaching strategies, such as sign language, communication keyboards, and the Picture Exchange Communication System (PECS; Bondy & Frost, 2001) are frequently employed to assist these youngsters in acquiring communication skills.

We can say that behavioral treatments have been empirically validated as effective in treating these children, since one feature of the behavioral approach is the continuous collection of objective data to determine treatment effects and limitations. Data are frequently collected not only with standardized assessments, but also via behavioral observation of the child in a variety of environments. These data are used to decide if the present course of intervention is effective or whether changes are indicated. Thus, treatment decisions are based on objective evaluation rather than subjective impressions.

A very important type of assessment used in the design of behavioral treatments is *functional assessment*, which involves a systematic evaluation of controlling variables for behavior. It is the understanding of these controlling variables that allows for an informed choice of treatment strategy. For example, Iwata, Dorsey, Slifer, Bauman, and Richman (1982) demonstrated how the challenging behaviors (e.g., self-injurious behavior, or SIB) of developmentally disabled children, while topographically similar, may indeed be under the control of very different environmental events. Thus, one child may engage in self-injury for the purpose of escaping an aversive situation, while another child may engage in self-injury to obtain social attention. Conducting brief analogue assessments of varying environmental events while observing the effects of the events on the target behavior allows the clinician to understand, on an individual basis, the controlling events for the behavior. Knowledge of these events allows for the design of specific treatment strategies that address the events. For one child, effective treatment for SIB would be not to allow the child to escape the aversive situation but rather to try to make the situation less aversive. For the second child, it would be appropriate not to provide social attention contingent on the SIB.

Along these same lines, Carr and colleagues (e.g., Carr and Durand, 1985) demonstrated that a functional analysis of disruptive behaviors allowed one to understand the communicative properties of the behavior, which would allow for training another, more appropriate but functionally similar behavior. For example, if a child engaged in aggression when educational tasks were too difficult, the clinician could teach the child another response that would allow escape from the task. The child might be taught to say, sign, or otherwise communicate, "Help me!" In such cases the child typically uses the more appropriate, but functionally equivalent, response.

While debates often occur over which type of behavioral strategy is overall superior, the fact is that no matter which of these strategies are employed, there is quite a bit of variability in treatment outcome. Thus, some of the children may improve a great deal, while others may improve minimally or not at all. This variability in treatment effect speaks to the action of other variables that are determining outcome. In fact, it is the case that the debate about which treatment is superior is ultimately of little help, since no one treatment is best for all children.

To address this issue, the behavioral treatment community is now focusing more on how to *individualize* treatments. Important child variables have been studied to determine a priori which treatments may in fact be most effective for a specific child. Sherer and Schreibman (2005) identified a behavioral profile that predicted the effectiveness of a particular naturalistic behavioral treatment, pivotal response training, for individual autistic children. While much more research will be required before we can prescribe specific treatments for the wide range of symptom presentation in autism, this is a start. This information is important since it essentially allows for treatment providers to be "right" the first time when providing treatment. Given the importance of early intervention, one certainly does not want to waste precious time providing an ineffective treatment. The overall goal is essentially to have a program of prescriptive treatments wherein we can conduct behavioral assessment of individual children and, based on this assessment, provide the best treatment. Frequent and comprehensive behavioral assessment will be essential because as the child's behaviors change, different treatments may be indicated.

CASE STUDY

IDENTIFICATION

Spencer's parents first voiced concern to their pediatrician at the 18-month well-child checkup. While Spencer had always been a fussy baby who had difficulty with new people and environments, this was becoming more obvious as they attempted to place him in toddler gym courses and other activities. He became upset in these settings, and did not appear to enjoy playing with other children his own age. Additionally, although at the 12-month visit they had reported the use of a few single words, these verbalizations had ceased by 18 months. Now Spencer used babbling and hand leading to show his parents what he wanted. He was a happy child much of the time and enjoyed playing on his own with his trains or videos. The pediatrician felt that Spencer was probably not interacting because of his lack of experience with other children, that he would be likely to gain language by age 3, and, though crying often during the visit, that he did look at the doctor. Spencer's parents attempted to provide their son with more opportunities to be around other children by enrolling him in a local preschool. At age 20 months his teachers suggested that a screening might be appropriate for Spencer because he did not like to join the group activities, spent a great deal of time wandering or playing with just a few specific toys, and was not yet talking or trying to communicate with the teachers. Although he was compliant and seemed happy, they felt that he was not as engaged as the other children and would become upset if a teacher or child tried to interact with him. At this time his parents requested a developmental evaluation with a psychologist knowledgeable in the area of autism.

PRESENTING COMPLAINTS

Spencer's parents were most concerned with his failure to develop language and with the loss of his first few words. They also had concerns about his difficulty in new environments, unusual sleep patterns, and apparent lack of interest in other children. According to his parents, Spencer's strengths included his attention to detail, as evidenced by his ability to play with a toy for extended periods and to find very small items hidden on the floor, his happy nature when he was home with his family, and his ability to identify letters and numbers at an early age.

HISTORY

Spencer had no siblings. He had an unremarkable birth history. He was born at 40 weeks with no complications, and the pregnancy had been normal. Spencer had been a difficult baby, not sleeping well and not easily comforted. He did enjoy music and movement as an infant, more than he enjoyed being held. He reached his motor skills milestones at typical ages, sitting up at 6 months and walking at 11 months. He became a very independent toddler, doing most things for himself when he could. He said his first word, "doggie," at 12 months and used it inconsistently. He used about five other single words, but by 18 months he was no longer using words to communicate. Parents reported no history of autism or mental retardation in the family; however, the paternal grandfather was described as an "eccentric loner." Spencer's mother reported having a 6-year-old niece who was receiving speech therapy for language delays. Spencer had a recent visit to the audiologist. He was unable to complete the behavioral assessment; however, the sedated BAER indicated normal hearing.

DEVELOPMENTAL ISSUES

Spencer was 22 months old when he arrived for his developmental evaluation. The parent interview and ADI-R portion of the evaluation were conducted prior to seeing him. This provided the psychologist with an understanding of his behavior at home and in other community environments. The child portion of the evaluation involved a cognitive assessment, an ADOS, and an additional play-based assessment. Spencer was assessed using the Mullen Scales of Early Learning in order to obtain separate scores for visual reception, fine motor skills, and receptive and expressive communication. Because of his young age, and difficulty with new environments, completing a standardized assessment was challenging. The psychologist conducted much of the assessment on the floor of the office, interspersing play and alone time between tasks. Spencer had a very uneven cognitive profile, which was to be interpreted with caution due to his age and attention level. He had the most difficulty in the area of expressive language, with an age equivalent of approximately 10 months. His receptive skills were slightly better, at the 15-month level. Spencer was much more willing to complete tasks that did not have a verbal component. He obtained an 18-month age-equivalent score on the visual task and was at age level in his fine motor skills. Although the ADOS can be used with children 18–24 months of age, Spencer's developmental level was younger than that in some areas. The psychologist chose to use the ADOS in order to obtain a sample of the Spencer's behavior that would allow for an assessment of an ASD; however, results would be interpreted with caution. Spencer did meet criteria for ASD on the ADOS. Spencer's communication and social skills were limited during the course of the ADOS activities. He did tend to play repetitively with specific toys, but no motor or verbal stereotypes were observed. Because of Spencer's young age and developmental delay as well as his lack of stereotypy, he was given a provisional diagnosis of autism, to be confirmed after age 4. It was recommended that services appropriate for children with autism be provided through early intervention.

PEER AND SCHOOL ISSUES

Spencer was referred to an early-intervention program. Goals included increasing his communication skills, increasing his ability to interact with peers, and reducing behavioral issues such as poor sleep patterns, difficulty in new environments, and resistance to demands. Spencer's visual/nonverbal skills and ability to engage in some cause-and-effect play on his own qualified him for an inclusion program. Spencer's parents felt this would enhance his peer interaction skills. Because of Spencer's young age, his peers in the program were relatively accepting of him. He did become somewhat aggressive if they approached in the beginning, and they began to shy away from him. His teachers in the program worked with him and the other children to gradually help Spencer tolerate having other children nearby. Additionally, the program used visual cues and routine to assist Spencer in participating in classroom activities. With the support of visual cues he was able to follow the routine. He learned to imitate, and when he understood the expectations he was able to complete activities. To improve his play the teachers gradually introduced new toys, rewarding that play with Spencer's favorite objects. As he became better able to play, his peers were more likely to join him, and he was also beginning to join in large motor imitative play. Spencer had begun to use single words and sometimes two-word phrases to communicate; however, he needed assistance to use his language.

Spencer's parents next needed to work with his school district to develop an appropriate plan for his transition at 36 months. The district did not offer a similar program, and his parents were concerned that Spencer might not obtain the structure and peer engagement that he needed to succeed. The district and the parents developed an individualized program specific to Spencer's needs that included highly structured learning time as well as time in a typical preschool, with an inclusion assistant to help Spencer with interaction and engagement. These issues would again need to be addressed at kindergarten, and solutions would vary based on Spencer's skill level, behavior and, symptomatology.

BEHAVIORAL ASSESSMENT RESULTS

Program personnel soon realized that some of Spencer's behavior problems were interfering with his progress in the educational program. His resistance to new tasks, tantrums, and aggression made working with him a challenge. Since it was felt he had good potential to do well in the program, the early-intervention team conducted various behavioral assessments to inform specific interventions aimed at reducing these behaviors. After objectively defining the behaviors and structuring an observation plan, program providers observed Spencer across several periods during the day and recorded his disruptive behaviors across the various activities. Results of these observations indicated that Spencer was most likely to tantrum or engage in aggression when confronted with tasks that he found difficult or if too many other children were close to him. In fact, the observational data suggested that the presence of other children was correlated with a decrease in teacher attention to Spencer.

Based on this information, the program personnel chose two specific interventions to implement. The first intervention was to give Spencer a functionally equivalent response that he could use to communicate that a task was too difficult for him and that he needed assistance (e.g., Carr & Durand, 1985). Thus, rather than tantrum and aggression when confronted with a new and difficult task, Spencer was first taught to sign and later to say, "I need help." As expected, when he was now confronted with a difficult task, he used the more appropriate, and functionally equivalent, response rather than disruptive behavior to communicate his needs.

The second intervention was aimed at reducing Spencer's tantrum and aggressive behavior when other children were present. Since the observational assessment indicated that such situations were associated with a loss of teacher attention, the teachers decided to ensure that Spencer received as much teacher attention as possible when other children were present. Over time, as Spencer tolerated the situation well, the teachers gradually reduced the amount of attention specifically aimed at Spencer.

ETHICAL AND LEGAL ISSUES

Due to Spencer's young age, a provisional diagnosis of autism was initially provided. As he continued to do well in his early-intervention program, there was the possibility that when he would leave the early-intervention program at age 3, he might not meet criteria for an autism diagnosis but rather a less severe diagnosis, such as PDD-NOS. Knowing that an autism diagnosis would likely lead to the availability of more intensive services than the PDD-NOS diagnosis, autism may be the "preferred" diagnosis. Certainly diagnosticians are aware of this, and the temptation to shade the diagnosis based on treatment availability may be an ethical issue that must be confronted.

SUMMARY

The pervasive developmental disorders are behaviorally defined syndromes characterized by specific patterns of behavioral characteristics. Given that these disorders are quite complex and affect virtually every area of functioning, it is the case that the development and utilization of assessment have proven to be most challenging. Accordingly, accurate, detailed, and comprehensive assessment has proven to be exceptionally important and has been the focus of a great deal of research. The development of diagnostic assessments has been particularly helpful, in that diagnostic precision is important for epidemiological studies, various areas of research, and the determination of appropriate services and placements. Diagnostic assessment typically includes interviews with parent or other caregiver, a medical evaluation, direct behavioral observation, cognitive assessment, and assessment of adaptive behavior. Ongoing research continues to improve our ability to diagnose these disorders accurately and at a younger age, which is essential, given the importance of early screening and early intervention. Assessments developed and used for these populations must reflect an appreciation for developmental issues that may affect their interpretation. Finally, appropriate and detailed assessment can be crucial to the identification of treatment and educational programming as well as the evaluation of such interventions.

REFERENCES AND RESOURCES

Akshoomoff, N. (submitted). Cognitive Assessment of Young Children with Autism spectrum disorder.

Akshoomoff, N., Pierce, K., & Courchesne, E. (2002). The neurobiological basis of autism from a developmental perspective. *Development and Psychopathology, 14,* 613–634.

Akshoomoff, N., Lord, C., Lincoln, A. J., Courchesne, R. Y., Carper, R. A., Townsend, J., et al. (2004). Outcome classification of preschoolers with autism spectrum disorders using MRI brain measures. *Journal of the American Academy of Child and Adolescent Psychiatry, 43,* 349–357.

American Academy of Pediatrics. (2000). *Fellows Survey*. Elk Grove Village, IL: Author.

American Psychiatric Association. (1994). *Diagnostic and statistical manual of mental disorders* (4th ed.). Washington, DC: Author.

Baird, G., Charman, T., Baron-Cohen, S., Cox, A., Swettenham, J., Wheelwright, S., et al. (2000). A screening instrument for autism at 18 months of age: A six-year follow-up study. *Journal of the American Academy of Child and Adolescent Psychiatry, 39,* 694–702.

Baird, G., Charman, T., Cox, A., Baron-Cohen, S., Swettenham, J., Wheelwright, S., et al. (2001). Screening and surveillance for autism and pervasive developmental disorders. *Archives of Diseases in Childhood, 84,* 468–475.

Baron-Cohen, S., Allen, J., & Gillberg, C. (1992). Can autism be detected at 18 months? The needle, the haystack, and the CHAT. *British Journal of Psychiatry, 161,* 839–843.

Baron-Cohen, S., Cox, A., Baird, G., Swettenham, J., Nightingale, N., Morgan, K., et al. (1996). Psychological markers in the detection of autism in infancy in a large population. *British Journal of Psychiatry, 168,* 158–163.

Bayley, N. (1993). *Bayley Scales of Infant Development* (2nd ed.). San Antonio, TX: Harcourt Brace.

Berument, S. K., Rutter, M., Lord, C., Pickles, A., & Bailey, A. (1999). Autism screening questionnaire: diagnostic validity. *British Journal of Psychiatry, 175,* 444–451.

Bishop, D. V. M., & Norbury, C. F. (2002). Exploring the borderlands of autistic disorder and specific language impairment: A study using standardized instruments. *Journal of Child Psychology & Psychiatry, 43,* 917–929.

Bondy, A., & Frost, L. (2001). The Picture Exchange Communication System. *Behavior Modification, 25,* 725–744.

Bristol-Power, M. M., & Spinella, G. (1999). Research on screening and diagnosis in autism: A work in progress. *Journal of Autism and Developmental Disorders, 29,* 435–438.

California Department of Developmental Services. (2002). *Autistic spectrum disorders: Best-practice guidelines for screening, diagnosis and assessment.* Sacramento, CA: Author.

California Departments of Education and Developmental Services. (1997). *Best practices for designing and delivering effective programs for individuals with autistic spectrum disorders.* Sacramento, CA: Author.

Campbell, S. B. (1990). *Behavior problems in preschool children: Clinical and developmental issues.* New York: Guilford Press.

Carr, E. G., & Durand, V. M. (1985). Reducing behavior problems through functional communication training. *Journal of Applied Behavior Analysis, 18,* 111–126.

Chakrabarti, S., & Fombonne, E. (2001). Pervasive developmental disorders in preschool children [Also see Comment, pp. 3141–3142]. *JAMA, 285*(24), 3093–3099.

Charman, T., & Baird, G. (2002). Practitioner review: Diagnosis of autism spectrum disorder in 2- and 3-year-old children. *Journal of Child Psychology & Psychiatry, 43,* 289–305.

Collacott, R. A., Cooper, S. A., Brandford, D., & McGrother, C. (1998). Epidemiology of self-injurious behavior in adults with learning disabilities. *British Journal of Psychiatry, 173,* 428–432.

Coplan, J. (2000). Counseling parents regarding prognosis in autistic spectrum disorder. *Pediatrics, 105,* E651–E653.

Cox, A., Klein, K., Charman, T., Baird, G., Baron-Cohen, S., Swettenham, J., et al. (1999). Autism spectrum disorders at 20 and 42 months of age: Stability of clinical and ADI-R diagnosis. *Journal of Child Psychology and Psychiatry and Allied Disciplines, 40,* 719–732.

DiLavore, P. C., Lord, C., & Rutter, M. (1995). The Prelinguistic Autism Diagnostic Observation Schedule. *Journal of Autism and Developmental Disorders, 25,* 355–379.

Dunn, L. M., & Dunn, L. M. (1997). *PPVT-III: Peabody Picture Vocabulary Test—Third Edition.* Circle Pines, MN: American Guidance Services.

Elliott, C. D. (1990). *Differential Ability Scales*. San Antonio, TX: Psychological Corporation.

Fecteau, S., Mottron, L., & Burack, J. A. (2003). Developmental changes of autistic symptoms. *Autism, 7,* 255–268.

Fenson, L., Dale, P. S., Reznick, J. S., Thal, D., Bates, E., Hartung, J. P., et al. (1993). *MacArthur Communicative Development Inventories: User's guide and technical manual.* San Diego, CA: Singular.

Filipek, P. A., Accardo, P. J., Baranek, G. T., Cook, E. H., Jr., Dawson, G., Gordon, B., et al. (1999). The screening and diagnosis of autistic spectrum disorders. *Journal of Autism and Developmental Disorders, 29,* 439–484.

Filipek, P. A., Accardo, P. J., Ashwal, S., Baranek, G. T., Cook, E. H., Jr., Dawson, G., et al. (2000). Practice parameter: Screening and diagnosis of autism: Report of the Quality Standards Subcommittee of the American Academy of Neurology and the Child Neurology Society. *Neurology, 55,* 468–479.

Gillberg, C., Ehlers, S., Schaumann, H., Jakobsson, G., Dahlgren, S. O., Lindblom, R., et al. (1990). Autism under age 3 years: A clinical study of 28 cases referred for autistic symptoms in infancy [also see Comments]. *Journal of Child Psychology & Psychiatry & Allied Disciplines, 31,* 921–934.

Gilliam, J. E. (1995). *Gilliam Autism Rating Scales*. Austin, TX: PRO-ED.

Gilliam, J. E. (2001). *Gilliam Asperger Disorder Scale (GADS)*. Austin, TX: PRO-ED.

Glascoe, F. (2000). Early detection of developmental and behavioral problems. *Pediatrics in Review, 21,* 272–280.

Halfon, N., Regaldo, M., McLearn, K. T., Kuo, A. A., & Wright, K. (2003). *Building a bridge from birth to school: Improving developmental and behavioral health services for young children.* New York: Commonwealth Fund.

Handleman, J. S., & Harris, S. L. (2001). *Preschool education programs for children with autism* (2nd ed.). Austin, TX: PRO-ED.

Iwata, B. A., Dorsey, M. F., Slifer, K. J., Bauman, K. E. & Richman, A. (1944). Toward a functional analysis of self-injury. *Journal of Applied Behavior Analysis, 27,* 197–209.

Joseph, R. M., Tager-Flusberg, H., & Lord, C. (2002). Cognitive profiles and social-communicative functioning in children with autism spectrum disorder. *Journal of Child Psychology and Psychiatry, 43,* 807–821.

Koegel, L. K., Koegel, R. L., & Smith, A. K. (1997). Variables related to differences in standardized test outcomes for children with autism. *Journal of Autism and Developmental Disorders, 27,* 233–243.

Krug, D. A., Arick, J. R., & Almond, P. J. (1980). Behavior checklist for identifying severely handicapped individuals with high levels of autistic behavior. *Journal of Child Psychology and Psychiatry, 21,* 221–229.

Lincoln, A. J., Courchesne, E., Kilman, B. A., Elmasian, R., & Allen, M. (1988). A study of intellectual abilities in high-functioning people with autism. *Journal of Autism and Developmental Disorders, 18,* 505–524.

Linder, T. W. (1993). *Transdisciplinary play-based assessment: A functional approach to working with young children* (Rev. ed.). Baltimore: Brookes.

Lord, C. (1995). Follow-up of two-year-olds referred for possible autism. *Journal of Child Psychology and Psychiatry, 36,* 1365–1382.

Lord, C., & Bailey, A. (2002). Autism spectrum disorders. In M. Rutter & E. Taylor (Eds.), *Child and adolescent psychiatry: Modern approaches* (4th ed., pp. 636–663). Oxford: Blackwell Publications.

Lord, C., Leventhal, B. L., & Cook, E. H., Jr. (2001). Quantifying the phenotype in autism spectrum disorders. *American Journal of Medical Genetics, 105,* 36–38.

Lord, C., & Risi, S. (1998). Frameworks and methods in diagnosing autism spectrum disorders. *Mental Retardation and Developmental Disabilities Research Reviews, 4,* 90–96.

Lord, C., & Risi, S. (2000). Diagnosis of autism spectrum disorders in young children. In A. Wetherby & B. Prizant (Eds.), *Autism spectrum disorders: A transactional developmental perspective* (pp. 167–190). Baltimore: Brookes.

Lord, C., Risi, S., Lambrecht, L., Cook Jr., E., Leventhal, B., DiLavore, P., et al. (2000). The Autism Diagnostic Observation Schedule—Generic: A standard measure of social and communication deficits associated with the spectrum of autism. *Journal of Autism and Developmental Disorders, 30,* 205–223.

Lord, C., Rutter, M., DiLavore, P. C., & Risi, S. (2001). *Autism Diagnostic Observation Schedule.* Los Angeles: Western Psychological Services.

Lord, C., Rutter, M., & Le Couteur, A. (1994). Autism Diagnostic Interview—Revised: A revised version of a diagnostic interview for caregivers of individuals with possible pervasive developmental disorders. *Journal of Autism and Developmental Disorders, 24,* 659–685.

Lord, C., Rutter, M., Goode, S., Heemsbergen, J., Jordan, H., Mawhood, L., et al. (1989). Autism Diagnostic Observation Schedule: A standardized observation of communicative and social behavior. *Journal of Autism and Developmental Disorders, 19,* 185–212.

Lord, C., Storoschuk, S., Rutter, M., & Pickles, A. (1993). Using the ADI—R to diagnose autism in preschool children. *Infant Mental Health Journal, 14,* 234–252.

Lord, C., Wagner, A., Rogers, S., Szatmari, P., Aman, M. G., & Charman, T. (in press). Challenges in evaluating psychosocial interventions for autistic spectrum disorders. *Journal of Autism and Developmental Disorders.*

Mars, A. E., Mauk, J. E., & Dowrick, P. W. (1998). Symptoms of pervasive developmental disorders as observed in prediagnostic home videos of infants and toddlers. *Journal of Pediatrics, 132,* 500–504.

Martin, N. T., Bibby, P., Midford, O. C., & Eikeseth, S. (2003). Toward the use of a standardized assessment for young children with autism. *Autism, 7,* 321–330.

Mullen, E. M. (1995). *Mullen Scales of Early Learning* (AGS ed.). Circle Pines, MN: American Guidance Service.

Murphy, G., Hall, S., Oliver, C., & Kissi-Debra, R. (1999). Identification of early self-injurious behavior in young children with intellectual disability. *Journal of Intellectual Disabilities Research, 43,* 149–163.

National Research Council. (2001). *Educating children with autism. Committee on Educational Interventions for Children with Autism. Division of Behavioral and Social Sciences and Education.* Washington, DC: National Academy Press.

Noland, R. M., & Gabriels, R. L. (2004). Screening and identifying children with autism spectrum disorders in the public school system: The development of a model process. *Journal of Autism and Developmental Disorders, 34,* 265–277.

Ozonoff, S., Rogers, S. J., & Hendren, R. L. (Eds.). (2003). *Autism spectrum disorders: A research review for practitioners.* Washington, DC: American Psychiatric Publishing.

Reynell, J. K., & Grueber, C. P. (1990). *The Reynell Developmental Language Scale* (U.S. ed.). Los Angeles: Western Psychological Services.

Robins, D. L. (2003). The Modified Checklist for Autism in Toddlers (M-CHAT): Early detection of autism spectrum disorders. *Dissertation Abstracts International: Section B: The Sciences & Engineering, 63(10-B),* 4922.

Robins, D. L., Fein, D., Barton, M. L., & Green, J. A. (2001). The Modified Checklist for Autism in Toddlers: An initial study investigating the early detection of autism and pervasive developmental disorders. *Journal of Autism and Developmental Disorders, 31,* 131–144.

Rogers, S. (2001). Diagnosis of autism before the age of 3. *International Review of Mental Retardation, 23,* 1–31.

Rutter, M., Bailey, A., & Lord, C. (2003). *Social Communication Questionnaire.* Los Angeles: Western Psychological Services.

Rutter, M., Le Couteur, A., & Lord, C. (2003). *ADI-R. Autism Diagnostic Interview—Revised* (WPS ed.). Los Angeles: Western Psychological Services.

Saemundsen, E., Magnusson, P., Smari, J., & Sigurdardottir, S. (2003). Autism Diagnostic Interview—Revised and the Childhood Autism Rating Scale: Convergence and discrepancy in diagnosing autism. *Journal of Autism and Developmental Disorders, 33,* 319–328.

Schopler, E., Reichler, R. J., & Rochen Renner, B. (1988). *The Childhood Autism Rating Scale*. Los Angeles: Western Psychological Services.

Semel, E., Wiig, E. H., & Secord, W. A. (2003). *Clinical Evaluation of Language Fundamentals—Fourth Edition (CELF-4)*. San Antonio, TX: Psychological Corporation.

Sherer, M. R., & Schreibman, L. (2005). Individual behavioral profiles and predictors of treatment effectiveness for children with autism. *Journal of Consulting and Clinical Psychology, 73,* 525–538.

Shriver, M. D., Allen, K. D., & Matthews, J. R. (1999). Effective assessment of the shared and unique characteristics of children with autism. *School Psychology Review, 28,* 538–558.

Siegel, B. (1999). *Detection of autism in the 2nd and 3rd years: The Pervasive Developmental Disorders Screening Test (PDDST)*. Paper presented at the biennial meeting of the Society for Research in Child Development, Albuquerque, NM.

Siegel, B. (2004). *Pervasive Developmental Disorders Screening Test—II (PDDST-II)*. San Antonio, TX: Harcourt.

Siegel, D. J., Minshew, N. J., & Goldstein, G. (1996). Wechsler IQ profiles in diagnosis of high-functioning autism [see Comments]. *Journal of Autism and Developmental Disorders, 26,* 389–406.

South, M., Williams, B. J., McMahon, W. M., Owley, T., Filipek, P. A., Shernoff, E., et al. (2002). Utility of the Gilliam Autism Rating Scale in research and clinical populations. *Journal of Autism and Developmental Disorders, 32,* 593–599.

Sparrow, S., Balla, D., & Cicchetti, D. (1984). *Vineland Scales of Adaptive Behavior: Interview edition, survey form*. Circle Pines, MN: American Guidance Service.

Stone, W. L., Lee, E. B., Ashford, L., Brissie, J., Hepburn, S. L., Coonrod, E. E., et al. (1999). Can autism be diagnosed accurately in children under 3 years? *Journal of Child Psychology and Psychiatry and Allied Disciplines, 40,* 219–226.

Teitelbaum, P., Teitelbaum, O., Nye, J., Fryman, J., & Maurer, R. G. (1998). Movement analysis in infancy may be useful for early diagnosis of autism. *Proceedings of the National Academy of Sciences, USA, 95,* 13982–13987.

Thorndike, R. L., Hagen, E. P., & Sattler, J. M. (1986). *The Stanford–Binet Intelligence Scale* (4th ed.). Chicago: Riverside.

Venter, A., Lord, C., & Schopler, E. (1992). A follow-up study of high-functioning autistic children. *Journal of Child Psychology and Psychiatry, 33,* 489–507.

Volkmar, F. R., Klin, A., Marans, W., & Cohen, D. J. (1996). The pervasive developmental disorders: Diagnosis and assessment. *Child & Adolescent Psychiatric Clinics of North America, 5,* 963–977.

Wechsler, D. (2003). *Manual for the Wechsler Memory Scale—Fourth Edition*. San Antonio, TX: Psychological Corporation.

Werner, E., Dawson, G., Osterling, J., & Dinno, N. (2000). Brief report: Recognition of autism spectrum disorder before one year of age: A retrospective study based on home videotapes. *Journal of Autism and Developmental Disorders, 30,* 157–162.

Wetherby, A. P. B. (1993). *Communication and Symbolic Behavior Scales* (Normed ed.). Chicago: Applied Symbolix.

Wiig, E. H., Secord, W. A., & Semel, E. (1992). *Clinical Evaluation of Language Fundamentals—Preschool (CELF-P)*. San Antonio, TX: Psychological Corporation.

21

Habit Disorders

Michael B. Himle
Christopher A. Flessner
Jordan T. Bonow
Douglas W. Woods

Department of Psychology
University of Wisconsin—Milwaukee
Milwaukee, Wisconsin

INTRODUCTION

The term *habit disorders* describes a broad class of disorders characterized by repetitive, unwanted behaviors that are distressing and often result in significant functional impairment. The two primary classes of habit disorders are tic disorders and body-focused repetitive behaviors (BFRBs). Whereas tic disorders are defined by the presence of one or more motor and/or vocal tics, the BFRB categorization involves a more broadly defined set of self-focused repetitive behaviors that cause physical harm or can result in harm if left untreated. Common examples of BFRBs include chronic hair pulling (trichotillomania; TTM), skin picking, and nail biting. Of these, only TTM is defined separately in the *DSM-IV*. Both tic disorders and BFRBs commonly begin in childhood.

DIAGNOSTIC CONSIDERATIONS FOR HABIT DISORDERS

Tic Disorders

Tics are defined as "sudden, rapid, recurrent, nonrhythmic, stereotyped motor movements or vocalizations" (American Psychiatric Association [APA], 2000, p. 108). There are three primary tic disorder diagnoses, each distinguished by the number of symptoms and their duration. Chronic tic disorder (CTD) involves the presence of one or more motor or vocal tics (but not both) for at least 1 year. In contrast, Tourette syndrome (TS) involves the presence of multiple motor tics *and* one or more vocal tics (not necessarily concurrently) that have been present for at least one year. If the tics have been present for less than one year but more than four weeks, then a diagnosis of transient tic disorder (TTD) is more appropriate. Tics typically begin at approximately 5–7 years of age, peak in early adolescence, and decline gradually, with a waxing and waning course (Leckman, King, & Cohen, 1999). Prevalence estimates suggest that 0.05% to 0.08% of the population meet criteria for TS and 3%–10% meet criteria for lifetime occurrence of CTD or TTD (for reviews see Hornesy, Banerjee, Zeitlin, & Robertson, 2001; Khalifa & von Knorring, 2003; Robertson, 2003). Across the spectrum, tic disorders appear to be more common in males (Khalifa & von Knorring).

Body-Focused Repetitive Behaviors

Except for TTM, no specific diagnostic category exists to classify body-focused repetitive behaviors. Sometimes BFRBs are classified as Stereotypic Movement Disorders and other times as Impulse-Control Disorders NOS. Nevertheless, researchers have begun to define a BFRB as a self-directed and repetitive behavior that occurs five or more times per day for at least four weeks and causes functional impairment or physical damage. Using these criteria, Teng, Woods, Twohig, and Marcks (2002) found that BFRBs were more common in females and occurred in approximately 14% of the general college population. Specific research on adults with TTM has consistently shown that the disorder is more common in females; and although estimates vary drastically, conservative estimates suggest that TTM is present in 0.6% to 2% of adults (APA, 2000; Christenson, Pyle, & Mitchell, 1991; McCarley, Spirrison, & Ceminsky, 2002; Rothbaum, Shaw, Morris, & Ninan, 1993). Although TTM may begin as early as 2–3 years, the typical age of onset for adultlike TTM is 13 years (Christenson, Mackenzie, & Mitchell, 1991). Adequate estimates of the prevalence of BFRBs in children are not currently available.

ASSESSMENT STRATEGIES AND RESEARCH BASIS

Tic disorders and BFRBs must be assessed across multiple domains. Establishing the diagnosis and assessing the physical dimensions and severity of the target behavior is of obvious importance, but other important domains should also be addressed. These include public and private maintaining variables, impairment in physical or social functioning, and the presence of comorbid conditions. A thorough assessment of habit disorders should utilize an assortment of instruments and methods, including unstructured and structured interviews, self-report inventories, self-monitoring, and direct observation. Each method addresses different features of the disorder, and each has varying levels of psychometric support. In this section, we review the different domains to be assessed and the different methods that may be useful and describe the research (if any) supporting their use.

ESTABLISHING A DIAGNOSIS, DESCRIBING THE BEHAVIOR, AND MEASURING SEVERITY

The first step in the assessment of habit disorders is to diagnose the condition and assess the various dimensions of the behavior and its severity. Well-conducted clinical interviews with a parent and a child can provide descriptive information about the topography, frequency, and severity of the habit. In addition, a skilled interviewer can obtain information about medical and psychological treatment history, pre- and postnatal development, family history (including medical and psychological), and educational and occupational history. Each of these domains is important for case conceptualization and treatment planning.

Tic Disorders

In diagnosing a tic disorder, it is important first to rule out the possibility that the symptoms can better be accounted for by another medical or alternative psychiatric condition (e.g., Obsessive-Compulsive Disorder, Sydenham's chorea, Huntington's disease, head injury, stereotypies associated with developmental disabilities). If a tic disorder is suspected, the interviewer should ascertain a complete list of both simple and complex tics along with their developmental course. In addition, the interviewer should inquire about suppressability or controllability of tics and patterns of waxing and waning. The Yale Tourette Syndrome Symptom List—Revised (TSSL; Cohen, Detlor, Young, & Shaywitz, 1980) can be useful in assessing the different types of tics that may be present, while the Yale Global Tic Severity Scale (YGTSS; Leckman et al., 1989) is a useful instrument for measuring tic severity. The YGTSS is a clinician-administered interview that provides separate severity ratings for motor and vocal tics across several domains, including number, complexity, intensity, and interference produced by the tics. In addition, it provides impairment and overall tic severity scores. In a sample consisting of mostly children and adolescents, the YGTSS demonstrated excellent internal consistency (item-subscale correlations range from $r = .66$ to $r = .84$) and correlated highly with comparable measures of tic severity, including the Tourette Syndrome Global Scale (TSGS; Harcherik, Leckman, Deltor, & Cohen, 1984, $r = .86$ and $r = .91$ for motor and phonic ratings, respectively), and the Tourette Symptoms Severity Scale (TSSS; Shapiro et al., 1989). The YGTSS has also demonstrated adequate discriminant validity and interrater reliability (see Leckman et al., 1989).

It should be noted that neither the TSSL nor the YGTSS has an identified minimum administration age, so the clinician must use clinical judgment to determine whether the parent, child, or both is the most appropriate respondent. It is our experience that for most children and adolescents, input from both the parent and child will be necessary to obtain the most adequate and useful information.

Self-report inventories have also been developed to aid in the assessment of tics. One example is the Motor Tic, Obsessions and Compulsions, Vocal Tic Evaluation Survey (MOVES; Gaffney, Sieg, & Hellings, 1994), which is a 20-item inventory that requires the child or parent to rate how often he/she has experienced the symptoms described in each of the statements on the inventory. The MOVES is designed to assess the severity of simple and complex motor and vocal tics as well as obsessive thoughts and compulsive rituals. Gaffney et al. reported that MOVES scores obtained by a sample of children with TS correlated highly with the YGTSS ($r = .75$) and that the MOVES was sensitive to clinical change. However, larger studies are needed to assess more adequately the psychometric properties of the MOVES.

Often used as an adjunct to the clinical interviews and standard severity measures, self-monitoring can provide information regarding the frequency, duration, severity, and environmental contexts in which tics are more (or less) likely to occur. Data sheets, handheld counters, checklists, or any other method of recording (e.g., tally marks on a sheet of paper) can be used to record self-monitoring data. Typically, this is done for fixed time periods between sessions (i.e., 15 minutes per day) in settings where the child is highly likely to tic and can be conducted by either the child or an adult observer, such as a parent or teacher.

The measures described so far rely on the child's or parent's account of the behavior, which creates several problems. First, children are often unaware of all of their tics. Second, children are vulnerable to many sources of bias when recording and reporting their symptoms. Third, it is unclear who may provide the most accurate information. Parents rarely observe their children at school, and teachers are not typically with the child after the school day ends. To overcome these concerns, direct observation procedures may be used.

Videotaping is the most common form of direct observation of tics. It is used to provide objective data on frequency, intensity, and variation in tic topography. Moreover, it allows for identification of tics not reported by the child or parent. Videotaping can occur in a variety of situations, but, whenever possible, we prefer to videotape covertly from behind a one-way mirror to prevent reactivity. Nevertheless, a clinician must use discretion when determining what method of taping to use to gain the most useful data while still respecting the rights of the child and parent.

Before a videotape is scored, a client's tics must be operationally defined. Three different methods of scoring can then be used for data collection. Frequency scoring (e.g., Chappell et al., 1994) involves recording the occurrence of each tic. This provides the total number of tics observed in a given time as well as the temporal distribution of those tics. When using frequency scoring, the length of the scored segment can vary, but a minimum segment of 5 minutes appears to be required to obtain a reliable short-term measure of a child's tics (Chappell et al.). In the partial interval scoring method (e.g., Woods, Miltenberger, & Lumley, 1996), the observation segment is divided into consecutive time intervals ranging from four to ten seconds. The examiner then records each interval that contained at least one tic. This information is used to determine the percentage of observation intervals that contained a tic. The Rush-Based Videotape Scoring System (Goetz, Tanner, Wilson, & Shannon, 1987) also utilizes frequency scoring but adds ratings of tic severity and topography to yield a composite tic severity score.

Each of the aforementioned methods will provide a direct measure of tic occurrence, and the choice of method employed will depend largely on examiner preference. However, a recent study evaluating the reliability and validity of direct observations methods for tic disorders found that partial interval (PI) scoring was highly correlated with frequency coding ($r = .89$) and that both methods were temporally stable at one week ($r = .90$ for both PI and frequency methods) and two-week ratings ($r = .87$ and $r = .91$ for the PI and frequency methods, respectively; Woods, Piacentini, Himle, & Chang, 2003). As such, it appears that partial interval coding is as valid and reliable as frequency coding and is easier to conduct.

Body-Focused Repetitive Behaviors

When diagnosing and establishing the severity of TTM or another BFRB, the clinician will need to consider possible underlying medical etiologies and rule out comorbid conditions. Because various medical etiologies could exist for TTM or other BFRBs, it is often recommended that a person with a potential diagnosis of TTM or BFRB be evaluated by a physician.

After alternative medical explanations have been ruled out, the diagnosis of TTM can be ascertained using the Trichotillomania Diagnostic Interview (TDI; Rothbaum & Ninan, 1994), which is a standardized clinician-administered interview based on *DSM-IV* criteria. Each of the *DSM-IV* diagnostic criteria for TTM are rated using a three-point scale, which also provides an overall index of confidence in TTM diagnosis. In terms of considering differential diagnoses, it is important to determine if the repetitive behavior is in reaction to some obsessive thought or image. If this is the case, a diagnosis of OCD must be considered.

In addition to considering the diagnostic issues, it is necessary for the clinician to adequately define and measure the behavioral topography involved in the BFRB. The actual act of pulling or picking can vary greatly across clients. Some children report that they pull/pick from single sites, use only their fingers to remove hairs or skin, and pull with little or no immediate awareness of their behavior. On the other hand, some children may pull/pick from several sites, use grooming implements, pull/pick while isolated and looking in a mirror, report an intense urge or drive to pull/pick and relief after the behavior has ceased, and can vividly recall their first pulling/picking episode. Although a particular duration of symptoms is not specified for diagnostic purposes, it is an important issue to consider. BFRBs are often transient. But if they occur for longer than four weeks and have a negative functional impact, a formal diagnosis may be warranted.

Clinician-rated measures can also be used in the assessment of BFRBs. Two clinician-rated measures we find useful in the assessment of TTM include the Psychiatric Institute Trichotillomania Scale (PITS; Winchel et al., 1992) and the National Institutes of Mental Health (NIMH) Trichotillomania Symptoms Severity and Impairment Scales (Swedo et al., 1989). Although these measures were developed and tested with adults, the instruments can easily be adapted for use with children and parents. In most cases, however, psychometric data are not available for children.

The PITS (Winchel et al., 1992) is a clinician-administered, semistructured interview designed to assess TTM along the following domains: number of sites from which a person pulls, the amount of time spent pulling daily, ability to resist pulling, interference, and distress from pulling, and amount of hair loss. Each item is rated on an eight-point scale (range 0–7). Ratings are then summed to obtain an overall symptom severity score. Stanley, Breckenridge, Snyder, and Novy (1999) utilized a small sample of adults with TTM and found that the interference, distress, and severity items on the PITS correlated highly with severity as measured by the Minnesota Trichotillomania Assessment Interview (MTAI; Christenson et al., 1991); however, site, duration, and resistance items showed low correlations. In addition, the overall score did not correlate with self-reported number of hairs pulled ($r = .10$), and the measure was shown to demonstrate questionable internal consistency ($\alpha = .59$).

The NIMH Trichotillomania Symptoms Severity and Impairment Scales (Swedo et al., 1989) is a clinician-administered semistructured interview designed to assess time consumed by pulling, ability to resist pulling, and interference and distress from pulling. Scores from each of the items are summed to provide an overall impairment score. In addition, the scale contains a single item designed to measure overall impairment based on severity and frequency of pulling, extent of hair loss, ability to resist pulling, functional impairment, and the client's subjective level of distress. This "Trich Global Scale" is a 0–10 rating, with higher scores indicating more impairment. To our knowledge, psychometric data are not yet available for the TDI or the NIMH scales.

The Massachusetts General Hospital Hairpulling Scale (MGH-HS; Keuthen et al., 1995; O'Sullivan et al., 1995) is the only available self-report measure specifically designed to assess TTM severity. The seven-item instrument assesses the frequency, intensity, and control of hair pulling urges along with the frequency, control of, and attempts to resist the actual act of pulling. One additional item targets pulling-related distress. Each item on the MGH-HS is rated on a scale of 0 (no symptoms) to 4 (extreme symptoms), and item scores are summed to produce a total score ranging from 0 to 28 (with higher scores representing more severe symptoms). With adults, the MGH-HS has shown adequate convergent and divergent validity, test–retest reliability, and sensitivity to change. Keuthen et al. (1995) and O'Sullivan et al. (1995) reported on a sample of 26 adults with TTM that showed the MGH-HS correlated highly with the PITS ($r = .63$) and Clinical Global Severity (CGS) scores ($r = .75$). In addition, the MGH-HS did not correlate highly with measures of depression ($r = .30$) or anxiety ($r = .10$), and change on the MGH-HS correlated highly with change on other measures of pulling severity. The scale was also shown to be internally consistent ($\alpha = .89$), and test–retest reliability was shown to be adequate ($r = .97$). It should be noted that some of the items on the MGH-HS are worded such that it may be difficult for young children to comprehend.

The only self-report measures available to assess other BFRBs are the Skin Picking Scale (SPS; Keuthen, Wilhelm et al., 2001) and the Skin Picking Impact Scale (SPIS; Keuthen, Deckersbach et al., 2001). The SPS is a six-item paper-and-pencil self-report that can be used to assess several domains of skin picking severity, including frequency and intensity of picking urges, duration, interference, avoidance, and distress from picking, and resistance and control over picking. Each item is rated on a four-point ordinal scale. In a preliminary analysis of adults with skin picking, the SPS demonstrated acceptable internal consistency ($\alpha = .80$) and the ability to specify injurious and noninjurious skin picking severity (Keuthen, Wilhelm et al., 2001). The SPIS is a 10-item paper-and-pencil scale that assesses the psychosocial ramifications of skin picking. In an initial analysis the SPIS demonstrated adequate internal consistency for both self-injurious ($\alpha = .93$) and non-self-injurious skin pickers ($\alpha = .88$). Like the MGH-HS, the wording of some of the items on the SPS and SPIS makes the measure questionable for use with young children.

In addition to the measures just described, three other assessment methods may be useful in assessing BFRBs. Self-monitoring can provide information on BFRB frequency, duration, and environmental contexts in which the behavior occurs more (or less) frequently. Self-monitoring is often used as the primary method of assessing the efficacy of treatment in clinical settings. Another method of assessing BFRB severity involves product recording. For TTM, this may involve having a child collect pulled hairs in a small bag or envelope; or for skin picking, this may involve collecting periodic photographs from damaged areas (e.g., Twohig & Woods, 2001).

The final strategy that may be used to measure BFRB severity is direct observation. Although this strategy can provide useful information, it is limited by the fact that hair pulling and other BFRBs usually occur when a child is alone and because children with these conditions are highly reactive to being observed. Two procedures that may be helpful in countering these concerns include time-sample recording and extended videotape recording. To conduct time-sample recording, a parent or other observer identifies rooms and contexts in which the child typically engages in the BFRB. The observer then enters the room at unpredictable times and records whether or not the child was engaging in the behavior, which yields a percentage of observations during which the child was engaged. A second method is the use of videotape recording via hidden cameras. Videotapes can later be watched and BFRBs can be recorded using frequency or duration measures. However, this approach poses obvious logistical problems and is rarely used.

PUBLIC AND PRIVATE MAINTAINING VARIABLES

As mentioned earlier, a comprehensive assessment of habit disorders must also consider the variables that may maintain the disorder, the functional impact of the behavior, and comorbid states. In the following sections, we address these issues.

Tic Disorders

Some children's tics are preceded by premonitory sensations (Leckman, Walker, & Cohen, 1993), commonly referred to as *premonitory urges*. These sensations can be uncomfortable, and some children may report them as being more distressing than the tics. Premonitory urges typically occur in localized muscle or body regions directly involved in the tic, but they can also occur globally across large body regions. Those who suffer from tics have described premonitory urges using both somatosensory terms (e.g., itch, tingle, tight, energetic) and/or cognitive terms (e.g., something is "not right"). Although the etiology of premonitory urges is unknown, urges appear to be functionally related to tics such that the urge precedes the onset of the tic and is temporarily alleviated contingent on the performance of the tic (Leckman et al., 1993). It is widely believed that attempts to resist or suppress tics result in a building of the urge, making tic performance inevitable. Although tics may be uncontrollable, recent research has suggested that some with tics view their symptoms as volitional acts that effectively (albeit temporarily) eliminate or reduce a premonitory urge (Kwak, Dat Vong, & Jankovik, 2003). Alternatively, not all children with tics report an urge. In fact, it has been suggested that the premonitory urge may be absent in young children (i.e., under 10 years) and develops over the course of the disorder (Leckman et al., 1999).

In addition to the use of informal interview strategies, the assessment of premonitory urge severity can be accomplished quickly though the use of short self-report instruments such as the Premonitory Urge for Tics Scale (PUTS; Woods, 2002), which contains a list of several urge descriptions commonly reported by individuals with tics. The PUTS asks children to rate the degree to which his/her tics are preceded by each of the listed urge descriptions (on a four-point scale). In an initial evaluation of 42 children with TS, the PUTS demonstrated good internal consistency ($\alpha = .81$) and acceptable one- and two-week test–retest reliability ($r = .79$ and $r = .86$, respectively; Woods, Piacentini, Himle, & Chang, in press), but the measure appears to be most valid for use with children over the age of 10 years.

Considerable evidence suggests that tics are the product of neurobiological dysfunction rather than a conditioning history (i.e., social reinforcement); and although the symptoms are not believed to be maintained exclusively by contextual variables, they are responsive to various environmental conditions. For example, Woods, Watson, Wolfe, Twohig, and Friman (2001) demonstrated that vocal tics increased in frequency during tic-related conversation in two individuals with TS. Similarly, Malatesta (1990) demonstrated that a boy's tics increased in frequency in the presence of his father, and Silva, Munoz, Barickman, and Friedhoff (1995) found that factors most likely to exacerbate tics in children with TS included events that increased anxiety or emotional "trauma" and fatigue. Factors reported to decrease symptoms included doctor visits, sleep, and talking to friends. Sedentary activities such as watching television and social gatherings were reported to markedly increase tics for some while decreasing tics for others.

A keen awareness of the potential for context-dependent symptom fluctuation has important clinical implications. A savvy clinician should possess the ability to identify conditions that exacerbate or ameliorate symptoms, for these factors can often be manipulated in the service of symptoms reduction. Clinical interviews, antecedent-behavior-consequence (ABC) self-monitoring, and existing functional assessment forms (e.g., Miltenberger, 2004, pp. 262–270) can easily be adapted to aid in the identification of antecedents (e.g., contexts and settings) and consequences (e.g., attention, avoidance) that may exacerbate or ameliorate tic severity.

Body-Focused Repetitive Behaviors

BFRBs are also preceded and influenced by a host of public and private events. For example, some children with TTM and chronic skin picking report a building of tension prior to pulling and relief of the tension after pulling (Christenson et al., 1991), a phenomenon similar to the premonitory urge associated with TS. In fact, sensations associated with BFRBs are often described using terms similar to those described in TS (e.g., anxiety, vague tension, an urge, an itch, pressure, tingle), and the sensation can occur either globally throughout the body or in the focal area where the BFRB is concentrated. Research has shown that not all individuals with BFRBs (especially children) describe these sensations. But when present, addressing them may be instrumental in conceptualizing and treating an individual with a BFRB.

There is increasing evidence that the maintenance of BFRBs may involve cognitive and emotional factors. For example, an individual with TTM may think that a hair is abnormal (e.g., too coarse, thick, rough, or curly) and believe that it should therefore be removed. Similarly, individuals with chronic skin picking may view a patch of skin, scab, or blemish as unsightly, thereby justifying picking (at least to the patient). Recent research on private events in BFRBs has shown that individuals with TTM are likely to report shame, guilt, and anger about pulling. Wilhelm et al. (1999) reported on 31 adults with chronic skin picking and found that many of them reported escalating feelings of being mesmerized and satisfaction from before to during picking; decreased satisfaction from during to after picking; increased shame, guilt, and pain from before to after picking; decreased tension from before to after picking; and decreased feelings of being mesmerized from during to after picking. Although no psychometrically sound instruments are currently available to assess private events associated with

BFRBs, an examiner can utilize structured and unstructured interviews to obtain this information. It also warrants mention that although much of the understanding of these private events comes from studies with adults, similar phenomena are often reported by children and adolescents.

Overt environmental events can also influence BFRBs. Specifically, such events can function to elicit or exacerbate private maintaining variables or may simply set the occasion for pulling to occur because they have been associated with past episodes of BFRBs. For example, Christenson, Ristvedt, and McKenzie (1993) explored several internal and external cues related to pulling in TTM. A factor analysis identified two primary components important to hair pulling: negative affective states (e.g., sadness, anxiety, frustration) and sedentary activities (reading, studying, watching television). The authors suggested that the former represented cues that influence cognitive and/or emotional variables, whereas the latter represented common circumstances under which pulling is likely to occur. Findings such as these have led some experts to suggest that there may be specific subtypes of BFRBs: those that are performed volitionally with awareness and intention (i.e., focused) and that function to eliminate, control, or otherwise alter private events, and those that occur habitually in the absence of immediate awareness (i.e., nonfocused pulling) and that are influenced primarily by contextual cues and maintained by automatic sensory reinforcement (e.g., tactile reinforcement produced by stroking pulled hair; Miltenberger, Long, Rapp, Lumley, & Elliot, 1998). Several existing measures described earlier in this chapter contain items designed to assess cognitive and contextual antecedents to BFRBs. Additional information can easily be ascertained during a clinical interview, via ABC self-monitoring, and/or via functional assessment forms frequently used in behavior modification protocols (e.g., Miltenberger, 2004, pp. 262–270). Functional assessment interviews are preferred because they provide a structured, relatively simple method for obtaining information about the antecedents and consequences (both public and private) that may maintain the behavior.

IMPAIRMENT

Tic Disorders

In addition to the physical damage that may be caused by tics, research suggests that children with tic disorders often experience impairment in socialization (Champion, Fulton, & Shady, 1988) and family functioning (Hubka, Fulton, Shady, Champion, & Wand, 1988). This research, however, is often confounded by the high prevalence of comorbid conditions, and the relative role of tic severity independent of comorbid symptoms remains unclear. Some research has suggested that tic symptoms can independently result in impaired functioning (e.g., Woods, Fuqua, & Outman, 1999), while other research has shown that comorbid conditions such as ADHD and depression are primarily responsible for impairment (e.g., Carter, O'Donnell, & Schultz, 2000; Woods, Himle, Smerz, & Osmon, in press). Given the difficulty in differentiating the relative contribution of tics independent of comorbid symptoms, an assessment should include an evaluation of adaptive functioning to assess for functional impairment regardless of comorbid status. A variety of self- and parent-report instruments exists for this purpose (e.g., Matson Evaluation of Social Skills with Youngsters; Matson, Rotatori, & Helsel, 1983; Impact on Family Scale; Stein & Reissmann, 1980), but a detailed discussion of them is beyond the scope of this chapter.

Body-Focused Repetitive Behaviors

Children with BFRBs experience a variety of physical and psychosocial difficulties as a result of their behavior. Trichobezoars (masses of hair and food that form in the gastrointestinal tract of individuals who ingest the hair they pull) can result in a failure to gain weight or weight loss, iron deficiency anemia, pain, vomiting, and a variety of other medical complications. In addition, they sometimes require surgery for removal (Phillips, Zaheer, & Drugas, 1998). Children with chronic skin picking frequently experience skin lesions that place them at risk for serious infection and other medical complications. Less serious medical complications can also result from BFRBs, including scalp and skin irritation, follicle damage, scarring, and an atypical regrowth of hair (Christenson & Mansueto, 1999).

Another primary concern for children with BFRBs is cosmetic. Not surprisingly, repeated hair pulling, skin picking, or nail biting can have an unfavorable effect on physical appearance. Individuals with BFRBs frequently report decreased levels of self-esteem, poor body image, embarrassment, and diminished self-confidence (Soriano et al., 1996). Although these intrapersonal experiences can be distressing themselves, their negative impact on a child with a BFRB is exaggerated by the social difficulties that often result. Children with visible damage (e.g., hair loss, open sores) may even avoid or refuse routine public activities such as school (Casati, Toner, & Yu, 2000). Likewise, families of children with BFRBs often attempt to cover the effects of the disorder by using garments (e.g., hats, loose clothing, and bandannas) and use cosmetic items such as wigs, makeup, and false eyelashes, which can consume a considerable amount of time and money (Casati et al., 2000).

COMMON COMORBID CONDITIONS

Tic Disorders

Tic disorders are frequently accompanied by comorbid psychiatric symptoms. As such, it is important to screen for common comorbid conditions, which include Attention-Deficit Hyperactivity Disorder (ADHD), Obsessive-Compulsive Disorder (OCD), Oppositional Defiant Disorder (ODD), Major Depressive Disorder (MDD), and a variety of other internalizing and externalizing conditions. The assessment of these conditions is beyond the scope of this chapter, but a variety of clinician-rated and self-report instruments are available, as are several structured clinical interviews.

One behavior worthy of special consideration is explosive anger outbursts, or "rage attacks," that sometimes occur in TS. These unpredictable and uncontrollable verbal and physical aggressions are often displayed (to varying degrees) by children with TS (Budman, Bruun, Park, Lesser, & Olson, 2000). The defining characteristic of these outbursts is the degree to which they are disproportionate given the provocation. Topographically, they appear as an extreme temper tantrum preceded by little buildup that is much more intense than is developmentally appropriate. When rage attacks are present, they are likely to come to the attention of the clinician because of their severity and intensity. Nevertheless, it is important to assess for explosive episodes in children with TS even if they are not a component of the presenting problem. To our knowledge, the only instrument available to screen for the presence of rage attacks is the Rage Attacks Questionaire (Budman, Rockmore, Stokes, & Sossin, 2003), a 22-item self-report (or parent report) measure that assesses for the presence/absence of rage. Budman et al. (2003) reported descriptive statistics and a factor analysis from a small sample of children with TS + rage, but the instrument has not yet undergone rigorous psychometric validation.

Body-Focused Repetitive Behaviors

BFRBs are often accompanied by a high occurrence of comorbid psychological conditions. Christenson et al. (1991) found that 55% of an adult sample had a history of major depression or some other affective disorder during their lifetimes, 57% of individuals had a history of anxiety disorders, 22% of individuals reported they had suffered from substance use disorders, and approximately 20% had experienced eating disorders. Overall, Christenson et al. (1991) found that 82% of adults in their TTM sample met current or lifetime criteria for a comorbid Axis I diagnosis. Again, the assessment of these conditions is beyond the scope of this chapter, but a variety of clinician-rated and self-report instruments are available, as are several structured clinical interviews.

CLINICAL UTILITY

The use of the entire aforementioned assessment strategy would yield the greatest, most complex field of information when assessing habit disorders. Nevertheless, use of such a comprehensive battery is often not practical in typical clinical settings. For this reason, we recommend the following assessment strategy for clinical practice. First, a clinical interview conducted with both child and parent(s) should involve a functional assessment to determine the external triggers and changes in internal phenomena (e.g., emotions, thoughts, etc.) that result from the behavior. The interview should also rule out other possible explanations for the behavior (e.g., OCD, underlying physical condition) and determine whether or not the behavior results in any secondary gains (e.g., results in attention or produces escape from an aversive situation). The therapist should also screen for possible comorbid conditions that may require more immediate attention.

This initial interview can be supplemented with the ABC form of self-monitoring. Utilizing this type of self-monitoring will not only provide the clinician with ongoing data regarding the frequency and severity of the behavior but will provide additional information to further support or modify the current functional conceptualization. Nevertheless, because children are not always reliable in their recording, it is recommended that concurrent monitoring be conducted by the parent and that alternative ongoing outcome assessments be conducted. We suggest the use of the MGH-HS and SPS for assessing TTM and skin picking severity, respectively. These measures are brief and have demonstrated adequate psychometric properties in assessing BFRB severity (at least with adults). For BFRBs other than hair pulling or skin picking, we recommend that the MGH-HS be reworded to assess the target behavior. For tic disorders, we recommend using the YGTSS.

Other methods of assessment, while valuable, are less likely to be useful in clinical settings. Direct observation is often expensive, time consuming, and difficult to coordinate. In addition it is our clinical experience that children with TTM are unlikely to engage in the behavior when they are being recorded. Product assessment is also sometimes used in evaluating TTM by having children collect the number of hairs they pull and return the pulled hairs to the therapists. Although such a method may be useful and may even lead to rapid and transient symptom reduction, it is often difficult to get participants to collect the hair, for reasons of forgetting or embarrassment. Likewise, it is often difficult to determine whether or not a child is actually collecting all of his/her hair, even if he/she is faithfully trying to do so.

DEVELOPMENTAL CONSIDERATIONS

Perhaps the most important developmental consideration in the assessment of habit disorders is the understanding that all of the BFRB child- and clinician-report instruments were developed with adult samples. Psychometric data on BFRB assessments in children are not available. For this reason, care must be taken in administering and interpreting measures such as the MGH-HS and the SPS.

Second, it is very important to include information from both the child and his/her parents during the assessment. Due to the discrete nature of many habit behaviors, parent reports may be unreliable, especially when assessing nonvisible tics, such as stomach tensing, toe-curling, and subtle vocal tics. Third, it is our clinical experience that younger children with BFRBs may be less reactive to videotaped observation than adolescents with the same behaviors. For this reason, videotaped observation may be a more viable option when assessing younger children.

Fourth, when conducting self-monitoring assignments, it is often difficult for the younger children to provide the antecedent and consequent information unless the procedure is made very simple. In such cases, we recommend modifying the monitoring forms to provide simple forced choices or to forego the structured functional monitoring in favor of a more simple frequency count. In such cases, it may be useful to have parents conduct function-based monitoring.

Finally, when conducting assessments with children and with even adolescents, it is important to understand the child's perspective on his or her habit disorder. Often, it may be the case that the parents see a problem where the child sees none. In such cases, it is necessary for the therapist not to create a greater problem for the child than currently exists by conducting an overly intrusive assessment process with a child who sees no problem.

ASSESSMENT, CONCEPTUALIZATION, AND TREATMENT PLANNING

Following a comprehensive assessment as just described, the case is conceptualized within a behavioral framework. Four specific factors are considered when formulating a conceptualization and subsequently developing a treatment strategy. First, in some cases, there is an obvious underlying and treatable physical concern. In cases where a treatable medical condition has been identified, medical management should be conducted before beginning behavior therapy. Second, attempts are made to determine and modify the environmental variables that either maintain or exacerbate the frequency of the repetitive behavior. For example, if the assessment reveals that being in a specific situation (e.g., watching television or playing video games) exacerbates tics, then an attempt is made to limit a child's exposure to such situations. Likewise, if it reveals that a parent consistently draws attention to a child's tics and it is believed that doing so may reinforce the behavior, then the parent's behavior should be modified. Also, if it is revealed that certain items make the repetitive behavior more likely to occur (e.g., presence of mirrors or tweezers make hair pulling more likely), then these stimuli can be removed from the environment. Such techniques have typically been called *stimulus control* techniques.

Third, as implied in the label *habit disorders*, tic disorders and BFRBs often involve a pattern of habitual motor behavior with no clear behavioral function. To disrupt this pattern, habit reversal is often used and has become a mainstay of behavioral interventions for the disorders. Habit reversal is a multicomponent treatment procedure developed by Azrin and Nunn (1973) to treat habits and tics. The treatment has been simplified and now includes three primary components: awareness training, competing-response training, and social support (Woods, Twohig, Flessner, & Roloff, 2003). Awareness training teaches the child to be aware of occurrences of the target behavior (e.g., tics, hair pulling, skin picking) by teaching the child to detect early warning signs of the behavior. In competing response training, the child is taught to engage in a competing response that is incompatible with the target behavior (e.g., clenching a fist instead of pulling hair). Friends or family members are recruited to provide social support, which includes praise for correct implementation of the competing response and reminders to use the competing response when the child misses an occurrence of the target behavior.

A final factor to consider is the negative reinforcement function that many tics and BFRBs seem to have (i.e., behavior alleviates an unpleasant urge or emotion). A treatment strategy that has seen more recent attention involves the inclusion of specific therapeutic strategies designed to actually reduce or modify the impact of the aversive internal private experiences (e.g., premonitory urge, cognition, or tension) that are reduced after the repetitive behavior. Typically, this has included procedures such as relaxation training and cognitive restructuring (Deckersbach, Wilhelm, Keuthen, Baer, & Jenike, 2002), but recent research has begun to use acceptance-based procedures for the same effect (Twohig & Woods, 2004). Unfortunately, none of this work has been done with children.

CASE STUDY

IDENTIFICATION AND PRESENTING COMPLAINTS

What follows is a brief case description of Katie and the assessment conducted by her therapist to establish a diagnosis of TTM and to plan for treatment implementation.

Katie is a 12-year-old Caucasian female who presented at the clinic due to concern about her hair pulling problem. Katie's mother indicated that Katie's developmental milestones had been reached appropriately. Both Katie and her mother denied any history of past physical or sexual abuse, and Katie's mother reported no previous history of mental health concerns in her family but did report that her husband frequently played with his hair. Katie and her mother agreed that Katie did well at school, had two best friends, and got along well with others. They also stated that Katie put a tremendous amount of pressure on herself to do well. After obtaining a brief developmental history, a functional assessment interview was conducted.

HISTORY AND PEER AND FAMILY ISSUES

During the interview, Katie's mother reported that Katie began pulling at age 8, shortly after she had been burned in a hair-styling incident. Katie mentioned that she only pulled from her scalp and eyebrows, and her mother confirmed this fact. There was visible hair loss on both areas. Her eyebrows were absent except for a few hairs, and there was a 2-inch-diameter patch of very thin hair on the crown of her head.

Katie noted that she pulled the same way each time. When probed further, Katie indicated that she only pulled when at home and never pulled in front of others. Katie described that she usually pulled when sitting in her favorite chair and only used her fingers. She reported being unaware of the pulling when it was occurring. On occasion, Katie noted pulling while watching television or reading a book, but she was still unaware that it was happening ("Sometimes when I watch TV I lose my hair, but, when that happens, it is like that hair just falls out. I don't pull it on purpose."). When probed further, Katie noted that she occasionally pulled before bedtime, at which time she had thoughts such as "I have a lot of stuff to do at school tomorrow" and "I have a test that is going to be really hard. I should have studied more." During these times, Katie reported feeling very tense and stated that pulling helps calm her down. Other than these vague descriptions of school-related tension or anxiety, Katie did not report specific cognitions about hair. Having obtained a comprehensive picture of where, when, and how Katie pulled her hair, the therapist proceeded to ask questions about the consequences of the pulling.

BEHAVIORAL ASSESSMENT RESULTS

Two consequences seemed significant with respect to Katie's pulling. First, after she pulled while sitting in her chair, she reported often finding herself stroking the hair against her face, suggesting a tactile reinforcement function. Second, as stated earlier, when she was anxious or tense about school, these feelings would dissipate during the pulling episode, suggesting a negative reinforcement function.

Katie was unable to estimate the longest period of time she had gone without pulling, but her mother noted that Katie's hair "seemed to grow quite a bit during the summer." Further questioning revealed that she pulled very infrequently or did not pull at all during the summer break. Katie's mother made mention that she frequently colored her daughter's hair to make bald spots less noticeable, styled her hair in a particular fashion, and applied eyeliner to Katie's eyebrows during the school year, "to prevent any teasing from other children." Katie denied ever being teased by her peers, but upon further inquiry it became apparent that Katie had experienced some social and academic impairment from her pulling. Katie noted that she did not study as much as she should have because of her pulling ("Instead of studying when I get anxious about school, I end up pulling."). Katie's mother noted that Katie was no longer as active as she was prior to the noticeable hair loss and that although she still socialized with friends, it occurred less frequently.

To further assess Katie's mental health concerns, the Diagnostic Interview Schedule for Children (DISC) was administered. Information obtained from the DISC did not point to any additional mental health concerns and her mother reported that a dermatologist had ruled out an underlying medical cause. Based on information obtained from the clinical interview and the DISC, Katie was given a diagnosis of Trichotillomania. After the initial interview and assessment were completed, a feedback session was scheduled, at which time Katie and her mother were provided with several treatment recommendations.

CONCEPTUALIZATION AND TREATMENT RECOMMENDATIONS

The clinical assessment of Katie's hair pulling revealed that she often felt anxious about school, and it appeared as though this anxiety exacerbated Katie's pulling (in both severity and frequency). Katie also pulled her hair while watching television, but these episodes were more habitual or automatic in nature and appeared to have a tactile reinforcing function. Based on the information collected, a three-pronged approach to treatment was initiated. First, to disrupt the habitual motor pattern, habit reversal (HR) was recommended. In addition, to decrease the tactile reinforcing value of the pulled hair, it was recommended that Katie carry a tactile stimulation replacement object (e.g., koosh ball) in high-risk situations (e.g., watching TV, in bed at night) that she could manipulate as needed. Finally, an attempt was made to teach Katie behavioral relaxation skills, and additional cognitive change procedures were used to target her overly perfectionistic academic expectations. These procedures were recommended as a strategy for reducing the anxiety/tension antecedent that seemed to contribute to at least some of the pulling.

SUMMARY

Habit disorders are a broad class of disorders characterized by repetitive, unwanted behaviors that cause impairment in functioning. These disorders typically develop in childhood and often persist into adulthood. The two primary classes of habit disorders are the tic disorders and BFRBs. Within these classes there is considerable variability in symptom presentation and impairment. A thorough assessment of habit disorders in children should include an evaluation of the following domains: ascertaining a diagnosis, assessing the physical dimensions and severity of the target behavior, investigating public and private events that may maintain the behavior, determining the level of impairment in physical, social, and familial functioning, and screening for the presence of comorbid conditions. A multifaceted assessment employing clinical interviews, child and parent reports, and direct observation measures is well suited to accomplish this goal. Structured and unstructured clinical and diagnostic interviews are an invaluable resource for gathering information regarding the background, topography, and severity of the condition and help to ensure an appropriate diagnosis. Child- and self-report instruments allow for more detailed information about the nature and severity of the target behavior, and direct observation provides an objective record of the frequency and severity of the condition without relying on retrospective accounts. The discussion outlines a variety of available procedures and measures (with varying levels of psychometric support) that will aid the examiner in conducting a thorough yet feasible assessment that will guide case conceptualization and treatment strategy.

REFERENCES AND RESOURCES

American Psychiatric Association. (2000). *Diagnostic and statistical manual of mental disorders* (4th ed., Text Rev.). Washington, DC: Author.

Azrin, N. H., & Nunn, R. G. (1973). Habit Reversal: A method of eliminating nervous habits and tics. *Behaviour Research and Therapy, 11,* 619–628.

Budman, C. L., Bruun, R. D., Park, K. S., Lesser, M., & Olson, M. (2000). Explosive outbursts in children with Tourette's Disorder. *Journal of the American Academy of Child and Adolescent Psychiatry, 39,* 1270–1276.

Budman, C. L., Rockmore, L., Stokes, J., & Sossin, M. (2003). Clinical phenomenology of episodic rage in children with Tourette syndrome. *Journal of Psychosomatic Research, 55,* 59–65.

Carter, A. S., O'Donnell, D. A., & Shultz, R. T. (2000). Social and emotional adjustment in children affected with Gilles de la Tourette's syndrome: Associations with ADHD and family functioning. *Journal of Child Psychology and Psychiatry, 41,* 215–223.

Casati, J., Toner, B. B., & Yu, B. (2000). Psychosocial issues for women with trichotillomania. *Comprehensive Psychiatry, 41,* 344–351.

Champion, L. M., Fulton, W. A., & Shady, G. A. (1988). Tourette syndrome and social functioning in a Canadian population. *Neuroscience and Biobehavioral Reviews, 12,* 255–257.

Chappell, P. B., McSwiggan-Hardin, M. T., Scahill, L., Rubenstein, M., et al. (1994). Videotape tic counts in the assessment of Tourette's syndrome: Stability, reliability, and validity. *Journal of the American Academy of Child and Adolescent Psychiatry, 33,* 386–393.

Christenson, G. A., Mackenzie, T. B., & Mitchell, J. E. (1991). Characteristics of 60 adult chronic hair pullers. *American Journal of Psychiatry, 148,* 365–370.

Christenson, G. A., & Mansueto, C. S. (1999). Trichotillomania: Descriptive characteristics and phenomenology. In D. J. Stein, G. A. Christenson, & E. Hollander (Eds.), *Trichotillomania* (pp. 1–42). Washington, DC: American Psychiatric Press.

Christenson, G. A., Pyle, R. L., & Mitchell, J. E. (1991). Estimated lifetime prevalence of trichotillomania in college students. *Journal of Clinical Psychiatry, 52,* 415–417.

Christenson, G. A., Ristvedt, S. L., & Mackenzie, T. B. (1993). Identification of trichotillomania profiles. *Behaviour Research and Therapy, 31,* 315–320.

Cohen, D. J., Detlor, J., Young, J. G., & Shaywitz, B. A. (1980). Clonidine ameliorates Gilles de la Tourette syndrome. *Archives of General Psychiatry, 37,* 1350–1357.

Deckersbach, T., Wilhelm, S., Keuthen, N. J., Baer, L., & Jenike, M. A. (2002). Cognitive-behavior therapy for self-injurious skin picking: A case series. *Behavior Modification, 26,* 361–377.

Gaffney, G. R., Sieg, K., & Hellings, J. (1994). The MOVES: A self-rating scale for Tourette's syndrome. *Journal of Child and Adolescent Psychopharmacology, 4,* 269–280.

Goetz, C. G., Tanner, C. M., Wilson, R. S., & Shannon, K. M. (1987). A rating scale for Gilles de la Tourette's syndrome: Description, reliability, and validity data. *Neurology, 37,* 1542–1544.

Harcherik, D. F., Leckman, J. F., Deltor, J., & Cohen, D. J. (1984). A new instrument for clinical studies of Tourette syndrome. *Journal of the American Academy of Child Psychiatry, 23,* 153–160.

Hornsey, H., Banerjee, S., Zeitlin, H., & Robertson, M. (2001). The prevalence of Tourette syndrome in 3–14-year-olds in mainstream schools. *Journal of Child Psychology and Psychiatry, 42,* 1035–1039.

Hubka, G. B., Fulton, W. A., Shady, G. A., Champion, L. C., & Wand, R. (1988). Tourette syndrome: Impact on Canadian family functioning. *Neuroscience and Biobehavioral Reviews, 12,* 259–261.

Keuthen, N. J., Deckersbach, T., Wilhelm, S., Engelhard, I., Forker, A., O'Sullivan, R. L., et al. (2001). The Skin Picking Impact Scale (SPIS): Scale development and psychometric analyses. *Psychosomatics, 42,* 397–403.

Keuthen, N. J., O'Sullivan, R. L., Ricciardi, J. N., Shera, D., Savage, C. R., Borgmann, A. S., et al. (1995). The Massachusetts General Hospital (MGH) Hairpulling Scale: 1. Development and factor analysis. *Psychotherapy and Psychosomatics, 64,* 141–145.

Keuthen, N. J., Wilhelm, S., Deckersbach, T., Engelhard, I., Forker, A. E., Baer, L., & Jenike, M. A. (2001). The Skin Picking Scale (SPS): Scale construction and psychometric analyses. *Journal of Psychosomatic Research, 50,* 337–341.

Khalifa, N., & Von Knorring A. L. (2003). Prevalence of tic disorders and Tourette syndrome in a Swedish school population. *Developmental Medicine and Child Neurology, 45,* 315–319.

Kwak, C., Dat Vong, K., & Jankovik, J. (2003). Premonitory sensory phenomenon in Tourette's syndrome. *Movement Disorders, 18,* 1530–1533.

Leckman, J. F., King, R. A., & Cohen, D. J. (1999). Tics and tic disorders. In J. F. Leckman and D. J. Cohen (Eds.), *Tourette syndrome: Tics, obsessions, compulsions—developmental psychopathology and clinical care* (pp. 23–42). New York: John Wiley & Sons.

Leckman, J. F., Walker, D. E., & Cohen, D. J. (1993). Premonitory urges in Tourette's syndrome. *American Journal of Psychiatry, 150,* 98–102.

Leckman, J. F., Riddle, M. A., Hardin, M., Ort, S. I., Swartz, K. L., Stevenson, J., et al. (1989). The Yale Global Tic Severity Scale: Initial testing of a clinician-rated scale of tic severity. *American Academy of Child and Adolescent Psychiatry, 28,* 566–573.

Malatesta, V. J. (1990). An experimental assessment study of transient tic disorder. *Journal of Psychopathology and Behavioral Assessment, 12,* 219–232.

Matson, J. L., Rotatori, A. F., & Helsel, W. J. (1983). Development of a rating scale to measure social skills in children: The Matson evaluation of social skills with youngsters. *Behaviour Research & Therapy, 21,* 335–340.

McCarley, N. G., Spirrison, C. L., & Ceminsky, J. L. (2002). Hair pulling behavior reported by African American and non-African American college students. *Journal of Psychopathology and Behavioral Assessment, 24,* 139–144.

Miltenberger, R. G. (2004). *Behavior modification: Principles and procedures* (3rd ed.). Belmont, CA: Wadsworth-Thompson.

Miltenberger, R. G., Long, E. S., Rapp, J. T., Lumley, V., & Elliot, A. J. (1998). Evaluating the function of hair pulling: A preliminary investigation. *Behavior Therapy, 29,* 211–219.

O'Sullivan, R. L., Keuthen, N. J., Ricciardi, J. N., Shera, D., Savage, C. R., Borgmann, A. S., et al. (1995). The Massachusetts General Hospital (MGH) Hairpulling Scale: 2. Reliability and validity. *Psychotherapy and Psychosomatics, 64,* 146–148.

Phillips, M. R., Zaheer, S., & Drugas, G. T. (1998). Gastric trichobezoar: Case report and literature review. *Mayo Clinic Proceedings, 73,* 653–656.

Robertson, M. M. (2003). Diagnosing Tourette syndrome: Is it a common disorder? *Journal of Psychosomatic Research, 55,* 3–6.

Rothbaum, B. O., & Ninan, P. T. (1994). The assessment of trichotillomania. *Behavior Research and Therapy, 32,* 651–662.

Rothbaum, B. O., Shaw, L., Morris, R., & Ninan, P. T. (1993). Prevalence of trichotillomania in a college freshman population. *Journal of Clinical Psychiatry, 54,* 72.

Shapiro, E., Shapiro, A. K., Fulop, G., Hubbard, M., Mandali, J., Nordlie, J., & Phillips, R. A. (1989). Controlled study of haloperidol, pimozide, and placebo for the treatment of Gilles de la Tourette's syndrome. *Archives of General Psychiatry, 46,* 722–730.

Silva, R. R., Munoz, D. M., Barickman, J., & Friedhoff, A. J. (1995). Environmental factors related to fluctuations of symptoms in children and adolescents with Tourette's disorder. *Journal of Child Psychology and Psychiatry, 36,* 305–312.

Soriano, J. L., O'Sullivan, R. L., Baer, L., Phillips, K. A., McNally, R. J., & Jenike, M. A. (1996). Trichotillomania and self-esteem: A survey of 62 female hair pullers. *Journal of Clinical Psychiatry, 57,* 77–82.

Stanley, M. A., Breckenridge, J. K., Snyder, A. G., & Novy, D. M. (1999). Clinician-rated measures of hairpulling: A preliminary psychometric evaluation. *Journal of Psychopathology and Behavioral Assessment, 21,* 157–170.

Stein, R. E. K., & Reissman, C. K. (1980). The development of an impact-on-family scale: Preliminary findings. *Medical Care, 18,* 465–472.

Swedo, S. E., Leonard, H. L., Rapoport, J. L., Lenane, M. C., Goldberger, L. L., & Cheslow, D. L. (1989). A double-blind comparison of clomipramine and desipramine in the treatment of trichotillomania (hair pulling). *New England Journal of Medicine, 321,* 497–501.

Teng, E. J., Woods, D. W., Twohig, M. P., & Marcks, B. A. (2002). Body-focused repetitive behavior problems: Prevalence in a nonreferred population and differences in perceived somatic activity. *Behavior Modification, 26,* 340–360.

Twohig, M. P., & Woods, D. W. (2001). Habit reversal as a treatment for chronic skin picking in typically developing adult male siblings. *Journal of Applied Behavior Analysis, 34,* 217–220.

Twohig, M. P., & Woods, D. W. (2004). A preliminary investigation of acceptance and commitment therapy and habit reversal as a treatment for trichotillomania. *Behavior Therapy, 35,* 803–820.

Wilhelm, S., Keuthen, N. J., Deckersbach, T., Engelhard, I. M., Forker, A. E., Baer, L., et al. (1999). Self-injurious skin picking: Clinical characteristics and comorbidity. *Journal of Clinical Psychiatry, 60,* 454–459.

Winchel, R. M., Jones, J. A., Molcho, A., Parsons, B., Stanley, B., & Stanley, M. (1992). The Psychiatric Institute Trichotillomania Scale (PITS). *Psychopharmacology Bulletin, 28,* 463–476.

Woods, D. W. (2002). *Premonitory Urge Scale.* Unpublished manuscript.

Woods, D. W., Fuqua, R. W., & Outman, R. C. (1999). Evaluating the social acceptability of individuals with habit disorders: The effects of frequency, topography, and gender manipulation. *Journal of Psychopathology and Behavioral Assessment, 21,* 1–18.

Woods, D. W., Himle, M. B., Smerz, J., & Osmon, D. (in press). The use of the Impact-on-Family Scale in children with Tourette syndrome. *Child and Family Behavior Therapy.*

Woods, D. W., Miltenberger, R. G., & Flach, A. D. (1996). Habits, tics, and stuttering: Prevalence and relation to anxiety and somatic awareness. *Behavior Modification, 20,* 216–225.

Woods, D. W., Miltenberger, R. G., & Lumley, V. A. (1996). Sequential application of major habit-reversal components to treat motor tics in children. *Journal of Applied Behavior Analysis, 29,* 483–493.

Woods, D. W., Piacentini, J., Himle, M. B., & Chang, S. (2003, May). *Evaluating the reliability and validity of a videotaped observation system for tics associated with Tourette's syndrome.* Poster presented at the annual meeting of the Association for Behavior Analysis, San Francisco.

Woods, D. W., Piacentini, J., Himle, M. B., & Chang, S. (in press) Premonitory Urge for Tics Scale (PUTS): Initial psychometric results and examination of the premonitory urge phenomenon in children with tic disorders. *Journal of Developmental & Behavioral Pediatrics.*

Woods, D. W., Twohig, M. P., Flessner, C. A., & Roloff, T. E. (2003). Treatment of vocal tics in children with Tourette syndrome: Investigating the efficacy of habit reversal. *Journal of Applied Behavior Analysis, 36,* 109–112.

Woods, D. W., Watson, T. S., Wolfe, E., Twohig, M. P., & Friman, P. C. (2001). Analyzing the influence of tic-related talk on vocal and motor tics in children with Tourette's syndrome. *Journal of Applied Behavior Analysis, 34,* 353–356.

PART III

SPECIAL ISSUES

22

CHILD ABUSE ASSESSMENT

DEBORAH WISE

School of Professional Psychology
Pacific University
Portland, Oregon

INTRODUCTION

Behavioral assessment of child abuse can be a complex process, for several reasons: child abuse assessment may be undertaken for different and potentially conflicting purposes; child abuse assessment may address psychological abuse, physical abuse, sexual abuse, neglect, or a combination of all of these types of abuse; and child abuse assessment may address a diverse range of symptoms. Prior to initiating a child abuse assessment, a clinician should clarify the goals of the assessment, be familiar with legal definitions of child abuse, and be knowledgeable about potential outcomes of different types of child abuse.

Assessment of child abuse is undertaken either to evaluate allegations of physical abuse, sexual abuse, and neglect, so as to contribute to legal decision making, or to determine psychological adjustment following abuse experiences. Given these potentially divergent purposes, it is essential to clarify the purpose of each child abuse assessment and the consequent role of the evaluator at the outset of the evaluation process (American Professional Society on the Abuse of Children [APSAC], 1997). Goals of forensic evaluations of child abuse include offering an opinion as to whether or not abuse has occurred, determining a child's competency to stand trial, and addressing a child's credibility related to testifying (Myers, 1998). On the other hand, goals of therapeutic evaluations include evaluating a child's level of psychological adjustment, informing treatment planning, and determining the effectiveness of treatments (Friedrich, 2002). Due to the potential ethical conflicts inherent in dual forensic and therapeutic roles, these roles should be kept separate (American Psychological Association [APA], 2003; Myers, 2002).

Lack of clarity and consistency of definitions of child abuse adds to the complexity of child abuse assessment. Child abuse may comprise several distinct incidents and may reflect different types of abuse (including psychological, physical, and sexual abuse) and neglect. Moreover, definitions of various types of child abuse vary widely. Child abuse is legally defined in each state, and therefore definitions of child abuse frequently vary between states and across studies of child abuse. It is important for clinicians to become familiar with the legal statutes of the states in which they practice so that they can understand the parameters of child abuse and their roles as mandated reporters. For the purpose of this chapter, child abuse will be defined in a manner consistent with the American Professional Society on the Abuse of Children (Berliner & Elliot, 2002; Hart, Brassard, Binggeli, & Davidson, 2002; Erickson & Egeland, 2002; Kolko, 2002).

Psychological maltreatment includes repeated acts of omission or commission that convey the message that caretakers do not value the child (Hart et al., 2002). Given the complexity of defining and identifying psychological maltreatment and the frequent overlap of psychological maltreatment with other modes of abuse (Binggeli, Hart, & Brassard, 2001), psychological abuse will not be addressed in this chapter (see Binggeli et al., 2001 for a review of the assessment of child psychological abuse).

Child physical abuse includes injury or risk of injury as a result of being hit by a hand or object or being kicked, shaken, thrown, burned, or stabbed by a parent or caretaker (Sedlak & Broadhurst, 1996). Child physical abuse is often the easiest type of maltreatment to identify because it may be evidenced by physical injury.

Child sexual abuse includes sexual activity with a child without the child's consent or when a significant difference in age, size or developmental stage precludes consent (Berliner & Elliot, 2002). Child sexual abuse includes sexual contact events, such as penetration and fondling the child's or the perpetrator's genitalia, and noncontact events, including exposure and voyeurism.

Child neglect is the failure by the caregiver to provide needed, age-appropriate care, given adequate financial resources (U.S. Department of Health and Human Services, Administration on Children, Youth and Families, 2003). There are several subtypes of neglect, including physical, emotional, medical, mental health, and educational neglect (Erickson & Egeland, 2002). Physical neglect is the failure to protect a child from physical harm or to provide adequate food, shelter, or clothing. Emotional neglect is the failure of a caretaker to provide for the basic emotional needs of the child. Although emotional neglect is clearly difficult to substantiate, this type of abuse can be devastating. Emotional neglect is implicated as one of the primary causes of nonorganic failure to thrive, which connotes lack of appropriate growth in infants (Iwaniac, 1997). Medical neglect is the failure to meet a child's medical needs, such as withholding immunizations, medications, surgeries, or other medical interventions (Erickson & Egeland, 2002). Mental health neglect refers to lack of compliance with mental health interventions. Finally, educational neglect includes failure to ensure school attendance.

Prevalence of these various types of abuse is surprisingly high. Based on reports to child protective services (CPS) agencies in the United States during 2001, approximately 903,000 children experienced or were at risk for child abuse and/or neglect (U.S. Department of Health and Human Services, Administration on Children, Youth and Families, 2003). Among these reports of child abuse, 59% of victims suffered neglect (including medical neglect), 19% were physically abused, 10% were sexually abused, and 7% were emotionally or psychologically abused. Given the high prevalence of child abuse, it is likely that clinicians will have some involvement in child abuse assessment at some point in their careers.

Unfortunately, actual rates of abuse may be much higher than the statistics reported by the U.S. Department of Health and Human Services, because not all suspected cases of abuse are reported to CPS (Finkelhor, Hotaling, Lewis, & Smith, 1990). In the Third National Incidence Study of Child Abuse and Neglect (NIS-3), data on child abuse prevalence was gathered from child protective service agencies and from community professionals (Sedlak & Broadhurst, 1996). Based on this survey, an estimated 1,553,800 children in the United States were abused or neglected in 1993. Among these numbers, approximately 381,700 were physically abused, 217,700 were sexually abused, 338,900 were physically neglected, and 212,800 were emotionally neglected. Given the likelihood that the prevalence of child abuse is higher than reports of abuse to CPS, teachers, therapists, doctors, and caregivers, the skillful assessment of child abuse is particularly important.

The sequelae of child abuse also highlight the importance of careful child abuse assessment. The impact of child abuse can be devastating. According to reports to CPS in 2001, 1300 children died from maltreatment; among these deaths, 26% were due to physical abuse and 35% were due to neglect (U.S. Department of Health and Human Services, Administration on Children, Youth and Families, 2003). Moreover, child abuse is associated with a wide range of psychological symptomatology. Physical abuse is associated with various difficulties, including physical injuries, heightened aggression, oppositionality, delinquency, substance abuse, depression, Posttraumatic Stress Disorder, academic achievement deficits, and interpersonal difficulties (Boney-McCoy & Finklehor, 1995; Eckenrode, Laird, & Doris, 1993; Hotaling, Straus, & Lincoln, 1990; Kaplan, Pelcovitz, Salzinger, Mandel, & Weiner, 1998; Kilpatrick, Saunders, & Smith, 2003; Kolko, Moser, & Weldy, 1990; Pelcovitz, Kaplan, Goldenberg, & Mandel, 1994; Rogosch, Cicchetti, & Abre, 1995; Sedlack & Broadhurst, 1996; Wolfe, Wekerle, Reitzel-Jaffe, & Lefebvre, 1998). Child sexual abuse is associated with a wide range of emotional and behavioral problems; however, Posttraumatic Stress Disorder and sexual-acting-out behaviors are among the most consistently reported (Kendall-Tackett, Williams, & Finkelhor, 1993; Paolucci, Genius, & Violato, 2001). Other sequelae of child sexual abuse include depression, anxiety, low self-esteem, running away, eating disorders, substance use, and academic and social problems (Boney-McCoy & Finkelhor, 1995; Hibbard, Ingersoll, & Orr, 1990; Kendall-Tackett et al., 1993; Kilpatrick et al., 2003;

McLeer, Deblinger, Atkins, Foa, & Ralphe, 1988; McLeer et al., 1998; Mannarino & Cohen, 1996a, 1996b). Neglect has been associated with attachment difficulties, attention problems, aggression, internalizing problems, social skills deficits, language delays, poor grades, and failure to thrive (Erickson & Egeland, 1996, 2002; Iwaniac, 1997; Katz, 1992; Kendall-Tackett & Eckenrode, 1996). It is important to be familiar with the sequelae of child abuse because a careful assessment of these domains of functioning should be part of evaluation processes when assessing the impact of child abuse.

Although a wide range of emotional, behavioral and physical symptoms has been observed among groups of children with histories of child abuse, it is important to retain an idiographic approach to child abuse assessment. Many symptoms that are commonly associated with abuse histories can also be observed among nonabused populations (Friedrich et al., 2001; Gordon, Schroeder, & Hawk, 1993). For example, although sexual acting out is commonly associated with experiences of sexual abuse (Kendall-Tackett et al., 1993), many sexual-acting-out behaviors are observed among nonabused populations (Friedrich et al.). Moreover, children who have experienced child abuse may also manifest symptoms that are commonly observed among nonabused populations. For example, although a child who has experienced child sexual abuse may have sleep difficulties, this symptom is commonly observed among children who have not been sexually abused (Horn & Dollinger, 1995). To further complicate the issue, many children who have experienced abuse appear to be asymptomatic (Caffaro-Rouget, Lang, & van Santen, 1989; Conte & Scheurman, 1987; Finkelhor & Berliner, 1995; Kendall-Tackett et al., 1993; Mannarino & Cohen, 1986). Finally, regardless of symptom presentation, children who have experienced child abuse may not admit to abuse experiences. For example, a child who has experienced sexual abuse may not admit to abuse experiences because of embarrassment, because of the feared consequences of admitting to the abuse, or because she does not have the vocabulary to accurately describe her experience. Clearly, an idiographic approach is essential for a reliable and valid child abuse assessment.

In summary, child abuse assessment can be a complex task. In initiating child abuse evaluations, clinicians should clearly define evaluation goals and their roles with respect to evaluations and be knowledgeable about definitions of child abuse as given by state statutes, laws on child abuse reporting, common sequelae of child abuse, and the idiographic aspects of a child's presentation.

ASSESSMENT STRATEGIES

Given the high prevalence of various types of maltreatment and the broad range of sequelae associated with child abuse, it is important to conduct comprehensive psychological assessments that incorporate multiple domains of functioning, use multiple informants, and employ multiple assessment measures. No single test will indicate child abuse or adequately assess the impact of child abuse, and therefore it is important to gather information from a variety of sources (APSAC, 1997; American Academy of Child and Adolescent Psychiatry [AACAP], 1988).

MULTIPLE DOMAINS

Child abuse may impact many domains of functioning. Given that children who have experienced abuse may have functional difficulties at school, at home, and among peers, it is important to assess each of these domains to obtain an accurate understanding of current functioning.

Across these domains, a child's functioning may be impacted by risk and protective factors among the child, the child's family, and related systems (Davies, 2004; Samaroff & Fiese, 2000; Werner, 2000). Certain factors may heighten the risk or impact of child maltreatment, whereas protective factors may reduce the risk or impact of child maltreatment. Risk factors include the child's vulnerabilities, such as mental retardation, medical problems, and lack of coping skills; the parent's vulnerabilities, such as impaired parenting due to familial conflict, psychopathology, substance abuse, inadequate parenting skills, and parental history of maltreatment; and the family system's vulnerabilities due to socioeconomic and institutional factors, such as poverty and exposure to community violence. Protective factors include the child's strengths, such as health, intelligence, and coping skills; the parent's strengths, such as household rules, structure and close monitoring of the child, stable familial relationships, appropriate expectations of the child, and good problem-solving skills; and the family system's strengths due to socioeconomic and institutional factors, such as economic resources, access to health care services, consistent employment, adequate housing, and the presence of an adequate social support network. For example, facing skeptical and adversarial attorneys or reliving abuse experiences in a court context may exacerbate a child's experience of stress and therefore may serve as a risk factor for deterioration in functioning (Higgins, 1988). Stress related to court experiences may be expressed differently across domains of functioning. Conversely, social support is associated with improved functioning (Everson, Hunter, Runyon, Edelsohn, & Coulter, 1991), and may comprise a protective factor in the child's functioning. A comprehensive assessment of child abuse should include an assessment of risk and protective factors across the child's domains of functioning.

A careful assessment of risk and protective factors is important in the development of treatment priorities. Treatment priorities can be conceptualized as a multistage process (Azar & Wolfe, 1998). First, to ensure the welfare of the child, risk factors that reflect ongoing threats to a child's physical and emotional safety should be assessed and addressed throughout the child abuse assessment process. Second, treatment goals should be developed so as to bolster protective factors and diminish risk factors. Assessing risk and protective factors can be important in the development of interventions for children who have experienced abuse

(Kolko, 1996). It is particularly important to assess risk and protective factors among the child, her family, and her community context because transactions between the child and her environment impact the course of development, and therefore the effects of these risk and protective factors may be far reaching (Cicchetti & Olson, 1990; Davies, 2004; Sroufe, 1997). Clearly, regardless of the goal of the child abuse assessment, assessment of risk and protective factors should play a central role in the assessment process.

MULTIPLE INFORMANTS

Comprehensive information can best be obtained through gathering information from multiple informants (APSAC, 1997; AACAP, 1988; Kaufman, Jones, Stieglitz, Vitulano, & Mannarino, 1994; Sternberg, Lamb, & Dawud-Noursi, 1998; Stockhammer, Salzinger, Feldman, Mojica, & Primavera, 2001). Child protective services records and child, parent, teacher, and other records may all offer valuable information.

Child protective services (CPS) are an important source of information for child abuse assessment. CPS records typically contain information about child maltreatment, including descriptions of alleged abuse experiences, time frames of alleged abuse experiences, and identities of alleged perpetrators. However, many incidents of child abuse are not reported to CPS (Waldfogel, 1998), and CPS workers may not have gathered all of the information relevant to referral questions (Sternberg et al., 1998; Stockhammer et al., 2001). For example, CPS records may lack information about family risk factors, such as domestic violence and substance abuse (Stockhammer et al., 2001). Therefore, it is important to garner information from other sources as well.

Children are one of the most important sources of information about abuse history and impact (Lamb, 1994). Children are highly reliable reporters of abuse. In fact, only between 4.7% and 7.6% of allegations of child abuse are estimated to be false (Everson & Boat, 1989). To increase reliability of reports, children should be interviewed in a developmentally appropriate manner, ensuring that questions are short and open-ended and that the meaning of terminology is understood by children and interviewers (see Bourg et al., 1999, for a more comprehensive discussion of interviewing children).

Parents or caretakers are another important source of information about child maltreatment, and they may know critical information beyond what can be described by children or what is contained in CPS records (Kaufman et al., 1994). Therefore, parents should be asked about child symptomatology and abuse experiences.

For several reasons, disparities between parent and child reports of abuse and of current functioning have been widely observed in studies of maltreated children (Cohen & Mannarino, 1988; Kiser, Heston, Millsap, & Pruitt, 1991;

Mannarino, Cohen, Smith, & Moore-Motily, 1991; Tong, Oates, & McDowell, 1987; Wolfe, Gentile, & Wolfe, 1989). First, both children and parents may have conscious motivation for not providing accurate reports. For children, feelings of shame or embarrassment may impede the reporting of their abuse experiences. Similarly, threats of physical violence or familial hardship often accompany child abuse, and therefore children may be fearful of reporting information about abuse experiences or problems with current functioning. Parents, on the other hand, may themselves have played a role in perpetrating the abuse and therefore may be reluctant to describe details of child abuse or associated symptomatology. Second, developmental issues may yield dissimilarity among parent and child reports of abuse experiences and levels of functioning. Differences in parent and child reports may reflect the child's deficits in verbal competency rather than symptom differences. For example, young children may not have the vocabulary to accurately describe their experiences. Parents also may be better equipped to describe complex abstract concepts associated with sexual abuse, such as perceptions of responsibility and efforts to avoid thoughts; these concepts are essential to assessing abuse-related attributions and posttraumatic stress symptoms. Third, differential access to information of abuse experiences and symptoms may also result in disparities between parent and child reports. Parents may not be aware of all of the important information on abuse experiences or may have difficulty accurately assessing and describing their children's internal states, and this information is necessary to providing accurate diagnostic information. For children, avoidant symptoms associated with PTSD may contribute to denials of abuse or subjective distress. Finally, errors by interviewers may result in distortions of children's recall of abuse experiences (Ceci & Bruck, 1995). These factors may result in under- or overreporting of symptoms.

Teachers are another important source of information of child abuse because they have extensive opportunities to observe children's functioning throughout the course of the school day. For example, teachers may be more likely than parents to report internalizing behaviors (Stockhammer et al., 2001). Teachers also have the opportunity to observe numerous children throughout the day and, due to this basis for comparison, may be particularly able to identify behaviors that are notably different from the behavior of other children at the same developmental level.

Finally, a careful review of other documentation may also provide important clues to better understand a child's level of functioning and to assess child abuse allegations. Medical records may contain information of injuries, lead poisoning, malnutrition, sexually transmitted diseases, and pregnancy, which may indicate various forms of child abuse. However, given that abuse may have occurred despite an absence of medical findings, medical records are not conclusive sources of information (Lamb, 1994). School records may also contain important information on child abuse. Frequent school absences can be indicative of neglect, physical abuse, or sexual abuse. In addition, previous psychological evaluations may provide important sources of information about abuse histories and changes in levels of functioning.

MULTIPLE METHODS

Assessment of child abuse is usually based on a combination of strategies, including direct observation, interviews, and psychometric tests and questionnaires. Using multiple methods of assessment may provide a more accurate assessment of the presence of child abuse and a more comprehensive understanding of the impact of child abuse on current functioning.

Direct observation can provide important information on the quality of the relationship between parent and child. Observations of family relationships should be noted throughout the assessment process. Upon greeting families in waiting rooms, clinicians should observe the distance between family members, the quality of verbal and nonverbal communication among family members, parenting skills, a child's response to parental interventions, and affect among various family members. Careful attention to familial interactions should proceed throughout the assessment process. Direct observation may also include formal observations of family members engaged in various activities (Friedrich, 2002; Tuteur, Ewigman, Peterson, & Hosokawa, 1995). In addition to observations of families in clinical contexts, direct observation of family members in their natural environments is necessary to assess allegations of neglect (Iwaniec, 1995). During sessions in the family's home, careful observations should be made as to living conditions, physical and emotional care, interactions among family members, parental expectations of their children, child-rearing practices, support systems available to the family, and family stressors, including psychopathology, substance abuse, financial hardship, housing problems, and employment concerns. Observations of the quality of physical care should include a careful assessment of a child's clothing, hygiene, sleeping arrangements, nutrition, access to dangerous objects, level of supervision, and presence of adequate access to medical support.

As previously described, interviewing children, parents, and collateral sources, such as social workers and teachers, can be particularly valuable for child abuse assessment. During the interview process, information should be gathered about the child's developmental history, current symptoms, systemic risk and protective factors, parental and child attributions related to abuse, and the nature of abuse experiences. In particular, information of abuse type(s), duration, frequency, age of abuse onset and cessation, abuse severity, level of force or coercion to maintain secrecy and participation in abuse, context of the abuse disclosure, and repercussions of abuse allegations on child and family functioning should be addressed. Many of these factors have been shown to be associated with functioning following child abuse (Kendall-Tackett et al., 1993), and these factors may need to be addressed during treatment.

Interviewers should be sensitive to the likelihood that following child abuse allegations, families are overwhelmed. The child and her family members may feel intense guilt, shame, and fear during the child abuse assessment. Moreover, consequences of child abuse allegations, including separation from family members, court involvement, and significant changes in the financial stability of the family, may impact the functioning of the child and her family members and may affect initial perceptions of the assessment process. Awareness of these issues may facilitate empathy among interviewers and hence increase the likelihood of developing rapport with the child and her family members.

Although anatomically correct dolls are often used in interviewing procedures in cases of allegations of sexual abuse, their use is controversial. Sexualized play with anatomically correct dolls has been observed among presumably nonabused children, which may reflect exposure to sexual knowledge from sources other than sexual abuse experiences (Everson & Boat, 1990; Jampole & Weber, 1987). Although sexualized play with anatomically correct dolls does not provide definitive evidence of sexual abuse, this procedure is recognized as a means to assist children in communicating experiences (Lamb, 1994; Everson & Boat, 1990). Children can use anatomically correct dolls to describe their knowledge of body parts, show abuse experiences, cue recall of abuse experiences, spontaneously demonstrate sexual knowledge, or become comfortable discussing sexual knowledge and experiences (APSAC, 1995). Given that sexualized play with anatomically correct dolls is not conclusively suggestive of sexual abuse experiences, their use should be combined with other assessment methods.

Both interviewing and direct observation can provide important information for the functional analysis of problematic behaviors. Careful analysis of the antecedents and consequences of problematic behaviors should inform interventions. For example, defiance is not an uncommon behavior among children who have experienced physical abuse, sexual abuse, or neglect (e.g., Boney-McCoy & Finkelhor, 1995; Kaplan et al., 1998; Erickson & Egeland, 1996, 2002; Iwaniac, 1997). Defiance may include a child's failure to initiate behaviors requested by an adult within a reasonable amount of time, failure to sustain compliance with a command until it has been fulfilled, or failure to follow previously taught rules of conduct (Barkley, 1997). Antecedents to defiance, such as a parent's not providing adequate structure or attention to the child or lacking skills to effectively communicate directives, may promote such behavior. Moreover, consequences to a child's defiance, such as yelling at the child and ignoring defiance due to feelings of guilt in relation to the child's abuse experiences, may actually heighten the frequency of that behavior. Clearly, antecedents and consequences to problematic behavior may heighten the risk of child maltreatment and may play a role in the development and maintenance of symptoms associated with child abuse. For these reasons, functional analysis should play a key role in risk assessment and treatment planning.

In addition to direct observation and interviewing, psychological testing may facilitate child abuse assessment. As previously noted, there is no psychological profile that is indicative of child abuse, and variability exists in symptom presentation among children who have been abused (APSAC, 1997). Nonetheless, results from psychological testing may have several advantages as compared to interviews. Psychological measures are potentially less leading than interviews. In addition, psychological measures may be standardized, and therefore symptoms can be compared to other abused and nonabused populations for research and assessment purposes. Finally, psychological measures can be repeatedly readministered to children throughout treatment to assess changes in symptomatology in response to interventions. Therefore, use of psychological measures may provide information essential to develop and modify treatment plans during the course of treatment.

It is important to assess several facets of child abuse (National Research Council, 1993). Following is a description of some of the useful measures related to the assessment of child neglect, sexual abuse, and physical abuse. Because results from these tests alone cannot provide proof of child abuse, these measures should be part of a comprehensive assessment process in which data are gathered from multiple reporters and in which multiple methods are employed (APSAC, 1997; AACAP, 1988).

Measures of Risk and Abuse

Several psychological measures have been designed to address details of abuse incidents and factors that heighten the risk of child maltreatment. These include the Abuse Dimensions Inventory (ADI; Chaffin, Wherry, Newlin, Crutchfield, & Dykman, 1997), the Child Abuse Potential Inventory (Milner, 1986), the Child Well-Being Scales (Magura & Moses, 1986), the Ontario Child Neglect Index (Trocome, 1996), and the Parenting Stress Index (Abidin, 1995).

The Abuse Dimensions Inventory (ADI; Chaffin et al., 1997) is a 15-scale semistructured interview designed to be administered to nonoffending parents or caretakers and to provide a measure of abuse characteristics and severity of physical and sexual abuse. This measure was not developed for forensic investigations of child abuse allegations or for risk assessment, but rather as a means for gathering information on substantiated abuse incidents. With this measure, information is gathered on abuse severity, duration, number of most severely rated incidents, number of total incidents, abuser reactions to disclosures, use of force or coercion to gain submission or compliance, use of force or coercion to gain secrecy, and the role relationship of the abuser to the victim. This measure has adequate reliability and validity.

The Child Abuse Potential Inventory (CAPI; Milner, 1986) is a 160-item measure designed to be completed by CPS workers for the detection of physical abuse. Using the CAPI, CPS workers can note levels of distress, rigidity, and unhappiness and problems with the child, family, and others. Three validity scales in the CAP address lying, random responding, and inconsistency. Scales on this measure have excellent reliability and validity (Milner, Gold, Ayoub, & Jacewitz, 1984).

The Child Well-Being Scales (Magura & Moses, 1986) and the Ontario Child Neglect Index (Trocome, 1996) are measures of the type and severity of neglect. These measures are often administered by CPS workers. Both measures have adequate reliability and validity (Gaudin, Polansky, & Kilpatrick, 1992; Trocome).

Finally, the Parenting Stress Index (PSI; Abidin, 1995) is a 120-item self-report measure of stress among parents of children ages 12 and younger. A short form with only 36 items is also available. Questions on the PSI address risk factors associated with child maltreatment, including parental perceptions of the child, and parent and situational characteristics that may pose a risk to familial functioning. Child domain subscales include the child's perceived temperament (Adaptability, Demandingness, Mood, and Distractibility/Hyperactivity) and perceptions of the fit between parent and child (Reinforces Parent, and Acceptability). Parent domain subscales include parent characteristics (Depression, Sense of Competence, and Parental Attachment) and situational aspects of parenting (Relationship with Spouse, Social Isolation, Parental Health, and Role Restriction). Situational stressors that are unrelated to the parent–child relationship are reflected by the Total Stress Scale. The PSI has good reliability and validity and can be used to identify risk factors for both child abuse assessment and treatment planning.

Overall, these measures can provide important information for forensic evaluations, risk assessment, or treatment planning. However, these measures do not adequately address a child's current functioning, an aspect of child abuse assessment that is essential for treatment planning.

Measures of the Child's Functioning

Standardized behavior problems checklists can provide a thorough overview of various domains of functioning. Given the wide range of symptoms that have been observed among children who have been abused, broadband measures are particularly helpful in providing information necessary to determine treatment needs. However, broadband measures do not provide adequate detail about symptoms that are often displayed by children who have experienced child abuse, such as Posttraumatic Stress Disorder or sexual-acting-out behaviors (Kendall-Tackett et al., 1993; Paolucci et al., 2001). In addition, other facets of functioning, such as cognitive attributions, have been associated with symptomatology following child abuse (Mannarino & Cohen, 1996a, 1996b; Wolfe, Sas, & Wekerle, 1994; Taska & Feiring, 2000). Thus, for the purposes of treatment planning, comprehensive child abuse assessments should address each of these facets of functioning. Following is a description of some of the measures that are widely used in the context of child abuse assessment.

The Child Behavior Checklist, a broadband measure of symptoms, is a checklist of internalizing and externalizing behaviors among children ages 2–18 (CBCL; Achenbach, 1991a). The CBCL provides a broad array of information on problems in the parent–child relationship, school behaviors, and developmental delays. Although efforts have been made to develop a PTSD scale from the CBCL, this scale has poor concurrent and discriminant validity (Ruggiero & McLeer, 2000). Nonetheless, given the range of behavioral disturbances that has been observed among children who have been abused, this measure may provide information important for treatment planning. For children ages 11 and older, a self-report version is available (Youth Self-Report; Achenbach, 1991c). To access information about the child's functioning in school, a version to be completed by the child's teachers is also available (Teacher's Report Form; Achenbach, 1991b).

Given prevalence of posttraumatic stress symptoms among children who have experienced abuse, information on these symptoms also should be gathered (Pelcovitz et al., 1994; Kendall-Tackett et al., 1993; Paolucci et al., 2001). The Trauma Symptom Checklist for Children (TSCC; Briere, 1996) is a 54-item self-report instrument for children ages 8–16 designed to measure posttraumatic distress and related symptomatology. The TSCC includes questions about sexual abuse experiences; the TSCC-A is an alternate form of this measure that excludes questions about sexual abuse experiences. The TSCC has two validity scales and six clinical scales that measure anxiety, depression, posttraumatic stress symptoms, anger, dissociation, and sexual concerns. The TSCC is standardized, has adequate reliability and validity, and is sensitive to changes across the course of treatment (Lanktree & Briere, 1995). Therefore, the use of the TSCC is particularly helpful in treatment planning.

Sexual-acting-out behaviors are common among children with histories of sexual abuse, and therefore the assessment of these behaviors is particularly important in cases of child sexual abuse (Friedrich et al., 2001; Kendall-Tackett et al., 1993). The Child Sexual Behavior Inventory (CSBI; Friedrich, 1997) is a 38-item measure in which parents of children ages 2–18 respond to questions about sexual behaviors during the previous 6 months. This measure addresses boundary problems, exhibitionism, gender role behavior, self-stimulation, sexual anxiety, sexual interest, sexual intrusiveness, sexual knowledge, and voyeuristic behavior and yields information on behaviors that are common and uncommon among nonabused populations. It is important to note that although sexually abused children commonly display unusual sexual-acting-out behaviors, these behaviors may also be due to exposure to sexual material rather than to sexual abuse (Elliot, O'Donohue, & Nickerson, 1993). This measure has good reliability and validity (Friedrich et al.).

Symptomatology among children who have experienced child abuse may be moderated by cognitive attributions. For example, among sexually abused children and adolescents, self-blame has been associated with heightened depression, anxiety, posttraumatic stress symptoms, and self-esteem problems (Mannarino & Cohen, 1996a, 1996b; Taska & Feiring, 2000; Wolfe et al., 1994). Therefore, careful assessment of cognitive attributions associated with child abuse experiences can be important for case conceptualization and treatment planning purposes. Two measures of cognitive attributions have been developed to address cognitive attributions associated with sexual abuse experiences. The Children's

Impact of Traumatic Events Scales—Revised (CITES-R; Wolfe, Gentile, Michienzi, Sas, & Wolfe, 1991) was developed to assess abuse-specific attributions and perceptions of post-traumatic stress symptoms among children ages 8–16. This measure comprises 78 items that relate to 11 subscales, including Intrusive Thoughts, Avoidance, Negative Reactions by Others, Social Support, Self-Blame and Guilt, Dangerous World, Empowerment, Personal Vulnerability, Sexual Anxiety, and Eroticism. This instrument has demonstrated good validity and adequate reliability (Wolfe, 1996). The Children's Attributions and Perceptions Scale (CAPS; Mannarino, Cohen, & Berman, 1994) is another self-report measure designed to assess abuse-related attributions and perceptions among sexually abused children ages 7–14. The CAPS is an 18-item scale that yields information on perceptions of feeling different from peers, personal attributions for negative events, perceived credibility, and interpersonal trust. Because these types of attributions are often targeted in therapy, this measure is appropriate for measuring treatment change.

In summary, gathering information from multiple reporters, addressing multiple domains of functioning, and employing multiple methods of assessment is the ideal approach to child abuse assessment for case conceptualization and treatment planning purposes. Using a combination of assessment methods may increase the likelihood of addressing the important facets of child abuse assessment, including current risk issues, current symptomatology, developmental history, and abuse-specific and other relevant information.

DEVELOPMENTAL AND CULTURAL CONSIDERATIONS

Child abuse assessment should be conducted within a culturally sensitive developmental framework. Developing cognitive and linguistic skills may impact children's ability to respond to the demands of an assessment situation, and, therefore, clinicians should be knowledgeable about normative development (Hewitt, 1999). Considerations of developmental level and culture should inform both the content and the structure of an assessment.

Cognitive developmental level impacts children's ability to accurately understand and hence report abuse experiences. Children may struggle with coordinating multiple aspects of relationships among people, events, and objects, and this may impair their ability to understand and describe complex social situations, such as experiences involving child abuse (Fischer & Pipp, 1984). For example, in cases of sexual abuse, due to their inability to comprehend abstractions, children lack the cognitive ability to differentiate between concrete acts of agreement and the abstract concept of informed consent (Celano, 1992). Moreover, because they maintain respect for rules and fair play (Piaget, 1965), children may blame themselves for participating in child sexual abuse because of "initial consent." As children get older and internalize standards of conduct for members of the community, they may feel ashamed for having participated in an act that society deems wrong (Celano, 1992). Difficulties with the complexity of abuse experiences and emerging self-blame and feelings of shame may impact the reporting of abuse experiences.

Language development may also impact the reporting of abuse experiences. Children may use language concepts before they comprehend their meaning (Walker, 1994). For example, a child may report that she was abused last year without fully understanding the meaning of the word *year*. In general, children younger than age 10 often struggle with estimates of time, kinship, dimensions, and quantity, and pre-school-age children often struggle with prepositions (Bourg et al., 1999; Walker, 1994). To address these issues, interviewers should carefully examine children's understanding and use of terminology to ensure that both the child and the interviewer share the same meaning. For example, although an interviewer may use the term *private parts*, a child may not know the parts of the body to which this refers (Goodman & Aman, 1990). In addition, interviewers should use short, open-ended questions that employ clear, concrete, and developmentally appropriate vocabulary.

Although children are credible sources of information, there is some evidence that children's recounting of events may be vulnerable to suggested information (Ceci & Bruck, 1995; Everson & Boat, 1989; Reed, 1996). Preschool children are more vulnerable to suggestion than school-age children or adults (Ceci & Bruck). Under certain conditions, children may be particularly vulnerable to suggestibility. For example, adult interviewers who employ leading questions and who repeat questions can impact children's reports of abuse experiences. In addition, children may be more susceptible to suggestibility when intimidated by the interviewer (Reed, 1996). To reduce the chance of reports being colored by processes of suggestibility, child abuse assessments should be conducted in settings that are comfortable for children. In addition, assessments should be conducted by interviewers who are friendly and who encourage children to tell the truth and to let them know when they are confused, do not know the answer to questions, disagree with the interviewer, or do not want to answer questions (Ceci & Bruck, 1995; Hewitt, 1999; Reed, 1996). Moreover, interviewers should avoid leading and suggestive questioning. Instead, interviewers should ask open-ended questions that are sensitive to the cognitive and linguistic developmental level of the child. Documenting interviews with audio- or videotape will diminish the number of interviews to which a child is exposed and may allow the interviewer to review the interview to assess for the presence of conditions that may heighten suggestibility (Gordon, Schroeder, Ornstein, & Baker-Ward, 1995).

Although adolescents' cognitive and language development promotes their ability to understand complex concepts and address questions imbued with abstractions and complex vocabulary, accurate self-assessment is particularly challenging during this period of cognitive development (Elkind, 1978). Adolescents have an increasing sense of self-awareness and self-evaluation. Therefore, they may critically evaluate their responsibility for the abuse. For example, a sexually abused adolescent may think that if she were less developed or less sexually curious, then abuse would not have occurred (Celano, 1992). Young adolescents cannot relate abstractions to fully comprehend concepts such as intentionality and responsibility. Instead, they tend to engage in self-blame for sexual abuse experiences. Additionally, because they often engage in all-or-none thinking, they have difficulty coping with conflicting perspectives about perpetrators. These cognitive developmental factors likely color an adolescent's perspective and reporting of abuse experiences.

The quality of child abuse assessments can also be impacted by cultural competence. Culture may impact child-rearing practices, reactions to child abuse and child abuse assessments, communication styles, the expression of symptoms, and approaches to mental health treatment (Azar & Benjet, 1994; Fontes, 1995). Culture may also inform beliefs related to child abuse, including beliefs about parent–child relationships, discipline practices, boundaries, sexuality, nudity, and virginity (Fontes, 1995). Cultural awareness and sensitivity should inform the choice of informants and psychological measures. For example, the importance of interviewing extended family members such as grandparents will vary by cultural and familial norms. Therefore, evaluators should endeavor to enhance their cultural competence by becoming familiar with the culture of the family being assessed, being knowledgeable with regard to issues of cultural oppression and consulting and referring as needed (APA, 1993).

Overall, an awareness of developmental and cultural norms should inform child abuse assessment. The extent to which child abuse assessment yields information that is useful for forensic or treatment planning purposes may hinge on these competencies.

SUMMARY

Regardless of whether a child abuse assessment is for forensic, research, or treatment planning purposes, the overarching goal of every child abuse assessment should be to promote the health and welfare of the child (APA, 1998). Consistent with this goal, an ongoing focus on risk and protective factors should inform every child abuse assessment. Comprehensive information on relevant risk and protective factors is most likely gleaned through gathering information on multiple domains of functioning and using multiple informants and assessment measures (APSAC, 1997; AACAP, 1988). Moreover, functional analysis of problematic behaviors and repeated assessment of psychological functioning should inform case conceptualization and treatment planning processes. To meet the demands of complex evaluations such as child abuse assessments, evaluators need to be knowledgeable about a wide range of topics, including state laws that are specific to child abuse, psychological problems associated with child abuse, relevant treatment-outcomes research, developmental norms, and cultural competence.

REFERENCES AND RESOURCES

Abidin, R. R. (1995). *Parenting Stress Inventory* (3rd ed.). Odessa, FL: Psychological Assessment Resources.

Achenbach, T. M. (1991a). *Manual for the Child Behavior Checklist/4-18 and 1991 profile.* Burlington, VT: University of Vermont, Department of Psychiatry.

Achenbach, T. M. (1991b). *Manual of the Teacher's Report Form and 1991 profile.* Burlington, VT: University of Vermont, Department of Psychiatry.

Achenbach, T. M. (1991c). *Manual for the Youth Self-Report and 1991 profile.* Burlington, VT: University of Vermont, Department of Psychiatry.

American Academy of Child and Adolescent Psychiatry. (1988). Guidelines for the clinical evaluation of child and adolescent sexual abuse. *American Academy of Child and Adolescent Psychiatry, 27,* 655–657.

American Professional Society on the Abuse of Children. (1995). *Practice guidelines: Use of anatomical dolls in child sexual abuse assessments.* Oklahoma City, OK: Author.

American Professional Society on the Abuse of Children. (1997). *Practice guidelines: Psychosocial evaluation of suspected sexual abuse in children* (2nd ed.). Oklahoma City, OK: Author.

American Psychological Association. (1993). Guidelines for providers of psychological services to ethnic, linguistic, and culturally diverse populations. *American Psychologist, 48,* 45–48.

American Psychological Association. (2002). Ethical principles of psychologists and code of conduct. *American Psychologist, 57,* 1060–1073.

American Psychological Association, Committee on Professional Practice and Standards. (1998). *Guidelines for psychological evaluations in child protection matters.* Washington, DC: American Psychological Association.

Azar, S. T., & Benjet, C. L. (1994). A cognitive perspective on ethnicity, race, and termination of parental rights. *Law & Human Behavior, 18,* 249–268.

Azar, S. T., & Wolfe, D. A. (1998). Child physical abuse and neglect. In E. J. Mash & R. A. Barkley (Eds.), *Treatment of childhood disorders* (pp. 501–544). New York: Guilford Press.

Barkley, R. A. (1997). *Defiant children: A clinician's manual for assessment and parent training* (2nd ed.). New York: Guilford Press.

Berliner, L., & Elliot, D. M. (2002). Sexual abuse of children. In J. Myers, L. Berliner, J. Briere, C. T. Hendrix, C. Jenny, & T. A. Reid (Eds.), *The APSAC Handbook on Child Maltreatment* (2nd ed., pp. 55–78). Thousand Oaks, CA: Sage Publications.

Binggeli, N. J., Hart, S. N., & Brassard, M. R. (2001). *Psychological maltreatment: A study guide.* Thousand Oaks, CA: Sage Publications.

Boney-McCoy, S., & Finklehor, D. (1995). Psychosocial sequelae of violent victimization in a national youth sample. *Journal of Consulting and Clinical Psychology, 63,* 726–736.

Bourg, W., Broderick, R., Flagor, R., Kelly, D. M., Ervin, D. L., & Butler, J. (1999). *A child interviewer's guidebook.* Thousand Oaks, CA: Sage Publications.

Caffaro-Rouget, A., Lang, R. A., & van Santen, V. (1989). The impact of child sexual abuse. *Annals of Sex Research, 2,* 29–47.

Ceci, S. J., & Bruck, M. (1995). *Jeopardy in the courtroom: A scientific analysis of children's testimony.* Washington, DC: American Psychological Association.

Celano, M. (1992). A developmental model of victims' internal attributions of responsibility for sexual abuse. *Journal of Interpersonal Violence, 7,* 57–69.

Chaffin, M., Wherry, J. N., Newlin, C., Crutchfield, A., & Dykman, R. (1997). The Abuse Dimensions Inventory: Initial data on a research measure of abuse severity. *Journal of Interpersonal Violence, 12,* 569–589.

Cicchetti, D., & Olson, K. (1990). The developmental psychopathology of child maltreatment. In M. Lewis & S. M. Miller (Eds.), *Handbook of developmental psychopathology* (pp. 261–279). New York: Plenum Press.

Cohen, J. A., & Mannarino, A. P. (1988). Psychological symptoms in sexually abused girls. *Child Abuse and Neglect, 12,* 571–577.

Conte, J. R., & Scheurman, J. R. (1987). The effects of sexual abuse on children: A multidimensional view. *Journal of Interpersonal Violence, 2,* 380–390.

Davies, D. (2004). *Child development: A practitioner's guide* (2nd ed.). New York: Guilford Press.

Eckenrode, J., Laird, M., & Doris, J. (1993). School performance and disciplinary problems among abused and neglected children. *Developmental Psychology, 29,* 63–77.

Elkind, D. (1978). Understanding the young adolescent. *Adolescence, 13,* 127–134.

Elliot, A. N., O'Donohue, W. T., & Nickerson, M. A. (1993). The use of sexually anatomically detailed dolls in the assessment of sexual abuse. *Clinical Psychology Review, 13,* 207–221.

Erickson, M. R., & Egeland, B. (1996). Child neglect. In J. Briere, L. Berliner, J. Bulkley, C. Jenney, & T. Reid (Eds.), *The APSAC handbook on child maltreatment* (pp. 4–20). Thousand Oaks, CA: Sage Publications.

Erickson, M. R., & Egeland, B. (2002). Child neglect. In J. Myers, L. Berliner, J. Briere, C. T. Hendrix, C. Jenny, & T. A. Reid (Eds.), *The APSAC handbook on child maltreatment* (2nd ed., pp. 3–20). Thousand Oaks, CA: Sage Publications.

Everson, M. D., & Boat, B. W. (1989). False allegations of sexual abuse by children and adolescents. *Journal of the American Academy of Child & Adolescent Psychiatry, 28,* 230–235.

Everson, M. D., & Boat, B. W. (1990). Sexualized doll play among young children: Implications of anatomical dolls in sexual abuse evaluations. *Journal of the American Academy of Child and Adolescent Psychiatry, 29,* 736–742.

Everson, M. D., Hunter, W. M., Runyon, D. K., Edelsohn, G. A., & Coulter, M. L. (1991). Maternal support following disclosure of incest. In S. Chess & M. E. Hertzig (Eds.), *Annual progress in child psychiatry and child development* (pp. 292–306). Philadelphia: Brunner/Mazel.

Finkelhor, D., & Berliner, L. (1995). Research on the treatment of sexually abused children: A review and recommendations. *Journal of the American Academy of Child & Adolescent Psychiatry, 34,* 1408–1423.

Finkelhor, D., Hotaling, G., Lewis, I. A., & Smith, C. (1990). Sexual abuse in a national survey of adult men and women: Prevalence, characteristics, and risk factors. *Child Abuse & Neglect, 14,* 19–28.

Fischer, K., & Pipp, S. (1984). Development of structures of unconscious thought. In K. Bowers & D. Meichenbaum (Eds.), *The unconscious reconsidered* (pp. 88–148). New York: John Wiley & Sons.

Fontes, L. A. (Ed.). (1995). *Sexual abuse in nine North American cultures: Treatment and prevention.* Thousand Oaks, CA: Sage Publications.

Friedrich, W. N. (1997). *Child Sexual Behavior Inventory.* Odessa, FL: Psychological Assessment Resources.

Friedrich, W. N. (2002). *Psychological assessment of sexually abused children and their families.* Thousand Oakes, CA: Sage Publications.

Friedrich, W. N., Fisher, J. L., Dittner, C. A., Acton, R., Berliner, L., Butler, J., et al. (2001). Child Sexual Behavior Inventory: Normative, psychiatric, and sexual abuse comparisons. *Child Maltreatment: Journal of the American Professional Society on the Abuse of Children, 6,* 37–49.

Gaudin, J. M., Polansky, N. A., & Kilpatrick, A. C. (1992). The Child Well-Being Scales: A field trial. *Child Welfare, 71,* 319–328.

Goodman, G. S., & Aman, C. (1990). Children's use of anatomically detailed dolls to recount an event. *Child Development, 61,* 1859–1871.

Gordon, B. N., Schroeder, C. S., & Hawk, B. (1993). Clinical problems of the preschool child. In C. E. Walker & M. C. Roberts (Eds.), *Handbook of clinical child psychology* (pp. 296–334). New York: John Wiley & Sons.

Gordon, B. N., Schroeder, C. S., Ornstein, P. A., & Baker-Ward, L. E. (1995). Clinical implications of research on memory development. In T. Ney (Ed.), *True and false allegations of child sexual abuse: Assessment and case management* (pp. 99–124). New York: Brunner/Mazel.

Hart, S. N., Brassard, M. R., Binggeli, N. J., & Davidson, H. A. (2002). Psychological maltreatment (pp. 79–103). In J. Myers, L. Berliner, J. Briere, C. T. Hendrix, C. Jenny, & T. A. Reid (Eds.), *The APSAC handbook on child maltreatment* (2nd ed., pp. 79–103). Thousand Oaks, CA: Sage Publications.

Hewitt, S. K. (1999). *Assessing allegations of sexual abuse in preschool children.* Thousand Oaks, CA: Sage Publications.

Hibbard, R. A., Ingersoll, G. M., & Orr, D. P. (1990). Behavior risk, emotional risk, and child abuse among adolescents in a nonclinical setting. *Pediatrics, 86,* 896–901.

Higgins, R. B. (1988). Child victims as witnesses. *Law & Psychology Review, 12,* 159–166.

Horn, J. L., & Dollinger, S. J. (1995). Sleep disturbances in children. In M. C. Roberts (Ed.), *Handbook of pediatric psychology* (2nd ed., pp. 575–588). New York: Guilford Press.

Hotaling, G. T., Straus, M. A., & Lincoln, A. J. (1990). Intrafamily violence and crime and violence outside the family. In M. A. Straus & R. J. Gelles (Eds.), *Physical violence in American families: Risk factors and adaptations to violence in 8,145 families* (pp. 431–470). New Brunswick, NJ: Transaction.

Iwaniec, D. (1995). *The emotionally abused and neglected child.* New York: John Wiley & Sons.

Iwaniec, D. (1997). An overview of emotional maltreatment and failure-to-thrive. *Child Abuse Review, 6,* 370–388.

Jampole, L., & Weber, K. (1987). The assessment of behavior of sexually abused and nonsexually abused children with anatomically correct dolls. *Child Abuse and Neglect, 11,* 187–192.

Kaplan, S., Pelcovitz, D., Salzinger, S., Mandel, F. S., & Weiner, M. (1998). Adolescent physical abuse: Risk for adolescent psychiatric disorders. *American Journal of Psychiatry, 36,* 799–808.

Katz, K. (1992). Communication problems in maltreated children: A tutorial. *Journal of Childhood Communication Disorders, 14,* 147–163.

Kaufman, J., Jones, B., Stieglitz, E., Vitulano, L., & Mannarino, A. P. (1994). The use of multiple informants to assess children's maltreatment experiences. *Journal of Family Violence, 9,* 227–248.

Kendall-Tackett, K. A., & Eckenrode, J. (1996). The effects of neglect on academic achievement and disciplinary problems: A developmental perspective. *Child Abuse and Neglect, 20,* 161–169.

Kendall-Tackett, K. A., Williams, L. M., & Finkelhor, D. (1993). Impact of sexual abuse on children: A review and synthesis of recent empirical studies. *Psychological Bulletin, 113,* 164–180.

Kilpatrick, D. G., Saunders, B. E., & Smith, D. (2003). *Youth victimization: Prevalence and implications.* Washington, DC: U.S. Department of Justice.

Kiser, L. J., Heston, J., Millsap, P. A., & Pruitt, D. B. (1991). Physical and sexual abuse in childhood: Relationship with Post-Traumatic Stress Disorder. *Journal of the American Academy of Child and Adolescent Psychiatry, 30,* 776–783.

Kolko, D. J. (1996). Individual cognitive behavioral treatment and family therapy for physically abused children and their offending parents: A comparison of clinical outcomes, *Child Maltreatment, 1,* 322–342.

Kolko, D. J. (2002). Child physical abuse. In J. Myers, L. Berliner, J. Briere, C. T. Hendrix, C. Jenny, & T. A. Reid (Eds.), *APSAC handbook on child maltreatment* (2nd ed., pp. 21–54). Thousand Oaks, CA: Sage Publications.

Kolko, D. J., Moser, J. T., & Weldy, S. R. (1990). Medical/health histories and physical evaluation of physically and sexually abused child psychiatric patients: A controlled study. *Journal of Family Violence, 5,* 249–267.

Lamb, M. E. (1994). The investigation of child sexual abuse: An interdisciplinary consensus statement. *Journal of Child Sexual Abuse, 3,* 93–106.

Lanktree, C. B., & Briere, J. (1995). Outcome for therapy for sexually abused children: A repeated-measures study. *Child Abuse & Neglect, 19,* 1145–1155.

Magura, S., & Moses, B. (1986). *Outcome measures for child welfare services.* Wahington, DC: National Association of Social Workers.

Mannarino, A. P., & Cohen, J. A. (1986). A clinical-demographic study of sexually abused children. *Child Abuse and Neglect, 10,* 17–23.

Mannarino, A. P., & Cohen, J. A. (1996a). Abuse-related attributions and perceptions, general attributions, and locus of control in sexually abused girls. *Journal of Interpersonal Violence, 11,* 162–180.

Mannarino, A. P., & Cohen, J. A. (1996b). A follow-up study of factors that mediate the development of psychological symptomatology in sexually abused girls. *Child Maltreatment, 1,* 246–260.

Mannarino, A. P., Cohen, J., & Berman, S. (1994). The children's attributions and perceptions scale: A new measure of sexual abuse–related factors. *Journal of Child Clinical Psychology, 23,* 204–211.

Mannarino, A. P., Cohen, J. A., Smith, J. A., & Moore-Motily, S. (1991). Six- and twelve-month follow-up of sexually abused girls. *Journal of Interpersonal Violence, 6,* 494–511.

McLeer, S. V., Deblinger, E., Atkins, M. S., Foa, E. B., & Ralphe, D. L. (1988). Post-traumatic Stress Disorder in sexually abused children. *Journal of the American Academy of Child and Adolescent Psychiatry, 27,* 650–654.

McLeer, S. V., Dixon, J. F., Henry, D., Ruggerio, K., Escovitz, K., Niedda, T., & Scholle, R. (1998). Psychopathology in non-clinically referred sexually abused children. *Journal of the American Academy of Child and Adolescent Psychiatry, 37,* 1326–1333.

Milner, J. S. (1986). *Child Abuse Potential Inventory.* Odessa, FL: Psychological Assessment Resources.

Milner, J. S., Gold, R. G., Ayoub, C., & Jacewitz, M. M. (1984). Predictive validity of the Child Abuse Potential Inventory. *Journal of Consulting and Clinical Psychology, 52,* 879–884.

Myers, J. E. B. (1998). *Legal issues in child abuse and neglect* (2nd ed.). Thousand Oakes, CA: Sage Publications.

Myers, J. E. B. (2002). Risk management for professionals working with maltreated children and adult survivors. In J. Myers, L. Berliner, J. Briere, C. T. Hendrix, C. Jenny, & T. A. Reid (Eds.), *The APSAC handbook on child maltreatment* (2nd ed., pp. 379–401). Thousand Oaks, CA: Sage Publications.

National Research Council, Commission on Behavioral and Social Sciences and Education, Panel on Research on Child Abuse and Neglect. (1993). *Understanding child abuse and neglect.* Washington, DC: National Academy Press.

Paolucci, E. O., Genuis, M. L., & Violato, C. (2001). A meta-analysis of the published research on the effects of child sexual abuse. *The Journal of Psychology, 135,* 17–36.

Pelcovitz, D., Kaplan, S., Goldenberg, B., & Mandel, F. (1994). Post-traumatic stress disorder in physically abused adolescents. *Journal of the American Academy of Child and Adolescent Psychiatry, 33,* 305–312.

Piaget, J. (1954). *The construction of reality in the child.* New York: Basic Books.

Reed, L. D. (1996). Findings from research on children's suggestibility and implications for conducting child interviews. *Child Maltreatment, 1,* 105–120.

Rogosch, F., Cicchetti, D., & Abre, J. L. (1995). The role of child maltreatment in early deviations in cognitive and affective processing abilities and later peer relationship problems. *Development and Psychopathology, 7,* 591–609.

Ruggiero, K. J., & McLeer, S. V. (2000). PTSD Scale of the Child Behavior Checklist: Concurrent and discriminant validity with non-clinic-referred sexually abused children. *Journal of Traumatic Stress, 13,* 287–299.

Sameroff, A. J., & Fiese, B. H. (2000). Transactional regulation: The developmental ecology of early intervention. In J. P. Shonkoff & S. J. Meisels (Eds.), *Handbook of early childhood intervention* (2nd ed., pp. 135–159). Cambridge, UK: Cambridge University Press.

Sedlack, A. J., & Broadhurst, D. D. (1996). *Executive summary of the Third National Incidence Study of Child Abuse and Neglect.* Washington, DC: U.S. Department of Health and Human Services.

Sroufe, L. A. (1997). Psychopathology as an outcome of development. *Development and Psychopathology, 9,* 251–268.

Sternberg, K. J., Lamb, M. E., & Dawud-Noursi, S. (1998). Using multiple informants to understand domestic violence and its effects. In G. W. Holden, R. Geffner, & E. W. Jouriles (Eds.), *Children exposed to marital violence* (pp. 121–156). Washington, DC: American Psychological Association.

Stockhammer, T. F., Salzinger, S., Feldman, R. S., Mojica, E., & Primavera, L. H. (2001). Assessment of the effect of physical child abuse within an ecological framework: Measurement issues. *Journal of Community Psychology, 29,* 319–344.

Taska, L., & Feiring, C. (2000). *Why do bad things happen? Attributions and symptom development following sexual abuse.* Paper presented at the San Diego Conference on Responding to Child Maltreatment, San Diego, CA.

Tong, L., Oates, K., & McDowell, M. (1987). Personality development following sexual abuse. *Child Abuse and Neglect, 11,* 371–383.

Trocome, N. (1996). Development and preliminary evaluation of the Ontario Child Neglect Index. *Child Maltreatment: Journal of the American Professional Society on the Abuse of Children, 1,* 145–155.

Tuteur, J. M., Ewigman, B. E., Peterson, L., & Hosokawa, M. C. (1995). The Maternal Observation Matrix and the Mother–Child Interaction Scale: Brief observational screening instruments for physically abusive mothers. *Journal of Clinical Child Psychology, 24,* 55–62.

U.S. Department of Health and Human Services, Administration on Children, Youth and Families. (2003). *Child maltreatment 2001.* Washington, DC: U.S. Government Printing Office.

Waldfogel, J. (1998). Rethinking the paradigm for child protection. *The Future of Children, 8,* 104–119.

Walker, A. G. (1994). *Handbook on questioning children: A linguistic perspective.* Washington, DC: American Bar Association Center on Children and the Law.

Werner, E. E. (2000). Protective factors and individual resilience. In J. P. Shonkoff & S. J. Meisels (Eds.), *Handbook of early childhood intervention* (2nd ed., pp. 115–132). Cambridge, UK: Cambridge University Press.

Wolfe, D. A., Sas, L., & Wekerle, C. (1994). Factors associated with the development of Post-Traumatic Stress Disorder among child victims of sexual abuse. *Child Abuse and Neglect, 18,* 37–50.

Wolfe, D., Wekerle, C., Reitzel-Jaffe, D., & Lefebvre, L. (1998). Factors associated with abusive relationships among maltreated and nonmaltreated youth. *Development and Psychopathology, 10,* 61–85.

Wolfe, V. V. (1996). Measuring Post-Traumatic Stress Disorder: The Children's Impact of Traumatic Events Scale—Revised. *The APSAC Advisor, 9,* 25–26.

Wolfe, V. V., Gentile, C., Michienzi, T., Sas, L., & Wolfe, D. L. (1991). The Children's Impact of Traumatic Events Scale: A measure of PTSD symptoms. *Behavioral Assessment, 13,* 359–383.

Wolfe, V. V., Gentile, C., & Wolfe, D. A. (1989). The impact of sexual abuse on children: A PTSD formulation. *Behavior Therapy, 20,* 215–228.

23

CLASSROOM ASSESSMENT

JANINE P. STICHTER
TIMOTHY J. LEWIS
Special Education
University of Missouri
Columbia, Missouri

INTRODUCTION

The need for effective instruction to ensure that students maximize their potential has been well documented (Berliner, 1985; Cotton, 1995). This is especially relevant in today's classroom, where the demand for accountability as measured through student achievement is federally mandated (U.S. Department of Education, 2002). Equally important is the impact effective instruction has on children's and youth's social behavioral outcomes (Scott, Nelson, & Liaupsin, 2001). Research has demonstrated that effective classrooms, those defined by high rates of specific behaviors and physical arrangements, lead to higher academic achievement, increased time on task, and reductions in problem behavior (e.g., Brophy & Good, 1986; DuPaul & Stoner, 1994; Gunter, Coutinho, & Cade, 2002; Gunter, Hummel, & Conroy, 1998). The research is also clear on the deleterious effects ineffective or poor instruction can have on students' academic and social behavioral outcomes (Greenbaum et al., 1998; Laczko-Kerr & Berliner, 2002; Sanders & Horn, 1998). While the connection between what occurs within the classroom and student outcomes has been well established, the ability to measure essential features and then to use this information to inform practices is less well documented.

The basic logic behind the effective-schools literature is the assumption that if teachers arrange classrooms in a predictable manner and engage in certain levels of behavior, students will achieve at higher rates. What is unknown is the degree to which any one environmental variable or teacher behavior or combination of these produces the optimum outcomes. The challenge can be characterized as attempting to equip educators with one- or two-dimensional skills for use in a three-dimensional classroom. Opportunities to respond are only effective if the students possess the skills and knowledge to respond. High rates of praise and positive statements will only be effective if students produce high rates of desirable behavior and only when the praise is contingent and meaningful for the student. Likewise, any instructional behavior the teacher may engage in will be lost, or at best present minimal impact, if the context in which the instruction occurs lacks predictableness and cohesion. It is the interplay between currently identified effective instructional practices and the context in which they occur that must guide classroom assessment efforts.

The purpose of this chapter is first to review the multifaceted strengths of the ecobehavioral approach to classroom assessment and second, based on this literature review, to outline a four-level "ecobehavioral" assessment model that includes the essential discrete skills within each level, as directed by the literature. Following a review of essential features that should be included in classroom assessments, implications for practice and research are presented.

ECOBEHAVIORAL CLASSROOM ASSESSMENT

Decades of research have consistently shown that active student responding and engagement are highly correlated with achievement on standardized tests as well as with academic gains and are a key factor in the prevention of school failure (Brophy & Good, 1986; Bulgren & Carta, 1993; Carta, Atwater, Schwartz, & Miller, 1990; Cooper and Speece, 1990; Englert, 1983; Greenwood, 1991; Gunter et al., 2002; Kamps, Leonard, Dugan, Boland, & Greenwood, 1991; Sindelar, Smith, Harriman, Hale, & Wilson, 1986). Therefore, most classroom assessments are designed to analyze one or more environmental variables that may affect the degree to which students are actively engaged and responding (Carta et al.; Englert & Sugai, 1981; Wallace, Anderson, Bartholomay, & Hupp, 2000; Stichter, Lewis, Johnson, & Trussell, 2004; Roberson, Woolsey, Seabrooks, & Williams, 2004). These types of assessments are frequently referred to as *ecobehavioral assessments*.

Ecobehavioral assessments are designed to assess the relationship between the environment, in this case educational context, and behavioral interactions (Greenwood, Carta, Kamps, & Arreaga-Mayer, 1990). In its most comprehensive form, an ecobehavioral assessment serves four purposes. The first is to identify and describe the classroom environment. These instructional contexts consist of physical setup and structure, routines and procedures, and amount, level, and type of instruction. These metrics are further explored in a subsequent section of this chapter. The second function of the ecobehavioral assessment is to describe and compare these context variables across classrooms (Brophy & Good, 1986). The third purpose is to identify the key existing variables associated with high levels of achievement and engagement (Gunter et al., 2002). The final purpose is to utilize the assessment to monitor changes within classrooms, by students and teachers, as a result of experimental manipulation of the key variables associated with high achievement (Stichter & Conroy, 2005).

The respective literature base on instructional variables linked to student achievement is replete with examples of the use of ecobehavioral assessments for the aforementioned purposes. One of the earlier studies was called the Beginning Teacher Evaluation Study (BTES) (Powell, 1980). This large study began as an initial planning grant to identify teacher competencies in the teaching of reading. The later field studies were designed to identify generic teacher competencies as well as to evaluate recent teacher graduates. The initial studies assessed 200 teachers across two grade levels in reading and math. This cross-classroom assessment identified general teacher competencies as well as key instructional factors; that is, teacher behaviors were identified as linked to higher student achievement. From this sample of "more effective" teachers, further investigation ensued to directly measure these key behaviors comprehensively against specific students across various measures of student achievement and ability (Powell). Simultaneously, Greenwood, Delquardi, and Hall (1984) were conducting a 10-year study assessing teacher behavior in relation to students' opportunity to respond. Their work, along with findings from the BTES and subsequent large-scale studies by Good, Grouws, and Ebmeier (1983), Englert (1983), and Brophy and Good (1986), helped lay the foundation for ongoing and more concentrated research on such variables as the amount and type of instructional talk and opportunities to respond provided to students (Roberson, Woolsey, Seabrooks, & Williams, 2004; Sutherland, Alder, & Gunter, 2003; Wallace et al., 2002).

Over time a variety of ecobehavioral assessment tools has been created to meet the various purposes of this type of assessment as well as in response to the particular user. The BTES developed an unnamed protocol to measure and analyze teacher data, subsequently identified as the academic learning time (ALT) framework, which was designed from a "process-product model as described by Doyle (1977)" (Romberg, 1980). The Direct Instruction Observation System (DIOS) was developed by Englert and Sugai (1981) to code the direct instruction behavior of teachers within classrooms. This tool was used in subsequent research to identify direct instruction variables of teacher trainers related to content coverage, feedback strategies, pupil accuracy, and maintenance of task involvement (Englert, 1983). The Teacher/Student Interaction Analysis was developed by Sugai and Lewis (1989) to track the type, amount, and timing of various instructional behaviors and student responses during classroom observations. The data were plotted to provide a visual representation of the teachers' behavior during the targeted observations. The Classroom Activity Recording Form (CARF) was developed to assess three areas of classroom instruction: (1) teacher direct instruction, (2) independent work, and (3) noninstructional work across a total of 16 behaviors (Sindelar et al., 1986). Analysis of this tool, as with many of the descriptive ecobehavioral assessment tools, utilizes a mean proportion of allocated time or frequency for each category. Similarly and more recently, the Setting Factors Assessment Tool (SFAT) was developed to assess 26 teacher and six corresponding student behaviors divided into four levels of assessment (Stichter et al., 2004). The levels are designed to mirror a macro- to micro-assessment strategy where level 1 represents more global classroom structural variables (e.g., noise and traffic flow) and level 2 identifies the nature of the instructional context (e.g., amount of large-group vs. small-group instruction). Level 3 focuses on specific teacher instructional cues (e.g., prompts, accessing background knowledge), and level 4 identifies student behaviors. The SFAT is designed to collect all levels simultaneously in real time or to separate levels out as needed. Therefore it can be analyzed by mean frequency and duration, utilizing statistical analysis or conditional probabilities.

The aforementioned examples of ecobehavioral assessments reflect a class of assessments that tend to be descriptive in design as well as macro in nature. Due to the large-scale measurement facets involved with these larger tools, they typically rely on descriptive methodologies. Yet there exists a subset of ecobehavioal assessments that employ both descriptive and/or experimental methodologies to focus on specific, or isolated, variables. Many of these tools have developed or been employed as a direct result of the larger-scale assessment results or to address very specific or micro-level purposes. For example, the previously cited BTES, which began with 200 teachers, followed up the original study with additional fieldwork with fewer teachers more directly focusing on variables associated with the amount of instructional talk provided to students (Powell, 1980). Subsequent investigations have followed similar methodologies by narrowing the point of interest to the effects of key variables, such as, the effect of choice on math work (Dyer, Dunlap, & Winterling, 1990; Jolivette, Wehby, & Hirsch, 1999) to the amount of work presented (Gunter & Denny, 1998), to the level of structure within the classroom setting (Stichter, Hudson, & Sasso, in press), and to desirable types and amounts of social interaction stimuli (Stichter & Conroy, in press). Some of these area-specific assessment tools are also descriptive in nature. For example, the Social Skills Interview (SSI; Asmus, Conroy, Ladwig, Boyd, & Sellers, 2004) and the Snapshot Assessment Tool (SAT; Conroy, Asmus, Ladwig, Sellers, & Boyd, 2004) are two informal assessment instruments specifically targeting social interaction variables of students with autism spectrum disorders. Together these tools assess contextual variables associated with the peer-related social skills of children with ASD, including (a) the child's current social behaviors and communication strategies (both appropriate and inappropriate), (b) opportunities for social interactions, (c) events that are likely to predict social behaviors, and (d) factors that may maintain social behaviors. One earlier and best-known form of these targeted descriptive assessments is the antecedents, behaviors, consequences (ABC; Bijou, Petersen, & Ault, 1968). The ABC identifies key student outcomes to be monitored and provides a mechanism by which to assess patterns of ecobehavioral patterns surrounding the student outcome. This tool is most often used as one of the key classroom assessment tools employed for school-based functional behavioral assessment (FBA; Horner, 1994; O'Neill et al., 1997; Scott et al., 2004). Patterns identified in the FBA process regarding teaching strategies, instructional management, and physical context that seem to precipitate specific outcomes are then incorporated into changes employed by educators to create an enhanced match between student needs and the learning environment (Dunlap et al., 1993; Kern, Childs, Dunlap, Clarke, & Falk, 1994).

An experimental methodology also designed to identify interactions between the specific classroom characteristics and student outcomes is the process of functional or structural analysis (Repp, 1994; Stichter, 2001; Stichter & Conroy, 2005). Functional and structural analyses serve as a subcategory of the larger functional assessment process. Both procedures directly and systematically manipulate variables suspected to affect academic or social behavior. Each procedure includes those variables that seem to precipitate specific student outcomes (e.g., presenting student with challenging tasks, or classroom noise level) as well as those that seem to maintain specific student outcomes (e.g., rates of positive teacher feedback). However, structural analyses more specifically concentrate on identifying those variables that in isolation or collectively set the stage for specific student outcomes, for example, the degree to which providing opportunities to respond increases the frequency and accuracy of student responses. Functional analysis, in contrast, typically emphasizes the manipulation and hence the identification of those variables that maintain the frequency and accuracy of student responses, such as teacher praise. Although, rigorously employed by researchers since the work of Skinner (1953) and Kantor (1959), both structural and functional analyses are the least common types of ecobehavioral assessments employed in classroom settings. Controlled conditions are typically necessary to conduct such an analysis, and experimental designs are employed in order to allow a determination of functional relationships between the target student behavior(s) and the variables influencing the behavior. Even though these analyses respond directly to one of the intended purposes of ecobehavioral assessment through experimental manipulation and verification of these functional relationships, this form of analysis (due to the level of control necessary) has only recently been examined in natural settings (Repp; Sasso et al., 1992; Stichter et al., 2004) and least often by practitioners themselves.

Educators, including teachers and administrators, have employed various forms of classroom-based ecobehavioral assessments as described earlier. The virtue of ecobehavioral assessments are that they are easily created and adapted and are amenable to a variety of measurement forms. It is for this reason that school districts may have one form of classroom assessment that superintendents use for "classroom walk-throughs" focusing on various classroom attributes that visually signal a curriculum-rich, engaging, and inviting learning environment, whereas building-level administrators may employ a very different form that emphasizes amounts of specific preventative behavior management strategies and time spent on literacy-based direct instruction. Educators involved in peer coaching may utilize or develop an assessment tool that assesses the interaction

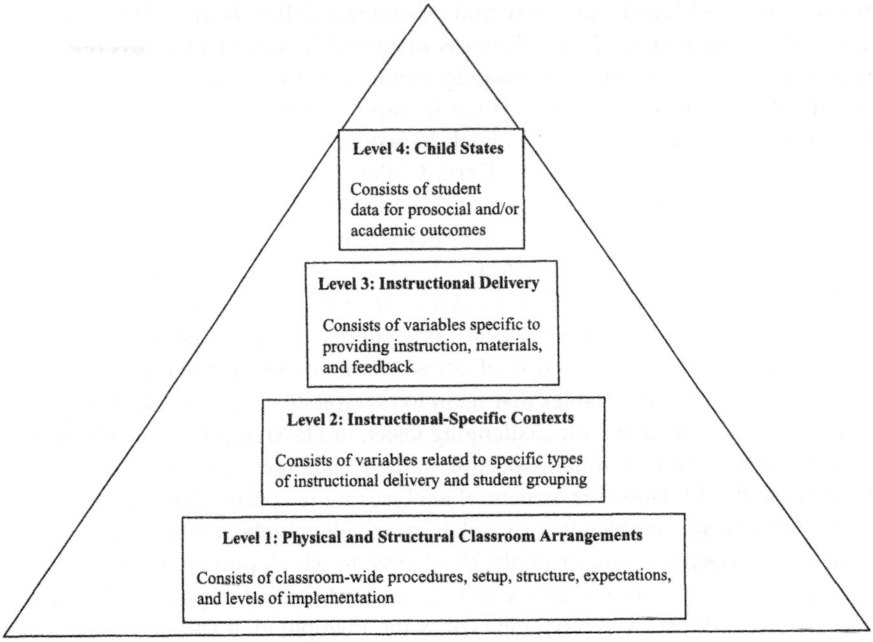

FIGURE 23.1 The four recommended levels of an ecobehavioral assessment model to examine effective instruction within classrooms.

between student grouping related to curriculum specific instruction and levels of student compliance and active responding.

Researchers and practitioners continue to collaborate to identify optimal forms of ecobehavioral assessments to best address various needs. Many of these formats and examples of corresponding tools were just described. The research employing ecobehavioral assessments has demonstrated consistent patterns regarding common metrics as well as related classifications for these variables (Conroy, Davis, Fox, & Brown, 2002; Carnine, 1976; Conroy & Stichter, 2003; Driscoll & Carter, 2004; Dyer et al., 1990; Fox & Conroy, 1995; Kameenui & Darsch, 1995; Kamps, Kravits, Rauch, Kamps, & Chung, 2000; Mayer, 1995; Marzano, 2003). Figure 23.1 provides a hierarchical representation of these classifications relative to level of specificity. The following section will further define each level.

COMMON CLASSROOM-BASED METRICS

The preceding section built the rationale for examining the classroom through an ecobehavioral perspective. Context, instructional behaviors, and student behaviors are ideally measured simultaneously to determine the optimal combination that leads to student learning. The remainder of this section focuses on those variables that the effective-instruction literature suggests as essential to include in any form of classroom assessment (Cotton, 1995).

PHYSICAL AND STRUCTURAL CLASSROOM ARRANGEMENTS

The broadest of the classroom assessment metrics is depicted as level 1 in the hierarchy triangle in Figure 23.1. Level 1 includes those measures that define classroom setup regarding physical properties as well as procedural properties designed to create various degrees of structure (Fox & Conroy, 1995; Stichter et al., 2004). The following are presented as a list of frequently used measures and general-purpose descriptors. In what combination and how these metrics are assessed is dependent on the purpose of the assessment.

- *Structural rating of classroom*: This item assesses the amount of structure that appears to be present in the classroom. Structure is defined by the level of material organization, clear seating arrangement, level of students who seem to be moving with purpose and who clearly understand current activities, as well as the level of noise.
- *Traffic patterns facilitate fluid movement:* This item reflects the ability to which students and teacher(s) can effectively move throughout the classroom without running into one another or interrupting one another's work or conversation when in transit. Additionally, it assesses the degree to which students can access their materials without similar disruptions. Does the spacial density and design of the room promote smooth transitions?
- *General classroom materials easily accessible:* This item assesses the degree to which students can independently access classroom materials as well as the age and activity appropriateness of the items. For example, are the classroom pencil sharpener, wastebasket, stapler, paper, computers, and necessary texts clearly visible, and do they appear accessible (i.e., the pencil sharpener is not behind the coat rack or wastebasket, which might therefore need to be moved to use the sharpener)?
- *Rules posted and visible for students:* This item reflects the degree to which students and outside observers can easily see school/classroom rules or expectations. That is, are these rules at a visible level that students could also easily see without having to specifically look for them (e.g., not above a 5-ft-high bookcase, for elementary students)?
- *Daily schedule posted and accessible:* This item should assess whether the schedule is posted and clearly visible to students in that classroom and whether the schedule reflects a predictable pattern that will assist in student learning (e.g., are low- and high-intensity activities rotated?).
- *Staffing patterns*: This should assess the student-to-staff ratio and the degree to which all adults in the classroom are actively aware of (a) the expectations and

routines of the classroom and (b) the behavior of all students across the room.

- *Procedures for classroom management established:* This item determines if there are specific and well-defined procedures for such regular activities as filing completed work, getting teacher assistance, responding to teacher queries (e.g., raising hand), re-entry to the classroom, access to the bathroom, getting completed homework, or any other procedure developmentally or curricular relevant (e.g., correct lab procedure for a science class). Evaluation procedures are also included in this metric, referencing common procedures understood by student and teacher for evaluating student progress and for provision of feedback.
- *Procedures observed:* This item determines if the articulated procedures are consistently implemented and followed through by the teacher.

INSTRUCTIONAL-SPECIFIC CONTEXTS

Level 2 of the hierarchy is, as depicted, associated with a more specific focus emphasizing variables related to specific types of instructional delivery and to student grouping. Pertinent here is research literature related to the degree to which teachers spend their time in whole-group discussion, small groups, or one on one and utilize peer-assisted learning instruction (McGill, Teer, Rye, and Hughes, 2003; Powell, 1980; Romberg, 1980).

- *Small Group:* What percentage of the time during curriculum instruction does the teacher spend working with more than one student and less than half of the entire class?
- *Large Group:* What percentage of the time during curriculum instruction does the teacher spend working with more than half of the students in the classroom?
- *One to One:* What percentage of the time does the teacher work one on one with various students? In this case, a student is working on a specific activity and the teacher is directly assisting the child in completing the activity. Distinction is made, however, between one-on-one assistance and providing intermittent prompts to a student during independent seatwork.
- *Independent Seatwork:* What percentage of the time are students engaged in independent seatwork? Typically this is loosely defined. For instance, if the target student is seated at a table with other children but is expected to work by him- or herself on a specific task and receives occasional attention from the teacher primarily to direct him back to work, but the teacher's attention is divided among all of the students, then this is typically considered independent seatwork and not group work. If the teacher begins to work with a small group while others are expected to do independent seatwork, then the small group might be considered a second activity.
- *Second Activity:* This measures how often while the teacher is in an instructional activity (e.g., small or large group) another subset of students is engaged

in a separate instructional activity with or without another adult (i.e., the teacher has most of the class engaged in a large-group activity, yet a subset of students is doing independent work at their desks with no direct teacher instruction/involvement).

- *Peer Collaboration:* What percentage of the time are students actively engaged in planned or encouraged collaboration with their peers on a project or activity?
- *Transition:* What percentage of the time are students engaged in transitions? How long do those transitions take to complete? Typically transitions begin when the teacher/adult signals the students to transition to another activity. They typically end when 90% of all students asked to engage in the next primary activity are doing so.

SPECIFIC INSTRUCTIONAL TECHNIQUES

Level 3 of the hierarchy pertains to specific instructional techniques employed by the teacher and consists of variables specific to providing instruction, materials, and feedback. Teacher-effectiveness literature on praise, lesson delivery, classroom management, and feedback are specifically pertinent to this section (Brophy & Good, 1986; Ellis & Worthington, 1994; Englert, 1983; Rowe, 2004).

- *Instructional Talk:* This is the amount of time the teacher provides instructional directions, explanations, or other information to the students regarding expectations of academic or general behavior.
- *Wait Time:* This is the amount of time the teacher waits for a student response or action following any form of prompt or feedback.
- *Downtime:* This is the amount of time during which no active instruction is occurring and students have been given no clear instructions, are waiting for further instructions, or are not being actively supervised. This will most often happen during transitions. For example, the teacher begins a lesson, then pauses and seems unclear about where to go next, begins to look for materials, and so forth. Meanwhile the students are not given a specific task to do and are waiting, by default. Another example: The teacher is engaged in large-group instruction when a student reenters the classroom, the teacher becomes engaged with that student and the remaining students are sitting waiting for his attention to return to their instruction.
- *Preview:* This involves any references made by the teacher to future activities or tasks that provide insight into upcoming lessons or that give a preview of an outcome desired for a task. For example, before instruction or a lesson begins, the teacher tells students that they are going to be writing a silly story for open house. They will be talking about their topics, creating an outline, and then writing a sloppy copy to be edited before a final copy is made.
- *Organizational Prompt:* This is a direction by the teacher that indicates next steps or suggestions for organization. For example, the teacher might say, "Class, you will be making a sloppy copy and a final copy, so you need to

put your good paper back in your desk until your sloppy copy has been edited."

- *Reference to Prior Knowledge:* This involves instances when a teacher refers to previous work or activity that the students have done as a means to link current activity, directions, or work. For instance, "Class, we are going to continue our editing from yesterday. What are the four key steps to editing we have been practicing all week?"
- *Instructional Model:* The teacher provides examples to show the students how to do an activity or request.
- *Student Model/Paraphrase*: When a teacher asks a student or group of students either to show or to restate the directions, indicating an understanding of the task or expected behavior.
- *Attention Signal:* The teacher utilizes a consistent and prior-taught signal designed to gain student attention. For example, she claps hands or holds up two fingers to signal the students to stop and look up.
- *Prompts:* These are defined as directives provided to the student by the teacher. Typically, prompts are measured as a ratio of positive or neutral prompts to negative. They can be specific (e.g., "Please provide the answer to this problem.") or nonspecific (e.g., "You need to think about your actions."). Specific negative prompts (e.g., "Do not get your materials out until I say go.") or nonspecific negative prompts (e.g., "Don't!") should be considerably less-than-positive prompts.
- *Feedback:* This is defined as verbal or nonverbal statements made by the teacher following student behavior and indicating approval or disapproval for either academic or social behavior. Positive or neutral feedback indicates appreciation or preference for a specific behavior. It can be specific (e.g., "I like the way everyone is listening so quietly.") or nonspecific (e.g., "Great job everyone!") and should exceed negative feedback (e.g., "I am not sure why everyone is talking; that is not what you were asked to do." or "This class is having some problems today!").

CHILD STATES

Level 4 of the classroom metric hierarchy model essentially translates into outcome measures. These are the academic and social behaviors exhibited by students, and they can be measured through permanent product as well as through a variety of social/behavioral formal and informal assessments. A variety of comprehensive as well as curriculum-specific research guides these metrics (Simmons & Kameenui, 1996; Rowe, 2004). The following simply serve as a representative subset of commonly used measures.

- *Verbal or Gestural, Positive:* This involves an appropriate vocalization or gesture (e.g., hand raising) by any student demonstrating active listening and corresponding response. It is a common measure of engagement.

- *Verbal or Gestural, Negative:* This is an inappropriate vocalization (e.g., "You are stupid" or "This sucks" or "I hate this work") to a teacher or peer or gesture by any student demonstrating nonengagement or difficulty with curricular materials and activities.
- *Student Entrance and Exits:* This measures the number of students who enter and exit the classroom during instruction for alternative reasons. These measures assess how many interruptions to class instruction occur as well as how much class instruction a student receives or misses for alternative instruction or nonessential activities (e.g., request to use the bathroom).
- *Student Instruction:* This involves the number of opportunities students have to share their work with the class or peers or to give instruction to the class on an activity or task. It reveals the ability of students to model and paraphrase instruction and new materials.
- *Feedback on Work Product:* Student work should be assessed to determine if there is feedback on the permanent product. Permanent product is defined as work that is submitted to the teacher for assessment.
- *Work Product Accuracy:* This is the mean accuracy percentage of students on independent as well as teacher-directed work tasks. Typical metrics for teacher-assisted tasks range from 70% to 80% accuracy and from 90% to 95% on independent work tasks.

IMPLICATIONS

IMPLICATIONS FOR PRACTICE

The optimal classroom assessment should provide an index of essential instructional behaviors but ensure that they are contextualized. While the literature is replete with the call for increased opportunities to respond (e.g., Sutherland & Wehby, 2001) and large ratios of positive to negative feedback statements (e.g., Ferguson & Houghton, 1992; Sutherland, Wehby, & Copeland, 2000), simply increasing discrete teaching behaviors without anchoring them in meaningful instruction and well-organized classrooms will probably not impact student achievement. The optimal classroom assessment strategy should provide practitioners with multilevel feedback and make sense of the amount and type of teaching behaviors engaged in relative to student academic and social behavior. By building a multilevel assessment, targeted feedback can be given that will allow educators to make alterations in classroom organization, instructional behaviors, or level and type of feedback that can then be directly mapped to student outcomes (Stichter et al., 2004).

While multilevel, multivariable classroom assessments yield the richest information that will allow educators to make meaningful adjustments in their classrooms, most current evaluation or teacher review practices do not approximate any of the previously outlined recommendations. What are needed are simple observation tools that allow administrators or teaching colleagues to make quick assessments on key factors likely to contribute the most to student outcomes. In our own work, along with colleagues, we hope to have statistical and clinical evidence pinpointing clear marker variables at each of the first three levels outlined (Stichter et al., 2004). In the meantime, practioners are encouraged to begin the review process using the logic of the four-level system while simultaneously examining the dynamic interactive features to get a better understanding of the interplay between effective instructional variables and their unique classroom context.

IMPLICATIONS FOR RESEARCH

The field of education has relied on the "effective-teaching" literature for the past two decades to target skills needed among preservice teachers and skills, ideally, on which to evaluate in-service teachers. Unfortunately, the field has not produced specific amounts or ratios of discrete teaching behaviors relative to the classroom context and student outcomes. Rather, to date, the "shotgun" approach is often recommended as "effective teachers," those whose students perform well on measures of achievement, engage in many or all of the behaviors (e.g., Brophy & Good, 1986).

Clearly more research in classroom assessment is warranted, at three levels. The first is to determine the optimum amount of a specific instructional behavior and the instructional circumstances under which it optimally leads to learner outcomes. For example, are there differences in the number and type of instructional prompts and the amount and type of feedback necessary during certain academic subjects, times of day, lesson setup versus lesson review? Logic and the descriptive database on effective teaching to date would say yes. However, we simply do not have the empirical or clinical database to answer. Understanding the optimal amount of specific instructional behaviors under specific instructional circumstances would allow the field to maximize in-service teacher impact and begin to streamline preservice teacher preparation to focus on the most parsimonious yet effective teaching skills.

The second level of research needed is a better understanding of the impact the instructional context has on the learner (Gunter, Coutinho, & Cade, 2002). What is needed at this level is an examination of "level 1" classroom variables and their impact on student performance. For example, in a study conducted by Stichter et al. (2004) it was shown that simple classroom modifications were sufficient to improve the social and academic behavior of a student with CIBD, whereas the typical response in both schools and the research community is to develop a specific plan to support the individual child. Additional research is needed to determine the "tipping point" between classroom structure and the need for individualized social and academic behavioral supports.

Finally, as underscored throughout this chapter, effective classroom assessment should be a complex dynamic process. Additional observational tools, including real-time computer analyses, are needed to capture the multiple and often simultaneous processes that occur in effective classrooms. Techniques used within small special education classrooms, such as the groundbreaking work by Shores, Gunter, Wehby and colleagues using lag sequential analyses to illustrate complex sequences of teacher and student behaviors, are needed across all classroom variables (Shores et al., 1993; Wehby, Symons, & Shores, 1995; Gunter & Coutinho, 1997). Using real-time data collected on computers, Shores and his colleagues were able to produce probability statements that when variable *X* happened, there was a high percentage likelihood that *Y* will follow (Gunter & Jack, 1993). Only by using sophisticated observational tools and equally sophisticated analyses will the field be able to demonstrate and pinpoint key instructional behaviors placed within contexts that lead to clear student outcomes.

SUMMARY

The purpose of this chapter was to describe a classroom assessment approach that captures the essential features of effective instruction and the contexts in which they occur. Using an ecobehavioral approach to classroom assessment, a four-level framework was provided. Within each of the levels, specific contexts, instructional variables, teacher behaviors, and student behaviors should be measured. Likewise, the interactions, connections, and sequences across each level should also be assessed. By examining patterns of behaviors within and across educational contexts, a picture of the amount and type of teacher behaviors emerges that will allow the field to discriminate effective from ineffective instruction. Measurable patterns of interactive behavioral sequences that have empirical and clinical significance have implications for practicing and preservice teachers and the larger research community. These implications were also discussed.

REFERENCES AND RESOURCES

Asmus, J. M., Conroy, M. A., Ladwig, C. N., Boyd, B., & Sellers, J. (2004). *Social skills interview.* Unpublished document.

Bijou, S. W., Peterson, R. F., & Ault, M. H. (1968). A method to integrate descriptive and experimental field studies at the level of data and empirical concepts. *Journal of Applied Behavior Analysis, 1,* 175–191.

Brophy, J. H., & Good, T. (1986). Teacher behavior and student achievement. In M. C. Wittrock (Ed.), *Handbook of research in teaching* (3rd ed., pp. 328–375). New York: Macmillan.

Bulgren, J. A., & Carta, J. J. (1993). Examining the instructional contexts of students with learning disabilities. *Exceptional Children, 59,* 182–191.

Carnine, D. W. (1976). Effects of two teacher-presentation rates on off-task behavior, answering correctly, and participation. *Journal of Applied Behavior Analysis, 9*(2), 199–206.

Carta, J. J., Atwater, J. B., Schwartz, I. S., & Miller, P. A. (1990). Applications of ecobehavioral analysis to the study of transitions across early childhood settings. *Education and Treatment of Children, 13,* 298–315.

Conroy, M. A., Asmus, J. M., Ladwig, C. N., Sellers, J., & Boyd, B. (2004). *The snapshot assessment tool.* Unpublished document.

Conroy, M. A., Davis, C. A., Fox, J. J., & Brown, W. H. (2002). Functional assessment of behavior and effective supports for young children with challenging behaviors. *Assessment for Effective Intervention, 27*(4), 35–47.

Conroy, M. A., & Stichter, J. P. (2003). The application of antecedents in the functional assessment process: Existing research, issues, and recommendations. *Journal of Special Education, 37*(1), 15–25.

Cooper, D. H., & Speece, D. L. (1990). Maintaining at-risk children in general education settings: Initial effects of individual differences and classroom environment. *Exceptional Children, 54,* 117–128.

Cotton, K. (1995). *Effective schooling practices: A research synthesis.* Portland, OR: Northwest Regional Education Laboratory.

Driscoll, C., & Carter, M. (2004). Spatial density as a setting event for the social interaction of preschool children. *International Journal of Disability, Development and Education, 51*(1), 7–37.

Doyle, W. (1977). Paradigms for Research on Teacher Effectiveness. In L. Schulman (Ed.), *Review of Research in Education 5.* Itasca, IL: F. E. Peacock.

Dunlap, G., Kern, L., DePerczel, M., Clarke, S., Wilson, D., Childs, K. E., et al. (1993). Functional analysis of classroom variables for students with emotional and behavioral disorders. *Behavioral Disorders, 18,* 275–291.

DuPaul, G. J., & Stoner, G. D. (1994). Classroom-based intervention strategies. In G. J. DuPaul & G. D. Stoner (Eds.), *ADHD in the schools: Assessment and intervention strategies* (pp. 96–134). New York: Guilford Press.

Dyer, K., Dunlap, G., & Winterling, V. (1990). Effects of choice making on the serious problem behaviors of students with severe handicaps. *Journal of Applied Behavior Analysis, 23,* 515–524.

Ellis, E. S., & Worthington, L. A. (1994). *Effective teaching principles and the design of quality tools for educators.* (Tech. Rep. No. 5). National Center to Improve the Tools of Educators, Eugene, University of Oregon.

Englert, C. S. (1983). Measuring special education teacher effectiveness. *Exceptional Children, 50*(3), 247–254.

Englert, C. S., & Sugai, G. (1981). *Direct Instruction Observation System (DIOS).* Lexington: University of Kentucky.

Ferguson, E., & Houghton, S. (1992). The effects of contingent teacher praise, as specified by Canter's Assertive Discipline program, on children's on-task behavior. *Educational Studies, 18,* 83–94.

Fox, J. J., & Conroy, M. A. (1995). Setting events and behavioral disorders of children and youth: An interbehavioral field analysis for research and practice. *Journal of Emotional and Behavioral Disorders, 3,* 130–140.

Good, T., Grouws, D., & Ebmeier, H. (1983). *Active mathematics teaching.* New York: Longman.

Greenbaum, P. E., Dedrick, R. F., Friedman, R. M., Kutash, K., Brown, E. C., Lardieri, S. P., & Pugh, M. (1998). National Adolescent and Child Treatment Study (NACTS): Outcomes for children with serious emotional and behavioral disturbance. In M. H. Epstein, K. Kutash, & A. Duchnowski (Eds.), *Outcomes for children and youth with emotional and behavioral disorders and their families: Programs and evaluation best practices* (pp. 21–54). Austin, TX: PRO-ED.

Greenwood, C. R. (1991). Longitudinal analysis of time, engagement and achievement in at-risk vs. nonrisk students. *Exceptional Children, 57,* 521–535.

Greenwood, C. R., Carta, J. J., Kamps, D., & Arreaga-Mayer, C. (1990). Ecobehavioral analysis of classroom instruction. In S. Schroeder (Ed.), *Ecobehavioral analysis and developmental disabilities* (pp. 33–63). Baltimore: Paul H. Brookes.

Greenwood, C. R., Delquadri, J. C., & Hall, R. V. (1984). Opportunity to respond and student academic performance. In W. L. Heward, T. E. Heron, D. S. Hill, & J. Trap-Porter (Eds.), *Focus on behavior analysis in education* (pp. 58–88). Columbus, OH: Charles E. Merrill.

Gunter, P. L., & Coutinho, M. J. (1997). Negative reinforcement in classrooms: What we're beginning to learn. *Teacher Education and Special Education, 20,* 249–264.

Gunter, P. L., Coutinho, M. J., & Cade, T. (2002). Classroom factors linked with academic gains among students with emotional and behavioral problems. *Preventing School Failure, 46*(3), 126–132.

Gunter, P. L., & Denny, R. K. (1998). Trends, issues, and research needs regarding academic instruction of students with emotional and behavioral disorders. *Behavioral Disorders, 24,* 44–50.

Gunter, P. L., Hummel, J. H., & Conroy, M. A. (1998). Increasing correct academic responding: An effective intervention strategy to decrease behavior problems. *Effective School Practices, 17*(2), 55–62.

Gunter, P. L., & Jack, S. L. (1993). Lag sequential analysis as a tool for functional analysis of student disruptive behavior in classrooms. *Journal of Emotional and Behavioral Disorders. 1,* 138–149.

Horner, R. H. (1994). Functional assessment: Contributions and future directions. *Journal of Applied Behavior Analysis, 27,* 401–404.

Jolivette, K., Wehby, J. H., & Hirsch, L. (1999). Academic strategy identification for students exhibiting inappropriate classroom behaviors. *Behavioral Disorders, 24,* 210–221.

Kameenui, E. J., & Darsch, C. B. (1995). *Instructional classroom management: A proactive approach to behavior management.* White Plains, NY: Longman.

Kamps, D. M., Kravits, T., Rauch, J., Kamps, J. L., & Chung, N. (2000). A prevention program for students with or at risk for ED: Moderating effects of variation in treatment and classroom structure. *Journal of Emotional and Behavioral Disorders, 8*(3), 141–154.

Kamps, D. M., Leonard, B. R., Dugan, E. P., Boland, B., & Greenwood, C. R. (1991). The use of ecobehavioral assessment to identify naturally occurring effective procedures in classrooms serving children with autism and other developmental disabilities. *Journal of Special Education, 1,* 367–397.

Kantor, J. R. (1959). *Interbehavioral psychology.* Granville, OH: Principia Press.

Kern, L., Childs, K., Dunlap, G., Clarke, S., & Falk, G. D. (1994). Using assessment-based curricular intervention to improve the classroom behavior of a student with emotional and behavioral challenges. *Journal of Applied Behavior Analysis, 27,* 7–19.

Laczko-Kerr, I., & Berliner, D. C. (2002, September 6). The effectiveness of "Teach for America" and other undercertified teachers on student academic achievement: A case of harmful public policy. *Education Policy Analysis Archives, 10*(37). Retrieved September 9, 2002, from http://epaa.asu.edu/epaa/v10n37/

Marzano, R. J. (2003). *What works in schools: Translating research into action.* Alexandria, VA: Association for Supervision and Curriculum Development.

Mayer, G. (1995). Preventing antisocial behavior in the schools. *Journal of Applied Behavior Analysis, 28,* 467–47.

McGill, P., Teer, K., Rye, L., & Hughes, D. (2003). Staff reports of setting events associated with challenging behavior. *Behavior Modification, 27*(2), 265–282.

O'Neill, R. E., Horner, R. H., Albin, R. W., Sprague, J. R., Storey, K., & Newton, J. S. (1997). *Functional assessment and program development for problem behavior: A practical handbook.* Pacific Grove, CA: Brooks/Cole.

Powell, M. (1980). The beginning teacher evaluation study: A brief history of a major research project. In C. Denham & A. Lieberman (Eds.), *Time to learn: A review of the Beginning Teacher Evaluation Study, conducted with funds provided by the National Institute of Education* (pp. 1–5). Washington, DC: U.S. Department of Education and National Institute of Education.

Repp, A. (1994). Comments on functional analysis procedures for school-based behavior problems. *Journal of Applied Behavior Analysis, 27,* 409–411.

Roberson, L., Woolsey, M. L., Seabrooks, J., & Williams, G. (2004). An ecobehaviroal assessment of the teaching behaviors of teacher candidates during their special education internship experiences. *Teacher Education and Special Education, 27,* 264–275.

Roberson, L., Woolsey, M. L., Seabrooks, J., & Williams, G. (2004). Data-Driven Assessment of Teacher Candidates During Their Internships in Deaf Education. *American Annals of the Deaf. 148*(5), 403–412.

Romberg, T. (1980). Salient features of the BTES framework of teacher behaviors. In C. Denham & A. Lieberman (Eds.), *Time to learn: A review of the Beginning Teacher Evaluation Study, conducted with funds provided by the National Institute of Education* (pp. 73–93). Washington, DC: U. S. Department of Education and National Institute of Education.

Rowe, K. (2004, August 26–27). *Ensuring better schooling by building teacher capacities that maximize the quality of teaching and learning provision—implication of findings from the international and Australian evidence-based research.* Paper presented at the Making Schools Better conference: A summit conference on the performance, management and funding of Australian schools. Melbourne Institute of Applied Economic and Social Research, in Association with the Australian and the Faculty of Education at the University of Melbourne.

Sanders, W. L., & Horn, S. P. (1998). Research findings from the Tennessee Value-Added Assessment System (TVAAS) database: Implications for educational evaluation and research. *Journal of Personnel Evaluation in Education, 12,* 247–256.

Sasso, G, Reimers, T., Cooper, L., Wacker, D., Berg, W., Kelly, L., & Allaire, A. (1992). Use of descriptive and experimental analyses to identify the functional properties of aberrant behavior in school settings. *Journal of Applied Behavior Analysis, 25,* 809–821.

Scott, T. M., Bucalos, A., Liaupsin, C., Nelson, C. M., Jolivette, K., & DeShea, L. (2004). Using functional behavioral assessment in general education settings: Making a case for effectiveness and efficiency. *Behavior Disorders, 29,* 189–201.

Scott, T. M., Nelson, C. M., & Liaupsin, C. J. (2001). Effective instruction: The forgotten component in preventing school violence. *Education & Treatment of Children. 24*(3), 309–322.

Shores, R. E., Jack, S. L., Gunter, P. L., Ellis, D. N., DeBriere, T. J., & Wehby, J. H. (1993). Classroom interactions of children with behavior disorders. *Journal of Emotional and Behavioral Disorders, 1,* 27–39.

Simmons, D. C., & Kameenui, E. J. (1996). A focus on curriculum design: When children fail. *Focus on Exceptional Children, 28*(7), 1–16.

Sindelar, P. T., Smith, M. A., Harriman, N. E., Hale, R. L., & Wilson, R. J. (1986). Teacher effectiveness in special education programs. *Journal of Special Education, 20,* 195–207.

Skinner, B. F. (1953). *Science and human behavior.* New York: Macmillan.

Stichter, J. P. (2001). Functional analysis: The use of analogues in applied settings. *Focus on Autism and Other Developmental Disabilities, 16,* 232–239.

Stichter, J., & Conroy, M. (2005). Using structural analysis in natural settings: A responsive functional assessment strategy. *Journal of Behavior Education, 14,* 19–34.

Stichter, J. P., & Conroy, M. A. (in press). *How to teach social skills and plan for peer social interactions with learners with autism spectrum disorders.* Schoal Creek, MD: Pro-Ed.

Stichter, J. P., Hudson, S., & Sasso, G. M. (in press). The use of structural analysis to identify setting events in applied settings for students with emotional/behavioral disorders. *Behavioral Disorders.*

Stichter, J. P., Lewis, T. J., Johnson, N., & Trussell, R. (2004). Toward a structural assessment: Analyzing the merits of an assessment tool for a student with E/BD. *Assessment for effective intervention. 30,* 25–40.

Sugai, G., & Lewis, T. (1989). Teacher/student interaction analysis. *Teacher Education and Special Education, 12,* 131–138.

Sutherland, K. S., Alder, N., & Gunter, P. L. (2003). The effect of varying rates of opportunities to respond to academic requests on the classroom behavior of students with EBD. *Journal of Emotional and Behavioral Disorders, 11,* 239–248.

Sutherland, K. S., & Wehby, J. H. (2001). Exploring the relationship between increased opportunities to respond to academic requests and the academic and behavioral outcomes of students with EBD. *Remedial and Special Education, 22,* 113–121.

Sutherland, K. S., Wehby, J. H., & Copeland, S. R. (2000). Effects of varying rates of behavior-specific praise on the on-task behavior of students with EBD. *Journal of Emotional & Behavioral Disorders, 8,* 2–9.

U.S. Department of Education. (2002). *No Child Left Behind executive summary.* Washington, DC: Author.

Wallace, T., Anderson, A. R., Bartholomay, T., & Hupp, S. (2002). An ecobehaviroal examination of high school classrooms that include students with disabilities. *Exceptional Children, 68,* 345–359.

Wehby, J. H., Symons, F. J., & Shores, R. E. (1995). A descriptive analysis of aggressive behavior in classrooms for children with emotional and behavioral disorders. *Behavioral Disorders, 20,* 87–105.

24

PEDIATRIC BEHAVIORAL NEUROPSYCHOLOGY

EILEEN B. FENNELL
Department of Clinical and Health Psychology
University of Florida
Gainesville, Florida

INTRODUCTION

Since 1980, pediatric neuropsychology has emerged as a subspecialty practice and research area in clinical neuropsychology. While examination of children by means of neuropsychological instruments has a longer history, beginning with mental health clinics, schools, and inpatient hospital settings in the 1950s, its current emphasis on understanding the effects of developmental disorders, pediatric neuropsychiatric disorders, and the consequences of CNS traumatic injuries has developed in the context of advances in assessment techniques, neuroimaging technologies, and genetics. These advances have greatly expanded our understanding of brain–behavior relationships in affected children (Baron, Fennell, & Voeller, 1995; Coffey & Brumback, 1998; Friedes, 2001; C. R. Reynolds & Fletcher-Janzen, 1997; Goldstein & Reynolds, 1999; Yeates, Ris, & Taylor, 2002). In addition, paralleling advances in adult assessment (Lezak, Howieson, & Loring, 2004), compendia of test measures and normative data are now available for children (Baron, 2004; Reitan & Wolfson, 1992).

The present chapter describes current approaches to assessment in pediatric neuropsychology as well as interview issues in the examinations, offers standard assessment instruments of the child's cognitive and emotional behavior, and presents a variety of parent-report instruments designed to assess aspects of both child behavior and family functioning. The chapter concludes with a discussion of recommended training for individuals who seek to pursue this specialty area.

OVERVIEW OF ISSUES UNIQUE TO ASSESSING CHILDREN

Unlike adult neuropsychology, clinicians who examine children are faced with understanding how a developing brain responds to the effects of potentially adverse events/conditions. Several important issues have been identified that distinguish adult and child assessment. First, the age at the time of the adverse event is especially important because an early-occurring lesion can affect not only brain functions already at full functional levels (e.g., motor systems), but also brain functions in the process of development or not yet ready for development (e.g., language areas). For example, a severe head trauma experienced by a 3-year-old child may affect subsequent development of higher-order language functions, acquisition of academic skills, and evolution of executive functions related to cognitive and social/emotional behavior and learning-to-learn abilities. Early trauma thus affects each of the domains of functioning awaiting further elaboration and refinement as the underlying brain structures mature. In addition, cognitive functions, such as memory, proceed to develop at different rates in conjunction with language development and other skills, such as visuoperception. As a result, the interpretation of deficits in children must take into account the normal acquisition of related skills, such as verbal and visual memory. This is less problematic when assessing the loss of fully developed skills in adult patients following a stroke.

Second, a similarly important factor is the differential impact on brain development of different types of lesions. For example, children who suffer a left hemisphere lateralized stroke in the perinatal period and who are often diagnosed with "cerebral palsy" around age 6 months may develop atypical language organization (unilateral right hemisphere language or bilateral language lateralization). Such reorganization of brain areas related to language functions subsequently impacts later acquisition of both reading and written language skills as well as typical visuospatial functions. This is captured in the description of children with "crowding" of right hemisphere skills (Baron et al., 1995). If the child also develops a seizure disorder due to the initial stroke, more global impairments may arise secondary to the effects of the seizure disorder and/or its treatment with antiepileptic drugs (Menkes, 1995).

Third, it is often difficult to clearly separate the different factors that present with medical conditions in children. Separating the primary, secondary, and tertiary effects of a medical condition suffered in childhood may be very complicated. For example, surgery, chemotherapy, or radiation therapy to treat childhood cancers can have both primary effects on the brain (e.g., surgical lesions excising tumors) and secondary effects on the brain (e.g., microscopic injuries to brain tissue, such as white matter pathways). In contrast, other medical disorders can exert negative tertiary effects on the brain (e.g., hypoxic injury due to non-brain/CNS disorders in cystic fibrosis, congenital heart defects). While the need to differentiate primary, secondary, and tertiary effects of medical disorders is not unique to pediatric neuropsychology, the fact that these effects are interacting with the brain and behavioral development complicates interpretations of clinical findings.

Fourth, although advances in test batteries were designed to specifically measure certain domains of child functioning, such as composite memory batteries or motor assessment tests, it is still the case that many conditions affecting children and adolescents have not been well described in terms of their neuropsychological typologies. As such, the field is still in development, and information beyond prototypical intellectual functioning and academic achievement is often lacking for many childhood disorders (Yeates et al., 2000).

Fifth, with techniques of different neuroimaging constantly developing, there are difficulties in applying these techniques to young children, with somewhat greater success in evaluating adolescents. There is a larger number of volumetric studies of neurological and neuropsychiatric disorders arising in childhood (e.g., autism, ADHD) than of fMRI studies of these same disorders, due to the technical demands of the differing imaging methodologies. With increased demand for inclusion of children and adolescents in NIH-sponsored studies and in clinical trials of treatment interventions, the need for large normative studies of brain volumes, brain structural development (e.g., DTI), and brain activation studies (e.g., SPECT, fMRI, MEEG) remains great if one is to understand even better the relationship between normal and abnormal brain functioning in childhood neurological and neuropsychiatric disorders. Achievement of these goals rests on development of testing procedures that are defined as low risk by institutional review boards (e.g., mock imaging training) and multicenter collaborations that utilize similar scanners and controls (e.g., phantoms) in order to generate normative data on brain development.

COMPONENTS OF A PEDIATRIC NEUROPSYCHOLOGICAL ASSESSMENT

Table 24.1 presents an outline of the typical components of a comprehensive neuropsychological assessment battery. In such a battery, information on behavioral functioning has four major sources:

1. Developmental history
2. Behavioral observations
3. Test behaviors
4. Parent and/or self-report questionnaires about problem behaviors

The goal of a comprehensive test battery assessing each of these sources of behavioral data is to determine the answer to several critical questions:

1. Is the behavior abnormal? That is, is there a pattern of behaviors that indicates some type of deviation from normal, age-appropriate functioning?

TABLE 24.1 Components of a Comprehensive Pediatric Neuropsychological Assessment Battery

I. Developmental interview
II. Neuropsychological tests
  a. Intellectual functioning
  b. Attention
  c. Memory—verbal and visual
  d. Language
  e. Visuospatial/visuoconstructional functions
  f. Visuomotor functions
  g. Sensory/motor functions
  h. Frontal/executive functions
III. Academic achievement
  a. Reading—single word, comprehension
  b. Arithmetic—computation, concepts, word problem solving
  c. Written language—spelling, grammar, content
IV. Emotional functioning
  a. Test-taking behaviors
  b. Self-report symptom questionnaires
  c. Parent report of problem behaviors
V. Adaptive functioning
  a. Developmental attainments
VI. Social-emotional

2. Do the behavioral problems noted by observation, testing performances, and parent–child questionnaires suggest a primary, secondary, or tertiary brain dysfunction?
3. Is there a pattern to the behavioral deficits/dysfunction that point to disruption of a higher cortical or subcortical functional brain system. And is the lesion diffuse or focal?
4. Does the pattern of test deficits and behavioral problems match the presenting problem or medical history of the child?
5. Are there other factors affecting the pattern of test results and behavioral complaints, such as testing conditions (e.g., bedside vs. clinic), state of the child (e.g., acute illness, post-treatment), emotional factors (e.g., anxiety, depression, low motivation, adjustment disorders, chronic neuropsychiatric conditions), and familial response to the child's behavioral and functional difficulties (e.g., parenting stress, limited resources, cultural/ethnic differences).
6. Are there appropriate interventions, remediation programs, or adaptive devices that may assist in the care and treatment of the child?
7. Should the child and family be referred to appropriate professionals (e.g., primary care physicians, pediatric neurologists, child psychiatrists), agencies (e.g., rehabilitation facilities, mental health clinics, special schools), and

community-based groups (e.g., Association of Retarded Citizens, sickle cell support groups) that may be helpful in the management of the child's needs?

THE DEVELOPMENTAL INTERVIEW

Table 24.2 provides the outline of a comprehensive developmental interview typically conducted with the parent(s)/caregiver(s) of a child referred for assessment. Ideally, all portions of the interview would be conducted on any given assessment. However, sometimes there are gaps in the interviewee's knowledge of the child's early history (Sections I and II), due to adoption, foster care placement, or referral source (juvenile justice system). In these instances, obtaining additional supplemental records that include that specific placement setting is recommended. Requests for release of records will need to be in compliance with HIPPA regulations for health information. Similarly, it is important to be able to review available school records that may include both standardized achievement scores and information developed in an IEP (Individual Education Plan), in referrals to ESE (Exceptional Student Education) placement, or in response to development of a Public Law 504 Plan for accommodations in the classroom for a child who does not meet state criteria for ESE placement (e.g., Specific Learning Disabilities). For professionals engaged in forensic practice, record reviews are a very important source of documentation of issues related to both civil suits (e.g., personal injury or malpractice) and criminal cases (e.g., competency to proceed, adjudication of delinquency). Sometimes there are discrepancies in parent recall of events, developmental trajectory, and pre- or postinjury changes and in behavioral problems that become apparent when past records are compared to interview data.

In addition to the individual developmental interview, a number of parent-report developmental questionnaires may also be administered as part of a pediatric neuropsychological assessment. For example, the BASC-2 (Behavioral Assessment System for Children; C. R. Reynolds & Kamphaus, 2004) also has a developmental interview format that can be completed by parents/caregivers. Similarly, Baron (2004) and Baron et al. (1995) provide examples of parent-report questionnaires that can be completed prior to the child's assessment.

STANDARD TESTS IN A COMPREHENSIVE EXAMINATION

Table 24.3 presents some standard tests that can be utilized to assess domains of functioning within a comprehensive pediatric neuropsychological assessment. The list is not meant to be exhaustive. Contained within each domain are selected tests that contain normative data for the ages of children typically evaluated by a pediatric neuropsychologist (ages 5–16). However, as can be seen from examining the table, the normative data available for differently aged children are still variable. In particular, there is a relative dearth of norms on many measures for adolescent children between the ages of 16 and 21. Some comprehensive testing

TABLE 24.2 Outline of a Developmental Interview for a Pediatric Neuropsychological Assessment

I. Prenatal, perinatal, and early postnatal history
  a. The history of the pregnancy—length, medical problems, trauma, hospitalizations by trimester, maternal age at birth
  b. The history of labor and delivery—vaginal delivery, forcepts, C-section
  c. Child's birth weight—comparison to other, prior deliveries, family history
  d. Apgar scores of child (1 minute, 5 minutes)
  e. Complications in the immediate postbirth period—breathing problems, medical problems (e.g., hypoglycemia, elevated bilirubin)

II. Medical history prior to the dates of clinic visit
  a. Birth to age 6 months—illnesses, immunizations, trauma/injuries
  b. Six months to 1 year—any recurrent problems: allergies, ear infections, asthma, new illnesses, trauma/injuries
  c. One year to 2 years—inquire same as point II.b
  d. Two years to 3 years—inquire same as point II.b
  e. Three years to 4 years—inquire same as point II.b
  f. Five years and each year thereafter to current age—inquire same as point II.b

III. Acquisition of age-related milestones
  a. Motor milestones—sits up without help, crawls, walks without help
  b. Language milestones—single repetitive words (mama, dada), two-word phrases, simple sentences
  c. Handedness—early hand preference

IV. School history
  a. Infancy and toddler-age child care
  b. Preschool experiences—formal school, play groups, child care
  c. Kindergarten—age of entry, problems, and progress (academic, social, behavioral)
  d. Elementary school—by grades: inquire re academic or social/behavioral problems
  e. Middle school—inquire same as point IV.d
  f. High school—inquire same as point IV.d

V. History of personality and social development
  a. Temperament as an infant and toddler—irritable, calm, activity level, cuddliness, soothability when upset, temper
  b. Ages 2.5–5 years—development of give-and-take play, aggression, imaginative play, social interests
  c. Ages 5–11 years—sports teams, clubs, other group activities, friendships
  d. Ages 11 years and into adolescence—development of interest in opposite sex, dating, school activities, sports
  e. Adolescence—dating, social groups, conflicts within the family, acting out

VI. Family history
  a. Parental history—length of marriage, number of children
  b. Parental demographics—ages, education, occupation
  c. Siblings—ages, school history, problems
  d. Family history of medical/developmental problems—seizures, language delays, developmental disabilities, mental retardation, drug or alcohol problems, psychiatric/psychological disorders requiring treatment, learning disabilities, ADHD, genetic disorders, inherited medical conditions, handedness

TABLE 24.2 *(continued)*

VII. History of the presenting problem
  a. Parental description of the problem—features of the problem, concerns about the problem
  b. Onset of the problem—when did it begin, initial presentation, comorbid disorders
  c. Duration of the problem—temporal history of the problem, fluctuations in timing, duration
  d. Interventions attempted—type, frequency, problems encountered, medications
  e. Prior assessments—school or community/hospital
  f. Parents' sense of the effects of the problem on the child and the family
  g. Parents' perception of the child's responses and understanding of the problem
  h. Child's view of the problem—obtained from the child

VIII. Expectations about the assessment visit
  a. What the parents hope to get out of the assessment
  b. Whom they expect to communicate with about the results
  c. Release of information

batteries have developed and published norms for this age group (e.g., Wide Range Assessment of Memory and Learning-2, WRAML-2; Adams & Sheslow, 2003; Delis–Kaplan Executive Function System, DKEFS; Delis, Kaplan, & Kramer, 2001). Many other composite batteries are applicable to younger children and adolescents (e.g., A Developmental Neuropsychological Assessment (ages 3–12), Korkman, Kirk, & Kemp, 1997 (NEPSY); Children's Memory Scale (ages 5–16), Cohen, 1997).

Within the domain of intellectual functioning, the composite Wechsler scales are examples of batteries that contain a variety of different subtests that tap both verbal and performance abilities. Other intellectual assessment instruments with multiple subtests available include the Stanford–Binet—IV (Thorndike, Hagen, & Sattler, 1986); however, most research studies in children tend to rely on the Wechsler scales or subtests from the Stanford–Binet that cross the age span from children to adults. Abbreviated intellectual assessment tests that also cross the age span, such as the relatively new WASI (Wechsler Abbreviated Intelligence Scale; Wechsler, 1999) have been developed to replace short forms of the standard scales, by retaining those types of subtests that predict most reliably to verbal, performance, and full-scale IQ estimates while taking relatively less time to administer. There is also a variety of so-called nonverbal tests of intelligence that may be utilized with children who may have significant deficits in language comprehension and/or expression. One example is the Test of Nonverbal Intelligence—3 (TONI-3; Brown, Sherbenon, & Johnson, 1997), which has a format somewhat similar to other visual reasoning tests, such as the Raven's Coloured Progressive Matrices (Ravens, 1998).

There is a variety of approaches to measuring attention, as noted in Table 24.3. Many of these developed from procedures initially utilized in adult neurological lesion studies, but they have been modified for studying children's performance.

TABLE 24.3 Standard Tests Utilized in Pediatric Neuropsychological Assessment[a]

Test Domains	Applicable Age Group (years)
Intellectual functions	
Wechsler Abbreviated Scale of Intelligence (WASI)	6–89
Wechsler Intelligence Scale for Children (WISC-III, IV)	6.0–16.11
Wechsler Preschool and Primary Scale of Intelligence (WPPSI-III)	2.6–7.3
Attentional functions	
Digit span	6+
Sentence repetition (MAE)	5–12.11
Conners CPT-II	6+
TEA-Ch	6–15.11
Paced Auditory Serial Attention Test (PASAT)	18+
Memory Functions	
Wide Range Assessment of Memory and Learning (WRAML-2)	5–90
Children's Memory Scale (CMS)	5–16
Tests of Memory and Learning (TOMAL)	5–19.11
Children's California Verbal Learning Test (C-CVLT)	5–16.11
Rey Osterrieth Complex Figure Test and Recognition Trial (ROCFT-R)	6–90
Wechsler Memory Scale III Visual Reproduction	16–89
Brief Visual Memory Test—Revised (BVMT-R)	18+
Language functions	
Boston Naming Test (BNT)	6+
Expressive One-Word Picture Vocabulary Test (EOWPVT)	2.0–18.11
Receptive One-Word Picture Vocabulary Test (ROWPVT)	2.0–18.11
Peabody Picture Vocabulary Test III (PPVT-III)	2.6–90
Expressive Picture Vocabulary Test (EVT)	2.6–18.11
Verbal Fluency Test (FAS, CFL)	6+
Clinical Evaluation of Language Fundamentals—4	5–21
Wepman's Auditory Discrimination Test (2nd ed.)	4–8
Visuospatial functions	
Judgment of Line Orientation (JOLO)	5–12.11
Benton Facial Recognition Test (BFRT)	5–12.11
Beery–Buktenica Visual Motor Integration Test (VMI)	2–Adult
Benton Visual Retention Test—5th ed.	8+
Raven's Coloured Progressive Matrices Test	3.6–11
Sensory motor functions	
Finger tapping	6–15
Groove Peg Board Test	6+
Frontal/executive functions	
Go No-Go Task	6+
Motor Programmes of Luria	6+
Trail Making Test (TMT)	6+
Wisconsin Card Sorting Test (WCST)	6.5–89
Stroop Color-Word Test (SCWT)	7–16
Academic achievement	
Wechsler Individual Achievement Test—2 (WIAT-2)	4–85
Wide Range Achievement Test—3	5–75
Woodcock Johnson Psychoeducational Battery III	2–90

TABLE 24.3 (*continued*)

Test Domains	Applicable Age Group (years)
Emotional functions	
Revised Children's Manifest Anxiety Scale (RCMAS)	6–19
State Trait Anxiety Inventory for Children (STAI-C)	9–12
Children's Depression Inventory (CDI)	7–17
Reynolds Adolescent Depression Scale—2 (RADS-2)	11–20
Conners–Wells Self-Report Scale for Adolescents	14–17
Conners' Parent Report Scale—Long Form (CPRS)	3–18
Behavior Report of Executive Functions (BRIEF)	5–18
Behavioral Assessment Scale for Children—2 (BASC-2)	2.5–18
Child Behavior Checklist (CBCL)	4–16
Adaptive functions	
Vineland Adaptive Behavior Scale—Revised	0–18.11
AAMR Adaptive Behavior Scale (2nd ed.)	3–18.11

[a]Bibliographic information on test publishers is given in the References section.

For example, cancellation tasks have been widely used in adult lesion studies to examine for problems of neglect and inattention to hemispace. Similarly, continuous performance tests of various types, including target signal detection, serial addition, and response-shifting paradigms, are well established in adult neuropsychological assessment of attention and are now frequently employed in child assessment as well. Fortunately, most of the available children's CPT tasks have reasonable normative data. However, intensive data on the performance of different childhood disorders, such as epilepsy, childhood brain tumors, cardiac anomalies, and organ failure (liver or lung transplant patients), is still lacking. In contrast, a CPT is more commonly used in the assessment of other childhood behavioral disorders, such as ADHD (Connors CPT) and traumatic brain injuries (TEA-Ch).

As mentioned previously, several composite memory batteries for children are available, such as the WRAML-2, the CMS, and the TOMAL, which have extensive normative data across the pediatric ages 5–19. However, here again, data available for various clinical groups are still limited (Baron, 2004). As a result, the pediatric neuropsychologist must depend on research findings from different clinical samples to determine both the patient's normative performance as well as comparing these test scores to comparable clinical case groups.

In the typical pediatric neuropsychological assessment, language functioning may only be screened. The clinician may use results of that screening to determine whether more extensive testing by a speech pathologist is preferred. This would be especially the case in certain childhood aphasias, in developmental language disorders such as pragmatics disorders, and in speech disorders secondary to CNS brain tumors and their treatment. For example, childhood mutism is sometimes an early symptom post-excision of lesions in the posterior fossa area of the brain. While this disorder is typically transient, treatment recommendations by a speech pathologist are particularly helpful in the postacute stages of recovery from surgery. Similarly, motor disorders of speech, the so-called speech apraxias, require specific types of therapeutic interventions that are typically beyond the expertise of the pediatric neuropsychologist. In my own clinical practice, the Speech and Communicative Services departments collaborate closely to enhance the appreciation of specific types of language development disorders and their remediation.

Use of measures of visuoperceptual processing and visuomotor functions has long been a part of the neuropsychological assessment of the pediatric patient. The goal of this aspect of the examination is to distinguish between perceptual disorders and motor programming output disorders. For this reason, tests that assess various aspects of visual processing by utilizing a visual match-to-sample paradigm are contrasted with visuomotor tasks (copying, constructing designs) and visual reasoning tasks. Typically comparisons are made in drawing or constructing simple versus complex stimulus designs in order to assess qualitatively the approaches used by the patient in planning, in use of space, and in monitoring motor output. These latter behaviors are within the realm of so-called executive functions.

A variety of tests of frontal and executive functions can be utilized in pediatric neuropsychological assessment. In a sense, these tests may "march forward" from the motor strip of prefrontal regions in order to assess a variety of domains of behavior, including behavioral fluency (motor, verbal), response shifting, response inhibition, processing speed, ability to maintain set, response monitoring, and abstract reasoning (verbal, visual). It is important, however, to acknowledge that an important concept in the examination of frontal systems and executive functions is that of "neighborhood signs." These signs refer to the expectation that problematic behaviors and behavioral deficits should both aggregate in neighboring frontal regions and be dissociable from lesions that cause some elements of the same behaviors but arise out of other brain systems. Thus, for example, a child who is very slow to complete Trails B and makes many errors of shifting from letters to numbers might also manifest loss of set in the Wisconsin Card Sorting Test or a verbal fluency test but may not exhibit evidence of an underlying language disorder or primary motor slowing.

Since children spend most of their early years in school settings, and success in the school setting is defined by the acquisition of various academic skills, assessment of achievement is a common part of a pediatric neuropsychological assessment. While it is obvious that this domain of functioning is a critical component in a learning disabilities assessment, negative consequences of primary neurological disorders as well as the CNS effects of various medical conditions and their treatment often include academic difficulties. It is helpful to compare results of school-based group-administered standardized achievement tests with individually administered tests in the pediatric neuropsychological assessment setting. Often, while the school assesses the grade or age-based levels of academic achievement of the patient, use of diagnostic testing by the neuropsychologist may be able to determine what factors in the child's attentional abilities, language development, memory functioning, motor and visuomotor skills, and/or executive functions may be contributing to academic difficulties. In addition, other confounding factors, such as comorbid disorders (ODD, Anxiety Disorders, Depression), adjustment disorders in response to an illness or injury, and even family stress, can negatively impact both classroom performance and standardized test scores. Social-emotional deficits, motor dyspraxias, and treatment-related side effects, such as attentional problems, sleepiness, fatigue, and physical changes, also are often factors that interfere with the affected child's ability to master age- or grade-appropriate academic skills. As a result, children who are experiencing these problems often do not match the phenotypical profile of the child with specific learning disabilities. Of similar concern, many schools utilize a restricted range of assessment instruments to determine eligibility for ESE services. Thus, the focus on achievement-intellectual discrepancies in many evaluations for learning disabilities services may be unable to "capture" subtle deficits in cognitive processing that contribute to academic difficulties for the child with a developmental or acquired neurological disorder.

Because the brain is responsible for both cognitive and emotional functioning and because emotional processing deficits may arise as a consequence of or in response to childhood neurological disorders or traumatic injuries, assessment of mood and psychiatric symptoms is an important part of a comprehensive pediatric neuropsychological assessment. There is a variety of self-report questionnaires that assess the child's and adolescent's awareness of problems in attention, impulsivity, and executive abilities. These can be compared to parent-report questionnaires of the same domains in order to develop a convergent and/or divergent picture of problematic behaviors that may be present. More experimental approaches to assessing emotional processing of pictures, faces prosody have been developed in adult neuropsychological assessment and are now being applied to research studies of groups of children with various developmental, neurological, and neuropsychiatric disorders (Baron, 2004; Goldstein & Reynolds, 1999; Rourke, 1995; Yeates et al., 2002). The impact of the child's illness on self-concept is also an important issue and may be assessed through self-report measures such as the Multidimensional Self-Concept Scale (Bracken, 1992). This scale is helpful in defining the child's perception of self in five functional domains: physical, social, competence, academic, and family functioning.

Finally, one important aspect of neuropsychological assessment is to understand the impact of a developmental or acquired neurological disorder on adaptive functioning. Traditionally, this can be assessed through a comprehensive interview such as the Vineland Adaptive Abilities Scale—2 (Sparrow, Balla, & Cichetti, 2005) or through a parent-report instrument such as the Adaptive Behavior Scales (Lambert, Nihira, & Leland, 1993). The goal of the domain of the examination is both to define the child's level of adaptive functioning and to determine the child's relative strengths and weaknesses when compared to children with comparable cognitive abilities. This type of information is particularly helpful in assessing children with developmental disabilities and/or mental retardation. The reader is referred to a recent compendium of normative data for neuropsychological assessment (Baron, 2004). Some normative data on children's tests are also found in an adult test compendium (Spreen & Strauss, 1998).

BEHAVIORAL OBSERVATIONS

Observations of a child's behavior can occur in several contexts:

1. In the waiting room with parents
2. Walking to and from the testing room
3. During the formal test taking
4. During informal observations of certain aspects of motor and sensory behavior

While waiting to be seen, the child may be observed playing alone with toys or books available in the waiting room of a clinical area or interacting with other children who are also waiting to be seen. This allows the examiner to observe for signs of potential behavior problems, such as hyperactivity, shyness or withdrawal, impulsivity, preferences to play with younger children, nature of interactive play with other children, aggression, social awkwardness, repetitive stereopathies, spontaneous language, and spontaneous emotional expressiveness. Tentative hypotheses about potential problematic behavior may develop from such behavioral observations. One can also sometimes get a sense of parent–child interactions, interjections of parental guidance in the child's play, the child's response to cautions or limit setting by the parent, and the child's inclusion of the parent in the free-form play activity. Older children may be more likely to be observed sitting beside the parent, actively looking at other children/adolescents in the waiting room, absorbed in handheld video games, reading a book, or engaged in pleasant or conflictual conversation with the parent. Again, this sometimes allows the examiner to develop tentative hypotheses about the social-emotional functioning and maturity/adaptability of the patient.

Observation of abnormalities of gait, posture, motor coordination, spontaneous language, and emotional expressiveness often occurs while walking patients to a testing room. The ease of separating from parents, their responses to rapport-building examiner behaviors, and even the evidence of initial motivational level (e.g., early complaints about how long the exam may take) may take place during this walk and entry into the testing room.

In addition, qualitative observation for so-called abnormal pathognomonic signs can take place. Overt behaviors, such as tics, movements, and lateralized weakness can occur. In addition, certain genetic syndromes or developmental disorders have typical physical features that indicate underlying neuropathology. For example, microcephaly, "electric hair," low-set ears, high palate, cutaneous tumors, and vascular hemangiomas and the like can be observed in the child's appearance.

Observations of behaviors relevant to formal testing are another source of data in the evaluation. Problems in maintaining attention, distractibility, anxiety about performance, fatigue, and the need for repeated redirection to the test procedures will often emerge over the course of a pediatric neuropsychological assessment. The impact of positive reinforcers (e.g., stickers, candy, and praise) and delayed rewards (e.g., a prize for completing the assessment) can also be assessed during the examination. Again, these data may be the basis for clinical inferences about the impact of problematic behavior on test scores obtained, as well as providing a window into similar problems that may arise in the school or home setting. Other significant observations may include seizures, stereotypes, perseverative behaviors, angry outbursts, tearfulness, comprehension difficulties, and oppositional or defiant behaviors that may support parent reports and other clinical data about the child's problematic behavior and/or developmental maturity.

Informal observations can also allow the clinician to develop inferences about the child's potential behavioral problems. For example, during a break in formal testing, the child may hurry to a water fountain in the hallway, and the clinician can observe the form of the child's walking/running, looking for such problems as toe running or walking, uneven arm swings, lateralized leg weakness, inability to rapidly alternate arm and leg movements, difficulties in initiating or stopping movement, and awareness of surroundings. Whether the child eagerly or reluctantly returns to the waiting area to talk to a parent or how the child proceeds to or has difficulty finding the testing room may again contribute to clinical inferences about the child's motor and sensory behaviors as well as motivational states, attention, and social interactions. However, when assessing a child who is an inpatient in a medical or psychiatric setting, nursing staff and therapists notes about the child's behavior may be a necessary additional source of data for clinical diagnostic inferences.

INTEGRATING SOURCES OF INFORMATION TO DEVELOP A CLINICAL DIAGNOSIS IN PEDIATRIC NEUROPSYCHOLOGICAL ASSESSMENT

The three main sources of behavioral data developed in a pediatric neuropsychological assessment are developmental history (including medical history), test results (including behavioral questionnaires), and behavioral observations over the course of the entirety of the neuropsychological assessment. These domains of behavioral data should be integrated in order to address the critical questions outlined earlier in the previous section on components of the comprehensive pediatric neuropsychological assessment. Specifically, comparisons to normal developmental indices and to normative test data allow a decision to be made about whether the findings indicate some abnormality of functioning. Second, data developed from parent report of medical history, along with behavior problems of the child, review of medical records, and developmental history, may suggest that the behavioral deficits found through observation and formal testing represent evidence of a primary, secondary, or tertiary brain dysfunction. Third, addressing the question of whether the behavioral deficits observed can be attributed to cortical or subcortical system deficits is important. Similarly, whether the pattern of behavioral deficits suggests diffuse or focal brain dysfunction should be included. Next, the report should address how well the description of the presenting problem (e.g., seizure disorder) matches the pattern of test deficits and behavioral problems documented in the neuropsychological examination. Other factors that may contribute to the clinical picture but not directly attributable to a primary brain disorder should be explained. Integration of these sources of information should lead to an initial clinical impression of the diagnosis and a clinical description of the domains of function affected by the disorder. Given the diagnosis, it would then be important to describe how well the individual child's pattern of impairment matches what is known about the behavioral phenotype of this disorder.

The final section of the report should include specific recommendations regarding:

1. Referral for any additional medical or other health professional evaluations relevant to the child's diagnosis
2. Possible referrals for additional therapies (e.g., pharmacotherapy, behavioral therapy)
3. Specific recommendations for interventions or strategies to maximize the child's performances in school and adaptations in the home environment.

In order for the assessment report to adequately address each of these questions, it is important for the examiner to have a background in both normal and abnormal development, knowledge of the different types of childhood disorders and their behavioral phenotypes, an appreciation of the sensitivity and specificity of the test measures in detecting both abnormal functioning and clinical group assignment, experience in obtaining information through a comprehensive clinical interview, an appreciation of the specificity of the various medical diagnostic procedures (physical and laboratory) that may be contained in the medical record, and some knowledge of both the commonalities and distinctiveness of the behavioral phenotypes of a wide variety of childhood developmental disorders and of acquired disorders.

Historically, the presence or absence of a brain lesion was the first question addressed in neuropsychological assessment of children or adults. More commonly, however, current emphasis is placed on description of the behavioral effects of a known disorder. A careful and comprehensive behavior description of the effects of a given brain disorder (whether developmental or acquired) complements the armamentarium of medical diagnostic tests such as EEGs, CT scans, and MRI scans that help define the structural integrity of the brain but cannot describe the complex behavioral consequences of structural or electrophysical deviations. It is in the richness of the behavioral depiction of the effects of brain structural or electrophysiological lesions that the neuropsychological examination can make its greatest contribution. And it is then on the basis of this behavioral phenotyping that preliminary interventions are developed and can be assessed for their efficiency. Knowledge of current advances in interventions, whether these involve environmental changes, teaching alternative strategies to improve performance, providing assistive devices to circumvent certain deficits, or direct therapeutic assault on a behavioral difficulty through pharmacological, physical, occupational, or speech therapies or more innovative behavioral strategies, including functional analysis of problematic behaviors, is an essential ingredient in the recommendations section of the report.

EDUCATIONAL TRAINING IN PEDIATRIC NEUROPSYCHOLOGY

Pediatric neuropsychology is an emerging subspecialty in clinical neuropsychology. Practitioners in the clinical area may first develop an interest in pediatric neuropsychology during their graduate school training. Master's research and doctoral dissertations on various topics in childhood developmental, neurological, and neuropsychiatric disorders are increasingly common. Through supervised practical experiences while in graduate training programs, the interested student may gain some experience in approaches to pediatric neuropsychology. However, such preinternship clinical and research experiences are not uniformly available in graduate programs in clinical psychology. Nor is there an accredited graduate program in clinical psychology or in clinical neuropsychology that offers an exclusive pediatric neuropsychology track. As a result, most advanced training in pediatric neuropsychology begins at the internship level and typically may continue in a clinical or research postdoctoral fellowship. In recognition of this area of clinical practice, specialty board certification for candidates who are pediatric neuropsychologists is available through two, sometimes competing credentialing boards: the American Board of Professional Psychology (ABPP) and the American Board of Professional Neuropsychology. However, neither board offers a specific subspecialty certification in pediatric neuropsychology at this time. As a result, basic knowledge in the methods and procedures in classical adult syndromes and current conceptualizations of clinical issues in adult neuropsychology remain part of the credentialing process. Both boards also require documentation of clinical and/or research training in clinical neuropsychology.

What general educational coursework in clinical or educational psychology is needed to specialize in pediatric neuropsychology? In addition to the required graduate school core courses in child development and in the behavioral bases of behavior, many pediatric neuropsychologists have had additional coursework in medical neuroanatomy as well as in developmental disorders, child neurology, and child psychopathology. Practicum experiences in clinical assessment of children and families are an essential early training ingredient. Advanced practica in settings that will expose the graduate student to specific populations of clinical groups is also critical to the development of professional level skills in pediatric neuropsychology. At the graduate level, research experiences and didactic coursework in assessing childhood medical, neurological, and behavioral disorders is also helpful to the student's development.

During the internship year, at a minimum some portion of the intern's training should take place in an outpatient clinic or inpatient setting where experiences in evaluations, consult-liaison activities, and intervention specific to children and their families occur. Postdoctoral training should be supervised by someone who specializes in pediatric neuropsychology. While this training may primarily emphasize research with children or clinical practice, exposure to the relevant research and clinical methodologies in examining acquired or developmental childhood disorders provides the postdoctoral fellow with the knowledge of how advances depend on clinical and experimental methodologies. If an individual seeks to emphasize practice and research with children but has not had the previously described background, it is unlikely that attending a workshop or assessing children will be sufficient to bridge the knowledge and experiential distance between studies of adults versus children. Continuing education on relevant topics in childhood disorders, as well as some supervision by an experienced pediatric neuropsychologist coupled with topical readings in the field, may help both to smooth the transition to a different practice area and to guarantee that the clinician is indeed practicing in his/her area of competence.

SUMMARY

As its current growth in terms of numbers of practitioners suggests, the specialty of pediatric neuropsychology is likely to continue to attract interested professionals. Future collaborations between pediatric neuropsychologists and pediatric medical subspecialties will continue to flourish. The parallel development of pediatric psychology in the assessment and treatment of children with a variety of congenital and acquired pediatric medical disorders has contributed to the growth of our understanding of the difficulties faced by children and families coping with medical and neurological disorders. Similarly, active research collaboration between pediatric neuropsychology, child psychiatry, and developmental pediatric specialists in the diagnosis and treatment of childhood behavioral disorders will continue to advance our appreciation of the role of brain functions in complex childhood neuropsychiatric disorders. As our knowledge of the genetic basis of common developmental disorders expands, it is likely that pediatric neuropsychology will continue to be able to extend our appreciation of these disorders and their treatments.

REFERENCES AND RESOURCES

Adams, W., & Sheslow, D. (2003). *Manual for the Wide Range Assessment of Memory and Learning* (2nd ed.). San Antonio, TX: Psychological Corporation.

Baron, I. S. (2004). *Neuropsychological evaluation of the child.* New York: Oxford University Press.

Baron, I. S., Fennel, E. B., & Voeller, K. (1995). *Pediatric neuropsychology in a medical setting.* New York: Oxford University Press.

Beery, K. E., Buktenica, N. A., & Beery, N. (2004). *Manual for the Beery–Buktenica Developmental Test of Visual Motor Integration* (5th ed.). Odessa, FL: Psychological Assessment Resources.

Benedict, R. H. B. (2001). *Manual for the Brief Visuospatial Memory Test—Revised.* Odessa, FL: Psychological Assessment Resources.

Benton, A., & Hamsher, K. (1983). *Multilingual Aphasia Examination.* Iowa City, IA: Department of Neurology, University of Iowa Hospital and Clinics.

Bracken, B. A. (1992). *Multidimensional Self-Concept Scale.* Austin, TX: Pro-Ed.

Brown, L., Sherbenou, R. J., & Johnson, S. K. (1997). *Examiner's manual for the Test of Nonverbal Intelligence* (3rd ed.). San Antonio, TX: Psychological Corporation.

Brownell, R. (2000a). *Expressive One-Word Picture Vocabulary Test—manual.* Los Angeles: Western Psychological Services.

Brownell, R. (2000b). *Receptive One-Word Picture Vocabulary Test—manual.* Los Angeles: Western Psychological Services.

Chelune, G. J., & Baer, R. A. (1986). Developmental norms for the Wisconsin Card Sorting Test. *Journal of Clinical and Experimental Neuropsychology, 8,* 219–228.

Coffey, C. E., & Brumback, B. A. (Eds.). (1998). *Textbook of Pediatric Neuropsychiatry.* Washington, DC: American Psychiatric Press.

Cohen, M. J. (1997). *Children's Memory Scale.* New York: Psychological Corporation.

Conners, K. C. (1996). *Manual for the Conners Rating Scales—Revised.* San Antonio, TX: Psychological Corporation.

Delis, D. C., Kaplan, E., & Kramer, J. H. (2001). *Delis–Kaplan Executive Functions System (DKEFS).* San Antonio, TX: Psychological Corporation.

Delis, D. C., Kramer, J. H., Kaplan, E., & Ober, B. A. (1994). *Manual for the California Verbal Learning Test: Children's Version.* San Antonio, TX: Psychological Corporation.

Dunn, L. M., & Dunn, L. M. (1997). *Examiner's manual for the Peabody Picture Vocabulary Test—III.* Circle Pines, MN: American Guidance Services.

Friedes, D. (2001). *Developmental Disabilities.* Malden, MA: Blackwell.

Gaddes, W. H., & Crockett, D. J. (1975). The Spreen–Benton aphasia tests: Normative data as a measure of language development. *Brain and Language, 2,* 257–280.

Gioia, G., Isquith, P. K., Guy, S. C., & Lenworthy, L. (2000). *Manual for the Behavior Rating Inventory of Executive Functions.* Odessa, FL: Psychological Assessment Resources.

Golden, C. J. (1978). *Stroop Color and Word Test manual for clinical and experimental uses.* Chicago: Stoelting.

Goldstein, S., & Reynolds, C. R. (1999). *Handbook of neurodevelopmental and genetic disorders in children.* New York: Guilford Press.

Grant, D. A., & Berg, E. A. (1993). *Wisconsin Card Sorting Test manual.* Odessa, FL: Psychological Assessment Resources.

Gronwall, D. M. A. (1994). *Administration manual for the Paced Auditory Serial Attention Test.* San Antonio, TX: Psychological Corporation.

Kaplan, E., Goodglass, H., & Weintraub, S. (1983). *Boston Naming Test—Revised.* Philadelphia: Lea & Febiger.

Korkman, K., Kirk, U., & Kemp, S. (1997). *NEPSY: A developmental neuropsychological assessment.* San Antonio, TX: Psychological Corporation.

Kovacs, M. (1992). *Children's Depression Inventory.* North Tonawanda, NY: Multi-Health Systems.

Lezak, M. D., Howieson, D. B., & Loring, D. W. (2004). *Neuropsychological assessment.* New York: Oxford University Press.

Manly, T., Robertson, I. H., Anderson, V., & Nimmo-Smith, I. (1998). *Manual for the Test of Everyday Attention for Children.* San Antonio, TX: Psychological Corporation.

Menkes, J. H. (1995). *Textbook of Child Neurology.* (5th ed.). Philadelphia: Lea and Febinger.

Meyers, J. E., & Meyers, K. R. (1996). *Manual for the Rey Osterrieth Complex Figure Test and Recognition Trial.* San Antonio, TX: Psychological Corporation.

Ravens, J. C. (1998). *Comprehensive technical manual for the Progressive Matrices.* San Antonio, TX: Psychological Corporation.

Reitan, R., & Davison, L. (1974). *Clinical neuropsychology: Current status and applications.* New York: Hemisphere.

Reynolds, C. R., & Bigler, E. D. (1994). *Test of Memory and Learning (TOMAL).* Austin, TX: Pro-Ed.

Reynolds, C. R., & Fletcher-Janzen, (Eds.). (1997). *Handbook of clinical child neuropsychology* (2nd ed.). New York: Plenum Press.

Reynolds, C. R., & Kamphaus, R. W. (2004). *Manual for the Behavioral Assessment System for Children—2.* Circle Pines, MN: American Guidance Services.

Reynolds, W. M. (1987). *Wepman's Auditory Discrimination Test—manual.* Los Angeles: Western Psychological Services.

Reynolds, W. M. (2002). *Reynolds Adolescent Depression Scale—Revised.* Odessa, FL: Psychological Assessment Resources.

Rourke, B. P. (Ed.) (1995). *Syndrome of Nonverbal Learning Disabilities.* New York: Guilford.

Semel, E., Wiig, E. H., & Secord, W. (2003). *Manual for the Clinical Evaluation of Language Fundamentals—4.* San Antonio, TX: Psychological Corporation.

Siven, A. B. (1991). *Manual for the fifth edition of the Benton Visual Retention Test.* San Antonio, TX: Psychological Corporation.

Sparrow, S., Balla, D., & Cichetti, D. (2005). *Vineland Adaptive Behavior Scales—II.* Circle Pines, MN: American Guidance Services.

Speilberger, C. D., Edwards, C. D., Lushene, R., Montuori, J., & Platzek, D. (1973). *State-Trait Anxiety Inventory for Children.* Odessa, FL: Psychological Assessment Resources.

Spreen, O., & Strauss, E. (1998). *A compendium of neuropsychological tests* (2nd ed.). New York: Oxford University Press.

Thorndike, R., Hagen, E. P., & Sattler, J. M. (1986). *Guide for administering and scoring for the Stanford–Binet Intelligence Scale* (4th ed.). Chicago: Riverside Press.

Wechsler, D. (1991). *Manual for the Wechsler Intelligence Scale for Children—III.* San Antonio, TX: Psychological Corporation.

Wechsler, D. (1997). *Manual for the Wechsler Memory Scale—III.* San Antonio, TX: Psychological Corporation.

Wechsler, D. (1999). *Manual for the Wechsler Abbreviated Scale of Intelligence (WASI).* San Antonio, TX: Psychological Corporation.

Wechsler, D. (2001). *Wechsler Individual Achievement Test* (2nd ed.). San Antonio, TX: Psychological Corporation.

Wechsler, D. (2003). *Manual for the Wechsler Preschool and Primary Scale of Intelligence—III.* San Antonio, TX: Psychological Corporation.

Wechsler, D. (2004). *Integrated and interpretative manual for the Wechsler Intelligence Scale for Children* (4th ed.). San Antonio, TX: Psychological Corporation.

Wilkinson, G. S. (1993). *Manual for the Wide Range Achievement Test—3.* San Antonio, TX: Psychological Corporation.

Williams, K. T. (1997). *Expressive Vocabulary Test manual.* Circle Pines, MN: American Guidance Services.

Woodcock, R., McGrew, K., & Mather, N. (2001). *Woodcock Johnson Psychoeducational Battery—III: Tests of achievement.* Circle Pines, MN: American Guidance Services.

Yeates, K. O., Ris, M. D., & Taylor, H. G. (2002). *Pediatric neuropsychology: Research, theory and practice.* New York: Guilford Press.

25

Academic Skills Problems

EDWARD S. SHAPIRO

Center for Promoting Research to Practice
Lehigh University
Bethlehem, Pennsylvania

MILENA A. KELLER

School Psychology Program
Lehigh University
Bethlehem, Pennsylvania

INTRODUCTION

The predominant reason that children are referred for assessment in schools relates to academic skill deficits. For example, Bramlett, Murphy, Johnson, and Wallingsford (2002) reported in a national survey of the practices of school psychologists that problems in reading or mathematics comprise 57% and 27% of total referrals, respectively. Referrals for behavior problems tended to make up less than 15% of those assessed. Others have reported similar findings, suggesting that academic skills problems represent the most significant problem referred to psychologists in schools (Reschly & Wilson, 1995). Such data are consistent with national longitudinal studies, which report that 17.5% of the nation's children will encounter reading problems in the crucial first three years of school (National Reading Panel, 2000). Approximately 75% of these children still have reading difficulties through the 9th grade (Francis, Shaywitz, Stuebing, Shaywitz, & Fletcher, 1996; Shaywitz et al., 1992).

Historically, the purpose of the school-based assessment process when students are referred because of academic skills problems is usually to determine whether they have the requisite discrepancy between cognitive ability and achievement that would qualify them as in need of special education for a learning disability. The typical methodology of assessment has been administration of individualized norm-referenced tests that cover multiple domains of academic skills problems. Outcomes from these measures are compared against the scores on a test of intellectual functioning, and if students show substantial differences between cognitive potential and academic achievement, they may be considered eligible for special education services under the category of learning disabled. A secondary purpose of the assessment of academic skills would be to identify strengths and weaknesses in students' academic profiles, which are designed to lead the evaluator toward making recommendations for potential intervention strategies to remediate these academic skill deficiencies.

Unfortunately, while the use of standardized achievement tests to conduct an assessment of a student referred for academic skills problems may lead to a diagnostic decision-making process to determine their prospective eligibility for special education services, the methodology does not meet the key ingredient of good assessment—the link to intervention. The roots of behavioral assessment lay in developing models that are linked closely to intervention planning and evaluation and that moved evaluators away from assessment predominately for diagnosis (e.g., Cone, 1978; Cone & Hawkins, 1977; Hartman, Roper, & Bradford, 1979; Hersen & Bellack, 1981). Since the mid-1980s, the methods embedded within behavioral assessment have been recognized as standard practice in conducting clinical assessments (Mash & Terdal, 1997; Shapiro & Kratochwill, 2000).

Parallel to the development of behavioral assessment as the accepted methodology for conducting assessments for students referred for behavioral or emotional problems, an identical process has emerged for assessing academic skills. The purpose of this chapter is to introduce readers to a methodology of assessing basic academic skills focused on problem solving that has been designed to evaluate a student's skills and performance that is linked to intervention development and that can be used dynamically to show responsiveness to instructional intervention. Specifically, the chapter introduces the reader to the concepts of *curriculum-based assessment* (CBA) and how these strategies are being used in the assessment of basic skill development of elementary students. A full description of these methods is beyond the scope of this chapter. Interested readers are encouraged to seek out sources such as Shapiro (2004a, 2004b), Shinn (1998), and the voluminous materials published by such authors as Doug and Lynn Fuchs and Stanley Deno.

ASSUMPTIONS AND PURPOSES OF ACADEMIC ASSESSMENT

Hartman et al. (1979), in the early development of the concepts of behavioral assessment, contrasted the basic differences in assumptions that underlie what they named as traditional versus behavioral models of assessment. The differences described by Hartman et al. illustrated the nature of behavioral assessment

TABLE 25.1 Comparison of Problem-Solving and Norm-Referenced Standardized Assessment Models for Academic Assessment

Area of Assumption	Problem-Solving Model	Norm-Referenced Standardized Tests Model
Conceptualization of learning process	Primarily environment/skills interaction	Primarily underlying psychological/neurological processes
Causes of behavior	Environment/skills interaction	Poor skills, information processing
Role of academic behavior	Sample skills under conditions of observation	Indexes underlying dysfunction
Role of history	Reinforcement history important	Important to explain observed dysfunction
Consistency	Performance problem/look for situational specificity	Assumed to be cross-situational
Uses of data	Target behavior; select intervention; monitor and evaluate treatment	Diagnostic; prescribe mode of instruction; match instruction with learning style
Level of inference	Low	High
Comparisons	Idiographic and local nomothetic	National nomothetic
Methods	Direct measurement	Indirect measurement
Timing	Ongoing	Pretest/post-test
Scope	Many variables, across situations, across skills	Global

as a method that emphasized the environmental context and situationally specific nature of behavior. They noted that behavioral assessment focused on idiographic over nomothetic interpretation as well as intervention development and evaluation over diagnosis. Although subsequent developments in behavioral assessment have resulted in an approach that blends idiographic and nomothetic interpretations (Cone, 1988; Mash & Terdal, 1997), the basic differences between behavioral and nonbehavioral models has yielded differences in the methods that underlie the assessment approach.

Table 25.1 compares the assumptions that underlie the problem-solving versus standardized norm-referenced assessment approaches to evaluating academic skills. Starting at the conceptualization of the academic skill deficit, the problem-solving model emphasizes the environment-by-skills interaction, over an emphasis on underlying neuropsychological processes. Likewise, academic skills problems are viewed as behavioral events that are specific to the conditions in which they occur, recognizing that many academic skills problems are as much a function of the instructional context as they are poor learning processes. Thus, in a problem-solving model, as much emphasis is placed on an assessment of the instructional environment as on an assessment of skill development (Lentz & Shapiro, 1986). Data in a problem-solving assessment are used to focus and direct the instructional process rather than to diagnose or identify the presence of learning problems, such as learning disabilities (Shinn, 1989). Inferences in a problem-solving model from the observed behavior to interpretation are low compared to standardized norm-referenced assessment, where the material actually assessed may not be as direct an assessment of what the child is actually being asked to learn. Finally, problem-solving approaches to assessment use direct rather then indirect measures of skills. Students who are referred for problems in reading will be assessed by asking them to read materials that are within or related to the curriculum of instruction. The nature of standardized norm-referenced assessment is such that the materials often included in the measures used for evaluation may be much less related to what students are actually being asked to do in classrooms.

Overall, a problem-solving method for assessing basic academic skills is viewed as closely linked to the foundations of a behavioral assessment methodology. Measures are direct, are focused on developing effective instructional strategies, consider both performance and skill deficits, and are capable of dynamic, ongoing evaluation of intervention development.

HISTORY OF CURRICULUM-BASED ASSESSMENT

Development of curriculum-based assessment (CBA) dates back primarily to the work of Stanley Deno and Phyllis Mirkin at the University of Minnesota, Institute for Research in Learning Disabilities, in the 1970s. These researchers and their team were looking for a method that could provide an efficient set of tools that would allow teachers to closely track the performance of students over time while instruction was being conducted. The measures were to be used to drive the instructional process and help teachers decide over short periods of time whether changes in instruction were being reflected in student performance. While teachers often pretest and posttest around an instructional change, Deno wanted a measure that could reflect overall growth toward long-term curriculum objectives. Likewise, the measures needed to be brief and have minimal impact on instructional time.

Researchers established that the measurement system needed to be standardized, repeatable over time, provide a direct assessment of the academic behavior of interest, and be sensitive to instruction. Over the course of many years and multiple research studies (e.g., Deno, 1985; Deno, Mirkin, & Chiang, 1982; L. S. Fuchs, Deno, & Marston, 1983; Shinn, 1989), Deno and colleagues developed the strategy known as curriculum-based measurement (CBM). Metrics were required to hold up to the psychometric properties of test–retest and internal reliability as well as concurrent and predictive validity that are expected of all norm-referenced standardized tests as established by national standards. However, CBM metrics were designed to be linked to the curriculum of instruction, were found to be sensitive to changes in instruction, and were found to have properties that allowed the measures to be used as a repeated assessment over time.

In the early years of development, Deno and his colleagues attempted to have teachers devise measures that were taken directly from the curriculum of instruction. These measures attempted to assess a student's acquisition of skills in the curriculum and to identify the points in the curriculum where skill deficits were evident. Instruction was very much tied to the outcomes of the measures; and as students acquired the skills being taught, new measures were developed that were keyed to the new objectives of the curriculum. Although this approach to assessment has considerable instructional validity, the measures failed to meet the technical adequacy standards expected of reliable and valid strategies. In addition, teachers needed to constantly develop new measures that would change when each objective was changed. What Deno and his colleagues found is that one could use a set of standardized measures that would be constant across the varied curricula offered by schools and that would meet the required properties of reliability and validity.

Use of the measures emerged predominantly within the special education literature, for the measures were found to be extremely valuable as a methodology for screening, identification, instructional decision making, and progress monitoring. Much of the research reported by Deno and those who were trained under his tutelage (Doug and Lynn Fuchs, Doug Marston, Mark Shinn, to name a few) continued to show that the measurement system had broad capability and applicability to general education students who were referred for academic skill problems but were not eligible for special education services (e.g., Deno, 2003; L. S. Fuchs, 2004). The efforts of Deno and his colleagues have led to the full acceptance of CBM as an empirically supported methodology for conducting academic assessments of basic skill areas such as reading, mathematics computation, mathematics concepts and applications, writing, and spelling (e.g., National Center on Student Progress Monitoring, 2005). Although there have been some attempts to extend this work to the secondary level and content-based instruction (e.g., Espin, Busch, Shin, & Krischwitz, 2001; Espin et al., 2000; Espin & Tindal, 1998), those efforts have not yielded the strong outcomes evident in assessing basic skills within the elementary levels.

Over the 20 years since the measures were first introduced, they have gained increasing interest and acceptability by education professionals (Shapiro, Angello, & Eckert, 2004; Shapiro & Eckert, 1994). Usage has been endorsed by major professional groups, including the Oregon Assessment Analysis, and most recently by the National Center on Student Progress Monitoring (http://www.studentprogress.org). Efforts have emerged to use the measures statewide for identification of special education eligibility (Iowa; Tilly, Reschly, & Grimes,

1999) as well as progress monitoring (PA) (Shapiro, Edwards, & Zigmond, 2005), and the measures have reached levels of national importance. Most recently, CBM has been viewed as a viable measure to be used when a response-to-intervention model is employed as an alternative to the discrepancy model in the process of conducting eligibility determination for learning disabilities (D. Fuchs & Reschly, 2004; Peterson & Shinn, 2002; Speece, Case, & Molloy, 2003).

MODELS OF CURRICULUM-BASED ASSESSMENT

Other researchers and practitioners developed models of assessment based on the original ideas of Deno and Mirkin. In particular, researchers developed measurement systems that would be derived directly from the curriculum of instruction, and the outcomes of these assessments would drive the ensuing instructional process. For example, Howell, Fox, and Morehead (1993) developed a measurement system entitled *curriculum-based evaluation* that would help teachers identify the strengths and weaknesses of the instructional process and focus the assessment process on determining responses to effective instruction. Others, such as Gickling and Havertape (1981) and Hargis (1995), likewise established models of curriculum-based assessment that would be focused on improving and informing the instructional process.

L. S. Fuchs and Deno (1991), in a seminal article, reviewed the identified models of CBA and divided all models into one of two categories—general outcomes measurement or specific subskill mastery. General outcomes measurement (GOM) systems use standardization across time. The measures themselves are not taken directly from the curriculum of instruction but are related to the behavioral outcomes expected from the skill under consideration. For example, GOM in reading involves students reading passages they have never seen before. The outcome behavior, that is, reading the passages aloud, becomes the measure of interest. Although students may not have seen the specific reading material before the assessment is conducted, their behavioral performance on the reading measure serves as the index of reading performance within the curriculum of instruction.

GOM is designed to determine student performance over the long-term period of instruction. Measures are used repeatedly, with alternate forms given at each assessment session. Measures are capable of being repeated as frequently as twice a week, without concern for practice effects. Research has shown these measures to be highly sensitive to instruction and to be a direct reflection of student acquisition of skills being taught through the instructional process. When student performance deviates from the expected level of performance, teachers and others using these measures are cued that the current instructional processes are ineffective and that changes are needed. Although the measures are not designed specifically to indicate the nature of the changes required, a GOM system offers opportunity for the evaluator to make reasonable educational hypotheses about what instructional changes may need to be made.

Material used in GOM models are always brief and timed measures of behavior. Rate (behavior change over time) is the key outcome variable, because this metric has been found consistently to be the most sensitive to student learning (Fuchs & Fuchs, 1999; Fuchs, Fuchs, Hamlett, Walz, & Germann, 1993). For example, if two students are asked to read the same 200-word passage, both read the passage without error, both correctly answer any questions about the material following reading, but one takes 2 minutes to complete the task and the other 5 minutes, it is clear that the student who took only 2 minutes to read the material would be deemed the better reader. Thus, rate rather than accuracy becomes the only metric that clearly differentiates the performance of these two students.

Among the types of GOM models, CBM represents the one with the most empirical support. The model has been widely validated for use in screening (Shinn, Shinn, Hamilton, & Clarke, 2002), determining special education eligibility (Shinn, 2002; Tilly et al., 1999), instructional decision making (Shinn et al., 2002), and progress monitoring (Marston & Tindal, 1995; Shinn, 1989, 1998). Indeed, as indicated previously, the model has attained widespread acceptability among teachers (Eckert, Shapiro, & Lutz, 1995), psychologists (Shapiro, Edwards, Lutz, & Keller, 2004), and other education professionals.

Specific subskill (SS) mastery models focus on the acquisition of skills that the student is being taught. This model of CBA breaks down the skill being taught into subskills that, when accumulated, reflect the learning process of the larger skill. Essentially, SS models view the learning process as the acquisition of a series of short-term objectives. For each of these objectives, a new measure is constructed that serves as a pre–post type of assessment on the skill development. Each test is seen as a criterion-referenced type of assessment that reflects how well students have learned that particular skill. Emphasis in measurement is on the accuracy of student performance, rather than rate, with most measures reporting the number or percentage of correct responses made on the assessment tool. The measurement system requires a defined skill hierarchy that guides the instructional process. Each time a new objective is defined, a new measure is developed and administered. The measures are not standardized, and typically they are teacher developed because they reflect the specifics of the teaching process.

An example will best illustrate this model of academic assessment. Suppose a teacher assesses and determines that a student who is struggling in spelling is having difficulties with vowel teams and blending. Deciding to begin teaching vowel teams (which is a skill earlier in the skill hierarchy than blending), the teacher administers an assessment of vowel teams and establishes the baseline levels of instruction. An instructional plan is implemented to teach the skill, and the student is reassessed once a week using an alternate form of the measure. Once the student achieves criterion on the skill of vowel teams, the teacher then turns her attention to blending. A new measure is developed and administered that assesses blending, and a new instructional plan is implemented as well. Repeated assessment of blending is conducted; when the student meets the criterion for blending, the teacher moves on to yet another skill.

Although there has been far less empirical development and support for the SS model of CBA, several efforts to offer validation of the measurement system have emerged. In particular, Burns and his colleagues (Burns, 2004; Burns, Tucker, Frame, Foley, & Hauser, 2000) have established that the measures can have reasonable levels of reliability, can be used as effective judgments of student performance, and can offer valid guides for directing the instructional process. The measures have shown themselves valid for the assessment of sight-word acquisition, retention, and reading comprehension (Burns et al., 2000; Burns, 2001).

Both of these broad models have components that are necessary for conducting an effective and full-scale assessment of academic skills problems. Whereas the GOM model is ideal for establishing a student's instructional placement against expected performance of peers as well as for determining the long-term outcomes of student progress toward instructional objectives, the SS model offers the evaluator an opportunity to establish short-term objectives and to examine student acquisition of skills targeted for instruction by the teacher. Likewise, both models offer opportunities for evaluators to identify areas in need of intervention as well as to suggest likely effective strategies to target the deficit skills. Unfortunately, neither the GOM nor the SS model focuses attention on the student's academic environment and the impact of the context of instruction on academic outcomes.

Shapiro (2004a) and Shapiro and Lentz (1985) have described a model of academic assessment that incorporates a four-step process linking the key components of an SS and a GOM model of CBA, but it also includes a full assessment of the academic environment as a critical aspect of the evaluation process. As illustrated in Figure 25.1, the model begins with an assessment of the academic environment (step 1), continues with an evaluation of determining a student's instructional level within the curriculum (step 2), the development and implementation of instructional strategies to improve academic skills (step 3), and finally progress monitoring (step 4) to determine the effectiveness of the interventions implemented in step 3. As seen in Figure 25.1, Shapiro's (2004a) approach to assessment includes aspects of the models described by the original work of Deno and Mirkin (1977), the SS models such as those described by Gickling (Gickling & Havertape, 1981; Gickling & Rosenfield, 1995) or Howell (Howell & Nolet, 1999), as well as the GOM model described by Deno (1985, 2003) and his many colleagues.

CBA is conceptualized as a form of behavioral assessment of academic skills. Like other behavioral assessment methods, the measures are outcomes of direct skills that represent the skill of interest. If the assessment is of a student's reading, then the skill assessed is whether the student can read. If the assessment is of a student's mathematics, the skill assessed is whether students can accurately com-

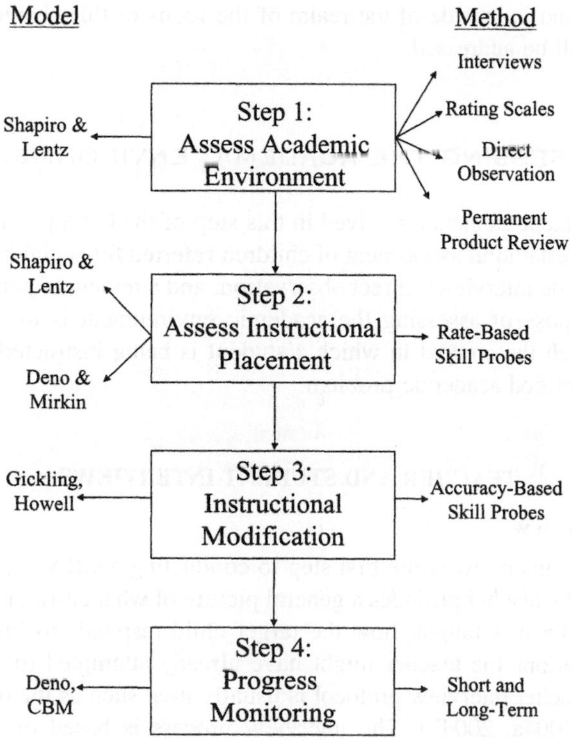

FIGURE 25.1 Integrated model of curriculum-based assessment. Adapted from Shapiro (1990, p. 331). Copyright 1990 by the National Association of School Psychologists. Adapted by permission of the author and reprinted from Shapiro (2004a).

plete problems in math computation and/or concepts. The key difference from more norm-referenced standardized measures is that the material students are being assessed on are clear representations of what they are being taught. Indeed, the link between what is tested and what is taught is extremely important in CBA models. Although in some models (GOM) the measures tested are not the same curriculum of instruction, such tested materials have a demonstrated link.

Like other behavioral assessment models, the methodology is multimodal and multidimensional. As indicated by Mash and Terdal (1997) and Shapiro and Kratochwill (2000), behavioral assessment has come to incorporate multiple perspectives and multiple sources of data. CBA has likewise used multiple sources and modes of evaluation. As indicated in the model described by Shapiro, one incorporates both direct and indirect sources of measurement (i.e., interviews with informants (teachers), students, direct observation, rating scales as needed, and an assessment of skills).

The remainder of this chapter offers a more detailed description of the methodology embedded in Shapiro's (2004a) model. Given that step 3, Instructional Modification, involves predominantly the work done by instructional consultants and teachers and is outside of the realm of the focus of this chapter, only steps 1, 2, and 4 will be addressed.

ASSESSING THE ACADEMIC ENVIRONMENT

The assessment elements involved in this step of the CBA process mirror the tools used in behavioral assessment of children referred for social/behavior problems and include interviews, direct observation, and a review of permanent products. The purpose of assessing the academic environment is to determine the degree to which the context in which a student is being instructed is contributing to the identified academic problem.

TEACHER AND STUDENT INTERVIEWS

Teacher Interview

The teacher interview is the first step to conducting a CBA. Gathering information from the teacher provides a general picture of what curriculum is used for instruction, how it is taught, how the target child responds to instruction, and what modifications the teacher might have already attempted to remediate the problem. A teacher interview protocol is usually used such as the one developed by Shapiro (2004a, 2004b). The interview process is based on the problem-identification portion of the behavioral consultation model, which involves identifying those environmental variables that may be impacting the problem (DiPerna & Elliott, 2002; Kratochwill & Bergan, 1990; Kratochwill, Elliott, & Stoiber, 2002). Through the interview all major academic areas are discussed, including reading, math, spelling, and writing, and it typically requires 15–20 minutes once the interviewer is fluent with the interview protocol (Shapiro, 2004a, 2004b).

The first portion of the teacher interview gathers information about the curriculum used and the target student's progress through the curriculum compared to the "typical" student in the class. It is also necessary to determine how instructional time is used (e.g., small groups based on reading levels or a large group) and what the expectations are for students during the various instructional settings. Specific skills in areas such as word attack, vocabulary, and comprehension (for the portion of the interview on reading) and how the target student's performance on these skills relates to peers at the same level are also discussed. Since it is likely that a student referred for instructional difficulties has been experiencing these problems for some time, the interventions that have already been used to address the referral concerns are explored and the frequency, intensity, and integrity of implementation are also determined. Finally, any salient competing behaviors that occur during reading instruction should be explored to determine the degree to which they impact the target student's learning.

The teacher interview specific to mathematics is similar to that for reading. Given that problems in mathematics occur in both computation and concepts/applications skills, an effective interview must explore both of these areas. In order to get an accurate picture of the target student's progress in the math curriculum, it is most informative to determine what basic computational skills he or she has developed. This can be accomplished using a list of computation objectives and an understanding of what concepts and applications skills (e.g., money, estimation, and graphing) are important for the particular grade level. Within the list of skills it is important to determine the skills in which the student is currently being instructed, which skills the student has accomplished, and which skills are frustrating for the student. It is beneficial to ask the same questions for the "average" student in the classroom, to serve as a comparison. The remaining questions related to mathematics instruction are similar to the reading teacher interview and gather information related to the instructional setting, assessment procedures, and interventions implemented.

Written language, including spelling and handwriting, are also addressed during the teacher interview. These skills are typically embedded in language arts instruction, so the portions of the teacher interview investigating this area are less involved but still address the salient characteristics of instruction and student performance.

In addition to interview data from the teacher, rating scales can be used to gather supplementary data regarding the target student's academic performance. Two such rating scales include the Academic Performance Rating Scale (APRS; DuPaul, Rapport, & Periello, 1991), which is designed to investigate teacher perceptions of student academic performance, and the Academic Competence Evaluation Scales (ACES; DiPerna & Elliott, 2002), designed to gather information about academic enablers, such as motivation, study skills, and academic engagement, from not only teachers but also parents and students.

Based on the interviews with the teacher, along with rating scales, a considerable amount of information is gathered to determine the academic tasks and settings that are most problematic for the target student and the environmental variables that are potentially influencing behavior. Indeed, teacher reports have consistently been found to be highly reliable sources of data on academic performance (e.g., Feinberg & Shapiro, 2003; Gerber & Semmel, 1984; Hoge & Coladarci, 1989) and often can serve as the springboard for attaining a full understanding of the nature of the academic environment.

Student Interview

The student interview is designed to assess the student's perspective on the classroom, the academic tasks assigned, and his or her own skills and behavior. It is important to obtain from the target student the degree to which he or she understands teacher instructions and expectations. The student interview can be initiated around a classroom observation, which provides the student with a concrete example to which to refer when answering questions related to how he or she feels about his or her own academic skills and abilities in the classroom. This information can be used not only to better understand the target student's areas of need but also to appropriately design interventions that will be effective.

Several formats for student interviews have been reported in the literature, including ones described by Shapiro (2004a, 2004b) and Ysseldyke and Christenson (2002). In these interviews, students are asked to provide an indication of how well they understood a teacher's instructions, to explain what they were expected to do on a particular task, to indicate the degree to which they felt they were going to be successful on the assigned task before they began, and their understanding of what they need to do if they have to seek help. These and similar types of questions offer the evaluator insight into the students' perspective on their own academic skill problems.

DIRECT OBSERVATION

Using the information from the teacher interview and rating scales, the next step in assessing the academic environment is conducting a direct observation of the target student. This step in assessing the academic environment provides a quantitative picture of academic behavior that may or may not be consistent with the other information gathered. Direct observation allows the assessor to gather data in the student's natural instructional environment in order to quantify how much time the student spends focused on academic tasks as well as the nature and frequency of opportunities to respond in the classroom (Greenwood, Horton, & Utley, 2002).

Prior to starting the classroom observation, the observer determines what tasks children will be involved in during the observation and what the teacher's expectations are for student behavior so that an accurate assessment of behavior can be made. It is most beneficial to observe during the instructional time and topic that is most problematic for the student. For example, if the target student is struggling with basic math skills and the teacher indicated that independent seatwork is particularly problematic, then that instructional time and setting should be observed. Although special attention should be paid to those settings noted by the teacher as problematic, it is also important to obtain a broad sample of behavior, and thus additional settings and subjects should be observed.

A valuable addition to the observation of the target student is inclusion of observational data on comparison children in the classroom. Observation of comparison children allows for a determination of how much the target student's behavior diverges from that of the typical student in the class. Teacher input can help to identify "average-performing" peers in the classroom that can be used as comparisons. Direct classroom observation serves to complement the information provided by the teacher interview.

Many structured observational codes exist that would be effective for an observation conducted as part of CBA. The reader is directed to Shapiro (2004a,

2004b) for a complete list of suitable observation protocols. One such code is the Behavioral Observation of Students in Schools (BOSS; Shapiro, 2004b). The BOSS allows for the recording of two types of on-task behavior, active and passive, as well as the observation of three types of off-task behavior, including verbal, motor, and passive behavior. Data are also collected as to whether the teacher is engaged in instruction toward the target student, and an observation of comparison children is integrated into the code every fifth interval. Each behavior observed using the BOSS is clearly defined, which results in quantified observational data that allow for the comparison of the target student's behavior across settings and academic subjects, a comparison of the target child to other children in the classroom, and a more complete understanding of how environmental variables impact the target student's learning. Software for the BOSS is also available for data collection on a personal digital assistant (PDA), making the data collection process relatively simple (Shapiro, 2003). For a more involved discussion of how to interpret BOSS data as part of CBA, the reader is directed to Shapiro (2004a, 2004b).

PERMANENT PRODUCT REVIEW

A permanent product review should include the materials completed by the target student during the direct classroom observation as well as recent work completed in the classroom, with special attention given to the subject of concern. The purpose of the permanent product review is to evaluate how the student performs on a typical day in the classroom. Reviewing student worksheets, quizzes, and everyday assignments can provide further information regarding relative strengths and weaknesses for the target child. Reviewing the task completed during direct classroom observation is particularly informative because it can either confirm or contradict the observation results. If a child were to be observed off-task for a large duration of the class period but he or she completed the assigned task, the conclusion would be different than if the child were to be observed on-task for most of the observation but only completed a small portion of the assignment. These two scenarios provide an example of how the data collected through two methods, direct observation and permanent product review, can work side by side for effective interpretation.

An assessment of the academic environment involves several components, including teacher interview and rating scales, direct classroom observation, student interview, and permanent product review. Taken together these pieces of assessment data serve to validate each other and to provide a complete picture of the student's performance in the classroom and what aspects of the instructional setting prove to be strengths and weaknesses. By identifying the components of the instructional environment that may be problematic, interventions can be developed during the instructional modification phase that target these components and result in improved academic performance.

ASSESSING INSTRUCTIONAL PLACEMENT

The next step in the four-step model of CBA is an assessment of instructional placement. Through the teacher interview, preliminary information is gathered regarding the target student's progress through the curriculum in all major subjects. With this background information gathered, instructional assessment of the student must take place using what was learned about the student's progress through the curriculum to select what skill levels to assess. The target student's skills are assessed through the use of CBM probes in all major academic subjects. The assessment methodology for each academic subject, to be addressed later, is based on Shapiro (2004a) and Shinn (1989). The reader is directed to these two resources for a more in-depth discussion of the procedures for assessing instructional placement.

READING

Today's elementary reading curricula are typically a compilation of existing literature selected on the basis of several criteria, including grade-level appropriateness, but are not always controlled for grade-level readability. Materials used to assess instructional level must have an established level of readability that is within the grade level of that which it has been labeled. Although it is possible to construct probes from the curriculum used in the classroom, the skill level and readability of the content of the curricula make it difficult to locate a passage appropriate for use in CBA. A better strategy than developing passages from the curriculum of instruction is for assessors to use passages with established readability, such as those commercially available from AIMSweb (http://www.aimsweb.com), Scholastic Fluency (http://teacher.scholastic.com), or similar sources. Interested readers can find a large number of free sets of passages at www.interventioncentral.org. For a more detailed discussion of how oral reading probes are actually constructed, the reader is directed to Shapiro (2004a) for assistance.

The purpose of assessing reading is to determine whether the student is placed at the instructional level in the curriculum and to provide initial, or baseline, reading skill levels that can be used to track student progress in response to instruction. Instructional level is defined as the level at which instruction is likely to be most effective. In contrast, if the student is being instructed at a frustrational level, then they are likely to fail, whereas if they are instructed at their mastery level, then they are not being sufficiently challenged.

Administration

Administering oral reading fluency probes involves several steps. The child should be informed that he or she will be asked to read aloud and should do his or her best. If reading comprehension will be assessed, the child should be told, prior to reading that passage, that questions will be asked about its content. The child can then be given a copy of the probe to read and the timer should be started. While the child reads aloud, errors are documented, including omitted words, mispronunciations, and substitutions. If the child inserts a word that is not in the passage, it is noted but not counted as an error. Repetitions and self-corrections are not counted as errors; and if the child pauses longer than 3 seconds, the assessor provides the word and counts the pause as an error. After 1 minute has elapsed, the assessor stops and marks where the child ended. The number of words read correctly and the number read incorrectly should be recorded. In situations where the child completes the passage early or if more than 1 minute is used, the rate of reading should be calculated by dividing the number of words (correct or incorrect) by the number of seconds read and multiplying that number by 60, which will provide the words per minute.

If comprehension questions are being asked, the child must read the entire probe, but the examiner must still note the number of words read during 1 minute. While comprehension questions are asked, the assessor should note if the child uses the passage to answer the questions. The percentage of questions correct should be calculated.

Starting at the level where the child is being instructed, the child is asked to read three probes from that level. Comprehension is usually checked on only one of the three probes. Once the reading probes for the target child's grade level have been administered, each probe is scored and the median (middle score) correct, the median incorrect, and the comprehension score are reported. Using primarily the data on the number of words correct per minute, the level of the child's reading is classified as frustrational, instructional, or mastery. The objective is to find the highest level at which the child is instructional. Based on the child's performance, the evaluator repeats the process by either administering the next level up or down in the series and continues until an instructional level followed by a frustrational level is found (e.g., Level 4 = Frustrational, Level 3 = Instructional, Level 2 = Instructional, Level 1 = Mastery). If two instructional levels are obtained, as in the example here, the highest instructional level is used. Determination as to what constitutes a frustrational, instructional, or mastery level in oral reading fluency is usually based on the collection of local norms, where instructional level is set as the 25th percentile or better of the grade in the district and mastery is usually set at the 75th percentile or better.

Interpretation

The reading assessment provides information related to the instructional level of the target student and what level of curricular materials would allow for the most learning opportunities, that is, a level that is both challenging and allows for growth. The instructional level determined during the reading assessment may also explain the target child's current difficulties with the material being presented in the classroom. If a child's instructional level is one or more grade levels behind the material currently used in instruction, it would be beneficial to talk with the classroom teacher about appropriate adjustments to level of material used such that the target child is able to fully benefit from instruction. Consistent with the purpose of the oral reading fluency assessment, the results can be used as guidelines for setting instructional goals to be achieved in the classroom.

MATH

The curriculum-based assessment of mathematics differs from that of reading in that the focus is on specific skill acquisition. A sequence of computation skill instruction should be obtained from the school district, or a generic list of skills can be used, as described by Shapiro (2004a, 2004b). Assessment of computational skills can be done through single-skill or multiple-skills probes, each with its own advantages. Single-skill probes are useful when determining what specific skills have been mastered and for providing detailed recommendations on how to improve skills. When constructing single-skill probes, it must be determined what skills should be evaluated through the skills survey done during the teacher interview. The probes should include 20–30 problems on a sheet for simple problems, allowing space for the student to work, and they should include a representative sample of problems and digits. Commercial and free electronic methods of constructing single skill math probes are available, including online services that generate probes, such as Aplus math (http://www.aplusmath.com) and Intervention Central (http://www.interventioncentral.com).

Multiple-skill mathematics computation probes are also valuable because they allow for the assessment of a larger number of skills at once. Several problems for each skill should be included, with two to three computational skills included in one probe. Multiple-skill probes can be constructed manually or accessed through the Web sites noted earlier.

As with the assessment of mathematics computation skills, the assessment of concepts and applications relies on the information provided by the teacher regarding the skills with which the student has become comfortable and those with which the student is struggling. Concepts and applications probes are most practically constructed to include multiple skills and are designated for various grade levels. Pro-Ed publishes a series of concepts and applications probes (L. S. Fuchs, Hamlett, & Fuchs, 1999a, 1999b, 1999c) that are suitable for the assessment of these skills.

Administration

The assessment and scoring of mathematics probes include two general steps. First, when using single-skill probes, only two probe sheets for each skill should be administered. The child is presented with the probe and told to solve each problem without skipping any and that if he or she does not know how to solve a problem, he or she can move to the next item. Addition and subtraction probes use a 2-minute time limit; probes that include multiplication and division use a 5-minute time limit. Students need to be monitored while working to ensure that they do not skip around to answer only those problems they know. Student performance is scored as the number of individual digits correct per minute.

The final step of scoring the probes includes counting the separate digits in an answer that are correct and incorrect. For computation probes, digits below the answer line are counted, except for long division problems. The number correct and the number incorrect are counted. If the child completes the entire probe prior to the time limit, the number of digits must be divided by the total number of seconds used to complete the probe and then multiplied by 60 to find the numbers of digits correct and incorrect per minute. For mathematics computation, the *mean* score for the probes assessing the same skill becomes the score for that skill. Although digits correct per minute is the metric used to determine math performance, it might also be valuable to compute the percentage of problems correct. The scoring of concepts and applications probes involves counting all the blanks on the page as one point and then computing the percentage of possible points earned. Using district normative data, instructional levels can be established, again using the 25th to 75th percentiles of the grade-based district performance. If the student scored at the mastery level, then a more difficult probe can be administered; if the student performed at the frustrational level of performance, a probe including easier skills can be used.

Interpretation

Determining the instructional placement of students with respect to mathematics skills is less important than it is in the assessment of reading. Instead, determining what skills the student has mastered and which skills he or she struggles with is more important from a practical perspective. The emphasis is on fluency, particularly with basic computational skills, because fluency is a foundational skill allowing for acquisition of more advanced skills. The same is true for development of concepts and applications skills; those students who are slow to solve problems will not be able to advance to more complex skills and concepts. A child's performance on the computation and on the concepts and applications math CBA probes can be used in ways similar to that suggested for reading, including setting goals and monitoring a student's progress toward the goals through repeated assessment.

WRITTEN EXPRESSION

The next skill area to be assessed is written expression. Its purpose, as with math and reading, is to identify the type of skills the target student has attained and the level of fluency displayed when using those skills.

Administration

Assessment of written expression involves the use of "story starters," short phrases that are used to give the target student an idea of what to write about. Story starters are typically narrative in nature and should be interesting to children. Two or three story starters can be used; as with the reading assessment, the median score is considered most representative of the student's performance. The story starter is presented to the child and read aloud. The assessor instructs the child to write a story using the story starter as the first sentence. Students are given 3 minutes to write their story after a minute of time to think about their story. Once the student has finished writing, the number of words written that can be deciphered are counted. The child's spelling does not have to be correct, and capitalization and punctuation are ignored. The number of correct and incorrect words produced during the 3-minute time period are calculated; if the child stops writing prior to the end of 3 minutes, the same calculation procedure used to determine the number of words correct per minute in reading should be used to determine the number of words written correctly. Normative data can be developed to establish acceptable levels for each grade.

Interpretation

The written expression probe offers a great deal of data for assessing the student's current skills, including spelling, writing mechanics, and grammar. The results of a written expression assessment can, like the other forms of instructional assessment, guide the setting of goals and be used to monitor progress. Another method of interpreting a student's written expression product is using the "correct word sequences" method suggested by Espin et al. (2000). The reader is directed to the aforementioned reference for additional information on this method.

SPELLING

The final instructional area to be assessed in the CBA process is spelling. This can be taken directly from the curriculum; as with the other subjects, the teacher interview information should be useful in determining how spelling is taught and the instructional materials used. Since the placement of spelling instruction and the curriculum used are often elusive, the assessment of spelling is most informational if a specially designed, grade-level-specific list of words is used. Such a list can be obtained from AIMSweb (http://www.aimsweb.com).

Administration

When assessing a child's spelling skills, three sets of words are used. The words are read to first- and second-grade students at a rate of about one word every 10 seconds and at a rate of one word every 7 seconds for those students in third grade and beyond. The grade level of the words administered should be adjusted until appropriate grade levels are obtained (20–39 letter sequences for grades 1–2 and 40–59 letter sequences correct for grades 3–6).

Letter sequences correct are counted to evaluate performance. In order to determine letter sequences correct, a "phantom" character is used at the beginning and end of each word; then the number of correct letters in order is determined. For example, the word _apple_ has six letter sequences, one at each end of the word and four between the letters. If the word apple is spelled as _aple_, it has five letter sequences correct, and so on for the variety of mistakes that children may make.

Interpretation

The interpretations that can be made with the results of a spelling assessment are fairly limited. It can be used to determine the specific mistakes a student is making, such as difficulty with ending sounds or the frequent use of phonetic spelling. Those skills can then be targeted for increased intervention and monitoring.

INSTRUCTIONAL MODIFICATION

After the assessment of the academic environment and the assessment of instructional placement have been completed, the next step in the CBA is to modify instruction to address student needs. The strategies used to modify instruction and address the skill needs identified through the assessment of instructional placement are outside the realm of this chapter, and the reader is directed to several resources (McCarney, Wunderlich, & Bauer, 1993; Rathvon, 1999; Shapiro, 1996a, 1996b, 2004a, 2004b; Shinn, Walker, & Stoner, 2002). Once the method of instruction is modified, CBA strategies should be used to assess the progress of the student in response to the interventions being implemented. Frequent assessments of the student's progress should be made and instruction adjusted accordingly.

PROGRESS MONITORING

The method used to evaluate a child's response to instructional modification and his or her growth toward reaching instructional goals is progress monitoring. Progress monitoring is a data-based process by which teachers can track student progress and make instructional decisions in response to the child's performance (Deno, Espin, & Fuchs, 2002; L. S. Fuchs, 1989; Shapiro, 2004a). Progress monitoring can be used to set both short- and long-term goals, is repeated over time, is a direct assessment of student skills, and is examined graphically so that data-based decisions can be made effectively. Progress monitoring can focus on specific-skill mastery in order to determine whether instruction on a very narrow topic (e.g., double-digit multiplication) is effective, or the monitoring can be more general and examine more broad goals, which involves the general outcomes measurement form of monitoring. This more general form of monitoring uses probes to examine a student's progress through the general curriculum for that academic year. Such probes are designed to include all the curricular objectives for that year. The focus of this discussion will be primarily on long-term monitoring, which represents the use of the GOM model of CBA.

GENERAL PRINCIPLES OF PROGRESS MONITORING

Several general principles cut across progress monitoring in the various subject areas. These characteristics include direct and repeated assessment over time, setting goals, graphic depiction of the data, and the use of decision rules through which instructional decisions and modifications can be made. Regardless of the instructional subject being monitored, the probes are direct assessments of the child's skills, and they can be administered repeatedly. In fact the probes can be administered about once a week, for a time span of weeks or months. Repeated collection of data allows for the assessment of growth over time toward a goal, as long as the probe data are depicted graphically (Marston & Tindal, 1995; Shinn, 1989, 1998).

When conducting progress monitoring, a specific goal must be set that represents the performance expected of the student in response to intervention. There are general principles for what is considered a well-established goal, including that the goal be clear and precise, sufficiently ambitious, and developed through a collaborative process (L. S. Fuchs, 2002). Specifically setting CBM goals can be done in several different ways. If local norms for the measure have been developed, goals can be set to achieve a certain level of performance, based on the performance of other students in the district at the same grade level (Fuchs, 2002; Shapiro, 2004a). General norms are also available if districts have not been able to establish their own norms (Hasbrouck & Tindal, 1992).

Another option for goal setting is the use of average learning rates, which emphasizes the amount of growth expected over the course of a year (Fuchs, 2002; Shapiro, Edwards, & Zigmond, 2005). This method then uses the amount of growth expected at each grade level to set individualized goals for students and to establish the slope at which a student's skills should improve.

The final method of setting instructional goals for progress monitoring is to use the criteria from the instructional placement phase to set a goal. For example, a second-grade student who performs at the upper end of the frustrational category could have a goal to reach the middle of the instructional category. Although this type of goal setting is a bit more crude than others, it still provides general guidelines for goal setting and allows for the monitoring of student progress over time.

Once the performance goal has been set and monitoring has begun, data collected must be depicted graphically (Deno, Espin, & Fuchs, 2002). Time is plotted on the horizontal axis, with student performance plotted on the vertical axis. The graph includes four pieces of information, including the student's baseline performance, the goal he or she is expected to reach, the aim line that depicts the student's expected rate of growth, and the monitoring data, which are plotted as they are collected. This process can be done with the use of computer programs, or it can be done on paper.

The graph is then used to make instructional decisions based on the student's performance (Fuchs & Deno, 1991). Instructional decisions are based on decision rules established prior to the start of monitoring. This is done either by examining data points (e.g., if four points fall below or above the aim line, then instructional modification and goal adjustment should take place) or by using a trend line (e.g., if the student data trend line is higher than the aim line, then the goal should be increased) (Deno et al., 2002).

Conducting progress monitoring can be used to identify children who are struggling in the development of basic skills, but it can also be used to track the progress and model the growth of average-performing and successful students (Shinn et al., 2002). This type of ongoing assessment, done while instruction takes place, is truly dynamic in nature, thus complementing and informing the instructional process (Deno et al., 2002; Shinn et al., 2002).

This was a very brief discussion of progress monitoring for academic skills. The reader is directed to more complete resources for more information (Deno et al., 2002; Shapiro, 2004a; Shinn, 1989, 1998).

SUMMARY

CBA has increasingly become a staple of the assessment process for students referred in schools for academic skills problems (Shapiro et al., 2004). The methodology draws on the foundations of behavioral assessment methodology and emphasizes measures that are frequent, repeatable, direct, and focused on the development and evaluation of instructional intervention. Use of graphic analysis is critical to interpretation. The data are useful for multiple purposes of assessment, including screening, eligibility determination, instructional development, and program evaluation. Although the measures are not designed to replace the use of published, norm-referenced achievement tests, the purposes of CBA meet the important philosophical function of being closely linked to intervention.

The use of CBA is very popular within the special education community. Increasingly, the methodology is coming to be recognized as a legitimate and valid approach for use with students in general education settings who are referred because they are struggling in basic academic skill development. In addition, the measures have been validly extended downward in the area of reading to students who are showing difficulty with preliteracy skills (Good & Kaminski, 2002) and, most recently, with students showing difficulties in developing basic numeracy skills (Chard et al., 2005; Clarke & Shinn, 2004). Although the measures are used less and have less developed research for students who struggle with academics at the secondary level, some attempts to extend CBA to this level of concern have been reported in the literature (e.g., Espin et al., 2000; Espin & Tindal, 1998).

Despite the strengths of CBA, the limitations of the measurement systems certainly are evident. Given that interpretations of these measures rely on local normative comparisons, the necessity for local normative development becomes critical. Unfortunately, many local education agencies have not made such an investment. Normative data reported in the literature do afford such local education agencies the opportunity to still use these metrics (e.g., Fuchs et al., 1993; Hasbrouck & Tindal, 1992; Shapiro, 2004a); however, the need to develop local norms still remains. Peterson and Shinn (2002) recently showed the importance of the local comparison in the decision-making process when eligibility for learning disabilities is determined, reemphasizing the importance of collecting local CBA norms.

Second, the acceptability of the content validity of the measure is still questioned by many teachers and other education professionals. Validation of CBA comes primarily from the multiple studies reported where concurrent and predictive validity were determined. In these studies, CBA data in reading and math have consistently shown moderate-to-strong correlations with standardized, norm-referenced tests of achievement, including high-stakes statewide achievement measures (Good, Simmons, & Kame'enui, 2001; McGlinchey & Hixon, 2004; Stage & Jacobsen, 2001; Shapiro, Edwards, Lutz, & Keller, 2004). Despite these data, when first exposed to the nature of the CBA data, teachers oftentimes are not convinced that a student's reading performance is fully reflected in the oral reading fluency scores obtained on passages with which they have little familiarity. In a sense, teachers often question the content validity of the metrics. Experience has shown that it takes multiple years and repeated use of these metrics before teachers become comfortable (e.g., Shapiro, Edwards, Zigmond, 2005).

Regardless of the potential limitations of the metric, CBA has indeed become a significant methodology for the assessment of academic skills problems. The measures have clear conceptual links to behavioral assessment methodologies, are directly tied to the interpretation of academic behavior problems, and are closely linked to the development of intervention strategies. Recent literature surrounding this topic has outlined goals for the future of the CBA research agenda, including the amelioration of some of the limitations discussed here. L. S. Fuchs (2004) suggests that the future of CBM research must delve into addressing some of the issues that have prevented the full acceptance of this metric. Research must focus on the nature of progress monitoring and the instructional utility of CBM in practical settings. Throughout this discussion, research addressing these two areas has been highlighted; however, more research is needed to facilitate the routine use of CBM by educators. Efforts to make these measures as easy as they are effective and relevant are clearly needed. Readers of this chapter who operate from a more clinical, private-practice orientation would be wise to learn more about this methodology, which is a dominant approach to assessment in school settings.

REFERENCES AND RESOURCES

Bramlett, R. K., Murphy, J. J., Johnson, J., & Wallingsford, L. (2002). Contemporary practices in school psychology: A national survey of roles and referral problems. *Psychology in the Schools, 39,* 327–335.

Burns, M. K. (2001). Measuring sight-word acquisition and retention rates with curriculum-based assessment. *Journal of Psychoeducational Assessment, 19,* 148–157.

Burns, M. K. (2004). Using curriculum-based assessment in consultation: A review of three levels of research. *Journal of Educational & Psychological Consultation, 15,* 63–78.

Burns, M. K., Tucker, J. A., Frame, J., Foley, S., & Hauser, A. (2000). Interscorer, alternate-form, internal consistency, and test–retest reliability of Gickling's model of curriculum-based assessment for reading. *Journal of Psychoeducational Assessment, 18,* 353–360.

Chard, D. J., Clarke, B., Baker, S., Otterstedt, J., Braun, D., & Katz, R. (2005). Using measures of number sense to screen for difficulties in mathematics: Preliminary findings. *Assessment for Effective Intervention, 30,* 3–14.

Clarke, B., & Shinn, M. R. (2004). A preliminary investigation into the identification and development of early mathematics curriculum-based measurement. *School Psychology Review 33*(2), 234–248.

Cone, J. D. (1978). The Behavioral Assessment Grid (BAG): A conceptual framework and a taxonomy. *Behavior Therapy, 9,* 882–888.

Cone, J. D. (1988). Psychometric considerations and the multiple models of behavioral assessment. In A. S. Bellack & M. Hersen (Eds.), *Behavioral assessment: A practical handbook* (3rd ed., pp. 42–66). New York: Pergamon Press.

Cone, J. D., & Hawkins, R. (1977). *Behavioral assessment: New directions in clinical psychology.* New York: Brunner/Mazel.

Deno, S. L. (1985). Curriculum-based measurement: The emerging alternative. *Exceptional Children, 52,* 219–232.

Deno, S. L. (2003). Developments in curriculum-based measurement. *Journal of Special Education Special Issue: What Is Special About Special Education? 37*(3), 184–192.

Deno, S. L., Espin, C. A., & Fuchs, L. S. (2002). Evaluation strategies for preventing and remediating basic skill deficits. In M. R. Shinn, H. M. Walker, & G. Stoner (Eds.), *Interventions for academic and behavior problems II: Preventative and remedial approaches* (pp. 213–241). Bethesda, MD: National Association of School Psychologists.

Deno, S. L., & Mirkin, P. K. (1977). *Data-based program modification: A manual.* Arlington, VA: Council for Exceptional Children.

Deno, S. L., Mirkin, P. K., & Chiang, B. (1982). Identifying valid measures of reading. *Exceptional Children, 49,* 36–47.

DiPerna, J. C., & Elliott, S. N. (1999). Development and validation of the Academic Competence Evaluation Scales. *Journal of Psychoeducational Assessment, 17,* 207–225.

DiPerna, J. C., & Elliott, S. N. (2002). Promoting academic enablers to improve student achievement: An introduction to the mini-series. *School Psychology Review, 31,* 293–297.

DuPaul, G. J., & Rapport, M. D., & Periello, L. M. (1991). Teacher ratings of academic skills: The development of the Academic Performance Rating Scale. *School Psychology Review, 20,* 284–300.

Eckert, T. L., Shapiro, E. S., & Lutz, J. G. (1995). Teachers' ratings of the acceptability of curriculum-based assessment methods. *School Psychology Review, 24,* 499–510.

Espin, C., Busch, T. W., Shin, J., & Kruschwitz, R. (2001). Curriculum-based measurement in the content areas: Validity of vocabulary-matching as an indicator of performance in social studies. *Learning Disabilities: Research and Practice, 16,* 142–151.

Espin, C. A., & Tindal, G. (1998). Curriculum-based measurement for secondary students. In M. R. Shinn (Ed.), *Advanced applications of curriculum-based measurement* (pp. 214–253). New York: Guilford Press.

Espin, C., Shin, J., Deno, S. L., Skare, S., Robinson, S., & Benner, B. (2000). Identifying indicators of written expression proficiency for middle school students. *Journal of Special Education, 34,* 140–153.

Feinberg, A. B., & Shapiro, E. S. (2003). Accuracy of teacher judgments in predicting oral reading fluency. *School Psychology Quarterly, 18*(1), 52–65.

Francis, D. J., Shaywitz, S. E., Stuebing, K. K., Shaywitz, B. A., & Fletcher, J. M. (1996). Developmental lag versus deficit models of reading disability: A longitudinal, individual growth curves analysis. *Journal of Educational Psychology, 88,* 3–17.

Fuchs, D., & Reschly, D. (2004). National research center on learning disabilities: Multimethod studies of identification and classification issues. *Learning Disabilities Quarterly, 27,* 189–195.

Fuchs, L. S. (1989). Evaluating solutions monitoring progress and revising intervention plans. In M. Shinn (Ed.), *Curriculum-based measurement: Assessing special children* (pp. 153–181). New York: Guilford Press.

Fuchs, L. S. (2002). Best practices in defining student goals and outcomes. In A. Thomas and J. Grimes (Eds.), *Best practices in school psychology,* Vol. 1 (4th ed., pp. 553–563). Bethesda, MD: National Association of School Psychologists.

Fuchs, L. S. (2004). The past, present, and future of curriculum-based measurement research. *School Psychology Review, 33*(2), 188–192.

Fuchs, L. S., & Deno, S. L. (1982). *Developing goals and objectives for education programs* [Teaching Guide]. Minneapolis: U.S. Department of Education Grant, Institute for Research in Learning Disabilities, University of Minnesota.

Fuchs, L. S., & Deno, S. L. (1991). Paradigmatic distinctions between instructionally relevant measurement models. *Exceptional Children, 57,* 488–500.

Fuchs, L. S., Deno, S. L., & Marston, D. (1983). Improving the reliability of curriculum-based measures of academic skills for psychoeducational decision making, *Diagnostique, 8,* 135–149.

Fuchs, L. S., & Fuchs, D. (1999). Monitoring student progress toward the development of reading competence: A review of three forms of classroom-based assessment. *School Psychology Review, 28*(4), 659–671.

Fuchs, L. S., Fuchs, D., Hamlett, C. L., Walz, L., & Germann, G. (1993). Formative evaluation of academic progress: How much growth can we expect? *School Psychology Review, 22*(1), 27–48.

Fuchs, L. S., Fuchs, D., Hosp, M. K., & Jenkins, J. R. (2001). Oral reading fluency as an indicator of reading competence: A theoretical, empirical, and historical analysis. *Scientific Studies of Reading, 5*(3), 239–256.

Fuchs, L. S., Hamlett, C. L., & Fuchs, D. (1999a). Monitoring Basic Skills Progress: Basic Math Computation (2nd ed.) [Computer software]. Austin, TX: Pro Ed.

Fuchs, L. S., Hamlett, C. L., & Fuchs, D. (1999b). Monitoring Basic Skills Progress: Basic Reading (2nd ed.) [Computer software]. Austin, TX: Pro Ed.

Fuchs, L. S., Hamlett, C. L., & Fuchs, D. (1999c). Monitoring Basic Skills Progress: Basic Math Concepts and Applications (2nd ed.) [Computer software]. Austin, TX: Pro Ed.

Gerber, M. M., & Semmel, M. I. (1984). Teacher as imperfect test: Reconceptualizing the referral process. *Educational Psychologist Special Issue: Special Education, 19*(3), 137–148.

Gickling, E., & Havertape, J. (1981). *Curriculum-based assessment.* Minneapolis, MN: National School Psychology Inservice Training Network.

Gickling, E., & Rosenfield, S. (1995). Best practices in curriculum-based assessment. In A. Thomas & J. Grimes (Eds.), *Best practices in school psychology III* (pp. 587–595). Washington, DC: National Association of School Psychologists.

Good, R. H., & Jefferson, G. (1998). Contemporary perspectives on curriculum-based measurement validity. In M. R. Shinn (Ed.), *Advanced applications of curriculum-based measurement* (pp. 61–88). New York: Guilford Press.

Good, R. H., III, & Kaminski, R. A. (2002). *Dynamic Indicators of Basic Early Literacy Skills* (6th ed.). Eugene, OR: Institute for the Development of Educational Achievement.

Good, R. H., Simmons, D. C., & Kame'enui, E. J. (2001). The importance and decision-making utility of a continuum of fluency-based indicators of foundational reading skills for third-grade high-stakes outcomes. *Scientific Studies of Reading, 5*(3), 257–288.

Greenwood, C. R., Horton, B. T., & Utley, C. A. (2002). Academic engagement: Current perspectives on research and practice. *School Psychology Review, 31,* 326–349.

Hargis, C. H. (1995). *Curriculum-based assessment: A primer* (2nd ed.). Springfield, IL: Charles C Thomas.

Hartman, D. P., Roper, B. L., & Bradford, D. C. (1979). Some relationships between behavioral and traditional assessment. *Journal of Behavioral Assessment, 1,* 3–21.

Hasbrouck, J. E., & Tindal, G. (1992). Curriculum-based oral reading fluency norms for students in grades 2 through 5. *Teaching Exceptional Children, 24*(3), 41–44.

Hersen, M., & Bellack, A. S. (Eds.). (1981). *Behavioral assessment: A practical handbook* (2nd ed.). Elmsford, NY: Pergamon Press.

Hintze, J. M., & Christ, T. J. (2004). An examination of variability as a function of passage variance in CBM progress monitoring. *School Psychology Review, 33*(2), 204–217.

Hoge, R. D., & Coladarci, T. (1989). Teacher-based judgment of academic achievement: A review of literature. *Review of Educational Research, 59*(3), 297–313.

Howell, K. W., Fox, S. L., & Morehead, M. K. (1993). *Curriculum-based evaluation: Teaching and decision making* (2nd ed.). Pacific Grove, CA: Brooks/Cole.

Howell, K. W., & Nolet, V. (1999). *Curriculum-based evaluation: Teaching and decision making* (3rd ed.). Belmont, CA: Wadsworth.

Kratochwill, T. R., & Bergan, J. R. (1990). *Behavioral consultation in applied settings: An individual guide.* New York: Plenum Press.

Kratochwill, T. R., Elliott, S. N., & Stoiber, K. (2002). Best practices in school-based problem-solving consultation. In A. Thomas and J. Grimes (Eds.), *Best practices in school psychology,* Vol. 1 (4th ed., pp. 583–608). Bethesda, MD: National Association of School Psychologists.

Lentz, R. E., & Shapiro, E. S. (1986). Functional assessment of the academic environment. *School Psychology Review, 15,* 346–357.

Marston, D., & Tindal, G. (1995). Best practices in performance monitoring. In A. Thomas & J. Grimes (Eds.), *Best practices in school psychology* (Vol. 3, pp. 597–607). Washington, DC: National Association of School Psychologists.

Mash, E., & Terdal, L. (1997). *Assessment of childhood disorders* (3rd ed.). New York: Guilford Press.

McCarney, S. B., Wunderlich, K. C., & Bauer, A. M. (1993). *Pre-referral intervention manual* (2nd ed.). Columbia, MO: Hawthorne.

McGlinchey, M. T., & Hixon, M. D. (2004). Using curriculum-based measurement to predict performance on state assessments in reading. *School Psychology Review, 33*(2), 193–203.

National Center on Student Progress Monitoring. (2005). Retrieved July 22, 2005 from http://www.studentprogress.org/

National Reading Panel. (2000). *Teaching children to read: An evidence-based assessment of the scientific research literature on reading and its implications for reading.* Retrieved July 22, 2005 from http://www.nichd.nih.gov/publications/nrp/smallbook.htm

Peterson, K. M. H., & Shinn, M. R. (2002). Severe discrepancy models: Which best explains school identification practices for learning disabilities? *School Psychology Review, 31,* 459–476.

Rathvon, N. (1999). *Effective school interventions: Strategies for enhancing academic achievement and social competence.* New York: Guilford Press.

Reschly, D. J., & Wilson, M. S. (1995). School psychology practitioners and faculty: 1986–1991–92 trends in demographics, roles, satisfaction, and system reform. *School Psychology Review, 24,* 62–80.

Shapiro, E. S. (1996a). *Academic skills problems: Direct assessment and intervention* (2nd ed.). New York: Guilford Press.

Shapiro, E. S. (1996b). *Academic skills workbook.* New York: Guilford Press.

Shapiro, E. S. (2003). Behavioral Observation of Students in Schools—BOSS [Computer software]. San Antonio, TX: Psychological Corporation.

Shapiro, E. S. (2004a). *Academic skills problems: Direct assessment and intervention* (3rd ed.). New York: Guilford Press.

Shapiro, E. S. (2004b). *Academic skills workbook* (2nd ed.). New York: Guilford Press.

Shapiro, E. S., Angello, L. M., & Eckert, T. L. (2004). Has curriculum-based assessment become a staple of school psychology practice? An update and extension of knowledge, use, and attitudes from 1990 to 2000. *School Psychology Review, 33,* 243–252.

Shapiro, E. S., & Eckert, T. L. (1994). Acceptability of curriculum-based assessment by school psychologists. *Journal of School Psychology, 32,* 167–184.

Shapiro, E. S., Edwards, L., Lutz, J. G., & Keller, M. A. (2004, March). *Curriculum-based measurement predicted outcomes on high-stakes testing: Reading and math outcomes in Pennsylvania.* Paper presented at the meeting of the National Association of School Psychologists Convention, Dallas, TX.

Shapiro, E. S., Edwards, K., & Zigmond, N. (2005). Progress monitoring of mathematics among students with learning disabilities. *Assessment for Effective Intervention, 30,* 15–32.

Shapiro, E. S., & Kratochwill, T. R. (Eds.). (2000). *Behavioral assessment in schools: Theory, research, and clinical foundations* (2nd ed.). New York: Guilford Press.

Shapiro, E. S., & Lentz, F. E. (1985). Assessing academic behavioral: A behavioral approach. *School Psychology Review, 14,* 325–338.

Shaywitz, S. E., Escobar, M. D., Shaywitz, B. A., Fletcher, J. M., & Makuch, R. (1992). Distribution and temporal stability of dyslexia in an epidemiological sample of 414 children followed longitudinally. *New England Journal of Medicine, 326,* 145–150.

Shinn, M. R. (Ed.). (1989). *Curriculum-based measurement: Assessing special children.* New York: Guilford Press.

Shinn, M. R. (Ed.). (1998). *Advanced applications of curriculum-based measurement.* New York: Guilford Press.

Shinn, M. R. (2002). Best practices in using curriculum-based measurement in a problem-solving model. In A. Thomas and J. Grimes (Eds.), *Best practices in school psychology,* Vol. 1 (4th ed., pp. 671–697). Bethesda, MD: National Association of School Psychologists.

Shinn, M. R., Shinn, M. M., Hamilton, C., & Clarke, B. (2002). Using curriculum-based measurement in general education classrooms to promote reading success. In M. R. Shinn, H. M. Walker, & G. Stoner (Eds.), *Interventions for academic and behavior problems II: Preventative and remedial approaches* (pp. 113–142). Bethesda, MD: National Association of School Psychologists.

Shinn, M. R., Walker, H. M., & Stoner, G. (Eds.). (2002). *Interventions for academic and behavior problems II: Preventive and remedial approaches.* Washington, DC: National Association of School Psychologists.

Speece, D. L., Case, L. P., & Molloy, D. E. (2003). Responsiveness to general education instruction as the first gate to learning disabilities identification. *Learning Disabilities Research & Practice, 18,* 147–156.

Stage, S. A., & Jacobsen, M. D. (2001). Predicting student success on a state-mandated performance-based assessment using oral reading fluency. *School Psychology Review, 30*(3), 407–419.

Tilly, W. D., Reschley, D. J., & Grimes, J. (1999). Disability determination in problem-solving systems: Conceptual foundations and critical components. In D. J. Reschly, W. D. Tilly, & J. P. Grimes (Eds.). *Special education in transition: Functional assessment and noncategorical programming* (pp. 221–254). Longmont, CO: Sopris West.

Ysseldyke, J. E., & Christenson, S. L. (2002). *Functional assessment of academic behavior: Creating successful learning environments.* Longmont, CO: Sopris West.

26

Ethical and Legal Issues

CATHERINE MILLER
School of Professional Psychology
Pacific University
Forest Grove, Oregon

INTRODUCTION

Assessment, considered a "defining practice" and a hallmark of psychology (Camera, Nathan, & Puente, 2000, p. 141), may be defined as "a conceptual, problem-solving process of gathering dependable, relevant information about an individual, group, or institution to make informed decisions" (Turner, DeMers, Fox, & Reed, 2001, p. 1100). The outcomes of child assessment, in particular, may be wide ranging and life altering, including placement of a child in a special education class, determination of custodial arrangements within a family, and modification of treatment of a child patient (Miller & Evans, 2004). Given the potential impacts of assessment results, it is not surprising that both ethical and legal dilemmas are inherent in the practice.

This chapter has two goals: to familiarize the reader with ethical issues in assessment and to sensitize the reader to potential legal dilemmas inherent in testing. To accomplish these goals, the major resources for psychologists are reviewed first, including ethics codes, practice guidelines, federal and state statutes, and case law. Next, common ethical and legal issues encountered when assessing children are discussed. Finally, seven specific recommendations for child assessors are outlined.

ASSESSMENT RESOURCES

ETHICS CODES

Ethics codes regulating professional behavior have been developed for every major mental health organization. The American Psychological Association

(APA) first published a general ethics code for psychologists in 1953 (Miller, 2002). There have been several revisions since that time, with the latest version of the ethics code being published in 2002 (APA, 2002a). The American Counseling Association (ACA) developed a similar set of ethical guidelines for counseling students and master's-level counselors (ACA, 1995). Mental health professionals should be familiar with the ethics code promulgated by their professional organization, for adhering to these codes often is a requirement of state licensing laws.

PRACTICE GUIDELINES

Practice guidelines are defined as "statements that suggest or recommend specific professional behavior, endeavors, or conduct for psychologists" (APA, 2002b). Several organizations have produced general and specific practice guidelines pertaining to assessment. A well-known general guideline is the *Standards for Educational and Psychological Testing* (SEPT) (Joint Committee of the American Educational Research Association, American Psychological Association, and the National Council on Measurement in Education, 1999), which discusses the importance of employing psychometrically sound assessment instruments. Other general guidelines discuss training recommendations for assessors (e.g., *APA's Guidelines for Test User Qualifications*; Turner et al., 2001), confidentiality limits in assessment (e.g., *Statement on the Disclosure of Test Data*; American Psychological Association's Committee on Psychological Tests and Assessment, 1996), and appropriate expectations of test takers (*Rights and Responsibilities of Test Takers*; American Psychological Association Working Group of the Joint Committee on Testing Practices, 1998). Specific practice guidelines discuss how to assess clients in particular situations. Examples of specific guidelines include the *Specialty Guidelines for Forensic Psychologists* (Committee on Ethical Guidelines for Forensic Psychologists, 1991), *Guidelines for Psychological Evaluations in Child Protection Matters* (American Psychological Association Committee on Professional Practice and Standards, 1998), and *Guidelines for Child Custody Evaluations in Divorce Proceedings* (APA, 1994).

Practice guidelines are aspirational rather than mandatory and are intended to facilitate the continued development of the profession (APA, 2002b). Therefore, professional organizations cannot hold psychologists accountable for not following these guidelines. However, it is important for psychologists to be familiar with practice guidelines, because they may be regarded in courts of law as part of the ever-evolving standard of care.

FEDERAL AND STATE STATUTES

Several federal statutes affect assessment practices, including the Health Insurance Portability and Accountability Act (HIPAA, 1996), the Family Education

Rights and Privacy Act (FERPA, 1974), and the Individuals with Disabilities Education Act (IDEA, 1975). In addition, each state may set its own laws regarding confidentiality, informed consent, and types of training required for professionals to conduct assessments. Although several of these laws are discussed in this chapter, it is imperative that psychologists acquaint themselves with all applicable state and federal laws.

CASE LAW

The written decisions produced by judges ruling on individual cases are referred to as case law. Often, case law provides specific interpretations of somewhat vague state or federal statutes. Although it may be difficult at times to obtain information on specific cases, psychologists must remain current on assessment case law in their own states in order to practice effectively. LexisNexis is a search engine that all law libraries and many university libraries subscribe to that enables psychologists to search for legal cases on specific topics, such as assessment. Alternatively, psychologists may obtain summaries of case law by joining their state psychological organizations or Internet Listservs dedicated to ethical and legal issues in psychology.

ETHICAL ISSUES IN CHILD ASSESSMENT

COMPETENCE

Weiner (1989) stated that "competence is prerequisite for ethicality," concluding that "although it is . . . possible in psychodiagnostic work to be competent without being ethical, it is not possible to be ethical without being competent" (p. 829). Clearly, competence should be the assessor's first consideration, and ethical dictates require that clients be referred elsewhere if the assessor is not competent to answer the referral question(s).

Competence in assessment implies that the psychologist has a sufficient level of knowledge and training to determine appropriate tests, how to administer them, and how to interpret them. It should be noted that competence is not dependent on the specific degree obtained; instead, competence is determined by relevant training and supervised experience (Anastasi, 1976). Psychologists are advised to employ only those tests they have been trained to administer and to avoid using instruments with which they have no training or experience (Adams & Luscher, 2003). In its ethics code, APA emphasized the importance of competence in Standard 2.01, stating that psychologists provide services only within the boundaries of their competence, based on their education, training, supervised experience, consultation, study, or professional experience (APA, 2002a). However, APA did not clearly define the professional qualifications necessary for competence in administering tests. With few guidelines available on requisite qualifications of testers, "psychologists are generally left to address this matter on the basis of their own awareness of their competencies and limitations" (Koocher & Keith-Spiegel, 1998, p. 156).

At a minimum, psychologists should acquire training and supervised experience on each and every test they want to administer and interpret. Training should include courses in psychometrics, statistics, and test interpretation. Turner and colleagues (2001) outlined three areas of training considered essential for all test users: (a) psychometrics, including reliability, validity, and norms; (b) effects of ethnic, racial, cultural, gender, age, and linguistic variables on administration of tests and interpretation of scores; and (c) effects of disabilities on administration of tests and interpretation of scores. SEPT (Joint Committee of the American Educational Research Association, American Psychological Association, and the National Council on Measurement in Education, 1999) discussed how to modify tests to accommodate minorities and disabled clients, recommending that test reports include any modifications and the presumed impact on scores.

Because "competence in the use of one test or one group of tests [does not] imply competence in any other test" (Welfel, 1998, p. 226), overall competence in assessment cannot be assumed. Instead, competence on each test must be obtained through supervised administration and scoring experience. Clearly, the amount of time required to become competent in administration and scoring will vary, for some tests, such as the revised Wechsler Adult Intelligence Test (WAIS-III; Wechsler, 1997) and the Rorschach Inkblot Test (Rorschach, 1942) are more difficult to learn. Therefore, "a specific prescribed format or mechanism for supervision cannot be described for each test user" (Turner et al., 2001, p. 1104). What is clear is that supervision should be continued until the supervisor judges that mastery of the test is attained.

Adams and Luscher (2003) cautioned psychologists that competence is an impermanent construct. To avoid ethical dilemmas, they stated that psychologists "must maintain some degree of awareness regarding their level of competency" (p. 276). More specifically, Adams and Luscher advised psychologists to maintain competence by "reading current literature, attending conventions, and involving oneself in other, related scholarly activities" (p. 276).

INFORMED CONSENT

Informed consent in assessment suggests that the person being assessed (or his/her legal guardian) has agreed to be evaluated prior to testing and after being given relevant information on assessment (APA Committee on Psychological Tests and Assessment, 1996). Such information should include the reasons for testing, intended uses of data, possible consequences (including risks and benefits), what information will be released (if any), and to whom the information will be released (APA Committee, 1996). APA's ethics code reviews informed consent in assessment in Standard 9.03. Additional information on informed consent generally and on therapy can be found in Standards 3.10 and 10.01, respectively (APA, 2002a).

The term *informed consent* implies that only information is necessary for consent to be given. However, consent actually consists of three separate aspects: information, voluntariness, and competence (Bersoff, 1999a; Everstine et al., 1980). Although all three must be present for consent to be valid, the third aspect (competence) is especially important in child cases.

First, sufficient information must be provided to allow the individual the opportunity to make an informed decision regarding his or her participation in assessment. While it is unnecessary (and perhaps impossible) to review all possible outcome scenarios with the client, it is necessary to provide facts a reasonable person would need in arriving at an informed decision (Miller & Evans, 2004). Welfel (1998) advised psychologists to inform clients how test results will be used in decision making and to whom copies of test reports will be disseminated. He also suggested that psychologists inform clients that they have the right to refuse testing or to withdraw at any time without penalty (Welfel). Following presentation of this information, common practice entails asking the client to state the concept in his own words. This practice gives the examiner some degree of certainty regarding the client's understanding of consent (Miller & Evans).

Second, voluntariness means that the psychologist must obtain the test taker's consent "without exercising coercion or causing duress, pressure, or undue excitement or influence" (Koocher & Keith-Spiegel, 1998, p. 417). Discounting fees for assessment, offering incentives to complete survey questionnaires, and making positive consequences contingent on completing an evaluation (e.g., reentry to school after suspension) are all situations where voluntariness should be carefully scrutinized.

Finally, the test taker must be considered legally competent to grant consent. Unless legally deemed incompetent, all adults are assumed competent to give consent (Bersoff, 1999b). Children, on the other hand, generally are not presumed to be competent to provide consent in most cases. When assessing children, substitute consent typically must be obtained from parents or legal guardians (Przwansky & Bersoff, 1978). However, a psychologist must be aware of his/her own state's statutes, for the legal age to give consent varies by state. For example, in Oregon, state statutes grant minors 14 years of age or older the ability to consent to mental health treatment (Right to Diagnosis or Treatment for Mental or Emotional Disorder or Chemical Dependency without Parental Consent, 2003).

In states where legal consent must be obtained only from a parent or legal guardian, Everstine and colleagues (1980) recommended that psychologists acquire consent from the parent and assent from the child. The term *assent* suggests that children may not completely understand the nature and purpose of assessment or their involvement in it (Keith-Spiegel, 1983). However, clinicians are encouraged to provide information to children in developmentally appropriate language about the particular tests employed (Keith-Spiegel; Miller & Evans,

2004). As part of assent, the clinician should attempt to ascertain the child's wishes about participating. In these situations, psychologists may find that what a parent desires and what a child needs may be in conflict. Courts have generally given parents the authority to consent to assessment, regardless of what the child wants (Bersoff, 1999b).

CONFIDENTIALITY

Koocher and Keith-Spiegel defined confidentiality as "a general standard of professional conduct that obliges a professional not to discuss information about a client with anyone" (1998, p. 116). APA emphasized the importance of confidentiality primarily in Standards 4.01 and 4.02, which require psychologists to inform test takers, prior to assessment, of any mandatory, as well as any likely, releases of information (APA, 2002a). Confidentiality may be viewed as the basis for candid and cooperative participation from the client in the assessment process (Miller & Evans, 2004). Without such client participation, assessment results may be considered unreliable and invalid (DeKraai & Sales, 1982).

Release of Information to the Test Taker

APA Working Group (1998) has stated that test takers have the right to feedback about testing results, unless this right is waived by the test taker prior to testing or prevented by law (e.g., when courts mandate testing for competency to stand trial). However, it appears that psychologists may not routinely provide feedback to test takers. As recently as 1983, Berndt's survey of 100 psychologists found that a majority favored only limited feedback to test takers, suggesting that most examiners viewed full disclosure on a regular basis as an unrealistic goal. At least one feedback session following assessment is recommended to serve two main purposes (Welfel, 1998). First, a feedback session allows the test taker an opportunity to respond to incorrect or misleading conclusions. Second, feedback may be therapeutic for the client, promoting symptom reduction and improved client–therapist rapport. Welfel recommended that psychologists "provide as full a description as time, interest, and test security allow, [only] omitting or postponing review of results that the counselor judges would be harmful to the client's current well-being" (p. 230). A description of the examiner's feedback policy always should be reviewed during the initial informed consent process.

Release of Information to Third Parties

Regardless of the age of the test taker, some information obtained during assessment may be released to third parties (e.g., insurance companies, referral agencies, state agencies). For example, information may be requested by insurance companies and health maintenance organizations (HMOs) in order to determine eligibility for coverage or reimbursement for services rendered. In addition, information may be requested by employers, legal representatives, and schools in order to determine eligibility for services (Miller & Evans, 2004). In general, psychologists should exercise extreme caution in releasing only the necessary information to satisfy the inquiry of the third party rather than releasing the entire contents of the client's chart.

Child test takers pose special dilemmas for examiners. As previously discussed, unless granted by law, children are not considered capable of consenting to assessment. Therefore, testing results may be shared with the legal guardian who consented to the child's participation in assessment. However, a good rule of thumb is to follow the same procedures utilized for release of information to third parties. In other words, examiners must clarify the limits of confidentiality with the child and legal guardian at the outset of testing and should only release relevant information to the legal guardian (Miller & Evans, 2004).

MULTIPLE ROLES

APA (2002a) defined two types of multiple relationships: engaging in more than one professional relationship with a client (e.g., therapist and business partner) and mixing social and professional relationships with a client (e.g., therapist and significant other). Furthermore, APA (2002a) stated that multiple relationships may be either concurrent or consecutive.

Although certain multiple relationships (i.e., sexual relationships with clients) are prohibited, APA recognized in Standard 3.05 that not all multiple relationships are unethical. Specifically, a multiple relationship is allowed as long as it meets two criteria: (a) the relationship could not reasonably be expected to impair the psychologist's objectivity, competence, or effectiveness in performing his/her functions as a psychologist; and (b) the relationship does not exploit or harm the client. APA emphasized that it is the psychologist who bears the burden of proving that the multiple relationship meets both of these criteria (APA, 2002a).

To fulfill their ethical obligations, psychologists must clarify their roles with clients at the outset of the professional relationship. Practice guidelines suggest that psychologists be cautious in switching roles between assessor and therapist (APA, 1994; APA Committee on Professional Practice and Standards, 1998; Committee on Ethical Guidelines for Forensic Psychologists, 1991), for two main reasons. First, the assessment role requires a level of objectivity and neutrality not found in the therapy role; attempting to switch from a therapist to an assessor may compromise the assessment process (Hedges, 2000). Second, switching roles may harm the therapist–client relationship, because the assessment role may require the psychologist to report data perceived as negative by the client (Bailey, 2003).

LEGAL ISSUES IN CHILD ASSESSMENT

In addition to ethical proscriptions, assessment activities are affected by the legal system. Bersoff (1981) claimed that "no activity performed by psychologists is so closely scrutinized by the legal system as testing," due to the fact that testing has the "potential for causing legally cognizable injury to test takers" (p. 1047). Confidentiality and educational testing are two major legal issues within child assessment.

CONFIDENTIALITY

Although confidentiality has been reviewed as an ethical issue, it is also frequently a legal concept. A recently enacted federal law called the Health Insurance Portability and Accountability Act (HIPAA, 1996) set a federal floor on confidentiality, requiring explicit client authorization for release of information. Consequences of violating HIPAA may be severe, including monetary fines and imprisonment. State statutes may set stricter confidentiality standards, but they may not be less stringent than the federal standard. States and the federal government have created statutes regulating several issues within confidentiality, including rights of noncustodial parents, release of test protocols to parents, and child abuse reporting.

Rights of Noncustodial Parents

As previously stated, the parent or legal guardian may have access to his/her child's assessment information. Some states have also granted the noncustodial parent the right to access such information. In Oregon, for example, as long as the parent's rights were not terminated by the court, the noncustodial parent has access to his/her child's mental health records, including assessment information (Authority of One Parent When Other Parent Granted Sole Custody of Child, 2003). Psychologists must stay informed about their own state statutes to enable them to fully inform clients at the outset of the assessment process whether or not noncustodial parents will have access to testing results.

Parent Access to Test Protocols

Although Standard 9.11 (APA, 2002a) requires that psychologists maintain the security of test materials (including the test manual, test protocol, and test questions or stimuli), a federal law called the Family Education Rights and Privacy Act (FERPA, 1974) provides, in part, that parents be allowed access to test protocols if those tests were utilized in any educational decision making (Bersoff, 1981). Psychologists must be aware of applicable laws pertaining to assessment and must not refuse parents access to test protocols if the request is legally enforceable (Abeles, 1992).

Child Abuse Reporting

As stated previously, clients or their legal guardians generally must explicitly consent to the release of assessment information to third parties. However, in some circumstances, client consent for release of information is not needed. For example, all 50 states have mandatory reporting laws that require disclosure of child abuse to state agencies such as police departments and Child Protective

Services (Miller & Evans, 2004). Clearly, clients must be fully informed of this exception to confidentiality prior to beginning the assessment process.

EDUCATIONAL LAW

In 1975, Congress passed Public Law 94-142, also known as the Individuals with Disabilities Education Act (IDEA). This federal law requires states, through their local school districts, to provide appropriate individualized educational plans in the least restrictive environment for all children identified with disabilities. Psychologists must be familiar with educational law prior to providing assessment services to school districts or to parents seeking an independent evaluation of their child. Two landmark cases on assessment illustrate the difficulty psychologists have in identifying children in need of special services in the school setting.

First, in *Larry P. v. Riles* (1979, Federal District Court in San Francisco), plaintiffs were several African American elementary school children who were placed in special education classes due to their low scores on standardized intelligence tests. Plaintiffs claimed that intelligence tests were biased against the culture and experience of African American children as a class. To prove their case, plaintiffs demonstrated racial imbalances in special education classrooms, showing that while African Americans made up only 29% of all students in the San Francisco school district, a full 66% of students in special education classrooms were African American. The federal court ruled that, whether intentionally or not, the result of utilizing standard intelligence tests was unequal placement. Therefore, the court ruled that intelligence tests could not be used with African American children to make educational placement decisions.

In contrast, in *People in Action on Special Education (PASE) v. Hannon* (1980, Federal District Court in Illinois), the court ruled that standardized intelligence tests may be used in educational decision making as long as resulting scores are not the sole criterion for placement decisions. Currently, most school districts allow the use of standardized intelligence tests in decision making but do not allow the scores to be used in isolation. Within school settings, psychologists must employ multiple data points prior to diagnosing a child or making placement recommendations.

RECOMMENDATIONS FOR CHILD ASSESSORS

Psychologists should strive to follow seven principles each time testing is conducted in order to ensure a reliable and valid assessment process: (a) Assess using psychometrically sound devices; (b) assess using relevant tests; (c) assess within a defined relationship; (d) integrate multiple sources of data; (e) supervise administration and interpretation of tests; (f) interpret using current data; and (g) write reports in language that is understandable to all parties.

First and foremost, psychologists should employ only those tests that are psychometrically sound (Joint Committee of the American Educational Research Association, American Psychological Association, and the National Council on Measurement in Education, 1999). It is important that psychologists only use tests that are reliable and that have been validated for the purpose at hand, because "a test that is reliable, valid, and quite useful for one purpose may be useless or inappropriate for another" (Koocher & Keith-Spiegel, 1998, p. 149). To ensure that reliability and validity coefficients retain their meaning, psychologists should do two things: (a) follow standardized administration procedures of each test, and (b) maintain strict security with testing protocols. Standardized administration is necessary to reduce the impact of error on test scores (Joint Committee). Test security is necessary to guarantee that client responses to tests are genuine, unrehearsed, and an accurate sample of behavior. Prior knowledge of test questions and understanding of test scoring and interpretation can serve to compromise the utility and validity of test results. A lack of test security results in "very concrete harm to the general public—loss of effective assessment tools" (APA Committee on Psychological Tests, 1996, p. 646). While many secure tests can be accessed to at least some extent by searches of university libraries or the Internet, protecting assessment instruments should remain a high priority for examiners. Therefore, psychologists should require that all tests be completed in a secure setting, such as the psychologist's office, rather than allowing the test taker to complete a test at home (Adams & Luscher, 2003).

Second, psychologists should not haphazardly select assessment instruments but instead should employ tests that are relevant to the needs of a particular client (Adams & Luscher, 2003; Anastasi, 1988). Regardless of the type of assessment being conducted, "implementation of any psychological instrument requires a clearly specified reason for its use" (Loveland, 1985, as cited in Adams & Luscher, p. 276). Specifically, psychologists must "define the purpose of using a particular testing measure [and] have viable reasons for its administration" (Adams & Luscher, p. 276). A client's right to privacy must be respected, because the "process of arriving at the diagnosis, of prodding the client for details of his or her experience, is in many ways an invasion of privacy no less severe than a physical examination by a medical doctor or an audit by the IRS" (Welfel, 1998, p. 218). In other words, testing must be given for a good reason, because "testing for its own sake, or because of an institutional mandate, is inappropriate" (Welfel, p. 226). To achieve this principle, psychologists should thoroughly review the research on each proposed test, in order to ensure each test's relevance to the referral question (Adams & Luscher).

Third, psychologists should assess only within a defined relationship (APA, 2002a). In other words, psychologists should resist any temptation to assess persons casually in social situations or to provide a diagnosis without having conducted an in-person evaluation. In defining the relationship, psychologists should always provide adequate information to the client, including information about the nature of the assessment and the use of the results. In addition, psychologists should obtain written informed consent for assessment from the client or legal guardian (Adams & Luscher, 2003). Documentation of informed consent should be reviewed verbally with the client in language appropriate to the client's level of understanding and free from technical jargon or colloquial terminology (Mann, 1994; Welfel, 1998). As a rule of thumb, consent forms should be written at no higher than a 7th-grade reading level (Miller, 2002). Additionally, the client should be given an opportunity to look over such documentation and ask questions before signing, in order to ensure understanding. Research conducted on the effects of written informed consent forms generally has found positive effects. For example, Handelsman (1990) found that the use of written consent forms increased clients' positive judgments of therapists' experience, likeability, and trustworthiness.

Fourth, psychologists must integrate multiple sources of data rather than relying on test scores as the sole criterion on which clinical, educational, or other decisions are made. Multiple methods of assessment are preferred, for no single measure will be sufficient to answer the referral question(s) (Kazdin, 1992). Interviews with collateral sources (e.g., parents, teachers), reviews of prior school and medical records, and direct observations of classroom and in-home behavior are necessary for a thorough, competent evaluation (Miller & Evans, 2004).

Fifth, psychologists should carefully supervise test administration and scoring. Regardless of who administers and scores tests, only trained and competent professionals should supervise the assessment process. Students or assistants may administer tests, and automated services may score tests, such as the Minnesota Multiphasic Personality Inventory—2 (MMPI-2; Butcher, Dahlstrom, Graham, Tellegen, & Kaemmer, 1989) and the Rorschach Inkblot Test (Rorschach, 1942). However, the trained professional is still responsible for appropriate administration and interpretation of scores (APA, 2002a).

Sixth, psychologists should interpret based on current data. APA (2002a) clearly requires that examiners refrain from basing recommendations or decisions on obsolete or outdated testing data. However, a survey of 100 psychologists by Berndt (1983) found that 91% kept old testing protocols in files. Berndt reported that the oldest records ranged from 2 to 35 years, with a mean of 12.8 years. Scores in these older records are likely invalid, because they may be based on outdated norms and may no longer be reflective of the client's current functioning. It is the psychologist's responsibility to ensure that only current, valid data are interpreted and utilized in decision making. How long a psychologist may rely on test scores depends primarily on the construct being measured (Welfel, 1998). Tests that measure rapidly changing constructs, such as depressed or anxious moods (e.g., Beck Depression Inventory—II; Beck, Steer, & Brown, 1996; Beck Anxiety Inventory; Beck & Steer, 1990) may be valid only for several days or weeks. Other tests that measure more stable personality constructs (e.g., MMPI-2; Butcher et al., 1989) may be valid for several months.

Finally, special care should be given in how written information is presented to the individual client or to third parties. For example, summary reports may be more beneficial to clients than raw test data, because such data may be complex and difficult to understand. In addition, any such report should be written in a manner that is clear and free of technical language in order to avoid misinterpretation and misunderstanding. As Koocher and Keith-Spiegel (1998) noted, "It is wisest to write reports with a directness and clarity that makes it possible to give copies of the report to the client" (p. 165).

SUMMARY

Assessment is a complex process that is affected by ethics codes as well as federal and state laws. In addition, several aspirational practice guidelines offer advice to psychologists engaged in the assessment process (e.g., APA Committee on Psychological Tests and Assessment, 1996; APA Working Group of the Joint Committee on Testing Practices, 1998). Considerable knowledge and training is necessary to competently complete assessment activities. At a minimum, psychologists should receive training in psychometrics and statistics and obtain supervised experience prior to administering and interpreting any test (Turner et al., 2001).

In summary, a competent assessor is one who employs psychometrically sound and relevant tests, along with other data sources, to answer specific assessment questions within a defined relationship (Miller & Evans, 2004). Ultimately, "knowing what one's tests can do—that is, what psychological functions they describe accurately, what diagnostic conclusions can be inferred from them with what degree of certainty, and what kinds of behavior they can be expected to predict—is the measure of the [psychologist's] competence" (Weiner, 1989, p. 829).

REFERENCES AND RESOURCES

Abeles, N. (1992). An ethical dilemma: Disclosure of test items to parents. *Psychotherapy in Private Practice, 10,* 23–26.

Adams, H. E., & Luscher, K. A. (2003). Ethical considerations in psychological assessment. In W. O'Donohue & K. Ferguson (Eds.), *Handbook of professional ethics for psychologists: Issues, questions, and controversies* (pp. 275–283). Thousand Oaks, CA: Sage Publications.

American Counseling Association. (1995). *Code of ethics and standards of practice.* Alexandria, VA: Author.

American Psychological Association. (1994). Guidelines for child custody evaluations in divorce proceedings. *American Psychologist, 49,* 677–680.

American Psychological Association. (2002a). Ethical principles of psychologists and code of conduct. *American Psychologist, 57,* 1060–1073.

American Psychological Association. (2002b). Criteria for practice guideline development and evaluation. *American Psychologist, 57,* 1048–1051.

American Psychological Association Committee on Professional Practice and Standards. (1998). *Guidelines for psychological evaluations in child protection matters*. Washington, DC: American Psychological Association.

American Psychological Association Committee on Psychological Tests and Assessment. (1996). Statement on the disclosure of test data. *American Psychologist, 51,* 644–648.

American Psychological Association Working Group of the Joint Committee on Testing Practices. (1998). *Rights and responsibilities of test takers: Guidelines and expectations*. Retrieved from http://www.apa.org/science/ttr.html

Anastasi, A. (1976). *Psychological testing* (4th ed.). New York: Macmillan.

Anastasi, A. (1988). *Psychological testing* (6th ed.). New York: Macmillan.

Authority of One Parent When Other Parent Granted Sole Custody of Child, Oregon Revised Statutes 107.154 (2003).

Bailey, D. S. (2003, October). Should you testify for your client? *Monitor on Psychology,* 72–73.

Beck, A. T., & Steer, R. A. (1990). *Beck Anxiety Inventory (BAI)*. San Antonio, TX: Psychological Corporation.

Beck, A. T., Steer, R. A., & Brown, G. K. (1996). *Beck Depression Inventory—II (BDI-II) manual.* San Antonio, TX: Psychological Corporation.

Berndt, D. J. (1983). Ethical and professional considerations in psychological assessment. *Professional Psychology: Research and Practice, 14*(5), 580–587.

Bersoff, D. N. (1981). Testing and the law. *American Psychologist, 36,* 1047–1056.

Bersoff, D. N. (Ed.). (1999a). *Ethical conflicts in psychology* (2nd ed.). Washington, DC: American Psychological Association.

Bersoff, D. N. (1999b). The legal regulation of school psychology. In C. R. Reynolds & T. B. Gutkin (Eds.), *The handbook of school psychology* (3rd ed., pp. 1043–1074). New York: John Wiley & Sons.

Butcher, J. N., Dahlstrom, W. G., Graham, J. R., Tellegen, A., & Kaemmer, B. (1989). *Minnesota Multiphasic Personality Inventory—2 (MMPI-2): Manual for administration and scoring.* Minneapolis: University of Minnesota Press.

Camera, W. J., Nathan, J. S., & Puente, A. E. (2000). Psychological test usage: Implications in professional psychology. *Professional Psychology: Research and Practice, 31*(2), 141–154.

Committee on Ethical Guidelines for Forensic Psychologists. (1991). Specialty guidelines for forensic psychologists. *Law and Human Behavior, 15*(6), 655–665.

DeKraai, M. B., & Sales, B. D. (1982). Privileged communications of psychologists. *Professional Psychology: Research and Practice, 13*(3), 372–388.

Everstine, L., Everstine, D. S., Heymann, G. M., True, R. H., Frey, D. H., Johnson, H. G., et al. (1980). Privacy and confidentiality in psychotherapy. *American Psychologist, 35,* 828–840.

Family Education Rights and Privacy Act (FERPA), 20 U.S.C. 1232g; 34 CFR Part 99 (1974).

Handelsman, M. M. (1990). Do written consent forms influence clients' first impressions of therapists? *Professional Psychology: Research and Practice, 21*(6), 451–454.

Health Insurance Portability and Accountability Act (HIPAA), Pub. L. No. 104–191 (1996).

Hedges, L. (2000). *Facing the challenges of liability in psychotherapy: Practicing defensively.* Northvale, NJ: Jason Aronson.

Individuals with Disabilities Education Act (IDEA), Pub. L. No. 94-142 (1975).

Joint Committee of the American Educational Research Association, the American Psychological Association, and the National Council on Measurement in Education. (1999). *Standards for educational and psychological testing*. Washington, DC: American Educational Research Association.

Kazdin, A. E. (Ed.). (1992). *Methodological issues and strategies in clinical research.* Washington, DC: American Psychological Association.

Keith-Spiegel, P. (1983). Children and consent to participate in research. In G. B. Melton, G. P. Koocher, & M. J. Saks (Eds.), *Children's competence to consent* (pp. 179–211). New York: Plenum Press.

Koocher, G. P., & Keith-Spiegel, P. (1998). *Ethics in psychology: Professional standards and cases* (2nd ed.). New York: Oxford University Press.
Larry P. v. Riles, 343 F. Supp. 1306 (1979).
Mann, T. (1994). Informed consent for psychological research: Do subjects comprehend consent forms and understand their legal rights? *Psychological Science, 5,* 140–143.
Miller, C. A. (2002, November). *Update on ethical and legal issues.* Workshop presented at Pacific University, Forest Grove, OR.
Miller, C. A., & Evans, B. B. (2004). Ethical issues in assessment. In M. Hersen (Ed.), Psychological assessment in clinical practice: A pragmatic guide (pp. 21–32). New York: Brunner-Routledge.
People in Action on Special Education v. Hannon, 506 F. Supp. 831 (N. D. Ill 1980).
Przwansky, W. B., & Bersoff, D. N. (1978). Parental consent for psychological evaluations: Legal, ethical, and practical consideration. *Journal of School Psychology, 16,* 274–281.
Right to Diagnosis or Treatment for Mental or Emotional Disorder or Chemical Dependency without Parental Consent, Oregon Revised Statute 109.675 (2003).
Rorschach, H. (1942). *Psychodiagnostics: A diagnostic test based on perception* (P. Lemkau & B. Kronenberg, Trans.). Berne, Switzerland: Huber. (1st German ed. published 1921; U.S. Distributor, Grune & Stratton)
Turner, S. M., DeMers, S. T., Fox, H. R., & Reed, G. M. (2001). APA's guidelines for test user qualifications. *American Psychologist, 56,* 1099–1113.
Wechsler, D. (1997). *Wechsler Adult Intelligence Scale—III (WAIS-III).* San Antonio, TX: Psychological Corporation.
Weiner, I. B. (1989). On competence and ethicality in psychodiagnostic assessment.
Welfel, E. R. (1998). *Ethics in counseling and psychotherapy.* Pacific Grove, CA: Brooks/Cole Publishing.

AUTHOR INDEX

C

F

Subject INDEX

Printed and bound by CPI Group (UK) Ltd, Croydon, CR0 4YY
03/10/2024
01040413-0010